Respiratory: An Integrated Approach to Disease

Human Organ Systems Series

Series Editor: Paul G. Schmitz, MD, FACP

Dr. Schmitz is a distinguished physician-scientist who has been listed as one of America's Best Doctors for over a decade. He has received over a dozen teaching awards spanning multiple levels of training, from preclinical medical students, to residents, fellows, and faculty. In 2003 he received the prestigious Missouri Governor's award from Governor William Holden for teaching excellence in higher education. He has been closely involved in the human organ systems curriculum at Saint Louis University School of Medicine. His learning philosophy stresses the scientific foundation of medicine, with a resolute commitment to bridging the gap between the basic sciences and clinical medicine.

Respiratory: An Integrated Approach to Disease

ANDREW J. LECHNER, PhD

Professor
Departments of Pharmacological & Physiological Science and Internal Medicine
Founding Director of the Respiratory Module, Year-2 Medical Curriculum
Director, Saint Louis University MD/PhD Physician Scientist Training Program
Saint Louis University School of Medicine
St. Louis, Missouri

GEORGE M. MATUSCHAK, MD

Professor
Departments of Internal Medicine and Pharmacological & Physiological Science
Director, Division of Pulmonary, Critical Care, and Sleep Medicine
Saint Louis University School of Medicine
St. Louis, Missouri

DAVID S. BRINK, MD

Associate Professor
Departments of Pathology and Pediatrics
Saint Louis University School of Medicine
Director, Saint Louis University Pathology Residency Training Program
St. Louis, Missouri

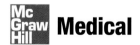

New York Chicago San Francisco Lisbon London Madrid Mexico City Milan
New Delhi San Juan Seoul Singapore Sydney Toronto

Respiratory: An Integrated Approach to Disease

Copyright © 2012 by The McGraw-Hill Companies, Inc. All rights reserved. Printed in China. Except as permitted under the United States Copyright Act of 1976, no part of this publication may be reproduced or distributed in any form or by any means, or stored in a data base or retrieval system, without the prior written permission of the publisher.

1 2 3 4 5 6 7 8 9 0   CTP/CTP   15 14 13 12 11

ISBN 978-0-07-163501-7
MHID 0-07-163501-7

This book was set in Times by Cenveo Publisher Services.
The editors were Michael Weitz and Regina Y. Brown.
The production supervisor was Catherine H. Saggese.
Project management was provided by Nidhi Chopra, Cenveo Publisher Services.
The designer was Elise Lansdon. The cover designer was Thomas DePierro. Cover art by SciePro Science Productions.
China Translation & Printing Services, Ltd. was printer and binder.

Cataloging-in-Publication Data is on file with the Library of Congress.

McGraw-Hill books are available at special quantity discounts to use as premiums and sales promotions, or for use in corporate training programs. To contact a representative please e-mail us at bulksales@mcgraw-hill.com.

*This book is respectfully
dedicated to our teachers
and to our students.*

AJL, GMM, and DSB

About the Authors

Drs. Lechner and Matuschak have been collaborators and friends at Saint Louis University since 1988. From then until now, they have co-authored at least 35 publications in the fields of acute lung injury, multiple systems organ failure, oxygen transport, and hypoxic regulation of cytokine gene expression. Dr. Brink joined their research efforts for the first time in 1991 as a medical student, and subsequently has provided his essential expertise in the pathology of pulmonary and renal diseases to that research. In 1995, they co-chaired the curriculum design committee to identify core topics for inclusion in the Respiratory Module that has been taught ever since to all second-year medical students at Saint Louis University School of Medicine. Their lifelong commitments to medical education are reflected in their various roles as directors of residency and fellowship programs and of their institution's medical scientist training program.

Contents

Contributors xi
Preface xiii
Acknowledgments xv

Abbreviations xvi

SECTION I **ANATOMY AND PHYSIOLOGY OF THE RESPIRATORY SYSTEM**

1. Respiratory System Nomenclature and Ambient Conditions / 3
   ANDREW J. LECHNER, PhD

2. Development and Functional Anatomy of the Lungs and Airways / 9
   DAVID S. BRINK, MD AND ANDREW J. LECHNER, PhD

3. Mechanisms of O_2 and CO_2 Transport by Erythrocytes / 23
   ANDREW J. LECHNER, PhD

4. Principles of Lung Ventilation and Spirometry / 31
   ANDREW J. LECHNER, PhD

5. Surfactant Biology and Lung Compliance / 39
   ANDREW J. LECHNER, PhD AND MARY M. MAYO, PhD

6. Integrated Respiratory System Compliance and the Work of Breathing / 47
   ANDREW J. LECHNER, PhD

7. Pulmonary Circulation and Capillary Fluid Dynamics / 55
   ANDREW J. LECHNER, PhD

8. Ventilation/Perfusion Matching and Estimating Alveolar Ventilation / 63
   ANDREW J. LECHNER, PhD

9. Alveolar O_2 and CO_2 Exchange, Physiological Shunt, and Acid-Base Balance / 71
   ANDREW J. LECHNER, PhD

10. Airway and Parenchymal Defense Mechanisms / 81
    ANDREW J. LECHNER, PhD AND GEORGE M. MATUSCHAK, MD

11. Central and Peripheral Neural Controls of Respiration / 93
    W. MICHAEL PANNETON, PhD AND ANDREW J. LECHNER, PhD

12. Importance and Derivation of Aerobic Capacity / 103
    GERALD S. ZAVORSKY, PhD AND ANDREW J. LECHNER, PhD

13. Respiratory Responses to Extreme Environments / 113
    GERALD S. ZAVORSKY, PhD AND ANDREW J. LECHNER, PhD

SECTION II **EVALUATING PATIENTS WITH RESPIRATORY DISEASES**

14. Conduct and Interpretation of the Basic Chest Exam / 125
    WILLIAM C. MOOTZ, MD AND GEORGE M. MATUSCHAK, MD

15. Interpreting Chest X-Rays, CT Scans, and MRIs / 133
    ASHUTOSH SACHDEVA, MD AND GEORGE M. MATUSCHAK, MD

16. Pulmonary Function Testing, Plethysmography, and Pulmonary Diffusing Capacity / 143
    GERALD S. ZAVORSKY, PhD AND ANDREW J. LECHNER, PhD

17. Blood Gas Analyses and Their Interpretation / 151
    MARY M. MAYO, PhD AND ANDREW J. LECHNER, PhD

18. Diagnostic Flexible Bronchoscopy / 159
    DAVID A. STOECKEL, MD AND GEORGE M. MATUSCHAK, MD

19. Evaluating Sputum and Pleural Effusions / 169
    MARY M. MAYO, PhD AND ANDREW J. LECHNER, PhD

SECTION III **OBSTRUCTIVE AND RESTRICTIVE LUNG DISEASES**

20. Pathology of Obstructive Pulmonary Diseases / 179
    DAVID S. BRINK, MD AND ANDREW J. LECHNER, PhD

21. Diagnosis and Management of Asthma / 189
    JOSEPH R. D. ESPIRITU, MD AND GEORGE M. MATUSCHAK, MD

22. **Management of Chronic Obstructive Pulmonary Diseases / 199**
    JOSEPH R. D. ESPIRITU, MD AND GEORGE M. MATUSCHAK, MD

23. **Pathology of Restrictive Lung Diseases / 207**
    DAVID S. BRINK, MD

24. **Management of Restrictive Lung Diseases / 221**
    RAVI P. NAYAK, MD AND GEORGE M. MATUSCHAK, MD

25. **Management of Sleep-Related Breathing Disorders / 231**
    JOSEPH R. D. ESPIRITU, MD AND GEORGE M. MATUSCHAK, MD

SECTION IV | **INFLAMMATORY, VASCULAR, AND PLEURAL DISEASES**

26. **Pathology of Atelectatic, Vascular, and Iatrogenic Diseases of the Lungs and Pleural Space / 245**
    DAVID S. BRINK, MD

27. **Pulmonary Embolism / 255**
    ASHUTOSH SACHDEVA, MD AND GEORGE M. MATUSCHAK, MD

28. **Acute Lung Injury and the Acute Respiratory Distress Syndrome: Pathophysiology and Treatment / 267**
    GEORGE M. MATUSCHAK, MD AND ANDREW J. LECHNER, PhD

29. **Pathophysiology and Diseases of the Pleural Space / 275**
    GEORGE M. MATUSCHAK, MD AND ANDREW J. LECHNER, PhD

30. **Principles and Goals of Mechanical Ventilation / 283**
    DAYTON DMELLO, MD AND GEORGE M. MATUSCHAK, MD

SECTION V | **CANCER AND RELATED LUNG MASSES**

31. **Pathology of Lung Tumors / 295**
    DAVID S. BRINK, MD

32. **Lung Cancer / 307**
    DAVID A. STOECKEL, MD AND GEORGE M. MATUSCHAK, MD

33. **Diseases of the Upper Airways and Sinuses / 319**
    DAVID S. BRINK, MD AND ANDREW J. LECHNER, PhD

SECTION VI | **INFECTIONS OF THE LUNG**

34. **Pathology of Lung Infections / 331**
    DAVID S. BRINK, MD

35. **Management of Pneumonias / 345**
    DAVID A. STOECKEL, MD AND GEORGE M. MATUSCHAK, MD

36. **Mycobacterial Diseases in the Lung / 353**
    ASHUTOSH SACHDEVA, MD AND GEORGE M. MATUSCHAK, MD

SECTION VII | **PEDIATRIC LUNG DISEASES**

37. **Congenital Anomalies of the Respiratory System / 365**
    GARY M. ALBERS, MD AND ANDREW J. LECHNER, PhD

38. **Presentation and Management of Cystic Fibrosis / 375**
    BLAKESLEE E. NOYES, MD AND ANDREW J. LECHNER, PhD

39. **Neonatal Respiratory Distress Syndrome and Sudden Infant Death Syndrome / 385**
    ROBERT E. FLEMING, MD, W. MICHAEL PANNETON, PhD, AND ANDREW J. LECHNER, PhD

40. **Lower Respiratory Tract Infections in Children / 397**
    BLAKESLEE E. NOYES, MD AND GEORGE M. MATUSCHAK, MD

Index 407

Contributors

Gary M. Albers, MD

Professor
Department of Pediatrics
Division of Pulmonary Medicine
Saint Louis University School of Medicine
St. Louis, Missouri

David S. Brink, MD

Associate Professor
Departments of Pathology and Pediatrics
Saint Louis University School of Medicine
Director, Saint Louis University Pathology Residency
    Training Program
St. Louis, Missouri

Dayton Dmello, MD, MBA

Adjunct Faculty
Saint Louis University School of Medicine
Critical Care & Pulmonary Associates
Skyridge Medical Center & The Medical Center of Aurora
Denver, Colorado

Joseph R. D. Espiritu, MD

Medical Director
SLUCare Sleep Disorders Center
Assistant Professor of Internal Medicine
Division of Pulmonary, Critical Care, and Sleep Medicine
Saint Louis University School of Medicine
St. Louis, Missouri

Robert E. Fleming, MD

Departments of Pediatrics and of Biochemistry &
    Molecular Biology
Saint Louis University School of Medicine
St. Louis, Missouri

Andrew J. Lechner, PhD

Professor
Departments of Pharmacological & Physiological
    Science and Internal Medicine
Founding Director of the Respiratory Module, Year-2
    Medical Curriculum
Director, Saint Louis University MD/PhD Physician
    Scientist Training Program
Saint Louis University School of Medicine
St. Louis, Missouri

George M. Matuschak, MD

Professor
Departments of Internal Medicine and Pharmacological
    & Physiological Science
Director, Division of Pulmonary, Critical Care, and
    Sleep Medicine
Saint Louis University School of Medicine
St. Louis, Missouri

Mary M. Mayo, PhD, DABCC

Associate Professor of Pathology
Saint Louis University School of Medicine
Director, Clinical Chemistry Laboratory
Saint Louis University Hospital
St. Louis, Missouri

William C. Mootz, MD

Professor
Department of Internal Medicine, Division of General
    Internal Medicine
Assistant Dean for Medical Curriculum
Saint Louis University School of Medicine
St. Louis, Missouri

Ravi P. Nayak, MD

Assistant Professor
Department of Internal Medicine, Division of
    Pulmonary, Critical Care, and Sleep
    Medicine
Saint Louis University School of Medicine
Medical Director of the Adult Cystic Fibrosis
    Program and the Pulmonary Function
    Laboratory
Saint Louis University Hospital
St. Louis, Missouri

Blakeslee E. Noyes, MD

Professor
Department of Pediatrics
Saint Louis University School of Medicine
Director, Division of Pulmonary Medicine
Cardinal Glennon Children's
    Medical Center
St. Louis, Missouri

W. Michael Panneton, PhD

Professor
Department of Pharmacological & Physiological Science
Saint Louis University School of Medicine
St. Louis, Missouri

Ashutosh Sachdeva, MD

Assistant Professor
Department of Internal Medicine
Director, Pulmonary Hypertension Program
Saint Louis University School of Medicine
St. Louis, Missouri

David A. Stoeckel, MD

Assistant Professor
Department of Internal Medicine
Division of Pulmonary, Critical Care and Sleep Medicine
Director, Minimally Invasive Lung Cancer Program
Saint Louis University School of Medicine
St. Louis, Missouri

Gerald S. Zavorsky, PhD

Associate Professor
College of Health and Human Services
Director, Human Physiology Laboratory
Marywood University
Adjunct Associate Professor of Physiology
The Commonwealth Medical College
Scranton, Pennsylvania

Preface

In the fall of 1994, Saint Louis University (SLU) School of Medicine was visited by the Liaison Committee for Medical Education (LCME) for its routine reaccreditation of our medical curriculum. Remarkably, SLU's entire second-year medical class had recently passed Step 1 of the United States Medical Licensure Exam (USMLE) boards on their first attempts the preceding summer. Such an outcome can powerfully reinforce the *status quo*: If it's not broken, why fix it? Despite that auspicious showing, we were confronted by the LCME criticism that our traditional discipline-based curriculum must be redesigned so that it would be governed by a cross-disciplinary committee of practicing physicians. The LCME's operational hypothesis seemed to be that such top-down management would free curricular content from the pedagogical constraints exerted by powerful academic departments in charge of individual courses like biochemistry, physiology, pathology, and medicine. We soon learned that other medical schools were hearing this same message.

To this institution's credit, its teaching faculty reinvented all four MD years over the next 18 months. When our new year one rolled out in the fall of 1997, it resembled the old only by starting with Gross Anatomy (now a 2-month introduction), followed by 7 months of what I came to call "one cell and less" biology, with short courses in intermediary metabolism, genetics, cell biology and cell pathology, and introductions to immunology, microbiology, and pharmacology. Our second MD year became all about "two cells and more" biology, in what has emerged as a common paradigm: organ system modules that at SLU follow the sequence of neural, cardiovascular, respiratory, renal, gastrointestinal, endocrine/reproduction, and skin/bone/joint. Then comes Step 1.

At this writing, SLU's Respiratory Module has grown through 13 years of trial and error, field-tested annually over 5 weeks each November and December on an increasingly sophisticated student body. The module syllabus has grown from <400 pages of mostly outlines to twice that length, now mostly full text. Because we cover all erythrocyte biology within Respiratory, the module includes 50 one-hour lectures and nine labs and/or small group activities, all team-taught to utilize the breadth and expertise of >20 devoted faculty members. This book represents our current state-of-art for at least the formal course content on the lung, if not all ancillary activities. Each chapter represents the material we cover in a 50-minute lecture. The book's associate editors Drs. George Matuschak and David Brink, my collaborators and friends for 20+ years, have very capably guided the module's design and implementation of its clinical presentations and pathology.

During the module's evolution, I was privileged to serve two "tours of duty" on the Physiology Test Item committee of the National Board of Medical Examiners that produces the questions for USMLE Step 1. That experience reinforced the importance of writing clear test items that are vignette-driven, have parallel answer foils, and evaluate higher learning skills beyond rote memorization. Each chapter here includes sample questions that we consider of the right depth for medical students at this level of training. We hope our student audience will use these items for structured self-testing, and will let us know when items need repair because they are ambiguous or incorrect.

The book is organized into subsections that reflect the general flow used with our students, but most chapters can be read out of sequence without difficulty once the introductory section is completed. Although there is not universal agreement on common phrases, terms, abbreviations, and acronyms, we have adopted those which we consider the most accepted in the fields of respiratory physiology and pulmonary medicine. The **Glossary** should help novices to decipher this sometimes bewildering array of terminology. Likewise, we are committed to a worthwhile **Index** so that readers can quickly identify the extent of coverage on topics of particular importance to them; **textual phrases in bold font** are indexed and usually represent their first appearances in the book or section. At our institution, the Respiratory Module has assumed "ownership" of specific multi-system diseases, such as cystic fibrosis, the systemic inflammatory response syndrome, and masses of the neck. Consequently, such topics achieve coverage here that others might consider more extensive than strictly necessary. Pedagogically, we also favor introducing medical students to contemporary methods of diagnosis in pulmonary medicine, both at the patient's bedside and in the clinical laboratory. Hence, specific chapters here on the basic chest exam, pulmonary function testing, lung imaging, interpreting blood gases, and diagnostic bronchoscopy may exceed another course director's desire for their inclusion. Be reassured that this material is well within the ability of medical students to learn, integrate, and master.

Among all the diagrams, tables, equations, and images in this book, we hope that students can still perceive the love of this subject and the passion to teach it well that characterize our mission. The lungs are among the most beautiful and complex organs in our bodies, but beauty and complexity should not be impediments that prevent every physician for understanding their many functions and treating their numerous ailments.

Although the primary audience for this book is likely to be the second-year medical student, we believe that interns, residents, junior attendings, and even seasoned practitioners will find the text useful as a refresher of pulmonary histology, physiology, pathology, and pharmacology. We admire and want to encourage our students' willingness to learn more about a subject for which we care deeply. Love your lungs.

To our faculty peers, forgive our errors of omission and commission, and let us know your thoughts on how we might improve this first effort in the future. We also want to extend an invitation to those of you whose own institutions are wrestling with similar curricular innovation. My colleagues and I would be happy to share specific details about successful implementation, including suggested course calendars, core lab and clinic facilities, and the requisite expertise and team size needed to achieve your goals.

—Dr. Andy Lechner, Editor
February, 2011

Acknowledgments

I am indebted to several individuals at Saint Louis University (SLU) for the completion of this project. In addition to Drs. George Matuschak and David Brink, my longtime colleagues and friends, special thanks are due Dr. Paul Schmitz for making this shared dream of an "organ systems bookshelf" a reality. My departmental chairman Dr. Tom Westfall encourages a commitment to teaching medical students what they need to know; he steadfastly fosters a nurturing environment for the many faculty members at SLU who share his passion for the wonderful dialogue that education engenders. Our managing editor at McGraw-Hill, Michael Weitz, has provided critical advice and just the right amount of energy to keep us on deadline. His colleagues Ms. Regina Y. Brown and Ms. Nidhi Chopra collectively supported us through the publications maze to produce what we can see is an attractive and carefully edited book; factual errors rest with us, the authors. Finally, I am forever indebted to my wife and best friend Victoria Salvato-Lechner, who with our children Melissa and Andrew, carried me through the trials and tribulations of these past two years with great humor and no complaints.

nitric oxide synthase (inducible)	NOS (iNOS)
nonsteroidal anti-inflammatory drug(s)	NSAID(s)
normal sterile saline (0.9% NaCl)	NS
nucleotide binding domain(s)	NBD(s)
oxygen, molecular	O_2
peroxynitrite	$ONOO^-$
phosphatidylethanolamine, in surfactant	PEt
phosphatidylglycerol, in surfactant	PG
phosphatidylinositol, in surfactant	PI
phosphatidylserine, in surfactant	PS
platelet activating factor	PAF
platelet-derived growth factor	PDGF
proton, free as in acid solution	H^+ or $[H^+]$
purified protein derivative (for TB skin test)	PPD
reactive nitrogen species	RNS
reactive oxygen species	ROS
recombinant tissue plasminogen activator	rt-PA
sex hormone binding globulin-1	SHBG-1
superoxide anion	$\cdot O_2^-$
surfactant associated proteins A, B, C, D	SP-A, SP-B, SP-C, SP-D
technetium, radiolabeled	^{99}Tc (most common radioisotope)
transforming growth factor-beta	TGF-β
tumor necrosis factor-alpha	TNF-α
2,3-diphosphoglycerate	2,3-DPG
unfractionated heparin	UFH or UF Heparin
xenon, inert gas, radiolabeled	^{133}Xe (most common radioisotope)

Blood, RBC, and hemoglobin-related

carbaminohemoglobin	$HbCO_2$
carboxyhemoglobin	HbCO
hemoglobin A, F, S, etc	Hb-A, Hb-F, Hb-S
hematocrit or packed red cell volume	hct (%)
hemoglobin concentration in blood	[Hb] (g/dL or g%)
mean red cell hemoglobin concentration	MCHC (%)
mean red cell hemoglobin content	MCH (pg/cell)
mean red cell volume	MCV (fL or μm^3)
methemoglobin	metHb
oxygen dissociation curve	ODC
pH, arterial or mixed venous	pH_a, $pH_{\bar{v}}$
red blood cell(s)	RBC(s)
red cell count in whole blood	#RBC/μL

Diagnostic techniques, procedures, professional entities, and locations

acid-fast bacillus (organisms), stain	AFB, AFB stain
activated partial thromboplastin time	aPTT (sec)
adaptive support servo-ventilation	ASV
American College of Sports Medicine	ACSM
American Thoracic Society (guidelines, etc)	ATS
anteriorñposterior or anteroposterior (as a view)	AP
anti-neutrophil cystoplasmic antibody (study)	ANCA
arterial blood gas sample	ABG(s)
average volume-assured pressure support vent	AVAPS

bilevel positive airway pressure ventilation	BiPAP
bronchoalveolar lavage (fluid)	BAL (BALF)
Centers for Disease Control and Prevention	CDC
colony-forming unit(s), as of bacteria	CFU
computed tomography	CT
continuous positive airway pressure ventilation	CPAP
directly observed therapy (as for TB treatment)	DOT
electrocardiogram, electrocardiography	ECG
emergency room, emergency department	ER, ED
Environmental Protection Agency	EPA
European Respiratory Society (guidelines, etc)	ERS
extracorporeal membrane oxygenation	ECMO
fluorescence polarization	FP
foam stability index (of surfactant)	FSI
fractional excretion of nitric oxide	F_eNO
genioglossus advancement + hyoid myotomy + suspension	GAHMS
Global Initiative for Obstructive Lung Disease	GOLD
high resolution computed tomography	HRCT
immunoreactive trypsinogen	IRT
inspiratory positive airway pressure ventilation	IPAP
intensive care unit	ICU
international normalized ratio (for coag assays)	INR
laser-assisted uvulopalatoplasty	LAUP
lecithin/sphingomyelin ratio (amniotic)	L/S
likelihood ratio, positive or negative	+LR, −LR
lower limit(s) of normal range	LLN
magnetic resonance imaging, functional	MRI, fMRI
mechanical ventilation	MV
[methacholine] inducing a 20% decline in FEV_1	PC_{20}
National Asthma Education & Prevention Program	NAEPP
National Health & Nutrition Examination Survey III	NHANES-III
non-invasive positive pressure ventilation	NIPPV
parts per billion (as for a rare gas species)	ppb
periodic acid-Schiff (reagent stain)	PAS
positron emission spectrometry	PET
positive end-expiratory pressure	PEEP
positive pressure during expiration ventilation	EPAP
posterior to anterior (as a view)	PA
Prospective Investigation of Pulmonary Embolism Diagnosis Trial	PIOPED Trial
prothrombin time	PT (sec)
pulmonary arterial catheter (Swan-Ganz)	PAC
pulmonary function test or testing(s)	PFT(s)
rapid shallow breathing index	RSBI
spontaneous breathing trial	SBT
saturation with oxygen, arterial by oximetry	S_aO_2 (%)
saturation with oxygen, mixed venous by oximetry	$S_{\bar{v}}O_2$ (%)
sustained-release (medications)	SR
transjugular intrahepatic portosystemic shunt	TIPS
uvulopalatopharyngoplasty	UPPP
ventilation/perfusion lung scan	V/Q scan
video-assisted thoracoscopic surgery	VATS
World Health Organization	WHO

Diseases, conditions, and syndromes

acute interstitial pneumonia	AIP
acute lung injury	ALI
acute mountain sickness	AMS
acute respiratory distress syndrome	ARDS
allergic bronchopulmonary aspergillosis	ABPA
benign asbestos pleural effusion	BAPE
bronchopulmonary dysplasia	BPD
carcinoma in situ	CIS
central sleep apnea	CSA
Cheyne-Stokes respiration	CSR
chronic obstructive pulmonary disease	COPD
coal worker's pneumoconiosis	CWP
community-acquired pneumonia	CAP
complete blood count	CBC
complex sleep apnea syndrome	CompSAS
congenital cystic adenomatoid malformation	CCAM
congenital central alveolar hypoventilation syndrome	CCAHS
congestive heart failure	CHF
cryptogenic organizing pneumonia	COP
cystic fibrosis	CF
cystic fibrosis-related diabetes mellitus	CFRDM
deep vein (or venous) thrombosis	DVT
desquamative interstitial pneumonitis	DIP
diffuse alveolar damage (a pathology diagnosis)	DAD
diffuse alveolar hemorrhage (a clinical diagnosis)	DAH
disseminated intravascular coagulation	DIC
distal intestinal obstruction syndrome	DIOS
environmental tobacco smoke	ETS
Epstein-Barr virus	EBV
heparin-induced thrombocytopenia	HIT
high altitude pulmonary edema	HAPE
human immunodeficiency virus	HIV
human papilloma virus	HPV
idiopathic pulmonary fibrosis	IPF
interstitial lung disease(s)	ILD(s)
Lambert-Eaton myasthenic syndrome	LEMS
lymphangioleiomyomatosis	LAM
lymphoid interstitial pneumonia	LIP
methicillin-resistant *Staphylococcus aureus*	MRSA
multiple drug resistant-organism	MDR-organism
multiple organ dysfunction syndrome	MODS
Mycobacterium avium complex	MAC
Mycobacterium tuberculosis	MTB
neonatal respiratory distress syndrome	neonatal RDS or nRDS
nonspecific interstitial pneumonia	NSIP
obesity-hypoventilation syndrome	OHS
obstructive sleep apnea	OSA
occupational asthma	OA
patent ductus arteriosus	PDA
patent foramen ovale	PFO
progressive massive fibrosis	PMF

pulmonary alveolar proteinosis	PAP
pulmonary arterial hypertension	PHT
pulmonary embolism, emboli	PE
respiratory bronchiolitis-interstitial lung disease	RB-ILD
respiratory syncytial virus	RSV
sleep-related hypoventilation/hypoxemic syndrome	SRH
squamous cell carcinoma	SCCA
syndrome of inappropriate antidiuretic hormone hypersecretion	SIADH
systemic inflammatory response syndrome	SIRS
systemic lupus erythematosus	SLE
thrombotic thrombocytopenic purpura	TTP
tuberculosis	TB
usual interstitial pneumonia	UIP
venous thromboembolism	VTE
ventilator-associated lung injury	VALI
ventilator-associated pneumonia	VAP

Physiological functions, processes, and measurements

acute hypoxic pressor response	AHPR
alveolar capillary endothelial surface area	S_C (in cm^2 or m^2)
alveolar epithelial surface area	S_A (in cm^2 or m^2)
alveolar septal barrier thickness, harmonic mean	τ_s (in μm)
alveolar ventilation rate	$\dot{V}_A$ (L/min)
alveolar ventilation/perfusion ratio	$\dot{V}_A/\dot{Q}$ (dimensionless)
anterior-posterior axis or direction (as an x-ray)	AP
apnea-hypopnea index	AHI (scorable events/h)
blood transfer conductance coefficient for CO	Θ_{CO}
body mass index, equal to weight/(height)^2	BMI (in SI units, kg/m^2)
body temperature/pressure (37°C, P_B,100% RH)	BTPS
carbon dioxide production rate	$\dot{V}_ACO_2$ (mL/min or L/h)
cardiac output	$\dot{Q}$ (L/min)
compliance, as of lung tissue or vasculature	$\Delta V/\Delta P$ (mL or L/mm Hg or cm H_2O)
dead space ventilation rate	$\dot{V}_D$ (L/min)
diffusivity, Krogh's coefficient for gas x	D_X
exercise-induced arterial hypoxemia	EIAH
filtration coefficient of permeability	K
fractional composition of gas "Xy"	F_{Xy} (a decimal from 0.0 to 1.0)
lung diffusive capacity for CO	DL_{CO}
maximal oxygen consumption rate	$\dot{V}O_{2max}$ (mL/min or L/h)
membrane diffusive capacity for CO	DM_{CO}
oxygen consumption rate	$\dot{V}O_2$ (mL/min or L/h)
peak expiratory flow (rate)	PEF(R) (mL or L/sec)
polysomnogram	PSG
protein reflection coefficient (Starling's equation)	σ (range = 0.0 – 1.0)
pulmonary vascular resistance	PVR (mm Hg/L/min)
rapid eye movement sleep, or non relative humidity	REM, NREM RH (%)
respiratory disturbance index	RDI (scorable events/h)
respiratory effort-related arousal(s)	RERA(s)
respiratory quotient	R
shunt fraction of cardiac output	$\dot{Q}_S/\dot{Q}_T$ (%)
six-minute walk test	6-MWT

standard temperature/pressure (0°C, 1 atm, dry)	STPD
surface tension, as in alveolus	T
systemic vascular resistance	SVR (mm Hg/L/min)
total ventilation rate, also "minute ventilation"	$\dot{V}_E$ (L/min)
viscosity, as of a gas in Poiseuille equation	η

Pressure (all types, in mm Hg or cm H_2O)

airway, critical opening	P_{CO}
airway, if "intratracheal" preferred	P_{IT}
airway, normal internal	P_{AW}
airway, peak as during MV	P_{PEAK}
airway, plateau as during MV	P_{PLAT}
airway, positive end-expiratory	PEEP
alveolar (total)	P_A
atmosphere (unit of pressure)	atm
barometric, ambient	P_B
carbon dioxide	P_{CO_2}
carbon dioxide, alveolar partial	P_ACO_2
carbon dioxide, arterial partial	P_aCO_2
carbon dioxide, end-expiratory partial	$P_{\acute{E}}CO_2$
carbon dioxide, expired	P_ECO_2
carbon dioxide, inspired	P_ICO_2
carbon dioxide, mean expiratory	$P_{\bar{E}}CO_2$
carbon dioxide, mixed venous blood	$P_{\bar{v}}CO_2$
colloid osmotic, of blood proteins	π_{MV}
colloid osmotic, of interstitial proteins	π_{PMV}
intrapleural	P_{IP}
nitrogen	PN_2
oxygen	PO_2
oxygen, alveolar–arterial gradient or difference	$(A-a)PO_2$
oxygen, alveolar capillary	P_cO_2
oxygen, alveolar end-capillary	$P_{c'}O_2$
oxygen, alveolar partial	P_AO_2
oxygen, arterial partial	P_aO_2
oxygen, arterial saturation by oximetry	S_aO_2 (%)
oxygen, inspired	P_IO_2
oxygen, mixed venous partial	$P_{\bar{v}}O_2$
oxygen, mixed venous saturation by oximetry	$S_{\bar{v}}O_2$ (%)
oxygen, to half-oxygenate Hb	P_{50}
pulmonary arterial blood	P_{PA}
pulmonary artery wedge (by PAC)	P_{PW}
pulmonary capillary or microvascular	P_{MV}
pulmonary peri-microvascular or interstitial	P_{PMV}
pulmonary venous blood	P_{PV}
systemic blood, diastolic	DP
systemic blood, mean	MAP
systemic blood, systolic	SP

Vital signs

cardiac output	$\dot{Q}$ (L/min)
heart or pulse rate	HR (b/min)
predicted body weight, often "ideal"	PBW (kg)

respiratory frequency	f (breaths/min) (note *italics*)
temperature, ambient environmental in Celsius	T_A (°C)
temperature, body or rectal in Celsius	T_B (°C)

Volume (all types) and related measurements

alveolar capillary blood	V_C (mL)
alveolar gas	V_A (mL or L)
dead space	V_D (mL or L)
dead space/tidal, ratio	V_D/V_T (dimensionless)
expiratory reserve	ERV (mL or L)
forced expiratory in "x" seconds	FEV_x, as in FEV_1 (mL or L)
forced vital capacity	FVC (mL or L)
functional residual capacity	FRC (mL or L)
inspiratory reserve	IRV (mL or L)
length of a structure, as an airway	l (note *italics*)
minimal lung tissue, collapsed and airless	V_{MIN} (mL or L)
radius of curvature, as an alveolus	r (note *italics*)
residual lung	RV (mL or L)
slow vital capacity	SVC (mL or L)
tidal	V_T (mL or L)
total lung capacity	TLC (mL or L)
vital capacity of the lung	VC (mL or L)

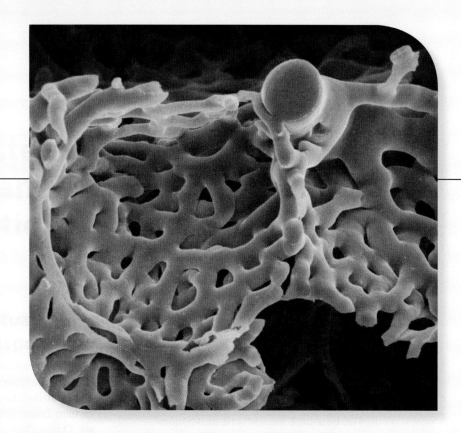

SECTION

I

ANATOMY AND PHYSIOLOGY OF THE RESPIRATORY SYSTEM

Overview of the O$_2$ Transport Cascade

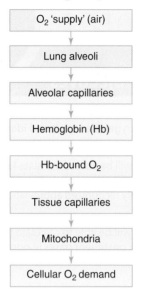

O$_2$ 'supply' (air)
↓
Lung alveoli
↓
Alveolar capillaries
↓
Hemoglobin (Hb)
↓
Hb-bound O$_2$
↓
Tissue capillaries
↓
Mitochondria
↓
Cellular O$_2$ demand

FIGURE 1.1 The oxygen transport cascade. See text for details.

P_Aco_2, with its most common units of mm Hg implied. Likewise, the phrase **fractional concentration of oxygen in the inspired gas mixture** reduces to F_Io_2. The proper labeling of respiratory gases begins with the notation of **F** (fractional concentration, as a decimal from 0.0-1.0), or **P** (for pressure in mm Hg, torr, kilopascals, etc). The second letter (often subscripted) states the source or location of the gas, if known, including: **A** = alveolar; **AW** = airway; **a** = arterial; **B** = ambient barometric; **c** = capillary; **ć** = end-capillary; **E** = expired or expiratory; $\overline{E}$ = mean expiratory; **É** = end-expiratory (sometimes called end-tidal); **I** = inspired; **IP** = intrapleural; **IT** = intratracheal; **v** = venous; and $\overline{v}$ = mixed or mean venous. Note that

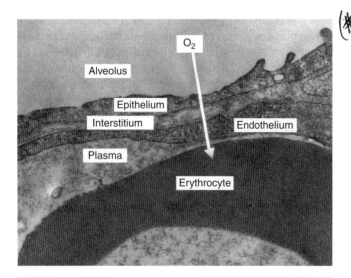

FIGURE 1.2 Representative electron micrograph of the air-tissue barrier to be traversed by diffusion if oxygenation is to succeed. In addition to the three tissue layers of alveolar septa, a thin fluid layer sits above the epithelium but was removed during intratracheal fixation.

conventional usage may specify upper versus lower case lettering to distinguish locations. The final designation is to the gas species: O$_2$, N$_2$, CO$_2$, H$_2$O, etc. Thus, the phrases $F_{\overline{E}}co_2 = 0.08$ and $P_ćo_2 = 105$ mm Hg indicate respectively that the average fractional CO$_2$ concentration in a sample of expired air is 8%, and that the partial pressure of O$_2$ in blood exiting an alveolar capillary to enter a pulmonary venule is 105 mm Hg.

Comparable examples of widely used abbreviations and acronyms for gas volumes in the lung, like V_T for tidal volume, will be introduced as needed. These and other terms for more complex functions are accompanied by units of measure that serve as helpful reminders to students of their derivation. For example, **pulmonary vascular resistance (PVR)** is a key measure of vascular tone across the lungs, usually expressed in **mm Hg/L/min**. This PVR is derived from the physiological restatement of Ohm's law (I = ΔV/R and thus R = ΔV/I). Thus, PVR is equal to the difference between pulmonary arterial and pulmonary venous pressures, divided by the **cardiac output** ($\dot{Q}$, in L/min). *Note: a dot placed over a symbol like $\dot{Q}$ is shorthand for a rate function, in this case the liters of blood pumped per minute by the right ventricle.*

Review of Basic Gas Laws
Dalton's Law

The total pressure of a gas mixture is equal to the sum of the partial pressures of individual gases in that mixture. The partial pressure of each gas is proportional to its fractional composition within such a mixture, and thus is the pressure each gas would exert if it alone occupied the total volume available. In ambient air, several gases comprise the total **barometric pressure (P_B)** [reported in mm Hg, torr, kilopascals, or atmospheres (atm) depending on local convention]:

$$P_B = Po_2 + Pco_2 + Pn_2 + Ph_2o$$

Boyle's Law

The pressure of a gas varies inversely with its volume. This relationship becomes critical when attempting to optimize mechanical ventilation to oxygenate patients whose thoracic and abdominal tissues naturally resist lung expansion.

Charles's Law

The volume of a gas varies directly with its temperature, due to changes in molecular energy as a closed gas system is heated or cooled. This principle has many ramifications in medicine, particularly when water vapor is present that displaces other gases (by Dalton's law) in a temperature-dependent manner. It also underlies **whole-body plethysmography**, an advanced form of **pulmonary function testing (PFT)** that will be described in Chap. 16. The technique utilizes gas expansion caused by the small differential between **ambient temperature (T_A)** and **body temperature (T_B)** to estimate inhaled volumes and intrapleural pressures (Chap. 6).

Historically, certain gas volumes in medicine, like oxygen consumption, are reported under **STPD** conditions of 0°C, 760 mm Hg (1 atm) of pressure, and $P_{H_2O} = 0$ mm Hg at 0% **relative humidity** (**RH**). Many other gas volumes are consistently expressed as **BTPS** conditions of actual T_B (often assumed as 37°C) and ambient P_B, and fully saturated with water vapor (100% RH) so that $P_{H_2O} = 47$ mm Hg, as exists throughout the normal respiratory system. This discordance between STPD data and those in BTPS occasionally requires clinicians and students to be able to convert from one set of units to the other. Recall the **General Gas** law which states that:

(#7)

$$P \cdot V = n \cdot R \cdot T$$

When the same molar amount (= n) of gas in a closed system under condition #1 (STPD or ambient) is heated, cooled, compressed, or decompressed to a new condition #2, it follows that:

$$(P_1 \cdot V_1)/T_1 = (P_2 \cdot V_2)/T_2$$

Thus, to convert a starting volume in STPD units into a final volume in BTPS units:

1. Assign STPD data the subscript 1, and assign BTPS data the subscript 2.
2. Rearrange terms: $V_2 = (P_1 \cdot V_1 \cdot T_2)/(P_2 \cdot T_1)$.
3. Substitute known terms: $V_{BTPS} = (760 \cdot V_{STPD} \cdot T_B)/[(P_B - 47) \cdot 273]$.
4. Solve for the desired volume. *Note: failing to make this correction will result in an average error of 22%-28%, arguably a consequential oversight.*

Henry's Law

The content or concentration of a gas dissolved in a liquid is proportional to its partial pressure that is in equilibrium above the liquid. In practice, this becomes:

$$[C_{Xy}] \text{ (in g or mL/L)} = K_{Xy} \cdot P_{Xy} \text{ (in mm Hg)}$$

where K_{Xy} = temperature-dependent solubility coefficient of gas Xy (in g or mL/L/mm Hg), and P_{Xy} = its equilibrium partial pressure by Dalton's law.

By this relationship, it is clear that twice as much O_2 would be dissolved in water that is equilibrated with two atmospheres of pure oxygen than water equilibrated with one atmosphere of 100% O_2. Importantly, the solubility coefficient in aqueous media for CO_2 is 20-30 times higher than that for O_2. Indeed, the metal-containing pigments like hemoglobin (Hb) and myoglobin (Mb) likely evolved specifically to increase the O_2 carried in solution by orders of magnitude over the dissolved amount alone. The greater solubility of CO_2, due to its ready combination with water to form carbonic acid, H_2CO_3, obviates the need for an analogous pigment system simply to excrete this waste gas. Henry's law finds several practical applications in pulmonary medicine, notably during calcula-

tion of the total **oxygen content of arterial blood** (C_aO_2) (Chap. 3) and the use of that number to estimate **physiological shunt** (**Qs**) (Chap. 9).

Ambient Atmospheric Conditions

The earth's atmosphere is detectable to a height of at least 80 km above sea level, and for at least 50 km closest to the earth it is of constant composition: 79.02% N_2; 20.93% O_2; 0.03% CO_2; plus trace quantities of inert and rare gases (helium, argon, ozone, etc) that collectively comprise <0.02%. When the total mass of this 80 km-deep atmosphere is multiplied by the acceleration of gravity, its barometric pressure, P_B (force or weight per unit area) is sufficient to displace a column of mercury (Hg) to a height of 760 mm (Fig. 1.3). In the English (nonmetric) units of measure common in America, the earth's atmosphere weighs about 14.2 lb/in² at sea level.

Although atmospheric composition is invariant, gravity compresses the air downward, making its density highest closest to earth. Data show that atmospheric density decreases by half every ~5,500 m (18,000 ft) of elevation gained above sea level. This means that hikers standing on the summit of Alaska's Mt. Denali (elev. 6,194 m) have more than half the atmosphere's molecules below them in the 5.5 km closest to the surface, and less than half of all atmospheric gas between their hats and deep space, a distance of at least 50 km. At 5,500 m elevation, P_B is ~380 mm Hg, or in English units ~7.1 lb/in². Similarly, at 11,000 m elevation (~36,000 ft) where commercial jets cruise, ambient P_B outside the plane's windows is ~190 mm Hg, only one-fourth the P_B at Los Angeles International Airport (Fig. 1.4). Thus, hikers breathing ambient air on Denali's summit and animals in a non-pressurized baggage compartment on the jet, all

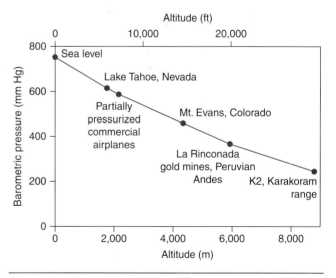

FIGURE 1.3 Barometric pressure P_B is reduced by half for every 5,500 m (18,000 ft) above sea level. *From West et al: High Altitude Medicine and Physiology. 4th ed. London, UK:Hodder-Arnold; 2007.*

#8

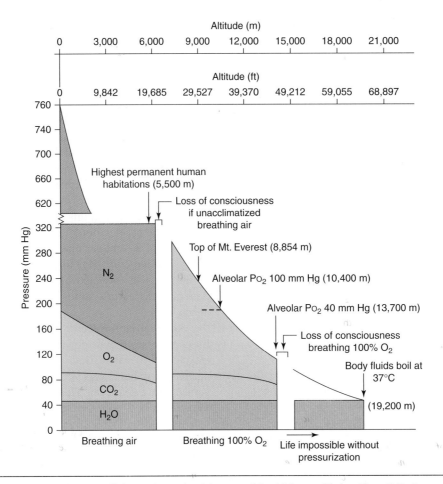

FIGURE 1.4 Decreasing P_B with altitude eventually lowers P_aO_2 to levels incompatible with human life (see Chap. 8). Native populations in the Andes of South America and the Himalayas of Tibet living at 5,500 m show physiological adaptations to altitude, both genetic and developmental. Mountaineering above this elevation by sea level natives is usually possible only for short durations and carries considerable risk.

experience "shortness of breath." They do so not because their F_IO_2 is less than at sea level, but because their P_IO_2 is less. We will see in Chap. 9 that it is this P_IO_2 and ultimately the **alveolar partial pressure for oxygen, P_AO_2** that drive the process of diffusive O_2 uptake in the alveoli.

▶▶ CLINICAL CORRELATION 1.1

This situation can be visualized as a thought experiment in which 100 people are stacked upon each other in the prone position. Everyone in the pile has essentially the same body composition as the person on top, but who is most likely to be squashed? In a relative sense, how will bodily distortion of the 75th person from the top compare to that of the 25th person from the top? Like a fluid-filled body, the atmosphere has real mass. Unlike those fluids, however, the atmosphere is compressible and conforms to the terrain around it, whether hill or hole.

Atmospheric water content varies over both time and space, often being very low and never approaching 100% RH globally. In addition, the atmosphere is generally much cooler than the human body at T_B of 37°C. Thus, atmospheric P_{H_2O} rarely exceeds the $P_{A_{H_2O}}$ of 47 mm Hg found within the warmer and fully humidified alveoli. Indeed, ventilation invariably represents a net loss of water to the body as a whole (Chap. 13). Putting all this information together with Dalton's law, we can calculate the partial pressures of ambient atmospheric gases in dry air at sea level to be: P_{O_2} = 159 mm Hg, P_{N_2} = 600 mm Hg, P_{CO_2} = 0.23 mm Hg, and P_{H_2O} = 0 mm Hg. As will be derived in Chap. 8, dilution of this ambient air during inspiration with the body's water vapor and CO_2 results in an alveolar P_AO_2 that cannot exceed about 110 mm Hg at sea level, with $P_{A_{N_2}}$ equal to ~560 mm Hg and $P_{A_{CO_2}}$ of ~40 mm Hg. All atmospheric values are reduced proportionally by altitude, so that the ambient P_{O_2} is ~80 mm Hg at 5,500 m, and P_AO_2 cannot exceed about 55 mm Hg at that elevation (Fig. 1.5). The consequences of such ambient **hypoxic hypoxia** (reduced P_AO_2) will be evident when the P_{O_2} required to fully oxygenate hemoglobin is formally considered (Chap. 3).

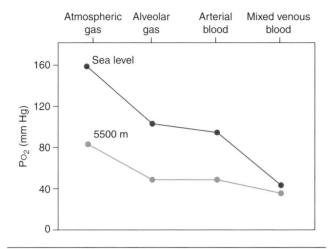

FIGURE 1.5 The unavoidable reductions in ambient P_{O_2} at altitude inevitably result in lower $P_{A_{O_2}}$, $P_{a_{O_2}}$, and reduced oxygen content in systemic capillaries. At 5,500 m elevation, $P_{a_{O_2}}$ is about 45 mm Hg, at which normal human hemoglobin is still >80% oxygenated. Compensatory increases in red cell mass and other elements of the O_2 transport cascade (Fig. 1.1) result in a mixed venous $P_{\bar{v}_{O_2}}$ that is only 7-10 mm Hg below that at sea level.

▶▶ **CLINICAL CORRELATION 1.2**

As implied in Fig. 1.5, the $P_{\bar{v}_{O_2}}$ of mixed venous blood rarely falls below 35-40 mm Hg in normal subjects at sea level. The P_{O_2} required to oxygenate 50% of hemoglobin's binding sites is only 26-27 mm Hg (Chap. 3). These observations indicate that systemic venous blood normally returns to the lungs for reoxygenation despite being still at ~75% of its binding capacity. Among other causes, both anemia and exercise will lower $P_{\bar{v}_{O_2}}$ slightly (Chap. 13) in otherwise healthy subjects. However, there appear to be other physiological constraints that prevent $P_{\bar{v}_{O_2}}$ from falling proportionally to the reductions in $P_{A_{O_2}}$ and $P_{a_{O_2}}$ that are unavoidable when breathing air at an altitude. These constraints may include tissue P_{O_2} levels in key organs like the heart and brain that cannot be lowered without causing irreversible injury by such blood-borne **hypoxemic hypoxia**.

Suggested Readings

1. West JB, Schoene RB, Milledge JS. *High Altitude Medicine and Physiology*. 4th ed. London, UK: Hodder-Arnold; 2007. *Each new edition of this highly rated text integrates the best of classic literature with the most recent findings in the field, with an excellent introduction to atmospheric conditions.*

2. Weinberger SE. *Principles of Pulmonary Medicine*. 2nd ed. Philadelphia, PA: WB Saunders; 1992. *One of the first attempts to combine within one text the fundamentals of respiratory physiology and the particulars of the many subcategories of pulmonary medicine.*

CASE STUDIES AND PRACTICE PROBLEMS

CASE 1.1 Which of the following statements is true or false, and why?

    a. The ambient $F_{I_{O_2}}$ decreases from sea level to the summit of Mt. Everest.

    b. P_B is greater at the bottom of a 2,000 m deep mine shaft than at the surface of the mine.

    c. The P_B in the passenger cabin of commercial airplanes is pressurized to sea level pressure.

    d. The $P_{I_{O_2}}$ of a scuba diver who is breathing compressed air under water at a depth of 30 m is higher than at sea level.

CASE 1.2 Ten different students attending New York University are each handed a 25°C glass of water open to the air, which they are instructed to stir continuously with a glass rod for 30 minutes. After stirring, a water sample from each glass is assessed for its P_{O_2} and compared to each student's own $P_{a_{O_2}}$ measured on blood drawn at that moment from their radial artery (these are brave students). On an average day, what percentage of these ten students will have a higher $P_{a_{O_2}}$ in their blood than the P_{O_2} of the water from their glass?

    Bonus question #1: Do the water and the subject's arterial blood have equal amounts of dissolved O_2 per mL?

    Bonus question #2: Which fluid has the greater total amount of O_2 per mL of each?

CASE 1.3 What is the expected clinical meaning of the following abbreviations, what are their likeliest units of measure, and where in the body would they be assayed?

    a. $P_{\bar{E}_{CO_2}}$

    b. $P_{\bar{v}_{O_2}}$

    c. $F_{IT_{N_2}}$

    d. $\dot{V}_{CO_2}$

Solutions to Case Studies and Practice Problems

CASE 1.1 The most appropriate answers to statements a-d are shown below, with at least a partial explanation:

a. **False**. Concentrations of atmospheric gases do not change appreciably with altitude, although their partial pressures decrease proportionally with the P_B.

b. **True**. Total atmospheric mass and thus its force (or weight and P_B) increase with total thickness or depth. The effect on P_B of this human-made increase in atmospheric depth (the mine shaft) would be most noticeable at or near the earth's surface where atmospheric density is highest.

c. **False**. It is difficult to make an aircraft as airtight as a can of soda. Their inherent leakiness permits a maximal pressurization to an effective P_B of 2,000-2,500 m when cruising at an actual elevation closer to 11,000 m. Most passengers do not note this modest degree of ambient **hypoxic hypoxia** in the aircraft cabin because they are resting rather than exercising vigorously.

d. **True**. The density of water is sufficient that its weight equals that of one atmosphere of air for every 10 m of water depth. Thus at 30 m, a diver's air-filled chest must be able to resist at least four atmospheres of total pressure (1 atm for the air + 3 atm for the water), or the airways and lungs will collapse from this external force. Remembering Dalton's law, the effective P_IO_2 for this diver would be four times that at the water surface.

CASE 1.2 0% (none).

The Po_2 in a glass of water is always higher for several reasons. First, there is no inherent barrier to O_2 diffusing into the water as there is for alveolar O_2 diffusing through the septal barrier to reach the blood. Thus, the Po_2 in the glass at sea level will equilibrate to that in the atmosphere, about 160 mm Hg at sea level where NYU is located. Second, there is very little CO_2 diffusing into or out of water in the glass that would reduce by Dalton's law the effective Po_2, as universally occurs in people. Third, there are no zones of "$\dot{V}_A/\dot{Q}$ mismatch" (nonequilibrium) in the glass as long as each student stirred as instructed, although even healthy people have a small difference between their P_AO_2 and P_aO_2 for this reason (Chap. 8). Fourth, the effective P_{H_2O} at the surface of the water glass at 25°C is about 31 mm Hg, considerably lower than the 47 mm Hg in a human at 37°C, which again by Dalton's law would reduce the effective Po_2. Thus, persons breathing air at sea level would have a P_AO_2 of ~100 mm Hg versus a Po_2 ~160 mm Hg in the glass of water they are holding.

Bonus question #1: Because of Henry's law, the water will contain more dissolved oxygen, owing to its higher Po_2.

Bonus question #2: The total content of oxygen per mL will always be higher in blood than in water (or plasma) because of the presence of hemoglobin. As will be covered in Chap. 3, the amount of oxygen carried in arterial blood as oxyhemoglobin will be several orders of magnitude larger than the dissolved fraction, unless P_B was very high.

CASE 1.3 The most appropriate answers for the four abbreviations are as follows:

a. $P_{\bar{E}}CO_2$ = the mean expiratory partial pressure of CO_2 in mm Hg, typically averaged at the mouthpiece over the course of a normal tidal volume V_T.

b. $P_{\bar{v}}O_2$ = the oxygen partial pressure of mixed venous blood in mm Hg, most often obtained from a central venous line or pulmonary artery catheter that is sampling from the right ventricle or main pulmonary artery.

c. $F_{IT}N_2$ = the decimal fraction of nitrogen gas within the trachea, nominally a value from 0.0 to 1.0 but likely to approximate the F_{N_2} in ambient air of 0.72-0.78, depending on its dilution by Dalton's law with airway CO_2 and water vapor.

d. $\dot{V}_{CO_2}$ = the whole-body rate of CO_2 production, usually in mL/min (STPD) and often corrected for subject body weight, that is, mL/min/kg. In practice, all expired gas is accumulated for several minutes, with its total volume calculated by anemometer and its average (CO_2) measured by infrared absorbance.

Development and Functional Anatomy of the Lungs and Airways

DAVID S. BRINK, MD AND ANDREW J. LECHNER, PhD

Introduction to Lung Structure

The respiratory system is classically divided into two parts, based on their structures and functions. The first is the **conducting zone**, being the organized array of progressively smaller airways through which air moves into and out of the lungs during **tidal ventilation**. The conducting zone starts at the nares (and/or mouth) and includes the **nasal cavities, pharynx, larynx, trachea, bronchi**, and **bronchioles**. The second part is the **respiratory parenchyma**, being the densely packed collection of membrane walls, thin enough to support **molecular diffusion** between the inspired air and blood coursing through the microvasculature of the lung (Fig. 2.1). Constituents of the respiratory parenchyma begin where the conducting zone ends and include the **respiratory bronchioles, alveolar ducts, alveolar sacs**, and **alveoli**. The gross and microscopic appearances of each component are the primary focus of this chapter, with the principal functions for each presented with more detail in subsequent chapters.

The major histologic features of each constituent of the respiratory tract are broadly summarized in Table 2.1. Within the lungs are blood and lymphatic vessels and nerves. The **pulmonary arteries** and their branches travel beside similarly sized airways, while **pulmonary veins** and **lymphatics** travel in the connective tissue septa that form the boundaries of each **lung lobule**. **Bronchial arteries** have narrower diameters and thicker walls than the pulmonary arteries, reflecting the smaller quantity of blood they carry (but under higher pressure). They also travel with airways but are inconspicuous due to their small size. Within the connective tissue surrounding larger airways are afferent and efferent nerve fibers. The external surface of the lung is covered by **mesothelium**, a simple squamous epithelium which normally is in contact with the mesothelial lining of the hemithoraces. The mesothelial layer that covers the entire outer surface of the lungs is called the **visceral pleura**, while the mesothelium that lines the hemithoraces is called the **parietal pleura**.

Principal Sections of the Respiratory Tract

The Nasal Cavities

The two nasal cavities are separated by a nasal septum composed of cartilage anteriorly and bone posteriorly. Each cavity is subdivided into three segments: the **vestibule**, the **respiratory segment**, and the **olfactory segment**. The vestibule is the short chamber just internal to the naris and is lined by stratified squamous epithelium. Externally, this epithelium is keratinized like skin before gradually transitioning to a nonkeratinizing form as in the oropharynx. Vestibular hairs, called **vibrissae**, filter large particulate matter. Within the **lamina propria** of the vestibule, as in the dermis, are hair follicles, eccrine glands, and sebaceous glands (Fig. 2.2).

Internal to each vestibule are the respiratory segments of the nasal cavities. Although they are parts of the conducting zone and not the diffusive respiratory parenchyma, their name reflects their lining of **respiratory mucosa**. Respiratory mucosa is common within the respiratory system and consists of a ciliated pseudo-stratified columnar **respiratory epithelium** overlying layers of dense irregular connective tissue, the **perichondrium** of cartilage and the **periosteum** of bone. Deeper within the respiratory system, this connective tissue layer consists of loose irregular connective tissue characteristic of **lamina propria**. The staggered vertical distribution of nuclei within the respiratory epithelium suggests that it is stratified into multiple layers. However, all of its cells touch the basement membrane, and thus the epithelium is pseudo-stratified. Within it are three main types of cells: **ciliated cells, goblet cells**, and **basal cells**. Ciliated cells exhibit coordinated

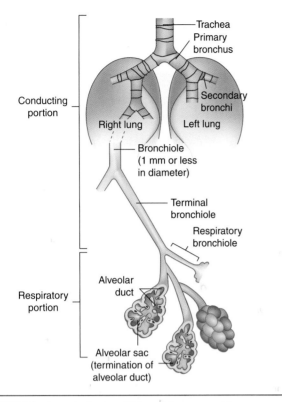

FIGURE 2.1 The main divisions of the respiratory tract. The structures illustrated are not drawn to scale. *From Junqueira et al. Basic Histology, 6th ed. Norkwalk, CT: Appleton & Lange; 1989.*

motility of their apical cilia to propel a sheet of mucus in retrograde direction over the surface of the epithelium, plus any particulate matter embedded within the mucus. Goblet cells are unicellular glands that produce copious quantities of mucus. Basal cells serve as progenitors that repopulate the epithelium as needed through mitosis and subsequent differentiation. Additional cell types that are less commonly noted within respiratory epithelium include **brush cells**, which are columnar in appearance and have apical microvilli rather than true cilia. There are also small granular **neuroendocrine cells** that rest upon the basement membrane (Fig. 2.3).

Extending from the lateral walls of the nasal cavity are three bony projections termed the superior, middle, and inferior **conchae**. The middle and inferior conchae are part of the vestibule and are lined by respiratory mucosa; the roof and superior concha comprise the olfactory segments of the nasal cavity. An olfactory segment consists of an **olfactory epithelium** overlying a lamina propria that contains **Bowman glands**, which are serous. The principal constituents within the olfactory epithelium are **olfactory cells** (or **bipolar neurosensory cells**). These are modified neurons with apical nonmotile cilia, which function as chemoreceptors, and basal afferent axons that join to form the olfactory nerves. In addition, the olfactory epithelium contains **supporting cells**, with apical microvilli that resemble the brush cells of respiratory epithelium, and regenerative **basal cells**, also similar to those in respiratory epithelium. Histologically, the olfactory epithelium

Table **2.1**   **Structural changes in the respiratory tract**

	Nasal cavity	Naso-pharynx	Larynx	Trachea	Bronchi Large	Bronchi Small	Bronchioles Regular	Bronchioles Terminal	Bronchioles Respiratory
epithelium	pseudo-stratified ciliated columnar[a]						pseudo-stratified ciliated columnar $\rightarrow$	transition simple ciliated columnar $\rightarrow$	simple ciliated cuboidal
goblet cells	abundant				present	few	scattered	none	
glands	abundant		present			few	none		
cartilage			complex	C-shaped rings	irregular rings	plates & islands	none		
smooth muscle	none			posterior spanning open ends of C-shaped rings		crisscrossing spiral bundles			
elastic fibers	none	present			abundant				

[a]The **vestibule** of the nasal cavity transitions from **keratinizing stratified squamous epithelium to nonkeratinizing stratified squamous** epithelium. Much of the epiglottis and the true vocal chords are lined by nonkeratinizing stratified squamous epithelium. *From* Basic Histology, *6th ed. Norwalk, CT: Appleton & Lange; 1989.*

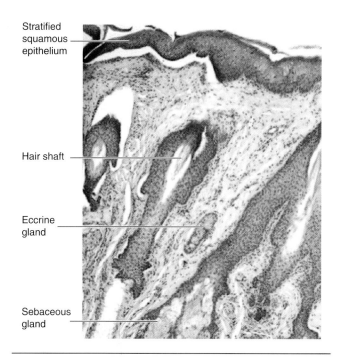

- Stratified squamous epithelium
- Hair shaft
- Eccrine gland
- Sebaceous gland

FIGURE 2.2 Histologically the nasal vestibule is very similar to skin, being lined by stratified squamous epithelium with eccrine sweat ducts and sebaceous glands associated with hair follicles. The vestibule is keratinized distally but not proximally.

is also termed pseudo-stratified: nuclei situated closest to the lumen belong to supporting cells; nuclei nearest the epithelium's basement membrane are basal cells; and nuclei located between these two other nuclear layers are those of the chemoreceptive olfactory cells (Fig. 2.4).

The Paranasal Sinuses

The paranasal sinuses are blind-ended cavities within the frontal, maxillary, ethmoid, and sphenoid bones. The sinuses open into the larger and more centrally located nasal cavities. As noted for the respiratory segments of the nasal cavities, the paranasal sinuses are lined by respiratory mucosa with abundant seromucinous glands. The motile cilia on their epithelial surfaces move mucus and any embedded particulate matter into the nasal cavity for subsequent expulsion.

The Pharynx

The pharynx is divided positionally into its nasal and oral portions. The **nasopharynx** is lined by the same general type of respiratory mucosa as the respiratory segments of the nasal cavities. In contrast, the **oropharynx** is covered by a nonkeratinizing stratified squamous epithelium, similar in appearance and function to epithelium that lines the internal nasal vestibule and much of the oral cavity (Fig. 2.5).

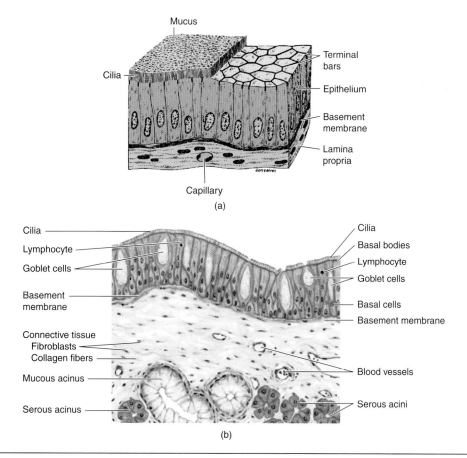

(a)

(b)

FIGURE 2.3 (a) Schematic of pseudo-stratified respiratory epithelium. Nuclei appear stratified, but all cells rest upon the basement membrane. *From Junqueria's Basic Histology, McGraw-Hill; 2009.* (b) Respiratory epithelium as it would appear with H&E staining. *From diFiore's Atlas of Histology with Functional Correlations, 10th ed. Lippincott; 2005.*

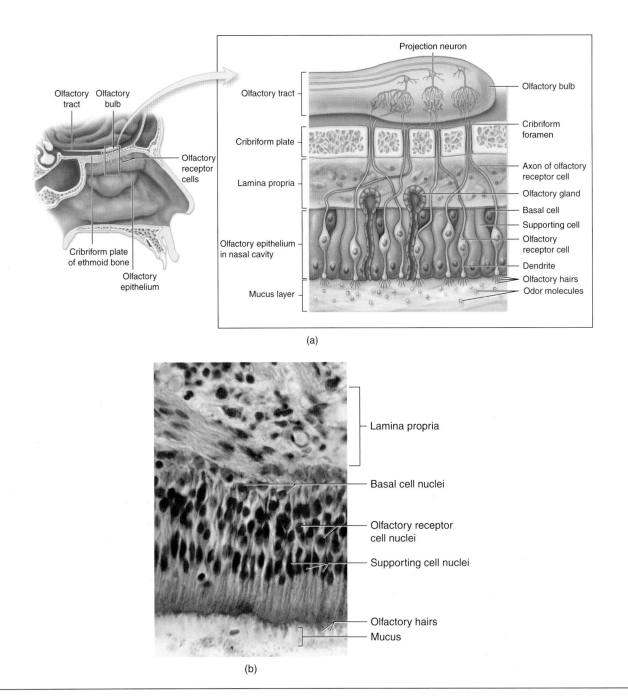

(a)

(b)

FIGURE 2.4 (a) and (b) Olfactory epithelium covers the roof of the nasal cavity and superior concha. Olfactory hairs are nonmotile cilia that function as chemoreceptors. Bowman olfactory glands secrete serous fluid. *From Junqueira's Basic Histology. New York, NY. McGraw-Hill; 2009.*

The Larynx 井13

The larynx connects the pharynx and trachea. Its most notable feature is the **epiglottis**, a movable boundary separating the respiratory tract from the digestive system. During swallowing, the epiglottis covers the laryngeal lumen to prevent aspiration of oropharyngeal materials and direct those materials into the esophagus. When breathing and/or speaking, the epiglottis is retracted anteriorly, allowing large volumes of air to travel into and out of the trachea. The core of the epiglottis is made of elastic cartilage that provides flexibility and strength.

The epiglottal surface is covered by stratified squamous epithelium on its anterosuperior/lingual portion and also on the superior segment of its inferior/laryngeal portion. On the laryngeal side of the epiglottis, the stratified squamous epithelium found apically makes a smooth transition into ciliated pseudo-stratified respiratory epithelium toward the base.

The larynx (Fig. 2.6) is generally arranged as an epithelium overlying sheets of fibrous connective tissue that contain abundant seromucinous glands and cartilage, all of which are surrounded by skeletal muscles. Inferior to the epiglottis are

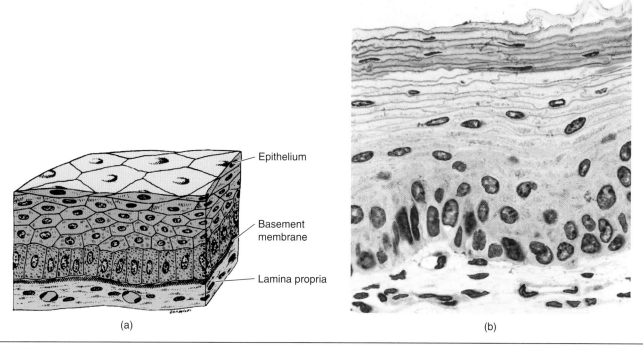

(a)   (b)

FIGURE 2.5 (a) Schematic of the stratified squamous epithelium lining the oropharynx and much of the oral cavity. (b) Histologic section (H&E stain) of nonkeratinizing stratified squamous epithelium. *From* Junqueira's Basic Histology. *New York, NY. McGraw-Hill; 2009.*

the **false vocal chords** (or **vestibular folds**). Inferior to the false chords are the **laryngeal ventricles**, blind-ended sacs that extend superolaterally from the laryngeal lumen. Beneath these ventricles are the **true vocal chords** (or **vocal folds**), a common reference point used to describe the position of masses and other objects within the larynx. In this sense, **supraglottic** refers to laryngeal locations that are superior to the true vocal chords, and **infraglottic** refers to laryngeal locations that are inferior to the true vocal chords.

Except for the true vocal chords and part of the epiglottis, the larynx is lined by true respiratory epithelium overlying perichondrium of any regional cartilage and overlying lamina propria in those areas lacking cartilage (Fig. 2.6). The lamina propria of the laryngeal ventricles contains lymphoid tissues that form an airway component of the **mucosa-associated lymphoid tissues (MALTs)**. Unlike most of the larynx, the true vocal chords are covered by nonkeratinizing stratified squamous epithelium that overlies a lamina propria containing the **vocalis muscle**, a skeletal muscle important in phonation. The shield-shaped **thyroid cartilage** and the signet ring-shaped **cricoid cartilage** are both composed of hyaline cartilage, while the epiglottis, **corniculate cartilages** and **cuneiform cartilages** are of the elastic form. The **arytenoid cartilages** that serve as insertions for the vocalis muscles contain both elastic and hyaline cartilage. Although these structures are collectively called the laryngeal cartilages, with age they can undergo ossification and become composites of cartilage and bone.

The Trachea and Bronchi

The trachea extends from the inferior-most cartilage of the larynx (the cricoid cartilage) to the primary bronchi and is lined

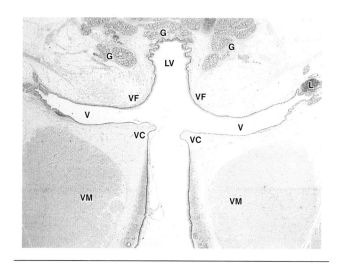

FIGURE 2.6 Coronal section of the larynx. Vestibular folds (VF) or false chords are superior to and separated from the true vocal chords (VC) by the laryngeal ventricles (V), whose lateral aspects are associated with lymphoid tissue (L). The vocalis muscle (VM) is a skeletal muscle in the VC under voluntary control and important for phonation. Seromucinous glands (G) surround the laryngeal vestibule (LV) superiorly. The VC are lined by nonkeratinizing stratified squamous epithelium, and all remaining structures by respiratory epithelium. *From* Junqueira's Basic Histology. *New York, NY. McGraw-Hill; 2009.*

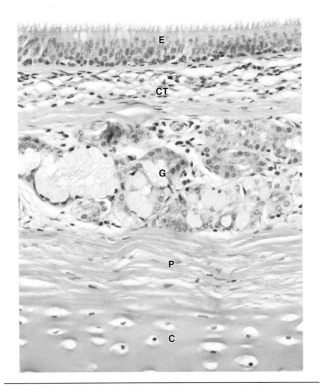

FIGURE 2.7 From luminal surface outward, tracheal wall consists of respiratory epithelium (E), a connective tissue (CT) lamina propria that contains seromucinous glands (G), and the perichondrium (P) overlying hyaline cartilage (C). The smooth muscle layer is not shown but is limited to the posterior tracheal wall and deep to the lamina propria. *From Junqueira's Basic Histology. New York, NY. McGraw-Hill; 2009.*

by the same respiratory mucosa described earlier. In the lamina propria of the tracheal mucosa are abundant seromucinous glands, below which are a series of C-shaped rings of hyaline cartilage (Fig. 2.7). The opening of each C-shaped tracheal ring is directed posteriorly, where the tracheal mucosa overlies smooth muscle that completes the wall of each ring. At the carina, the trachea bifurcates into right and left mainstem or **primary bronchi**, each of which dichotomously branches 9-12 times. Each generation of these deeper branches becomes successively shorter and narrower. From inside to out, bronchial walls consist of respiratory epithelium, with fewer goblet cells than in trachea, overlying a lamina propria that sits upon crisscrossing bands of smooth muscle comprising the **muscularis mucosae**. Beneath the muscularis mucosae is a submucosal layer with fewer seromucinous glands than the trachea. The submucosal layer overlies hyaline cartilage, which is itself surrounded by a diffuse adventitia of fibrous connective tissue (Fig. 2.8).

Proximally, bronchial cartilage forms a series of rings; distally, the bronchial cartilage consists of islands and plates. Moving from the proximal to distal bronchi, the relative densities of both goblet cells and seromucinous glands decrease (Fig. 2.8).

The Bronchioles

As these dichotomously branching airways become smaller, they contain less cartilage and fewer submucosal glands. Indeed, a **bronchiole** is defined as a distal airway devoid of cartilage and

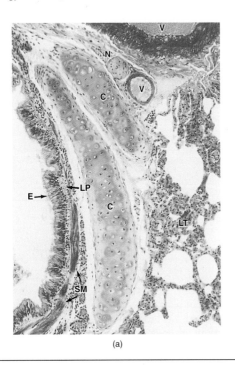

(a)

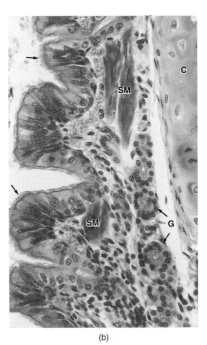

(b)

FIGURE 2.8 Histological sections of a large bronchus (a) and smaller bronchus (b) both by H&E staining. Bronchi are lined by respiratory epithelium (E) overlying a lamina propria (LP), crisscrossing bands of smooth muscle (SM), seromucinous glands (G), and hyaline cartilage (C). In mainstem bronchi, such cartilage forms complete rings; more distally the cartilage is not annular but rather is insular or plate-like. The presence of SM between the epithelium and cartilage layers is a useful distinguishing feature between bronchus and trachea. Moving distally, bronchi have fewer goblet cells and glands. Also shown are a nerve (N), several blood vessels (V), and adjacent alveolar lung tissue (LT). *From Junqueira's Basic Histology. New York, NY. McGraw-Hill; 2009.*

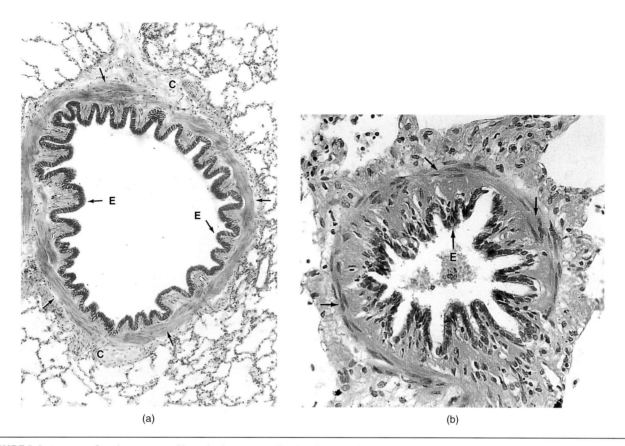

(a)   (b)

FIGURE 2.9 In moving from large proximal bronchioles (a) to smaller distal bronchioles (b), the epithelium transitions from pseudo-stratified ciliated columnar to simple ciliated cuboidal epithelia. Deep to these epithelia is the lamina propria, surrounded by thinning layers of smooth muscle (arrows). In contrast to bronchi, the bronchioles lack seromucinous glands and cartilage. Both sections shown are with H&E staining. *From* Junqueira's Basic Histology. *New York, NY. McGraw-Hill; 2009.*

submucosal glands. A bronchiole that subtends or abuts a lung acinus is termed a **terminal bronchiole**. When alveoli are seen histologically to project outward from the lumen of a bronchiole, that airway is called a **respiratory bronchiole**. Functionally, this is an important distinction because such a respiratory bronchiole signifies the beginning of the respiratory parenchyma, where at least limited diffusive gas exchange occurs (Chaps. 4 and 9). Bronchiolar epithelium changes in thickness over its proximal to distal length, from pseudo-stratified ciliated columnar epithelium (where the airway is widest) to a **simple ciliated columnar epithelium**, and then to **simple ciliated cuboidal epithelium** (where the airway is narrowest). While proximal bronchioles contain scattered goblet cells, the terminal and respiratory bronchioles normally contain none. The crisscrossing smooth muscle layers of the muscularis mucosae that are such prominent features of upper bronchi also diminish distally, being nearly absent in respiratory bronchioles (Fig. 2.9).

Alveolar Ducts, Alveolar Sacs, and Alveoli

Alveolar ducts arise from distal respiratory bronchioles but are difficult to recognize histologically due to their narrow

lumens and random orientation in a tissue plane. Students should remember to translate the flat images of lung they see on slides into what such a section must look like in three dimensions (Fig. 2.10). Thus, the wall of an alveolar duct often appears to be just two-three rows of openings into adjacent alveoli, separated by pillars of smooth muscle and elastin that function as tiny sphincters and maintain structural integrity.

Alveolar ducts and their surrounding alveoli are lined by a simple squamous epithelium composed of **type 1 pneumocytes** that account for ~95% of total alveolar surface area. Interspersed among type 1 cells and often situated in alveolar corners are cuboidal **type 2 pneumocytes** that cover ~5% of alveolar surfaces. As presented in Chap. 9, most diffusive gas exchange occurs from alveolar air spaces through type 1 pneumocytes, whose basement membranes are fused to the basement membrane of capillary endothelial cells (Fig. 2.11). Type 2 pneumocytes secrete **surfactant**, a mixture of phospholipids and proteins that reduces surface tension and promotes alveolar stability at low lung volumes (Chap. 5). While alveoli are often visualized as blind-ended sacs, their walls contain **pores of Kohn** to facilitate pressure equilibration and cellular communication among adjacent alveoli (Chap. 10).

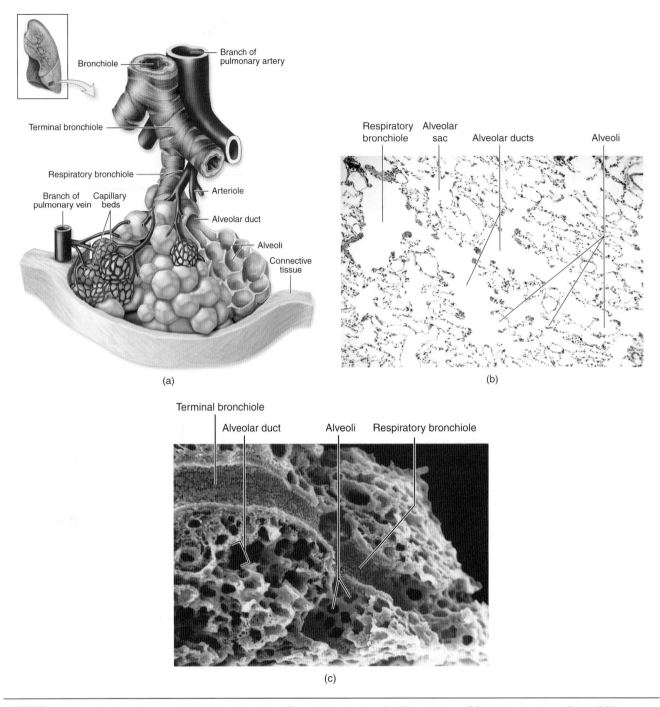

(a)

(b)

(c)

FIGURE 2.10 (a) Schematic diagram showing the relationship of bronchioles to more distal components of the respiratory parenchyma. (b) A respiratory bronchiole resembles a terminal bronchiole except that its wall is interrupted by occasional alveoli. Alveolar ducts may be difficult to distinguish due to the small amounts of smooth muscle in their walls. (c) Scanning electron microscopy is useful in showing the three-dimensional structure of respiratory bronchioles, alveolar ducts, and the alveoli distal to them. *From* Junqueira's Basic Histology. *New York, NY. McGraw-Hill; 2009.*

Organization of the Lung

A **lung lobule** is defined as the smallest subunit of respiratory parenchyma bounded by the connective tissue sheath of an **interlobular septum** (Fig. 2.12). A typical lung lobule is about 2 cm in diameter, and its boundary layer of connective tissue normally is very thin and difficult to see macroscopically. In certain pathologic conditions, these interlobular septa are thickened and more readily seen. In this context, a lung lobule is the smallest *anatomical* unit of lung that has its own major airway and innervation, and it receives blood from both ventricles. In contrast, the **lung acinus** is the smallest

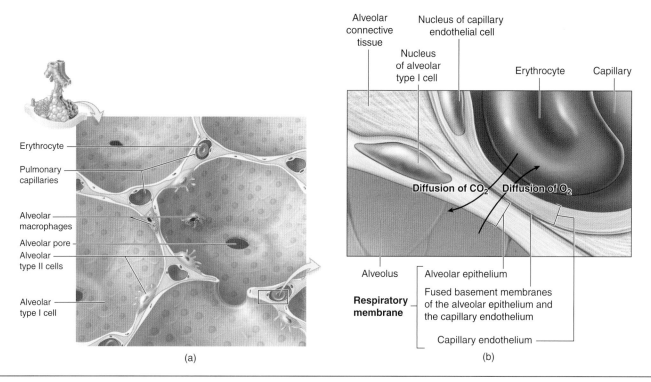

FIGURE 2.11 Alveoli are the sites of diffusional gas exchange. (a) Schematic representation of the three-dimensional structure of alveoli. (b) Diagram of the intimate relationship between a type 1 pneumocyte and the adjacent capillary endothelial cell. *From* Junqueira's Basic Histology. *New York, NY. McGraw-Hill; 2009.*

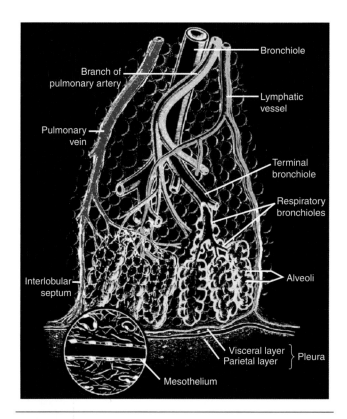

FIGURE 2.12 Organization of the lung into lobules. Lobules are bounded by connective tissue septa through which run pulmonary veins and lymphatic vessels. Between septa bounding the lobule are 3-10 acini. Note that pulmonary arteries travel with the airways and not with the pulmonary veins. Bronchial arteries (not shown) are much smaller and also travel with the airways. *From* Junqueira's Basic Histology. *New York, NY. McGraw-Hill; 2009.*

functional unit of the lung, consisting of all the respiratory parenchyma distal to one terminal bronchiole. Each lung lobule contains 3-10 acini.

Pulmonary arteries travel besides conducting zone airways, often being quite similar in diameters. These pulmonary arteries transport deoxygenated blood from the right ventricle to alveolar capillaries via pulmonary arterioles (Chaps. 7 and 9). In turn, alveolar capillaries drain reoxygenated blood into pulmonary venules, which merge into pulmonary veins and then fill the left atrium. While most arteries seen in lung tissue sections are pulmonary arteries from the right heart, smaller **bronchial arteries** can sometimes be distinguished. These represent aortic branches and carry oxygenated blood and other nutrients to the respiratory parenchyma. Such blood from bronchial arteries is delivered at higher perfusion pressures than those within pulmonary arteries (Chap. 7). Interestingly, bronchial arterial blood also drains into the pulmonary veins, since there are no distinct bronchial veins. This mixing of venous bloods with potentially very different oxygen contents contributes to **physiological shunt** (Chap. 9).

The lymphatic vessels of the lung as well as the main pulmonary veins do not travel along the principal airways but rather are found in the interlobular septa that define the lung lobules. Within the connective tissue adventitia that surrounds larger airways are efferent parasympathetic fibers (from the vagus nerve), which cause bronchial constriction, as well as efferent sympathetic nerves, which cause bronchial dilation. Also within this connective tissue zone are the smaller afferent visceral nerves that transmit sensations associated with airway caliber and pain (Chap. 11).

Development of the Respiratory System *(#14)*

During the third week of gestation, a groove in the primitive foregut originates, and, by week 4, the primordial single lung bud bifurcates. During weeks 5-6, the primary bronchi continue to elongate and divide, so that by the end of week 6 there are usually 10 segmental bronchi on the right and 8-9 segmental bronchi on the left. This entire period of lung development from gestational days 26 through 42 is known as the **embryonic stage** (Fig. 2.13).

During gestational weeks 6-16, in the **pseudoglandular stage** of lung development, many additional airways are formed, usually to the level of the terminal bronchioles (Fig. 2.14). During this phase, the first ciliated cells appear in the airways (week 10), followed by the first recognizable goblet cells (weeks 13-14), and then development of the more convoluted seromucinous glands of the submucosal layer (weeks 15-16).

During gestational weeks 17-28, the **canalicular stage** (or acinar stage) of lung development occurs, forming the fundamental gas-exchanging architecture of the lung acini (Fig. 2.15). During this phase, type 1 and type 2 pneumocytes appear (week 20), and by week 24 cartilage extends to the most distal bronchi.

During gestational weeks 28-34, the **saccular stage** of lung development occurs in which alveolar saccules form by subdividing existing acinar compartments into smaller spaces, and by elaboration of their associated capillary networks. By gestational week 35 and continuing after birth, the **alveolar stage** of development has begun in earnest, usually evident as an explosive increase of epithelial surface area and a corresponding thinning of the alveolar septal membranes to the dimensions seen in adult lungs.

Throughout gestation, lung vasculature forms concurrently with airway development and is fundamentally an intrauterine process. Major airways and their associated vessels are formed by week 16, although they continue to expand in length and diameter with subsequent growth. Although alveolar development begins in utero, most alveoli in the adult lung form postnatally. At birth, there are ~50 million alveoli. Within several years and presuming a normal growth pattern for a child, the number of alveoli grows to 300-600 million. Subsequent lung growth is predominantly related to modest increases in the diameters of alveoli (that increase respiratory parenchymal volume to the third power of such a change in diameter) rather than vastly increasing the numbers of alveoli.

All epithelial components of the respiratory system are **endodermal** in origin, while the cartilaginous and muscular components derive from the **splanchnic mesoderm** that surrounds the fetal foregut. Laryngeal muscles originate from the fourth and sixth **branchial arches** and are innervated by branches of the vagus nerve (cranial nerve X). Muscles that are derivatives of the fourth branchial arch, including the **cricothyroid**, **levator palatini**, and **pharyngeal constrictors**, are innervated by the **superior laryngeal nerve**. Muscles derived from the sixth branchial arch, notably the **intrinsic laryngeal muscles**, are innervated by the **recurrent laryngeal nerve**.

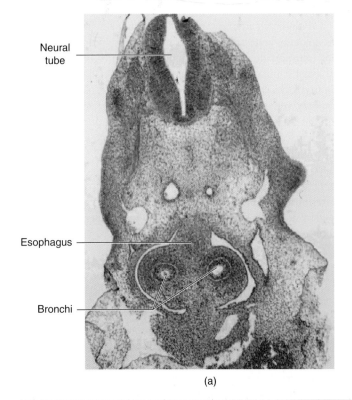

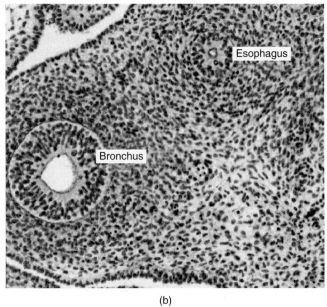

(a)   (b)

FIGURE 2.13 (a) The embryonic stage of early lung development in a 32-day fetus. (b) The developing bronchi at higher magnification. *From deMello and Reid.* Pediat Develop Path. *2000;3:439-449.*

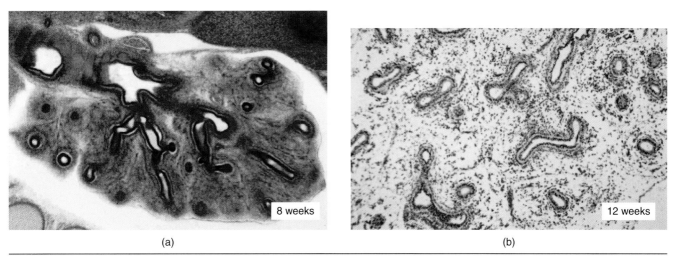

FIGURE 2.14 The pseudoglandular stage of early lung development in these two midterm fetuses at 8 weeks gestation (a) and 12 weeks gestation (b). *From deMello and Reid.* Pediat Develop Path. *2000;3:439-449.*

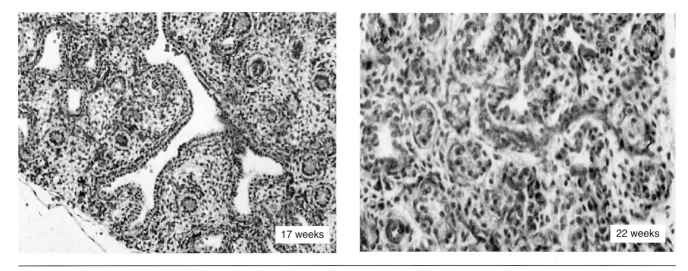

FIGURE 2.15 During the canalicular stage of lung development, airways continue to mature and the first acini appear, including the beginnings of their capillary networks. *From deMello and Reid.* Pediat Develop Path. *2000;3:439-449.*

Suggested Readings

1. Weibel ER. *Morphometry of the Human Lung.* New York, NY: Academic Press; 1965. *An excellent introduction to the design and dimensions of the alveolar compartment, Professor Weibel put the Anatomical Institute in Bern on the map.*

2. Reid L. The embryology of the lung. In: DeReuck AVS and Porter R, eds. *Development of the Lung.* London, UK: Churchill; 1967:109-124. *Most consider Dr Reid to be the mother of*

neonatal lung physiology, having taught two generations of students about the development of the human gas exchanger.*

3. Thurlbeck WM. Postnatal growth and development of the lung. *Am Rev Respir Dis.* 1975;111:803-844. *A pivotal paper in the field, in which the notion was first espoused that not all mammals are born with lungs at the same degree of maturation, and that alveolarization began in utero.*

CASE STUDIES AND PRACTICE PROBLEMS

CASE 2.1 The H&E stained tissue shown below was obtained by lobar biopsy and fixed in the inflated state by its major airway. The asterisk (*) is in what type of structure?

   a. Respiratory bronchiole

   b. Alveolar duct

   c. Terminal bronchiole

   d. Alveolus

   e. Lymphatic vessel

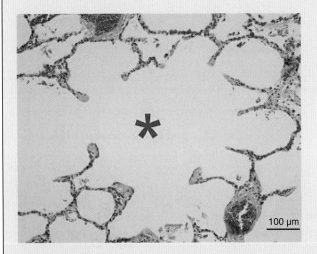

100 μm

CASE 2.2 Which of the following structures travel within the fibrous connective tissue septa between lung lobules?

   a. Pulmonary veins and pulmonary arteries

   b. Pulmonary veins and bronchial arteries

   c. Bronchial veins and bronchial arteries

   d. Pulmonary veins and lymphatics

   e. Pulmonary arteries and lymphatics

CASE 2.3 The H&E stained tissue shown in upper right column was obtained by lung biopsy from a healthy donor. The asterisk (*) is in the lumen of what type of structure?

   a. Pulmonary artery

   b. Pulmonary vein

   c. Bronchial artery

   d. Bronchial vein

   e. Large lymphatic vessel

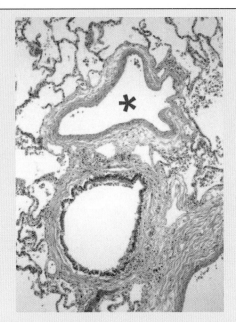

CASE 2.4 Shown below is a photomicrograph of an H&E stained section of normal adult lung tissue. The asterisk (*) is in the lumen of which type of structure?

   a. Larynx above the ventricle

   b. Larynx below the ventricle

   c. Bronchus

   d. Trachea

   e. Bronchiole

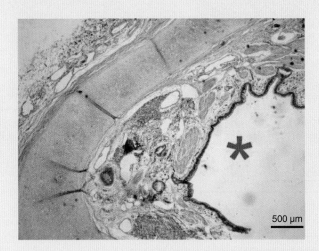

500 μm

Solutions to Case Studies and Practice Problems

CASE 2.1 The most correct answer is b, alveolar duct.

Note in this image the circumferential orientation of many alveolar openings around the central conduit or opening in the center, which itself has poorly defined walls that are interrupted by the pillar-like posts at the proximal ends of each.

CASE 2.2 The most correct answer is d, pulmonary veins and lymphatics.

Pulmonary arteries and bronchial arteries travel together adjacent to airways, although pulmonary arteries are much more commonly seen. Bronchial veins have never been convincingly demonstrated in the human lung.

CASE 2.3 The most correct answer is a, pulmonary artery.

Noting the prominent airway below the structure in question with its pseudo-stratified columnar epithelium, only one other structure listed among the possible answers could be correct (*answer c*), but this would be a very large bronchial artery. All other choices either travel along the interlobular septa (*answers b and e*) or do not exist (*answer d*).

CASE 2.4 The most correct answer is c, bronchus.

The presence of a smooth muscle layer that is deep to the epithelium rules out *choices a, b,* and *d*. The external muscles of the larynx as well as the vocalis muscle are all skeletal muscles. Note that the structure in question has cartilage (left side of image) and a few seromucinous glands, both of which rule out *choice e*.

Chapter 3

Mechanisms of O$_2$ and CO$_2$ Transport by Erythrocytes

ANDREW J. LECHNER, PhD

Learning Objectives

- The student will be able to define and derive the six standard erythrocyte indices as evaluated in a complete blood count.
- The student will be able to calculate dissolved and bound O$_2$ contents of blood when given data for its Po$_2$, percent oxygenation, and hemoglobin concentration ([Hb]).
- The student will be able to identify basic features of an HbO$_2$ dissociation curve including its P$_{50}$, and the effects of pH, Pco$_2$, [2,3-DPG], temperature, carbon monoxide, and common genetic changes on the P$_{50}$.
- The student will be able to describe the major mechanisms by which erythrocytes promote CO$_2$ transport, and estimate the compartment sizes of CO$_2$ carried in dissolved, Hb-bound, or dissociated states.

Introduction #18

The major function of **erythrocytes** or red blood cells (RBCs) is transport of the respiratory pigment **hemoglobin (Hb)**. In their mature form, erythrocytes are biconcave discs 7-8 μm in diameter, with thickness of 0.5-2.0 μm, and an average volume of 80-90 μm^3 or fL. Whole blood contains large numbers of RBCs, typically 4.5-6.0 × 10^6/μL. Although living cells, mature erythrocytes are anucleate and contain few organelles. During a typical functional life span of 120 days, each RBC may travel 1,000 km from synthesis in the marrow until #19 destruction in liver, spleen, or other site. Factors that regulate RBC production and longevity are beyond the scope of this book, except as they influence O$_2$ and CO$_2$ movements across alveolar septa and into blood vessels that originate in the right ventricle and traverse the lungs before returning to the left ventricle.

The Six Standard Erythrocyte (#20) Indices

As part of a **complete blood count** (CBC) done on each hospital admission, the following three indices are routinely measured on a patient's RBCs:

Hematocrit—the fraction of whole blood that is composed of erythrocytes, most commonly expressed in percent. Historically, blood was placed in glass capillary tubes and centrifuged until the erythrocytes sedimented together at the bottom, with a "buffy coat" of leukocytes and platelets above them, and clear, amber-colored plasma on top. Normal values for hematocrit (Hct) vary with age and sex over predictable ranges (Fig. 3.1).

Hemoglobin Concentration—the quantity of hemoglobin (Hb) per unit of blood, usually expressed as g/dL or simply g%. Historically, hemoglobin concentration ([Hb]) was determined by diluting whole blood with potassium ferricyanide to lyse the RBCs and oxidize ferrous ions (Fe^{2+}) to ferric ions (Fe^{3+}), thus converting normal Hb into **methemoglobin (metHb)** that cannot bind O$_2$. MetHb combines with cyanide ions to form a quantifiable color product, **cyanomethemoglobin**. [Hb] also varies with age and sex (Fig. 3.1).

Red Blood Cell Count—the density of erythrocytes in whole blood, typically reported as ×10^6/μL. Due to their great numbers and small size, whole blood is first diluted with 0.9% NaCl (**normal saline**). Historically, erythrocytes were counted manually by microscope on a calibrated glass slide (**hemacytometer**). Contemporary automated channel counters draw dilute red blood cell (RBC) suspensions through a narrow orifice, recording changes in saline conductivity between electrodes caused by passing erythrocytes. RBCs are both counted and sized in this way, yielding a histogram of diameters that is also reported as part of the CBC (Fig. 3.1).

These measured results for Hct, [Hb], and the number of RBCs from a patient's CBC are then used to calculate three additional derived indices that describe various features of an average erythrocyte and establish useful normal ranges for each:

Mean Cell Volume—the average volume of an erythrocyte, reported in fL (10^{-15} L) or μm^3 per RBC. Mean cell value (MCV) is computed by dividing the Hct of whole blood by the number of RBCs in that sample, with appropriate corrections made for differences in units. Among healthy adults, the **Normal Range for MCV = 80-90 fL**.

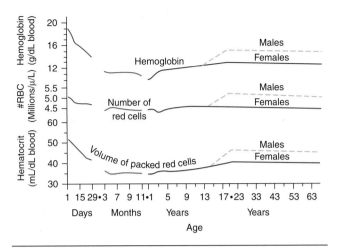

FIGURE 3.1 Relationship of age and sex to [Hb], number of RBCs, and Hct of the peripheral blood. *From Guyton.* Textbook of Medical Physiology; *1986.*

(#21)

Mean Cell Hemoglobin Content—the average mass of Hb in an erythrocyte, reported in pg. Mean cell hemoglobin content (MCH) is computed by dividing the [Hb] of whole blood by the number of RBCs in the sample, again correcting for differences in units. Among healthy adults, the **Normal Range for MCH = 25-30 pg**.

Mean Cell Hemoglobin Concentration—the average [Hb] inside erythrocytes, properly reported as the g Hb/100 mL RBCs, or more conventionally just as a percent. Mean cell hemoglobin concentration (MCHC) is computed by dividing the [Hb] of a blood sample by its Hct, corrected as needed for differences in units. Among healthy adults, the **Normal Range for MCHC = 32%-35%**.

Based upon the CBC results for millions of presumably healthy adults, the erythrocyte dimensions mentioned above and the Hb content of typical mature RBC populations vary little with postnatal age. In other words, the calculated indices of MCV, MCH, and MCHC are remarkably constant across the broad population. Thus, most observed changes in a person's Hct or [Hb] represent simple parallel variations in their number of RBC/μL, unless a specific genetic, biochemical, or physiological explanation is found.

Role of Erythrocytes in Oxygen Transport

Tetrameric Hb contains four ferrous (Fe^{2+}) atoms, each of which can reversibly combine with one molecule of O_2 (Fig. 3.2). Under optimal conditions, one mole (M) of Hb can combine with 4 M of O_2. With a molecular weight of 64,458 g, Hb can reversibly bind approximately 1.39 mL of O_2/g Hb [derived from = (4) • (22.4 L O_2/M O_2)/(64,458 g/M Hb)]. This factor of 1.39 is used to compute the maximal **O_2 carrying capacity** of a sample when its [Hb] is known, assuming 100% oxygenation.

What is the physiological significance of 1.39 mL O_2/g Hb? Consider that at 37°C the maximal amount of dissolved

Hemoglobin

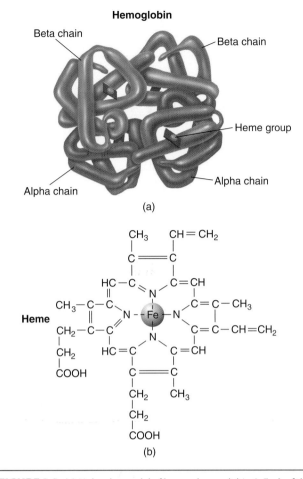

(a)

Heme

(b)

FIGURE 3.2 (a) Molecular model of human hemoglobin A. Each of the two α and two β globulin chains has an associated heme molecule. (b) Structure of a heme molecule with a central bound Fe^{2+} iron atom. *From Fox. Human Physiology, 10th ed.; 2008.*

O_2 = 2.33 mL O_2/dL blood/atm of pure O_2 **(1 atm = 760 mm Hg)**. At sea level and by **Dalton's law of partial pressures** (Chap. 1), we know that the ambient P_{O_2} in dry air = F_IO_2 • (barometric pressure, P_B) = (0.209) • (760) = 160 mm Hg. Thus, one deciliter of blood containing 15 g Hb/dL and equilibrated with air at sea level would contain **0.5 mL dissolved O_2** [= (2.33 mL O_2/dL blood/atm P_{O_2}) • (160/760)], plus **20.8 mL O_2 reversibly bound to Hb**.

The total O_2 content of any solution (including blood) depends upon the ambient P_{O_2} acting as the driving pressure. For saline and plasma, dissolved O_2 is proportional to ambient P_{O_2}: Plasma equilibrated with 2 atm of O_2 contains twice as much dissolved O_2 as plasma equilibrated with 1 atm of O_2 at the same temperature. Respiratory pigments like Hb are different in two important ways. First, Hb binds and releases O_2 in a nonlinear manner. Second, oxygenation of Hb is saturable, so that once maximized, any further elevations in ambient P_{O_2} increase only the dissolved O_2 fraction, which is both linear and nonsaturable under normal clinical conditions that are encountered.

These phenomena are best studied by first equilibrating a blood sample to a gaseous environment containing no O_2,

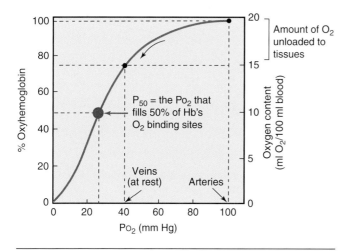

FIGURE 3.3 Basic features of hemoglobin-oxygen binding, the HbO_2 dissociation curve. Note the large difference in the amounts of oxygen transported by being bound to Hb versus carried only as a dissolved gas. *From Fox.* Human Physiology, *10th ed.; 2008.*

causing its Hb to become completely **deoxygenated** (less correctly termed "desaturated" or "unsaturated"). A suitable gas for this purpose is 95% N_2/5% CO_2, which yields by Dalton's law a clinically meaningful **partial pressure of CO_2 (Pco_2) =** 40 mm Hg. As we then increase the Po_2 to which the blood is equilibrated (holding Pco_2 at 40 mm Hg), its O_2 content increases both in absolute terms (mL O_2/dL blood) and as a percent of maximal Hb oxygenation. The resulting **oxygen dissociation curve (ODC)** for whole blood is sigmoidal (Fig. 3.3). When comparing the ODC within or across species, the Po_2 required to half-oxygenate the blood is termed its P_{50}, a bit of physiological shorthand that has gained wide acceptance.

The sigmoidal nature of the ODC is due to changes in the shape of Hb molecules that occur with their binding of sequential O_2 molecules. Binding of the first O_2 (ie, 25% oxygenation)

induces conformational changes within heme and globin subunits that facilitate **cooperative binding** of the second and third O_2 molecules (ie, 50% and 75% oxygenation). The symmetrical arrangement of the four heme sites suggests no preferential binding sequence, while binding of the fourth O_2 exhibits a more gradual approach to full Hb oxygenation. This cooperativity of binding causes the central portion of an ODC to be steeply sloped, so that large fluctuations in percentage of oxygenation and overall blood O_2 content can occur around the P_{50} with only small changes in ambient Po_2. **Myoglobin (Mb),** an intracellular pigment with one Fe^{2+} and the mass of one-fourth of a Hb molecule, exhibits a simple saturable approach to 100% oxygenation, but with higher affinity and thus a lower P_{50} (Fig. 3.4). The higher O_2 affinity of Mb illustrates an important physiological event: Oxygenated pigments with low affinity (high P_{50}) will surrender O_2 to any pigments of higher affinity that are not fully oxygenated. In this instance, oxygenated Hb will lose bound O_2 to deoxygenated Mb.

Endogenous Modulators of HbO_2 Affinity

The shape, slope, and P_{50} of an ODC are influenced by several physiologically important parameters. The most significant of these are pH and Pco_2, whose effects are related if not identical (Fig. 3.5). Acidification of blood with protons (hydrogen ion, H^+) from any metabolic source reduces HbO_2 affinity and increases the measured P_{50}, the so-called **acid Bohr effect.** Indeed, fluctuations in P_{50} due to Pco_2 are mediated primarily by pH changes caused when dissolved CO_2 interacts with H_2O to form weakly dissociative **carbonic acid, H_2CO_3.** Such Bohr effects are critical physiologically, since high hydrogen ion concentration ($[H^+]$) and CO_2 levels in tissues acidify the arriving arterial blood, increasing its P_{50} and facilitating dissociation of Hb-bound O_2. This O_2 transfer would occur even if tissue Po_2 equaled arterial Po_2, when in fact it is much lower.

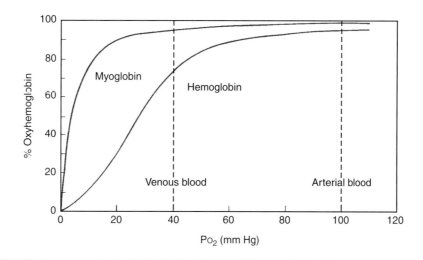

FIGURE 3.4 Hemoglobin-bound O_2 is easily transferred to intracellular myoglobin (Mb), due to the higher O_2 affinity (lower P_{50}) of Mb. *From Fox.* Human Physiology, *10th ed.; 2008.*

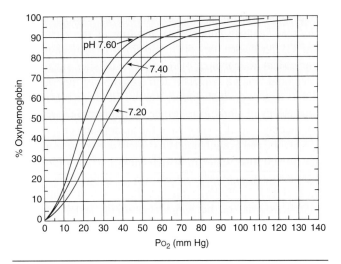

FIGURE 3.5 HbO_2 affinity is reversibly affected by the allosteric modulators CO_2 and H^+ (from any source), known as the Bohr effect. *From Fox. Human Physiology, 10th ed.; 2008.*

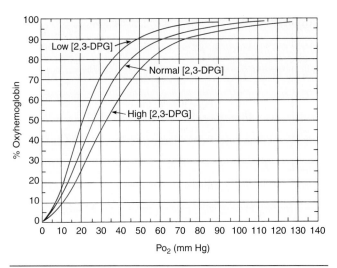

FIGURE 3.6 HbO_2 affinity is allosterically affected by the intracellular modulator 2,3-diphosphoglycerate ([2,3-DPG]), a product of erythrocyte metabolism. *Modified by Lechner from Fox. Human Physiology, 10th ed.; 2008.*

The reverse situation occurs as blood returns to the lungs. There, the high tissue CO_2 that caused acidification of venous blood is excreted, causing blood pH to rise. The P_{50} decreases as a result, signifying higher HbO_2 affinity (**alkaline Bohr effect**) and a greater ability of Hb to bind alveolar O_2.

Interestingly, fluctuations in CO_2 levels also affect P_{50} even if blood pH is held constant, causing what some authors have termed a pure CO_2 **Bohr effect**. In any case, the basis for the Bohr effects of both molecular CO_2 and protons is **allosteric competition**: $[H^+]$ and CO_2 both can bind reversibly to specific residues on Hb proteins that are remote from heme-coordinated Fe^{2+} binding sites for O_2. Association of $[H^+]$ or molecular CO_2 at those sites induces conformational changes in Hb that reduce its affinity of Fe^{2+} sites for O_2. As might be expected, the reverse of this allosteric competition is also true: Oxygenation of hemoglobin induces conformational shifts in the protein subunits that decrease their affinity for $[H^+]$. Consequently, Hb becomes a stronger acid as it is oxygenated, a protein that more readily dissociates its bound H^+. This **Haldane effect** is important in the lungs, where Hb oxygenation causes localized release of $[H^+]$ that are then available to combine with plasma and erythrocytic HCO_3^- to reform H_2CO_3 and then gaseous CO_2.

Another important regulator of HbO_2 affinity in vivo is the erythrocytic intracellular concentration of the glycolytic intermediate, 2,3-diphosphoglycerate ([2,3-DPG]). At a normal concentration within RBCs of about 0.8 mol 2,3-DPG/mol Hb, the [2,3-DPG] reversibly binds with α-amino groups on β-globulin chains, having an allosteric effect analogous to those of CO_2 and $[H^+]$ by reducing HbO_2 affinity and raising the P_{50} (Fig. 3.6). However, increased levels of intracellular [2,3-DPG] also makes O_2 uptake more difficult in the lungs, since [2,3-DPG] levels persist breath-to-breath, unlike CO_2 and $[H^+]$. Thus, when [2,3-DPG] increases as sea-level inhabitants ascend rapidly to altitude, it does not facilitate O_2 uptake to the extent postulated when first described in 1968. More likely, acute altitude probably evokes the normal response

to tissue hypoxia evident at sea level to increase erythrocyte [2,3-DPG] and improve tissue O_2 delivery without presuming a decline in inspired Po_2 as does occur at altitude. In some mammals lacking a distinct fetal Hb, the P_{50} of fetal blood is kept below that of maternal blood by maintaining fetal erythrocytes at a low [2,3-DPG]. Thus, O_2 moves readily into the fetal circulation with its higher-affinity blood from the lower-affinity maternal circulation.

Core temperature is a final variable that influences HbO_2 affinity. As blood temperature increases, so does its P_{50}, analogous to the effect that thermal energy has on other chemical processes like the dissociation of weak acids. Although temperature gradients exist in the human body at rest and during exercise, it may be erroneous to attach much adaptive significance to this effect. In true poikilothermic (cold-blooded) vertebrates, however, such temperature effects have striking implications on seasonal patterns of ventilation and acid-base regulation.

Genetic Effects on HbO₂ Affinity

A number of permanent changes in P_{50} have been discovered that are due to minor changes in the globin chains of Hb. Most notable among these is that between fetal and maternal hemoglobins. In humans, the P_{50} of whole blood composed of Hb-A is 26-27 mm Hg, while the P_{50} of Hb-F in the fetus is about 20 mm Hg. Recent evidence suggests that most of this 6-7 mm Hg differential occurs because Hb-F is not modulated allosterically by [2,3-DPG]. In addition to such normal physiological shifts in P_{50}, there are scores of described hemoglobin variants in humans with altered P_{50}'s attributable to amino acid substitutions in the globin chains. Certain variants, including **sickle cell hemoglobin (Hb-S)** and **hemoglobin Kansas**, have abnormally low O_2 affinity and high P_{50}'s. Other mutations like those causing **hemoglobin Rainier** and **hemoglobin Capetown** show exceptionally high oxygen affinity and low P_{50}'s. Except where an amino acid substitution produces a specific functional abnormality in the tetramer, for example, the precipitative tendency of homozygous Hb-S at low Po_2, it remains unclear what impact such altered P_{50}'s have on systemic oxygen delivery.

Confounding Variables of HbO_2 Affinity and O_2 Content

Several final comments should be made concerning Hb and its O_2 transport capacity. While 1 g of Hb can theoretically combine with 1.39 mL O_2, the observed O_2 content of well-oxygenated blood seldom exceeds 97% of that predicted by the [Hb]. This is due to the occurrence of circulating Hb that cannot bind O_2 due to the presence of a competitive molecule at the O_2 binding site, or a modification of the site itself. An example of the former is carbon monoxide (CO) that reversibly binds to the normal HbO_2 site as **carboxyhemoglobin (HbCO)**, but with very high affinity (P_{50} ~1 mm Hg). Even low concentrations of inspired CO can effectively block O_2 transport by Hb. A different type of interference with Hb function is caused by strong oxidants like cyanide that convert Fe^{2+} to Fe^{3+} (see earlier discussion of [Hb] assay). The oxidized product **methemoglobin (metHb)** remains within erythrocytes but cannot reversibly bind O_2. Indeed, the conversion of Hb to metHb by common environmental oxidants like ozone is normally maintained at <2% of total [Hb] by the erythrocytic enzyme **methemoglobin reductase**. In poisoning cases, the production rate of metHb obviously exceeds the capacity of this reducing enzyme to reverse an ongoing oxidative process.

▶▶ **CLINICAL CORRELATION 3.1**

The brilliant red color of HbCO is responsible for the ruby lips and ruddy complexion of CO-poisoned victims, who typically show 40%-60% of their hemoglobin as HbCO. Urban dwellers normally possess 1%-2% HbCO, which can rise to 8%-10% in automotive workers, cigarette smokers, and miners. Clinically elevated levels of HbCO are also common in developing countries where indigent populations are exposed to CO-bearing smoke and toxic fumes as they rely upon scrap wood, dung, or charcoal for indoor cooking, heating, and metalworking. Treatment options for CO poisoning are limited, but include hyperbaric chambers in which patients can be exposed to 2-3 atm of pure oxygen.

Role of Erythrocytes in Carbon Dioxide Transport

CO_2 produced by metabolically active cells must enter the vascular space as dissolved gas, with the majority entering the erythrocyte (Fig. 3.7). Once inside an RBC, CO_2 may: (1) remain dissolved as a gas for transport to the lungs (2) combine with intracellular water to form **carbonic acid, H_2CO_3** that reversibly dissociates into **bicarbonate anion, HCO_3^-** and free **protons, H^+** or (3) combine reversibly with Hb to form **carbaminohemoglobin, $HbCO_2$**. During these potential excretion pathways for CO_2 created in active tissues, the

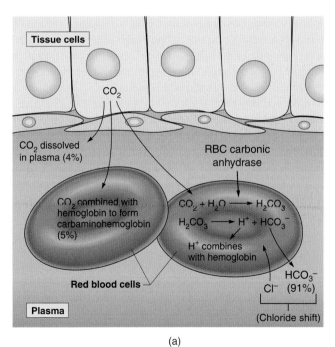

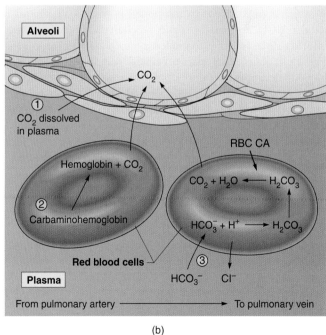

(a)   (b)

FIGURE 3.7 (a) Uptake and transport mechanisms for metabolic CO_2 in venous blood, with emphasis on the multiple roles of RBCs that maximize total CO_2 content. (b) The same biochemical processes to absorb CO_2 in active tissues are reversed in pulmonary capillaries during the excretion of CO_2 from, and the oxygenation of, the venous blood. *From Fox. Human Physiology, 10th ed.; 2008.*

Table **3.1** O_2 and CO_2 contents for paired arterial and mixed venous blood estimated at 37°C with Hct = 42% and [Hb] = 14 g/dL

Parameter	Arterial	Mixed Venous	A – V Difference
Whole blood, 1.0 L			
Po_2, mm Hg (% Oxy-Hb)	100 (100%)	40 (75%)	– 60 (25%)
Pco_2, mm Hg	39	45	+ 6
Total O_2, mM	8.82	6.62	– 2.20
Total CO_2, mM	22.40	24.23	+ 1.83
Erythrocytes, 0.420 L			
Total CO_2, mM	6.54	7.30	+ 0.76
Bicarbonate, mM	5.39	5.88	+ 0.49
Dissolved CO_2, mM	0.41	0.47	+ 0.06
Carbamino CO_2, mM	0.74	0.95	+ 0.21
Plasma, 0.580 L			
Total CO_2, mM	15.86	16.93	+ 1.07
Bicarbonate, mM	15.16	16.13	+ 0.97
Dissolved CO_2, mM	0.70	0.80	+ 0.10

erythrocyte provides: (1) the enzyme **carbonic anhydrase (CA)** to accelerate H_2CO_3 formation; (2) an exchange medium by which formed HCO_3^- is transported in plasma after intracellular HCO_3^- exchanges for extracellular Cl^-, termed the **chloride shift**, favoring continued intracellular HCO_3^- formation while maintaining electrochemical neutrality; (3) Hb as a **proton acceptor** to buffer H^+ produced with HCO_3^-; and (4) Hb to act as a reversible sink for molecular CO_2 bound as $HbCO_2$. The last reaction simultaneously decreases HbO_2 affinity by the CO_2 Bohr effect. These several processes are reversed in the lungs as CO_2 is expired.

In absolute terms, about 91% of the CO_2 in mixed venous blood exists as HCO_3^-, with an additional 5% as $HbCO_2$ and 4% as dissolved gaseous CO_2 (Table 3.1). To determine how each of these pools contributes to the CO_2 excreted from the lungs, consider the data on differences in CO_2 contents between arterial and venous blood presented in this table. One critical point is quickly apparent: Although the total CO_2 content of venous blood is large, the amount actually excreted during a single passage through the lungs is small, here 1.83 mM or about 7% of the total. As will become apparent in Chaps. 9 and 17, the residual 93% of the blood's total CO_2 constitutes an important source of labile (volatile) blood buffer. The plasma loss of HCO_3^- as venous blood traverses pulmonary capillaries to become oxygenated arterial blood is 0.97 mM, with the HCO_3^- loss from erythrocytes equal to an additional 0.49 mM.

Thus, the total amount of CO_2 excreted as HCO_3^- from erythrocytes and plasma during alveolar perfusion is 1.46 mM, or roughly 80% of all CO_2 exchanged during ventilation. The remaining CO_2 excreted is about 11% as $HbCO_2$, and 9% via dissolved CO_2 from erythrocytes and plasma. Since Cl^- ions move between the erythrocyte interior and plasma in the opposite directions to these shifts in HCO_3^- (Fig. 3.7), the fundamental contribution of RBCs to CO_2 transport is to accelerate HCO_3^- production via intra-erythrocytic carbonic anhydrase, with Hb molecules acting as proton donors or acceptors. The contribution of $HbCO_2$ formation to overall CO_2 excretion is minor, but that benefit is magnified due to the advantageous shift in P_{50} that occurs simultaneously whenever $HbCO_2$ is formed or dissociated (Haldane effect).

Two additional points are worth emphasizing from the data in Table 3.1. First, the amount of O_2 extracted from a liter of arterial blood, 2.20 mM, is of the same magnitude as the amount of CO_2 added to a liter of venous blood, 1.83 mM. In fact, these two numbers reflect the whole-body rates of **O_2 consumption, $\dot{V}o_2$** and **CO_2 production, $\dot{V}co_2$**, respectively. (As mentioned in Chap. 1, placing a dot over a letter like V indicates a rate function, such as mL O_2 consumed per minute here.) The ratio $\dot{V}co_2/\dot{V}o_2$ is the **respiratory quotient (R)**, here equal to (1.83/2.20) = 0.83. This topic will recur in Chap. 9. Second, the partial pressure gradient between arterial and venous bloods that drives this volume of O_2 into the body by diffusion is 60 mm Hg, or 10 times higher than the partial pressure gradient needed for a nearly equivalent amount of CO_2 to diffuse out of the body, here 6 mm Hg. This impressive difference in diffusional gradients is due to the 20- to 30-fold greater solubility of CO_2 in fluid and tissues versus O_2. That greater solubility derives from the reaction, $CO_2 + H_2O \leftrightarrow H_2CO_3$, that is propelled forward as long as H_2CO_3 continues to dissociate into H^+ and HCO_3^-.

Suggested Readings

1. Burton AC. *Physiology and Biophysics of the Circulation*, 2nd ed. Chicago, IL: Year Book Medical; 1972. *Classic introduction to red cell biology and the first serious effort to address relationships between erythrocyte dimensions and the microcirculatory constraints to flow posed by capillaries.*

2. Kaushansky K, Lichtman MA, Beutler E, Kipps TJ, Prchal J, Seligsohn U. *Williams Hematology*, 8th ed. New York, NY: McGraw-Hill; 2010. *Widely considered the definitive resource on all matters dealing with blood; the interested reader can find expert chapters devoted to erythrocyte production, degradation, iron metabolism, porphyrias, and hemoglobinopathies.*

CASE STUDIES AND PRACTICE PROBLEMS

CASE 3.1 Paired blood samples from left radial arteries and veins are drawn on healthy subjects who are 23-61 years old. Each individual breathes room air while resting quietly as samples are obtained. Lab results indicate their total CO$_2$ contents average 21.5 mM in arterial samples and 24.3 mM in venous samples. Which of the following provides the single largest amount of CO$_2$ excreted from their venous bloods?

  a. CO$_2$ bound as carbaminohemoglobin
  b. Dissolved CO$_2$ in the plasma
  c. Dissolved CO$_2$ within erythrocytes
  d. HCO$_3^-$ transported in the plasma
  e. HCO$_3^-$ transported within erythrocytes

CASE 3.2 The whole-blood P$_{50}$ for a healthy 25-year-old woman is found to be 27 mm Hg at pH = 7.40 when fully equilibrated with a range of gas mixtures from 0% O$_2$/5% CO$_2$/95% N$_2$ through 16% O$_2$/5% CO$_2$/79% N$_2$. Which of the following manipulations would cause the P$_{50}$ of this blood sample to decrease?

  a. Warming the blood from 20°C to 37°C before measurement

  b. Reducing this sample's pH by 0.3 units using lactic acid
  c. Increasing the concentration of [2,3-DPG] in these erythrocytes
  d. Equilibrating this blood sample with 16% O$_2$/12% CO$_2$/72% N$_2$
  e. Mixing her sample 1:1 with cord blood from a normal neonate

CASE 3.3 A patient is being admitted to the ICU of a hospital in Los Angeles. While a 3.0 mL arterial blood specimen is being drawn into a glass syringe, 0.8 mL air is accidentally introduced and not discovered until 30 minutes later as the sample is prepared for analysis. What effect will this bubble have on the blood gas results being reported?

  a. None if the specimen has been stored on ice until analyzed
  b. Increased P$_a$CO$_2$, decreased P$_a$O$_2$ with decreased pH
  c. Decreased P$_a$CO$_2$, increased P$_a$O$_2$ with increased pH
  d. Decreased P$_a$CO$_2$, increased P$_a$O$_2$ with no change in pH
  e. Increased P$_a$CO$_2$, increased P$_a$O$_2$ with decreased pH

Solutions to Case Studies and Practice Problems

CASE 3.1 The most correct answer is d.
While all listed choices contribute to CO$_2$ excretion from alveolar capillaries, the largest single fraction is plasma HCO$_3^-$ the instant before being exhaled (Table 3.1). Such data support a prominent role for an isoform of carbonic anhydrase expressed by capillary endothelia that can facilitate direct formation of H$_2$CO$_3$ from plasma H$^+$ and HCO$_3^-$, yielding a rapid rise in plasma dissolved CO$_2$ that then diffuses into alveolar airspaces.

CASE 3.2 The most correct answer is e.
A decrease in P$_{50}$ is equivalent to a leftward shift in the ODC and increased HbO$_2$ affinity. Of the choices offered, only mixing bloods containing normal Hb-A with normal Hb-F will achieve this, while all remaining choices would decrease HbO$_2$ affinity,

whether by temperature (*answer a*), acid Bohr effect (*answer b*), augmented [2,3-DPG] (*answer c*), or CO$_2$ Bohr effect (*answer d*).

CASE 3.3 The most correct answer is c.
Arterial blood drawn for gas analysis must be kept free of contaminating room air that contains high levels of O$_2$ and almost no CO$_2$. Failure to exclude such a large air bubble allows both gases to diffuse down their partial pressure gradients to raise the sample's P$_a$O$_2$ and reduce its P$_a$CO$_2$, causing a corresponding alkalosis (↑ pH). While good lab practice is always to store such samples on ice until analyzed, even that precaution (against continued aerobic metabolism by any leukocytes and platelets, and anaerobic acidification by the RBCs) will not prevent these artifactual changes in P$_a$O$_2$ and P$_a$CO$_2$ caused by air bubbles.

Chapter 4

Principles of Lung Ventilation and Spirometry

ANDREW J. LECHNER, PhD

Learning Objectives

- The student will be able to distinguish between the conducting zone where ventilation occurs, and the respiratory parenchyma where diffusion occurs.

- The student will be able to define terms for normal lung volumes, including tidal volume, dead space, total lung capacity, vital capacity, functional residual capacity, inspiratory and expiratory reserve volumes, and residual volume.

- The student will be able to describe the basic procedures used in routine pulmonary function testing, particularly bench top spirometry.

- The student will be able to describe two techniques to quantify residual volume and functional residual capacity, including underlying assumptions of each.

- The student will be able to explain the origin and maintenance of negative intrapleural pressures that are caused by elastic recoil forces within normal lung tissues and the chest wall/diaphragm complex.

Introduction

Respiration consists of two critical and nonoverlapping processes, **ventilation** and **diffusion**. Ventilation is the bulk movement of gases in and out of the lungs via the large and intermediate airways that collectively are termed the **conducting zone**. Here, inspired gas is warmed to 37°C, humidified to 100% relative humidity (RH), and cleansed of most airborne particulates, but its molecular composition is changed only by addition of water vapor. This is because conducting zone airways are too wide and their walls are too thick to allow appreciable molecular diffusion of O_2 and CO_2 between inspired air and the pulmonary arterial blood coursing through alveolar capillaries. On the other hand, the delicate alveolar membranes of the **respiratory parenchyma** are thin and have an enormous aggregate surface area. As will be formally introduced in Chap. 9, molecular diffusion requires such large, thin surfaces to maximize O_2 and CO_2 exchange. The remainder of this chapter will focus on ventilation, and the forces and constraints that make it more or less effective. It is worth noting now that the conducting zone volume is nearly constant during normal breathing, while respiratory parenchymal volume changes very dramatically as the depth of breathing is adjusted.

Normal Lung Volumes and Spirometry

Despite the histological complexity of lung tissue (Chap. 2), its key elements can be represented by a simple line drawing (Fig. 4.1). The many branching airways of the conducting zone that support ventilation are shown as a single tube comprising the **anatomic dead space (V_D)** (Fig. 4.2). V_D is normally ~2 mL/kg of ideal body weight, or about 160 mL in a normal adult. In Fig. 4.1, the respiratory parenchyma where diffusion occurs is shown as one contiguous compartment, the **alveolar gas volume (V_A)**, here 3.0 L. We define **tidal volume (V_T)** as the total volume of a typical inspiration, but clearly only a portion of each breath reaches the parenchyma while the remainder occupies V_D.

#22

Thus, in this example where V_D = 160 mL, only 440 mL of a 600 mL V_T reaches alveoli of the respiratory parenchyma, or 740 mL of a 900 mL V_T. Further, we define **total ventilation**, $\dot{V}_E$ (L/min) as the product of V_T and **respiratory frequency**, f (breaths/min). Using the data of Fig. 4.1, $\dot{V}_E$ = 9.0 L/min (= 0.60 L/breath × 15 breaths/min). Consequently, **alveolar ventilation**, $\dot{V}_A$ (L/min) equals $(V_T - V_D) \times f$. Using volumes in Fig. 4.1, we can compute that at a resting f = 15 breaths/min and V_T = 0.60 L, the resulting $\dot{V}_A$ of 6.6 L/min will exchange a V_A of 3.0 L about twice each minute.

> ▶▶ CLINICAL CORRELATION 4.1
>
> Virtually all patients requiring **mechanical ventilation** will experience an increase in dead space due to the added volume of endotracheal tubing, valves, and associated hardware needed to use the ventilator effectively.

Based on lung tissue morphometry, **alveolar capillary volume (V_C)** contains perhaps 70-100 mL of blood at any instant. Since baseline cardiac output ($\dot{Q}$) is ~6 L/min, a subject's V_C is typically replenished with mixed venous blood via the pulmonary arterioles at least once per second at rest [(6,000 mL/min)/70 mL] and more frequently during exercise. Thus, erythrocytes spend less than a second traversing a

31

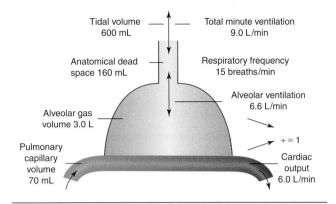

Tidal volume
600 mL

Total minute ventilation
9.0 L/min

Anatomical dead
space 160 mL

Respiratory frequency
15 breaths/min

Alveolar ventilation
6.6 L/min

Alveolar gas
volume 3.0 L

$\div \approx 1$

Pulmonary
capillary
volume
70 mL

Cardiac
output
6.0 L/min

FIGURE 4.1 Diagram of typical lung volumes and pulmonary blood flows. Considerable variation occurs around these values due to age, sex, and body size. *Modified from West* Respiratory Physiology - the Essentials. *6th ed. Williams & Wilkins; 2005.*

pulmonary capillary that is sufficiently close to alveolar air for diffusive gas exchange. We can also estimate that for an ideal lung with homogeneous architecture from apex to base, the **alveolar ventilation/perfusion ratio,** $\dot{V}_A/\dot{Q}$ is ~1.0 (ie, 6.6 L/6.0 L). Whether an ideal $\dot{V}_A/\dot{Q}$ ratio of 1.0 actually occurs in normal lung will be discussed in Chap. 8.

Most lung volumes are measured directly by **spirometry**, an apparatus originally consisting of an inverted, water-sealed bell filled with 100% O_2 from which a subject breathes through a mouthpiece while wearing nose clips (Fig. 4.3). As gases move in and out of the bell, pen tracings record volume changes

even as expired CO_2 is trapped chemically by an internal canister of soda lime. Thus, the eventual decline in bell height (superimposed on ventilatory pen movements) reflects $\dot{V}o_2$. Routine spirometry provides multiple lung volumes plus the rate functions $\dot{V}_E$ and $\dot{V}o_2$.

Most spirometric volumes are self-explanatory. A **capacity** is the sum of two or more volumes. After a normal expiration, the amount of gas remaining in the lungs is called the **functional residual capacity (FRC)**, an important reference value and the standard starting point for other pulmonary function measurements. By forcefully exhaling as much gas as possible beyond a normal V_T, we see that FRC is really the sum of the **expiratory reserve volume (ERV)**, plus the **residual volume, RV**. Thus, RV is a gas that cannot be expired from the lungs, as long as the chest wall and diaphragm remain intact. Then by inspiring maximally after the end of a normal inspiration, we utilize our **inspiratory reserve volume (IRV)** to achieve **total lung capacity (TLC)**. By beginning at TLC and exhaling maximally to RV, we achieve our normal **vital capacity (VC)**. Subjects are commonly asked to perform this maximal expiratory effort as quickly as possible (TLC → RV) to measure the time in seconds needed to expel their **forced vital capacity (FVC)** or **forced expiratory volume (FEV)**. As will be discussed in Chap. 6, carefully measuring the time required to complete an FEV maneuver can objectively estimate the severity of many pulmonary disorders. All terms and abbreviations presented in this section are used clinically and should be remembered (Table 4.1).

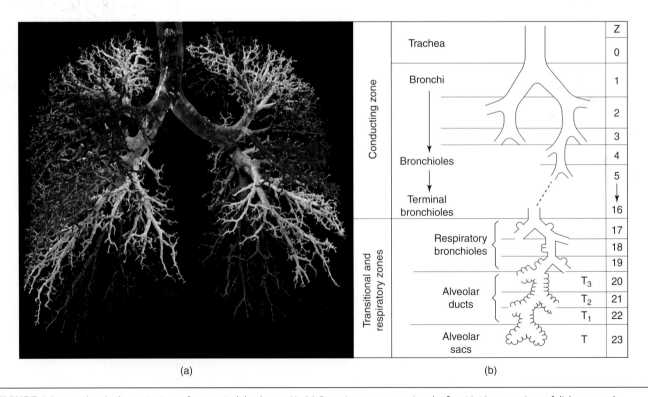

(a)

(b)

FIGURE 4.2 Actual and schematic views of anatomical dead space V_D. (a) Corrosion cast preserving the first 10-12 generations of dichotomously branched human airways. Surrounding lung tissue was dissolved with alkali after liquid plastic instilled into the airways had hardened. (b) Diagram of airways that terminate in true alveoli; the estimate of 22-23 generations was first made by Ewald Weibel in 1962. (a): *From Fox.* Human Physiology, *10th ed.; 2008.* (b): *From West* Respiratory Physiology - the Essentials. *6th ed. Williams & Wilkins; 2005.*

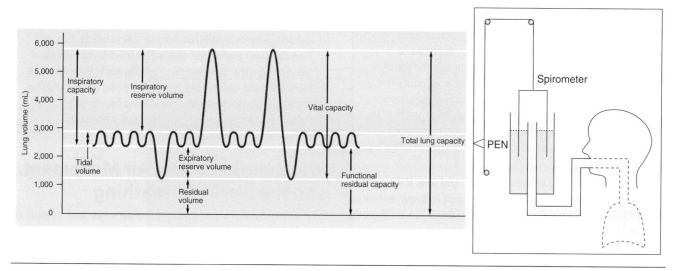

FIGURE 4.3 Lung volumes recorded by spirometry. Note that functional residual capacity **FRC** and residual volume **RV** cannot be measured directly with this apparatus alone. **IRV** and **ERV** are inspiratory and expiratory reserve volumes respectively. *Left: From Fox*. Human Physiology, *11th ed.; 2009.*

#23

Table **4.1 Terms ued to describe lung volumes and capacities**

Term	Definition
Lung Volumes	The four nonoverlapping components of the total lung capacity
Tidal volume	The volume of gas inspired or expired in an unforced respiratory cycle
Inspiratory reserve volume	The maximum volume of gas that can be inspired during forced breathing in addition to tidal volume
Expiratory reserve volume	The maximum volume of gas that can be expired during forced breathing in addition to tidal volume
Residual volume	The volume of gas remaining in the lungs after a maximum expiration
Lung Capacities	Measurements that are the sum of two or more lung volumes
Total lung capacity	The total amount of gas in the lungs after a maximum inspiration
Vital capacity	The maximum amount of gas that can be expired after a maximum inspiration
Inspiratory capacity	The maximum amount of gas that can be inspired after a normal tidal expiration
Functional residual capacity	The amount of gas remaining in the lungs after a normal tidal expiration

From Fox. Human Physiology, *10th ed. 2008.*

Since residual volume cannot be exhaled, RV and critical capacities like FRC and TLC that include it cannot be measured by spirometry alone. However, several non-invasive procedures estimate RV, or more correctly they measure FRC

so that RV is obtained by subtracting ERV from FRC. The **helium dilution** technique works because inert gases have low aqueous solubility and are not readily absorbed from the alveoli airspaces into surrounding fluids and tissues. A low F_{He} mixed with O_2 (eg, 0.8%/99.2%) is inspired from a spirometer by a subject breathing room air until the test begins through a side valve (Fig. 4.4). As the subject pauses at FRC, the valve is turned and the He/O_2 mixture enters their lungs. After 2-3 minutes of re-breathing, a lower F_{He} results within the total system (V_1, the spirometer + V_2, the patient's FRC). Using this equilibrium F_{He}, total system volume is computed using simple algebra and presuming conservation of mass [$F_1 \cdot V_1 = F_2(V_1 + V_2)$]. The accuracy of this RV measurement depends on starting the test at a reproducible FRC, having also accurately measured ERV.

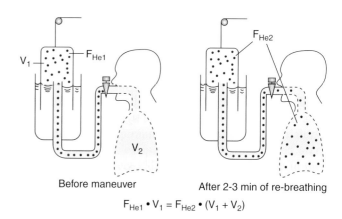

$$F_{He1} \bullet V_1 = F_{He2} \bullet (V_1 + V_2)$$

FIGURE 4.4 Like other inert gases, He diffuses slowly from alveolar airspaces into pulmonary capillary blood. Its dilution in the first 2-3 minutes of re-breathing will estimate an unknown recipient volume V_2, here equal to a subject's FRC.

Chapter 6

Integrated Respiratory System Compliance and the Work of Breathing

ANDREW J. LECHNER, PhD

Introduction

The **tissue elastic** and **surface tension** recoil forces that provide inherent compliance to normal lung tissue were reviewed in Chaps. 4 and 5. For excised lungs, these forces can be examined as if they operated independently of constraints placed on lung expansion by bones and muscles of the thorax. However, the **chest wall** and **airways** strongly influence lung distension and the work of breathing (Fig. 6.1). Incorporating these factors into a broad model of ventilation will facilitate understanding of the major categories of lung disorders, the **obstructive diseases** and **restrictive diseases**.

Elastic Properties of the Intact Thorax

The chest wall and diaphragm normally oppose the recoil forces of lung tissue elasticity and surface tension. Thus, the negative P_{IP} at functional residual capacity (FRC) (see Fig. 4.6) represents the equilibrium when these musculoskeletal elements are bowed inwardly by lung recoil. Since this balance is not intuitive, consider a bilateral pneumothorax when $P_{IP} = P_B$ (Fig. 6.2). When P_{IP} increases from −5 to 0 cm H_2O, healthy lungs recoil toward their minimal volume, while the chest walls spring outward and the diaphragm drops toward the abdominal viscera. Indeed, the volume of the open chest when $P_{IP} = P_B$ is about 80% of a subject's normal total lung capacity (TLC), implying that musculoskeletal elements will oppose all forces attempting to make the chest either larger or smaller than about 80% of TLC.

Thus, an in situ compliance curve for the entire lung-thorax system is the algebraic sum of the compliance curves for each component. Such a composite compliance curve can be obtained by having a subject perform a **relaxation pressure-volume maneuver** (Fig. 6.3) using a specialized apparatus for **whole-body plethysmography** (Chap. 16). While simultaneously monitoring P_{IT} in the airway and intraesophageal pressure to approximate P_{IP}, subjects inspire or expire to a series of lung

volumes between RV and TLC, and then are locked momentarily at that volume by a valve so they can completely relax their chest wall. Under these conditions, the maneuver begins and the subject's FRC is empirically defined as that volume when $P_{IT} = P_B = 0$ at the mouthpiece. This FRC also is the volume where inwardly directed lung recoil forces are equal and opposite to outwardly directed forces exerted by the chest wall plus diaphragm.

When subjects who are at FRC expire toward RV, their P_{IT} is less than P_B and a sensation of suction is felt as the thoracic structures are increasingly deviated inward from their preferred resting positions seen with a pneumothorax. Conversely, when the subject inspires to lung volumes above FRC and toward TLC, P_{IT} exceeds P_B and a sensation of chest compression develops as lung elastic and tension recoil forces increase. Indeed, the subject's sensation of chest tightness will maximize at lung volumes >80% of TLC (ie, the size of the thoracic space after a pneumothorax) since the chest wall and diaphragm will also then be exerting inwardly directed positive pressures that augment the positive pressure created by lung recoil.

From this explanation, it becomes apparent that if a subject breathes at lung volumes between FRC and about 80% of TLC, each inhalation to inflate the lungs is achieved in part by utilizing potential energy stored in the chest wall and diaphragm as they were pulled inward during the preceding exhalation. By the same argument, every exhalation uses potential energy stored in the inflated lungs to expel the tidal breath, while simultaneously storing potential energy in musculoskeletal elements being bowed inward. Thus, it is not accurate to consider normal inhalation to be entirely "active" or normal exhalation to be entirely "passive". Rather, normal breathing is

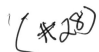

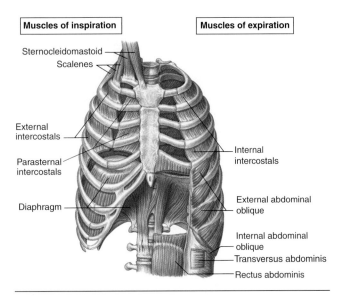

FIGURE 6.1 The diaphragm is normally the main inspiratory motor during respiration; its caudal excursions create negative pressures that expand the lungs. The intercostals and other accessory muscles enlarge the anterior-posterior and lateral chest diameters. *From Fox.* Human Physiology, *10th ed.; 2008.*

carefully controlled to oscillate around the midrange of available lung volumes so that inhalation consumes less energy than one might think, but exhalation also costs energy.

▶▶ **CLINICAL CORRELATION 6.1**

In contrast to this normal pattern, many patients with obstructive lung diseases (eg, emphysema, asthma) will struggle to exhale fully between breaths. They may become hyper-inflated, still breathing tidally but much closer to their TLC. Their work of breathing is vastly increased, since every inhalation will require distending both the lung tissues and the thoracic elements surrounding them. You can experience this phenomenon by first taking a deep breath, and then resume taking small tidal breaths but without allowing yourself to exhale to FRC each time.

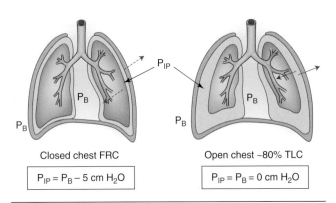

FIGURE 6.2 At FRC, lung recoil forces are opposed by thoracic elements and P_{IP} = −5 to −10 cm H_2O. A pneumothorax allows lung to collapse and chest volume to approach TLC as ribs spring outward and the diaphragm moves caudally.

Airway Resistance and Dynamic Lung Compliance

To this point, models of **static lung and chest wall compliance** have been used to estimate resistances to ventilation that are generated by surface and tissue recoil of lung tissue, and by thoracic musculoskeletal elements. However, additional resistance to ventilation also occurs in the airways during flow, only to disappear under no-flow conditions such as FRC. Such **dynamic airway resistance** is nevertheless a powerful determinant of the pattern, energetic cost, and overall efficiency of ventilation. Thus, **dynamic airway compliance** measurements are made to directly determine in-line resistances due to the airways. Such measurements have shown that most dynamic airway resistance resides in the upper airways (generations 1-7) because their flow rates tend to be high, their end-to-end pressure changes are large, and their aggregate cross-sectional areas are small. By the same argument, the smaller peripheral airways usually contribute less resistance despite having smaller individual diameters, due to their shorter lengths and their exponentially larger cross-sectional areas (Fig. 6.4).

To appreciate the role that airway dimensions play in creating resistance to ventilation and thereby add to the work of breathing, recall **Ohm's law**:

$$I = \Delta V/R$$

where I = current, ΔV = voltage potential, and R = resistance

In airways and other tubes, this becomes a generalized **flux equation**:

$$Air\ Flow = \Delta P/R$$

where ΔP = pressure differential, either end-to-end or end-to-side, and

R = resistance due to airway dimensions and gas viscosity, and thus:

$$R = (8 \cdot \eta \cdot l)/(\pi \cdot r^4)$$

where r = airway radius, η = viscosity, and l = airway segment length

Substituting terms gives the well-known **Poiseuille equation**:

$$Air\ flow = (\Delta P \cdot \pi \cdot r^4)/(8 \cdot \eta \cdot l)$$

Considering the dependence of resistance on radius to the fourth power, the importance of even a small change in airway radius is apparent. It will be shown in later chapters that many respiratory diseases pivot on this aspect of airway resistance, versus a lesser dependence on airway length or viscosity.

Applying the Poiseuille equation to human ventilation presumes an idealized laminar flow pattern, but evidence is not persuasive as to how often and how distally such flow exists in the airways (Fig. 6.5). Most bronchial airways are too wide, too frequently bifurcated, or too short before branching to promote consistent laminar flow. Rather, it seems likely transitional flow patterns predominate at rest, that deteriorate

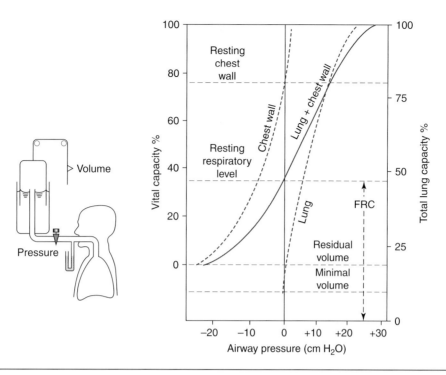

FIGURE 6.3 Relaxation pressure-volume curves obtained by spirometry combined with whole-body plethysmography. The solid line "lung + chest wall" recorded in the subject's airways must equal the algebraic sum of compliance curves for excised lungs (right) and the empty thorax (left). Minimal volume = lung volume without alveolar air. *From West.* Respiratory Physiology; *2005.*

to turbulent patterns during exercise and other associated with hyperventilation.

Clinically, airway resistance is calculated using the pressure gradient from trachea to alveolus divided by flow rate; the subject's tracheal pressure and flow rate are estimated at the

mouth by anemometer, and alveolar pressure by esophageal transducer or plethysmography (Chap. 16). When the in vivo volume/pressure changes are plotted for such a **dynamic compliance maneuver**, the area between the inflation and deflation curves representing hysteresis is larger than for excised lungs

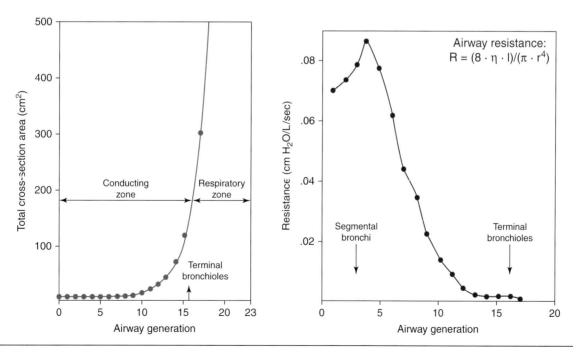

FIGURE 6.4 Total airway cross-sectional area increases exponentially plotted versus airway generation number. Although distal generations are both narrower and shorter, overall airway resistance is highest in the intermediate airways.

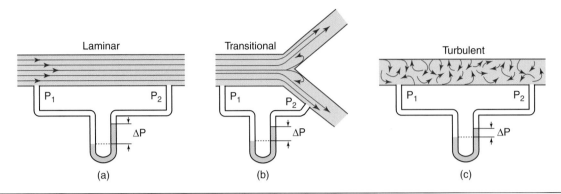

FIGURE 6.5 Flow patterns through tubes. In laminar flow (a), fast-moving cylinders of fluid occur near the vessel's center. Transitional flow (b) has laminar elements, but eddies form at smaller branch points. Turbulent flow (c) is least efficient, with wasted lateral energy. By Ohm's law, Resistance = $(P_1 - P_2)$/flow rate.

of the same size (see Fig. 5.2). Most importantly, this increased area represents additional nonrecoverable work during both inflation and deflation to overcome airway resistance.

In summary, the **total work of breathing** in a healthy adult can be partitioned into energy that must be applied to overcome:

- *Static lung resistance* caused by tissue elasticity and surface tension forces that must be overcome regardless of dynamic resistance, normally **65%-70%** but higher when pathologies involving surfactant or the respiratory parenchyma are present;

- *Dynamic airway resistance* that exists only when gas is moving, normally **25%-30%** and mostly in the upper 10 generations, but much higher in patients with obstructive disorders; and

- *Tissue viscous drag* due to physical abrasion and friction between pleural surfaces of the lung and chest, normally **5%** but can become fatally high if adhesions, congenital anomalies, or effusions are present.

Obstructive versus Restrictive Lung Diseases

The rationale for devoting such attention to the work of breathing and determination of lung compliance is that most respiratory diseases arise in patients who present with impaired ventilation characterized as an **obstructive airway disease** or a **restrictive lung disease**. In general, a disease is obstructive if there is an increased resistance to airflow, most evident during expiration but also detectable upon inspiration. Specific examples include asthma, bronchitis, and emphysema. Patients with restrictive lung diseases do not necessarily show airflow obstruction, but their ventilation is impaired due to restrictions in the maximal size or movement of the lungs or chest wall (or both). **Restrictive chest wall diseases** include kyphoscoliosis, neuromuscular disorders, and spinal trauma. **Restrictive lung diseases** include interstitial fibrosis, sarcoidosis, scarring after pneumonia or tuberculosis, bronchopulmonary dysplasia, and alveolar edema due to congestive heart failure. Patients can show features of both obstructive and restrictive lung diseases.

In Chap. 4, procedures to measure forced vital capacity (FVC) and forced expiratory volume (FEV) were introduced, in which patients on a spirometer or flowmeter inhale to TLC and then exhale as quickly as possible as volume and flow rate are recorded (Fig. 6.6). Exhaled volumes are reported as FVC (= TLC − RV) in liters, and as percentages of the actual FVC that are expired within the first second (FEV_1), first two seconds (FEV_2), and first three seconds (FEV_3) of the maneuver. For a healthy adult with FVC = 6 L, an FEV_1 = 5 L or 83% FVC would be normal; an FEV_2 of ~95% and FEV_3 of ~99% would also be expected.

In patients with obstructive airway diseases (Fig. 6.6), both FVC and FEV_1 are lower than predicted based on age, gender, and size. However, the patient's TLC is often larger than predicted because low expiratory flow rates lead to **peripheral gas trapping** that increases RV. As RV expands with disease severity, such patients will be forced to use their principal ventilatory muscles at distinct mechanical disadvantages. Indeed, the resulting hyperinflation of the chest as RV and FRC increase eventually flattens the diaphragm, so that its contraction fails to increase intra-thoracic volume. In contrast, a patient with restrictive lung disease shows lower FVC and TLC than predicted by age, gender, and size, due to physical limits imposed on lung and/or chest volumes (Fig. 6.6). Of note, given the smaller lung or thoracic volumes in such patients, the FEV_1 may be normal or even increased as a percent of FVC unless airway obstruction is also present.

Flow rate (in L/sec) is measured at the mouth continuously during an FVC test to obtain an expiratory flow-volume loop, with airflow plotted versus lung volume from TLC to RV on the abscissa (Fig. 6.7). The expiratory flow rate in healthy subjects quickly reaches a maximum that corresponds to the steepest portion of a conventional spirometer tracing (Fig. 6.6). Despite continued maximal effort by the subject, airways with high flow rates begin to collapse because pressures within parenchyma surrounding the airways soon exceed airway pressures themselves. This effect can be explained by principles developed by the mathematician and physician Bernoulli. The eventual decline in flow rate as a forceful exhalation proceeds is termed **effort-independent**: no matter how forcefully the subject attempts to exhale, their **volume-dependent airway compression** during dynamic conditions limits maximal flow rate.

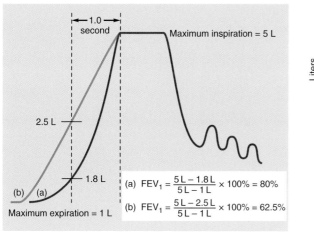
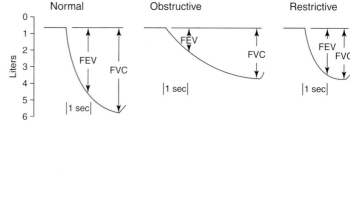

(a) $FEV_1 = \dfrac{5\,L - 1.8\,L}{5\,L - 1\,L} \times 100\% = 80\%$

(b) $FEV_1 = \dfrac{5\,L - 2.5\,L}{5\,L - 1\,L} \times 100\% = 62.5\%$

FIGURE 6.6   Normal, obstructive, and restrictive flow patterns during a forced vital capacity (FVC) maneuver. Here, FEV$_1$ is the amount of gas expelled in one second, expressed in absolute volume (L) and as a percentage of FVC. Note differences in both FVC and FEV$_1$ in various disease types. Left: *From Fox. Human Physiology, 10th ed. 2008.*

In fact, even if subjects exert a submaximal effort initially and then a maximal effort later, the effort-independent portion of their flow-volume loop is not displaced upward or to the right.

When compared to healthy subjects, individuals with obstructive or restrictive disease patterns show distinctive shapes for their flow-volume loops (Fig. 6.8). Patients with **obstructive airway disease** often begin an FEV maneuver at an abnormally higher TLC due to hyperinflation, and end the maneuver at a substantially increased RV. Such patients also take longer to achieve maximal flow rates, which are lower than expected, and their effort-independent region may be distinctly concave as they approach RV. Patients with **restrictive lung or chest disease** have a low or normal RV, depending on the nature of their disorder. By definition, such patients have abnormally low total lung capacities. However, their peak flow rates often resemble the effort-independent portion of normal subjects, if airway caliber is not a prominent feature of their disease.

When patients are being mechanically ventilated, it is common to monitor their inspiratory and expiratory flow-volume loops at the bedside. These data permit the clinical team to assess ongoing changes in dynamic airway resistance and in lung and chest wall compliances as these are altered by disease course or by interventions during hospitalization. This topic is discussed further in Chaps. 28 and 30.

Regional Lung Differences in Ventilation and Compliance

It has been assumed to this point that the lungs are uniformly ventilated, and that their compliance shows no regional heterogeneity. However, lungs are air-filled organs suspended in a partial vacuum within a body cavity susceptible to the effects of gravity. Lungs also have progressively smaller airways and blood vessels, moving distally from the trachea and pulmonary artery. These anatomical and physical conditions create a situation that is far from ideal. Indeed, when an upright subject breathes air containing trace amounts of ^{133}**Xenon**

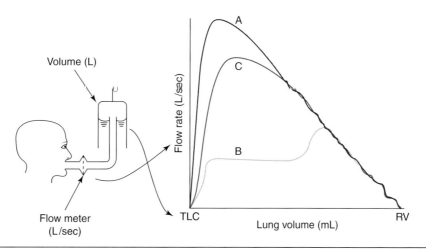

FIGURE 6.7   Maximal expirations during an FVC maneuver, with flow recorded at the mouth. Whether a normal subject expires with maximal force (A), or starts slowly and then maximizes effort (B), or never gives a maximal effort (C), all three curves converge near RV due to volume-dependent constraints on airway radii and transmural pressures.

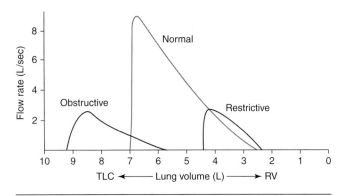

FIGURE 6.8 Normal, obstructive, and restrictive diseases detected by analyzing expiratory flow rates in an FVC maneuver. As airway collapse begins, peak flow rate is dictated more by airway dimensions and surrounding parenchymal pressure than by a subject's effort. Flow rates are plotted versus TLC, but TLC cannot be measured by a single expiration. Note the large TLC with obstructive disease, despite a smaller vital capacity (VC).

[which, like helium (He), is poorly soluble in fluid] while the chest is scanned with appropriate detectors, it is found that more inhaled ^{133}Xe goes to the lung base than to its apex. This result is not due simply to the greater volume of the lung bases. Rather, the inhaled tracer is always observed to distribute preferentially to **dependent lung zones**, defined as those regions lowest in the gravitational field. So when subjects inhale ^{133}Xe while standing on their head or lying supine, the tracer preferentially enters apical alveoli or those nearest the spine, respectively.

These nonintuitive results occur because at any instant, P_{IP} is not uniform for the entire lung but varies from the gravitational top of the lungs to their bottom within the thoracic space. When upright, P_{IP} is most negative at the thoracic apex, due to the hanging weight of the lungs as they maintain contact with adjacent apical pleural surfaces. In the same upright position, P_{IP} at the lung base is less negative or may even be positive, because here the lungs pull less on basal pleural membranes, or may even push against them. Such gradients in P_{IP} exist for a subject in any assumed body position and persist throughout a ventilation cycle. Thus, individual alveoli in more dependent regions are smaller at any lung volume, due to the less negative P_{IP} they are experiencing versus alveoli above them that are more distended due to the more negative P_{IP} adjacent to them in the same gravitational field.

At the same time, all alveoli in the lung still experience nearly identical levels of P_{IT} and P_A throughout a ventilation cycle since they are connected via common airways from primary bronchi to the most distal airspaces (Fig. 6.9). Consequently, all alveoli experience the same ΔP_{IT} and ΔP_A during inhalation, but those in the more dependent zones will inflate more easily because they are nearer to their own RV and thus more compliant (see Fig. 4.6). At the same instant, alveoli in gravitationally higher regions inflate less since they are already closer to their own TLC, and thus less compliant. Analogous gravitational effects that act upon the pulmonary arteries and the patency of alveolar capillaries will be discussed in Chap. 7.

There are significant clinical consequences to these regional differences in ventilation. In a subject at FRC (Fig. 6.9), basal alveoli are more easily ventilated because they are on

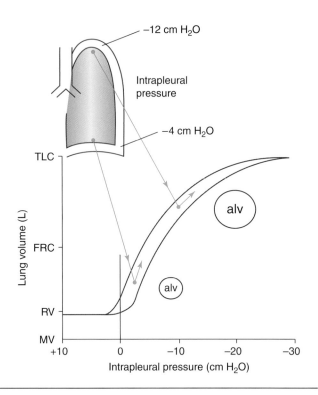

FIGURE 6.9 Zonal gradients in inhaled gas distribution during ventilation reflect gravitational effects on initial alveolar (alv) volumes. When upright and at FRC as shown here, $P_{IP} = -12$ cm H_2O in the apex versus -4 cm H_2O at the base because the lung's entire weight pulls downward from below. Thus, apical alveoli are well distended even at FRC, while basal alveoli in the so-called **dependent zone** are smaller due to compression from above. Such dependent zone alveoli will show a much greater increase in volume during inspiration.

the steepest portion of their individual compliance curves. However, if the same lungs are studied at a low lung volume like RV instead, perhaps in a comatose patient, the P_{IP} at the lung base is positive, and little or no alveolar expansion occurs during a typical tidal breath of only 0.5-0.7 L. Such situations also develop rather commonly in sedated patients, whose spontaneous ventilation may not prevent collapse of their dependent alveoli, particularly when an otherwise desirable increase in F_IO_2 accelerates this effect by **absorption atelectasis** (Chap. 30). In an awake and healthy subject, alveolar collapse is prevented or reversed by periodic **sighs**, with a sigh operationally defined as three times a subject's normal tidal volume (V_T).

▶▶ **CLINICAL CORRELATION 6.2**

During mechanical ventilation, in vivo compliance is optimized by judiciously applying **positive end-expiratory pressure (PEEP)** to increase the patient's effective RV. PEEP can allow a physician to offset a patient's undesirably low P_{IP}, recruit previously collapsed alveoli, and provide an 'air stent' to retard atelectasis of other dependent alveoli. A PEEP setting of 5-10 cm H_2O may suffice to achieve these goals without increasing intrathoracic pressure to levels that reduce venous return. More on these subjects will be covered in Chaps. 28 and 30.

Suggested Readings

1. Milic-Emili J, Henderson JA, Dolovich MB, Trop D, Kaneko K. Regional distribution of inspired gas in the lung. *J Appl Physiol.* 1966;21:749-759. *Insights gained from these authors' use of ^{133}Xe remain exciting and stimulating even today.*

2. Hankinson J, Odencrantz J, Fedan K. Spirometric reference values from a sample of the general US population. *Am J Respir Crit Care Med.*1999; 159:179-187; *and* Enright P,

Beck K, Sherrill D. Repeatability in spirometry in 18,000 adult patients. *Am J Respir Crit Care Med.* 2004; 169:235-238. *The notion that spirometric data can be reliably predicted by algorithms using patient's age, gender, height, and weight required the comprehensive accumulations of real data that studies like these represent.*

CASE STUDIES AND PRACTICE PROBLEMS

CASE 6.1 A nonsmoking 24-year-old man with no significant past medical history presents with a chief complaint of productive cough in the past 48 hours. Physical examination reveals an expiratory wheeze and his chest x-ray is consistent with a right middle lobe infection; lab results on a yellow-green sputum sample obtained for culture are pending. Compared with this patient's normal lung function, which of the following is most likely occurring during this phase of his illness?

a. Hyperinflation and peripheral gas trapping

b. Decreased functional residual capacity

c. Reduced respiratory frequency (breaths/min)

d. Elevated FEV_1 during a forced vital capacity maneuver

e. Increased expiratory reserve volume

CASE 6.2 A 27-year-old female patient performs spirometry and a forced vital capacity (FVC) procedure in her physician's office with the following results: RV = 600 mL; V_T = 700 mL; vital capacity = 5.00 L; f = 12 breaths/min; FEV_1 = 75%; FEV_2 = 90%; FEV_3 = 99%. What volume did she expire during the first two seconds of the FVC maneuver?

a. 3.5 L

b. 3.8 L

c. 4.0 L

d. 4.5 L

e. 5.0 L

CASE 6.3 A previously healthy 12-year-old boy becomes trapped horizontally in a ventilation shaft while exploring a building under construction. First-responders determine that he has no obvious bodily injuries, can say his name and age, and laughs in response to a joke, but is short of breath with both arms pressed tightly to his sides. Until he can be extricated, what is the most likely explanation for his respiratory distress?

a. Increased airway resistance due to anxiety

b. Acute reduction in inspiratory reserve volume

c. Elevated RV due to peripheral gas trapping

d. Compression of primary and secondary bronchi

e. Occult (undetected) pneumothorax

Solutions to Case Studies and Practice Problems

CASE 6.1 The most correct answer is a.

When otherwise healthy individuals develop an acute respiratory infection as this man apparently has done, most symptoms of respiratory distress including tachypnea (*answer c*) are attributable to secretions that obstruct intermediate airways. Until cleared, these secretions will promote peripheral gas trapping that reduces the man's ERV (*answer e*), expands his FRC (*answer b*), and limits his peak air flow rates (*answer d*).

CASE 6.2 The correct answer is d.

The woman's FEV_2 = 90%, which when multiplied by her vital capacity of 5.0 L yields 4.5 L of gas exhaled in the first two seconds of her FVC test.

CASE 6.3 The most correct answer is b.

His shortness of breath is likely due to an acute restrictive chest disorder limiting thoracic expansion and thus his vital capacity. Although, the boy will need a complete exam after this ordeal to rule out chest contusion or penetration (*answer e*), bronchial cartilage would generally prevent their collapse (*answer d*). He can vocalize without an apparent wheeze (*answer a*) and thus, is not likely experiencing airway obstruction that would expand his RV (*answer c*).

Chapter 7

Pulmonary Circulation and Capillary Fluid Dynamics

ANDREW J. LECHNER, PhD

Learning Objectives

- The student will be able to quantify and contrast the pulmonary and systemic circulations with respect to pressures, flow rates, and vascular resistances.
- The student will be able to describe the several vascular perfusion zones of lungs and the forces affecting flow in each.
- The student will be able to use Starling's law of the capillary to explain how interstitial and alveolar edemas occur.
- The student will be able to distinguish features and mechanisms underlying cardiogenic, noncardiogenic, and high altitude forms of pulmonary edema.

Introduction

The rate at which the right ventricle pumps blood, its **cardiac output** ($\dot{Q}$) (L/min), must equal that of the left ventricle to avoid an imbalanced distribution of blood volume within the systemic and pulmonary circulations. However, normal **pulmonary arterial blood pressure (P_{PA})** averages just 12-16 mm Hg, or about one-eighth of the average blood pressure in the dorsal aorta. Because Ohm's law states that flow = $\Delta P/R$ (Chap. 6), total **pulmonary vascular resistance (PVR)** normally is also a small fraction of vascular resistance in the much larger systemic circulation. (Diseases for which PVR is significantly increased will be presented elsewhere in this book.) This chapter will focus on factors that affect PVR and thus P_{PA}, realizing that increases in P_{PA} will increase the work required of the right ventricle and the gradient for fluid constituents of the blood to leak out of alveolar capillaries into the surrounding interstitium and airspaces.

Pressures and Resistances to Flow in the Pulmonary Vasculature

The basic features of the adult pulmonary circulation are shown in Fig. 7.1, which emphasizes its parallel nature to systemic flow patterns. A subject's average P_{PA} is most usually equated to their **diastolic pressure (DP)** plus one third of the difference between **systolic pressure (SP)** and the DP:

$$\text{mean } P_{PA} = DP + [(SP - DP)/3] \quad \#30$$

Pulmonary arterial blood flows through the alveolar microvasculature to drain as pulmonary venous blood into the left heart at a left atrial filling pressure = 4-6 mm Hg. Assuming a resting value for $\dot{Q}$ = 6 L/min and re-arranging Ohm's law ($\dot{Q} = \Delta P/R$), normal resting PVR = (16 mm Hg − 4 mm Hg)/6 L, or about 2 mm Hg/L of blood flow. Contrast this value for PVR of 2 mm Hg/L in the low-resistance pulmonary circulation with a resting value for **systemic vascular resistance (SVR)**. This SVR is calculated using the same resting $\dot{Q}$ and rearrangement of Ohm's law while estimating mean arterial and venous pressures to be 100 and 4 mm Hg, respectively: SVR = (100 mm Hg − 4 mm Hg)/6 L, or about 16 mm Hg/L of blood flow.

Development of the **pulmonary artery catheter (PAC)** provided the first direct measure of pulmonary vascular pressures. The standard PAC is 110 cm long and when used for an adult patient is about 2 mm in external diameter. Once the NS-filled PAC is inserted percutaneously through a jugular, femoral, or brachial vein, it is advanced through the right atrium and ventricle until the distal tip rests in a primary branch of the pulmonary artery, while monitoring blood pressure as a guide to tip location (Fig. 7.2). A properly positioned PAC directly measures P_{PA} and, if fitted with a thermistor at the distal tip, estimates $\dot{Q}$ by the principle of **thermal dilution** when saline boluses of known volume and temperature are infused through the proximal port. A small circumferential balloon located 1-2 cm from the distal tip can be inflated with about 1.5 mL of air to wedge the PAC tip in the pulmonary arterial branch. Since newly arriving arterial blood cannot flow past a properly wedged PAC, any blood within the arterial segment that is beyond the balloon will flow toward the left heart until its pressure equals that in the draining pulmonary vein. Within 1-2 seconds, the wedged catheter tip measures the pressure in the larger pulmonary veins. Hence, **pulmonary wedge pressure (P_{PW})** is equal to **pulmonary venous pressure (P_{PV})** which also can be defined functionally as the **left atrial filling pressure** that was mentioned above.

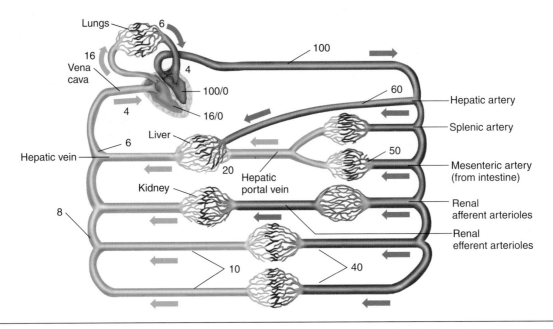

FIGURE 7.1 Comparison of perfusion pressures (mm Hg) in the pulmonary and systemic circulations. *From Fox,* Human Physiology; *2008, with Lechner's modifications shown to add typical mean blood pressure values as a function of location.*

▶▶CLINICAL CORRELATION 7.1

P_{PW} represents **left ventricular preload**, and is a sensitive diagnostic tool to assess left ventricular decompensation in patients with **congestive heart failure**. As will be discussed in Chap. 28, a P_{PW} >15-18 mm Hg indicates a low left ventricular stroke volume, causing pulmonary venous blood to stagnate in the left atrium. The previously healthy lung also is affected by elevations in left atrial filling pressure, since increased back pressure in the pulmonary capillaries leads to interstitial swelling and edema within the alveolar compartment.

Pulmonary Capillary Responses to Cardiac Output and Gravity

Systemic perfusion pressures and flow rates through specific organs fluctuate to meet changing needs in work output (muscle), digestion (gut), temperature (skin), or filtration (kidney). Through auto-regulation, these tissues rarely maintain their blood flow as a constant percentage of $\dot{Q}$ which might range from 5 to 20 L/min. However, such a response is not feasible for the lung, which must accept the entire output of the right ventricle regardless of factors that cause $\dot{Q}$ to rise or fall.

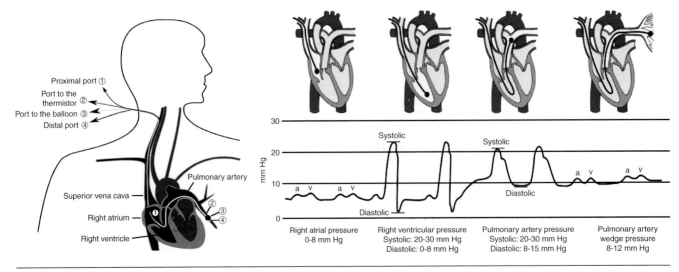

FIGURE 7.2 Blood pressure measured as a function of anatomic location using a pulmonary artery catheter (PAC). Specific pressure waveforms exist for the right atrium (RA), right ventricle (RV), and main pulmonary artery (PA), as well as for the pulmonary veins (PVs) when the catheter's balloon is inflated to wedge the PAC tip. *Left drawing from Wikipedia open access site; right drawing is from ScribD Web site, also open access.*

(#31)

As required by Ohm's law ($\dot{Q} = \Delta P/PVR$), the resistance of pulmonary blood vessels must decrease as $\dot{Q}$ increases if **pulmonary hypertension** is to be avoided. Studies show that when $\dot{Q}$ rises, PVR decreases by further **distension** of previously open arterioles and capillaries, and by **recruitment** of vessels that are collapsed when $\dot{Q}$ is lower. Such changes reflect the exceptional compliance of the thin-walled pulmonary vasculature. Thus when $\dot{Q}$ is low, many pulmonary arterioles and alveolar capillaries either are closed or are flowing at less than maximal diameters. To appreciate this effect requires understanding **transmural pressure**, the difference between air or fluid forces directed inwardly and outwardly that will attempt to collapse or open a vessel, respectively. Because alveolar capillaries are surrounded mostly by airspace, changes in P_A during ventilation will strongly affect this transmural pressure balance and resulting blood flow.

The real-time distribution of lung blood flow has been estimated by a technique similar to that using ^{133}Xenon (^{133}Xe) in airways (Chap. 6). In this case ^{133}Xe dissolved in saline is infused as a bolus via a PAC in the upright subject. When the bolus of dissolved ^{133}Xe reaches alveolar capillaries, labeled Xe rapidly escapes into alveolar air due to its low tissue solubility. Scintillation counters placed at various chest heights detect the ^{133}Xe, showing that pulmonary arterial flow (mL blood/ mL lung tissue) is high in the lung bases but low or nonexistent in the lung apices. As for the gravitational gradient of inhaled air, this regional distribution of blood flow is a top-to-bottom or nondependent/dependent phenomenon. As might be expected, apical under-perfusion is reduced with increases in $\dot{Q}$ as occur during exercise. Thus, alveolar blood perfusion is highest to the best ventilated lung regions, so that the **alveolar ventilation/perfusion $\dot{V}_A/\dot{Q}$ ratio** is normally well matched. How does gravity cause or modulate such a perfusion gradient?

Remember that pulmonary capillaries are compliant vessels surrounded by a fluctuating P_A while perfused by a relatively low P_{PA}. In the most widely accepted model of the pulmonary circulation described in 1963 as the **vascular waterfall** (Fig. 7.3), three zones of perfusion can be identified for the upright lung. In **Zone 1**, P_{PA} simply is too low to perfuse the lung apices, while P_A exceeds both P_{PA} and P_{PV}. Such Zone 1 capillaries are collapsed and have flow rates of zero. In **Zone 2**, P_{PA} exceeds P_A but P_{PV} does not. Such Zone 2 capillaries have flow rates proportional to the difference between P_{PA} and P_A, while P_{PV} has no direct effect on their flow. Extending the model, capillaries high in Zone 2 (near Zone 1) will open or closed with each pulse as P_{PA} rises during systole to exceed P_A, declining during diastole to fall below P_A. Capillaries lower in Zone 2 would remain open longer during each systolic cycle of pressure than would capillaries above them within the gravitational gradient. In **Zone 3**, alveolar capillaries presumably behave like those in the systemic circulation, since both P_{PA} and P_{PV} exceed P_A throughout the cardiac cycle. Additionally, alveolar capillary blood flow increases slightly with depth in Zone 3 due to progressively greater capillary distension (Fig. 7.3).

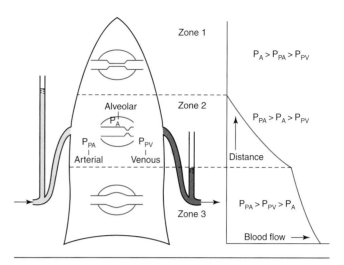

FIGURE 7.3 The "vascular waterfall" model is used to explain distribution of blood flow in the lung, based upon the intravascular and transmural airway pressures affecting the alveolar capillaries. *Modified from West,* Respiratory Physiology; *2005.*

These zonal boundaries of lung perfusion are not fixed in time or space, but fluctuate depending upon posture and changes in P_A, P_{PA}, or P_{PV} with exercise, disease, etc. For example, it is unlikely that Zone 1 conditions exist in the lungs of a healthy adult with normal chest size, cardiac output, and P_{PA}. However, Zone 1 conditions quickly arise in subjects holding their breath while swimming, as well as in patients being mechanically ventilated and in whom P_A increases dramatically during inspiration (Chap. 30). One can also appreciate how Zone 3 perfusion conditions would exist in the lung apex of a subject doing a handstand, or would move closest to the bed mattress in a supine patient. Consideration of these frequent adjustments in transmural capillary pressures makes the lung's elegant "vascular waterfall" an intelligible and useful working model to explain the easily observed and dynamic differences in regional pulmonary blood flow. Understanding the challenge of maintaining good $\dot{V}_A/\dot{Q}$ matching in the face of such fluctuating regional gradients in air and blood flow is the primary subject of Chap. 8.

▶▶ CLINICAL CORRELATION 7.2

Making the successful transition to air breathing that every fetus encounters goes beyond the adequacy of surfactant synthesis described in Chap. 5. As shown in Fig. 7.4, the fetal heart employs both the interatrial **foramen ovale** and the **ductus arteriosus (DA)** to shunt most right ventricular blood flow around the lungs and back into the systemic circulation. Shortly after birth, the neonate's systemic **arterial oxygen pressure (P_{aO_2})** rises dramatically above fetal levels if the lungs are adequately inflating with air. That increased P_{aO_2} causes reflexive contraction of smooth muscle cells in the DA wall, closing the bypass route and usually completing isolation of the two circulations. Interestingly, the incidence of a persistently open or

patent ductus arteriosus (PDA) is significantly higher among infants born at high altitude, presumably because their postnatal rise in P_aO_2 is insufficient to initiate closure of the ductal sphincter (see Chap. 13). Although autopsies for other reasons suggest that a **patent foramen ovale (PFO)** is more common in adults than is PDA, the amount of right-to-left shunting of blood that they allow is normally small given the trivial pressure differential between the two atria. However, the PFO may convert from benign to malignant in patients with pulmonary hypertension (Chap. 27).

Pulmonary Capillary Fluid Balance and Formation of Alveolar Edema

All pressures mentioned to this point have been hydrostatic, whether alveolar, vascular, or intrapleural. Hydrostatic pressures within blood vessels are only partially opposed by interstitial hydrostatic pressure of the delicate alveolar parenchyma. This imbalance would rapidly move blood water out of the vascular spaces by **ultrafiltration**, if capillary hydrostatic pressures were not opposed by **colloid osmotic pressure** exerted by blood proteins (Fig. 7.5). Formally presented, **Starling's law of the capillary** states that:

$$F = K \cdot [(P_{MV} - P_{PMV}) - \sigma\,(\pi_{MV} - \pi_{PMV})]$$

where: F = net **extravasation** or transvascular fluid movement
K = filtration coefficient for permeability of the capillary endothelium

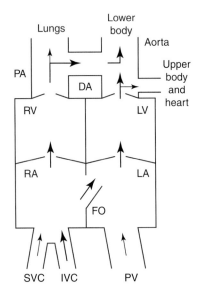

FIGURE 7.4 A unique situation exists in the perinatal timeframe when two fetal channels, the ductus arteriosus (DA) and the foramen ovale (FO), are available for venous return to shunt blood directly into the systemic circulation without first perfusing the pulmonary circulation. At birth, anatomical and physiological changes normally close the shunts or reduce their importance as bypass circuits.

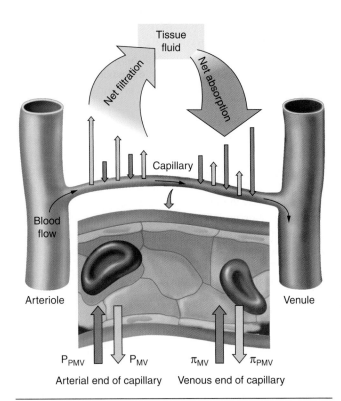

FIGURE 7.5 Blood fluids tend to **extravasate**, that is, leave a capillary at its arterial end to form **lymph**. Most lymph returns to the capillary by reabsorption at its venous end. Net fluid loss is normal and collects in adjacent lymphatics. Extravasation that exceeds lymphatic capacity to remove it causes **edema**. *From Fox,* Human Physiology, *10th ed.; 2008.*

P_{MV} = hydrostatic pressure within lung microvessels (~10 mm Hg)
P_{PMV} = hydrostatic pressure in perimicrovascular space (0 to −10 mm Hg)
σ = protein reflection coefficient, normally 1.0 (in arbitrary units)
π_{MV} = protein colloid osmotic pressure in the circulation (~28 mm Hg)
π_{PMV} = protein colloid osmotic pressure in peri-microvascular space (~20 mm Hg)

The hydrostatic pressure P_{MV} within the blood vessel causing fluid to extravasate from lung capillaries into the septal interstitium is mostly unopposed by any rise in P_{PMV}, because the delicate alveolar epithelial membranes cannot resist increases in interstitial volume as can occur systemically in tissues like skeletal muscle. Rather, the septal interstitial compartment expands with this capillary ultrafiltrate that drains into blind-ended pulmonary lymphatic capillaries. However, if lymphatic drainage cannot remove the ultrafiltrate at a sufficient rate, **interstitial edema** will occur that can progress to **alveolar edema** accompanied by disruption of epithelial layers (Fig. 7.6). Maximal lung lymphatic drainage is probably 2-3 times the normal flow rate of 20 mL/h.

The protein colloid osmotic pressure π_{MV} of blood in the alveolar capillaries is relatively constant as in systemic capillaries, except in diseases like **Kwashiorkor** or **liver failure**

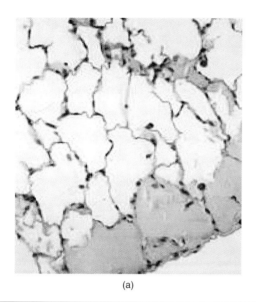
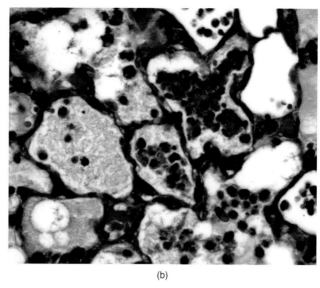

(a)   (b)

FIGURE 7.6 (a) Peripheral alveoli are filled with acellular ultrafiltrate in this specimen of endotoxemic lung tissue. (b) Neutrophil-rich edema and alveolar exudates in a rat with gram-negative pneumonia.

that reduce plasma [albumin]. Likewise, π_{PMV} is generally considered constant unless interstitial [protein] declines by dilution with water from the blood (ie, ongoing edema) or from within the airspaces (eg, near-drowning in fresh water). Smoke or fume inhalation, aspiration of stomach contents or toxic chemicals, and blood-borne diseases like gram-negative endotoxemia alter the endothelial K or σ such that net fluid flow out of alveolar capillaries increases and edema occurs, even if P_{MV}, P_{PMV}, π_{MV}, and π_{PMV} are all normal.

In practice, factors in Starling's equation are most likely to become unbalanced in two main ways to initiate interstitial and then often alveolar edema. The first occurs when P_{MV} becomes elevated due to systemic hypertension, generally rising in parallel with increases in P_{PA} and P_{PV}. The resulting leak is termed **cardiogenic edema** since its cause is usually congestive heart failure or mitral valve dysfunction (Table 7.1). In this type of edema, the endothelial barrier to protein movement is usually intact (ie, K and σ are normal), and the resulting edema fluid has a [protein] lower than that of plasma.

The second major type of pulmonary edema occurs despite normal hydrostatic forces and is considered **noncardiogenic** in etiology. It commonly begins as an increased permeability (K and/or σ) of the capillary endothelial or alveolar epithelial layers, often following direct cellular injuries. Plasma proteins can now leak out directly between adjacent barrier cells, so that such edema fluids have a higher [protein]. Indeed in severe cases, intact formed blood elements can appear within the interstitial or alveolar spaces as well, yielding a **hemorrhagic edema** (Fig. 7.7). Such severe forms of edema are a characteristic feature of **acute lung injury (ALI)** and the **acute respiratory distress syndrome (ARDS)**. How these disruptive changes in pulmonary endothelial or epithelial permeability occur in the previously healthy lung, and the impact they have on diffusional gas exchange will be discussed at length in Chap. 28.

▶▶ **CLINICAL CORRELATION 7.3** *(#32)*

Pulmonary edema is conventionally viewed as an acute **restrictive lung disease** (Chap. 6) because fluids within the alveolar septa and distal airspaces reduce the functional parenchymal volume available for ventilation. However, such edema also has a propensity to accumulate within the interstitial spaces surrounding larger airways and blood vessels (Fig. 7.7). Such edematous **cuffing** creates a sleeve of fluid that prevents dilatation along the length of such vessels, even if smooth muscle cells within their walls are relaxed. The resulting **bronchiolar edema** is an **acute obstructive lung disease** that will adversely affect peak expiratory flow rates and increase dynamic airway resistance. Thus, a patient with ALI or ARDS would have a **mixed respiratory disorder** that clinically has both a complex etiology and an uncertain outcome (Chaps. 26 and 28).

Table **7.1** Primary categories of pulmonary edema

Feature	Cardiogenic	Noncardiogenic
Most common etiologies	Left heart failure, mitral stenosis	ALI, ARDS[*]
Lung capillary pressure P_{MV}	Increased	Normal
Lung capillary K and σ	Normal	Increased
[Protein] of edema fluid	<< plasma [protein]	< or = plasma [protein]

[*]ALI, acute lung injury; ARDS, acute respiratory distress syndrome.

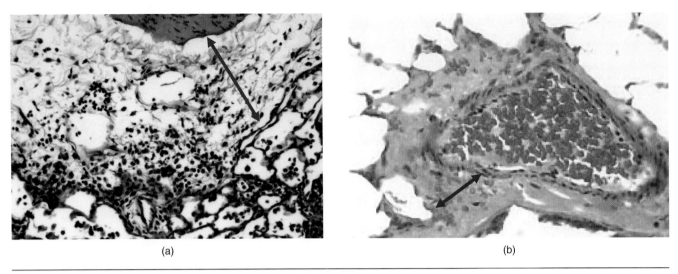

(a)   (b)

FIGURE 7.7 Interstitial edema around airways and blood vessels (double-headed arrows) decreases their diameters and increases resistances to flow. Such edematous **cuffs** or sleeves also reduce traction that can be exerted by elastic elements in the parenchyma. (a) Rat lung 72 hours after induction of plague pneumonia by intratracheal instillation of *Yersinia pestis*; neutrophils predominate the interstitial infiltrate below a large artery. (b) Rat lung 24 hours after acute IV (intravenous) infection with *Candida albicans*; numerous erythrocytes in the interstitial space of the arteriole are typical of this often hemorrhagic edema.

The specific causes of pulmonary edema are multiple (Table 7.2), and a complete discussion is beyond the scope of this introduction to the topic. However, it is evident that perturbations to virtually all terms within Starling's equation occur clinically, although not all result in cases of equal severity or duration. Of interest to the general public is the sudden and often unpredictable development of **high altitude pulmonary edema, HAPE** in some travelers to elevations above their normal residences. By poorly understood mechanisms, severe hypoxia reduces active Na^+ transport that normally drives the reabsorption of capillary ultrafiltrate and thereby keeps alveolar membranes moist but free of excess fluid. This uncleared alveolar fluid, whose formation is invariably accelerated by the increased P_{PA} and P_{MV} that are also caused by hypoxia (Chap. 8), leads to acute HAPE in susceptible individuals. What makes some climbers sensitive to this serious side effect of even moderate altitude exposure, while their climbing partners may be unaffected, remains an intriguing and unsolved question in the field (Chap. 13). In any case, resolution of their often hemorrhagic edema is rapid and reversible if a descent to lower elevations can be achieved in time.

Table **7.2** **Causes of pulmonary edema sorted by Starling's equation defect**

Altered Parameter	Diseases or Processes Affecting the Parameter
increased P_{MV}	congestive heart failure; mitral stenosis; myocardial infarct
increased P_{PMV}	reduced lymphatic drainage from lymphangitis or neoplasia
decreased P_{PMV}	alveolar overdistension (neurogenic or mechanical); hypoxia?
increased σ	endotoxemia; sepsis; inhalation injury; drug toxicity; prolonged hyperoxia
decreased π_{MV}	hemodilution; hypoalbuminemia; Kwashiorkor
decreased π_{PMV}	near-drowning in fresh water; evolving interstitial edema; high altitude?

Suggested Readings

1. Permutt S, Riley RL. Hemodynamics of collapsible vessels with tone: the vascular waterfall. *J Appl Physiol.* 1963;18:924-932. *As this papers' subtitle suggests, the model of lung perfusion first proposed by these authors has left an indelible mark in pulmonary medicine.*

2. West JB, Dollery CT, Naimark A. Distribution of blood flow in isolated lung: relation to vascular and alveolar pressures. *J Appl Physiol.* 1964;19:713-724. *This nearly contemporaneous paper to the article by Permutt and Riley stimulated much early thinking about the overarching importance of alveolar air pressure to venous return.*

3. Ashbaugh DG, Bigelow DB, Petty TL, Levine BE. Acute respiratory distress in adults. *Lancet. 1967;2:319-323; and:* Fowler AA, Hamman RF, Good JT, Benson KN, Baird M, Eberle DJ, Petty TL, Hyers TM. Adult respiratory distress syndrome: risk with common predispositions. *Ann Internal Med.* 1983;98:593-597. *These two papers make clear why researchers of pulmonary edema often trace the field's origins to Dr. Petty and his collaborators at the University of Colorado School of Medicine.*

4. Houston CA. Acute pulmonary edema of high altitude. *N Engl J Med.* 1960;263:478-480. *Six years after leading the first American assault on K2 (making it to nearly 8,000 m), Dr. Houston saves the life of a 21 year-old climber in the Maroon Bells above Aspen and publishes the first chest x-ray of HAPE. Exciting stuff.*

CASE STUDIES AND PRACTICE PROBLEMS

CASE 7.1 A previously healthy 25-year-old woman is brought to the ER 0.5 hours after extraction from a motor vehicle accident. Radial pulse is rapid and faint, breathing is shallow and intermittent, the abdomen is bruised and swollen, and thigh skin is pale and cool. A pulmonary artery catheter (PAC) inserted into the right brachial vein indicates $\dot{Q}$ = 3.0 L/min and heart rate (HR) = 100 b/min, with mean P_{PA} = 35 mm Hg and P_{PW} = 5 mm Hg. Brisk IV infusion of lactated Ringer's is begun while units of packed RBCs are typed and cross-matched. New PAC data 0.2 hours later (before transfusion) show that $\dot{Q}$ = 6 L/min at a HR = 80 b/min, with mean P_{PA} = 28 mm Hg, and P_{PW} = 4 mm Hg. Summarize the patient's initial status and the effects on her of the first emergent intervention.

CASE 7.2 A 61-year-old man presents with shortness of breath. His temperature and other vital signs are normal. The patient has a long history of aortic valvular insufficiency. His spouse reports that the patient takes all prescribed medications regularly. He has never smoked and denies any history of lung disease, but pulmonary function testing now shows an obstructive pattern. A new chest radiograph shows an enlarged heart and evidence of bilateral pulmonary edema. What mechanism most likely accounts for the airway obstruction in this patient?

a. Increased cardiac dimensions

b. Previously undiagnosed pneumonia

c. Excessive mucus production

d. Loss of elastin from upper airways

e. Bronchial and bronchiolar edema

CASE 7.3 A group of sixth-graders who all play on the same soccer team gather on the playground to judge by acclamation who is likely to be the best swimmer when they attend summer camp in a week. All agree to pinch their nostrils closed, take a deep breath at the same instant, and then hold it as long as possible. One child collapses to the ground within 15 seconds, immediately attracting the attention of a nearby teacher and scattering the rest of the children. What primary physiological effect best explains what occurred in the child who has apparently fainted?

a. Undiagnosed PDA

b. Grand mal epileptic seizure

c. Acute asthma attack

d. Cerebral anoxia or ischemia

e. Unilateral pneumothorax

Solutions to Case Studies and Practice Problems

CASE 7.1 The patient's symptoms suggest internal hemorrhage, hypovolemic shock, reduced cutaneous blood flow, and possible suppression of respiratory reflexes. Her low $\dot{Q}$ and stroke volume of 30 mL/beat (= 3.0 L/100 b/min) are likely sustainable only through intense peripheral vasoconstriction as well as an impressive elevation in PVR of 10 mm Hg/L (= 30 mm Hg/3.0 L). Rapid re-expansion of her plasma compartment with IV fluid improves ventricular preload, causing $\dot{Q}$ to increase as stroke volume normalizes to 75 mL/beat (= 6.0 L/80 b/min). **Lactated Ringer solution** is a sterile, non-pyrogenic solution for IV fluid and electrolyte replenishment containing NaCl, Na-lactate, $CaCl_2$, and KCl. This emergent volume expansion allows some relaxation of the prior vasoconstriction, so that PVR is now 4 mm Hg/L (= 24 mm Hg/6.0 L).

CASE 7.2 The most correct answer is e.

The man's aortic insufficiency has worsened to now distend the left atrium and pulmonary veins, and initiate cardiogenic edema that increases airway resistance. Because he does not smoke, is not febrile, and his sputum production is not remarkable, he likely does not have pneumonia (*answers b and c*) or emphysema (*answer d*). Increased cardiac dimensions (*answer a*) are more common in patients with congestive heart failure secondary to systemic hypertension; in any case such cardiomegaly would rarely reduce the diameters of conducting airways directly.

CASE 7.3 The most correct answer is d.

The single most consistent effect of a forced breath hold begun at or near total lung capacity is an acute increase in P_{AW} that will create global Zone 1 conditions throughout the respiratory parenchyma. The resulting rapid fall in pulmonary perfusion, and thus in venous return to the left ventricle, invariably reduces aortic blood flow. The appropriate autonomic response to such an abrupt reduction in left heart $\dot{Q}$ is to increase heart rate and peripheral vasoconstriction via the carotid baroreceptor reflex, but light-headedness and a brain-protective episode of **syncope** will still occur in many individuals. While *answers a, b, c,* and *e* are certainly possible in pediatric patients, those choices are farther down on a differential diagnosis among active children who were in no apparent distress before their little experiment. Interested readers can explore much more about such interactions between the cardiovascular and respiratory systems by researching the **Valsalva maneuver**, a historically important test of sympathetic autonomic function.

Chapter 8

Ventilation/ Perfusion Matching and Estimating Alveolar Ventilation

ANDREW J. LECHNER, PhD

Learning Objectives

- The student will be able to explain why the ratio of alveolar ventilation to lung vascular perfusion increases apically in lungs of an upright subject.

- The student will be able to distinguish between the anatomical and physiological concepts of dead space and shunt.

- The student will be able to explain the circumstances that elicit the acute hypoxic pressor response and its effect on pulmonary arterial pressure.

- The student will be able to apply multiple inert gas data to distinguish normal subjects versus diseased patients with increased shunt or dead space.

- The student will be able to use relevant equations to estimate alveolar versus dead space ventilations, and calculate alveolar P_{O_2} from patient data.

Introduction to Ventilation/ Perfusion Matching

In the normal upright lung, both ventilation and perfusion favor dependent lung regions (Chaps. 6 and 7). These relationships will be explored here to develop a fuller understanding of their normal ranges and perturbations having clinical importance (Fig. 8.1). Since both $\dot{V}_A$ and $\dot{Q}$ change with lung height, their alveolar ventilation perfusion ratio $\dot{V}_A/\dot{Q}$ increases exponentially from lung base to apex. In this situation, $\dot{V}_A/\dot{Q} < 1$ at the level of the diaphragm due to the heavy blood flow through Zone 3 capillaries. With increasing height above the heart of the upright lung, the $\dot{V}_A/\dot{Q}$ ratio rapidly passes through 1.0 toward higher values that could theoretically approach infinity (ie, the denominator = 0) if apical alveolar capillaries are actually in Zone 1 conditions.

Regardless of their cause, inequalities in $\dot{V}_A/\dot{Q}$ have a direct bearing on the efficiency of ventilation and the adequacy of perfusion. In simplified form, the extreme range of possible situations is shown in Fig. 8.2. The structures shown represent individual alveoli and their capillaries, or entire lung lobes, with several basic principles the same. First, inspired gas is well mixed and normally provides a suitable P_{O_2} even when diluted with alveolar air. Second, pulmonary arterial blood is also homogenous as it enters the lungs with respect to its **mixed venous O_2 content, $C_{\bar{v}}O_2$.** Under these conditions, the open airway and patent blood vessel serving the central gas exchange structure in this diagram offer no serious impediments to ventilation or perfusion, and thus its $\dot{V}_A/\dot{Q} = 1$.

The lung unit to the left in Fig. 8.2 has normal, unimpeded blood perfusion, but its ventilation is low, due perhaps to mucus, edema, or other cause for a narrowed airway. The end result of this unit with low $\dot{V}_A/\dot{Q}$ (1/10) is wasted cardiac output and a decrease in **pulmonary venous blood O_2 content, $C_{pv}O_2$.** Such wasted blood flow is termed **physiological shunt**, with the end result no different than if this blood had passed through an anatomical shunt between the right ventricle and left atrium. The lung segment to the right in Fig. 8.2 shows adequate (even excessive) ventilation compared to its reduced perfusion. The consequence of a high $\dot{V}_A/\dot{Q}$ (10/1) is enriched O_2 content in pulmonary veins (or at least no reduction), although significant ventilation is wasted and contributes to **physiological dead space**. Such vascular occlusion might occur by an embolism, clot, or other obstructive effect within the blood vessel.

Later sections of this chapter and Chap. 9 present equations to calculate a patient's **physiological dead space** and **physiological shunt**. It is important to emphasize that such physiological estimates are made on living subjects and include any anatomical defects that are only quantifiable by autopsy. Thus, a calculated physiological dead space includes the anatomical dead space of conducting zone airways (Chap. 4) plus the volume of all alveoli whose ventilation vastly exceeds their blood flow, that is $\dot{V}_A/\dot{Q} > 100$ (Table 8.1). Likewise, a calculated physiological shunt as detailed in Chap. 9 includes actual extra-pulmonary anatomical defects like **PDA** or **PFO** (Chap. 7) that allow systemic blood to bypass the pulmonary circulation plus any pulmonary arterial blood flowing through alveoli with inadequate ventilation, that is, $\dot{V}_A/\dot{Q} < 0.01$ (Table 8.1). By these definitions, healthy subjects are those whose physiological dead space and shunt do not exceed their anatomical dead space and shunt.

Beyond such large-scale adjustments between ventilation and perfusion, pulmonary arterioles constrict directly in response to reduced $P_{A}O_2$. This **acute hypoxic pressor response (AHPR)** is a reflex unique to the pulmonary circulation, evident even in isolated lungs (Fig. 8.3). AHPR adaptively

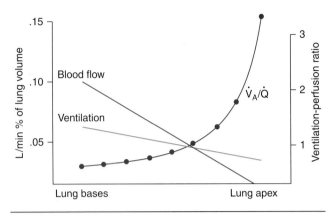

FIGURE 8.1 Distribution of ventilation and blood flow in the upright lung. The ventilation/perfusion ratio decreases toward the lung bases. *From West, Respiratory Physiology; 2005.*

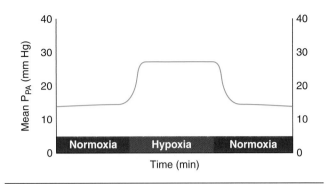

FIGURE 8.3 Demonstration of the pulmonary **acute hypoxic pressor response, AHPR**. Isolated lungs are first ventilated with normoxic gas (21% O_2/5% CO_2/74% N_2) while perfused with blood. When ventilation begins with hypoxic gas (10% O_2/5% CO_2/85% N_2), mean pulmonary artery pressure P_{PA} promptly increases, but returns to baseline when normoxic ventilation resumes.

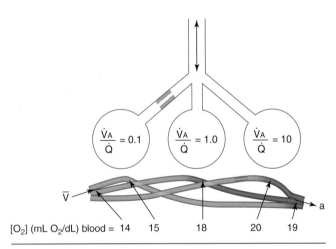

FIGURE 8.2 Mechanisms that alter systemic P_aO_2 by well-matched or poorly matched ventilation and pulmonary arterial blood. Lung units with high $\dot{V}_A/\dot{Q}$ (right) add relatively little O_2 overall to blood because blood flow is low; such regions contribute to **physiological dead space**. Lung units with low $\dot{V}_A/\dot{Q}$ (left) add little oxygen because they are under ventilated; such regions contribute to **physiological shunt**. *From West, Respiratory Physiology; 2005.*

diverts blood from hypoxic alveoli to improve local $\dot{V}_A/\dot{Q}$ matching and minimize arterial hypoxemia for the entire lung.

The degree of flow diversion attributable to the AHPR diminishes when the entire lung is experiencing hypoxia. Hypoxic foci that are small or limited to particular lobes, as during pneumonia, receive little perfusion because the AHPR shunts their blood supply to less hypoxic alveoli. In such cases, PVR may be normal for the lungs as a whole, P_{PA} need not increase to maintain $\dot{Q}$, and so the risk of edema is low (Chap. 7). However, when alveolar hypoxia involves the entire lung, as at altitude, the AHPR affects all alveolar units and PVR increases substantially. In that situation, right heart output and lung blood flow can only be maintained by large increases in P_{PA}. If persistent, the resulting pulmonary hypertension can lead to vascular remodeling, enlargement of the right ventricle, and **cor pulmonale**, topics that will be discussed in Chaps. 13 and 26.

Quantifying Abnormalities in Ventilation/Perfusion Matching

Advances in gas analyses allowed development of the **multiple inert gas technique** to estimate $\dot{V}_A/\dot{Q}$ distributions. In this research test, six tracer gases dissolved in saline (Table 8.2) are infused into the right ventricle at known rates. They have a range of molecular weights and thus differing diffusion rates as gases, and variable solubilities in blood and tissue as described by Henry's law. These properties affect how quickly each gas leaves the blood and enters alveolar air to be collected as expired air, where concentrations are measured by mass spectrometry. Less soluble gases leave blood quickly, enter alveolar airspaces and are not reabsorbed. Once there, their rates of free diffusion determine the speed at which they are expired. These clearance data are compiled to estimate the proportion of ventilation and perfusion going to alveolar units having various $\dot{V}_A/\dot{Q}$ ratios, plotted on a log scale from 0.01 to 100 (Fig. 8.4).

The area under either curve must equal the entire $\dot{V}_A$ or $\dot{Q}$ per minute. Thus, the apex of the ventilation curve indicates

Table **8.1** **Working definitions of $\dot{V}_A/\dot{Q}$ matching**

Accepted Terminology	Measured $\dot{V}_A/\dot{Q}$ Ratios
"Deadspace Ventilation"	$\dot{V}_A/\dot{Q} > 100$
"High $\dot{V}_A/\dot{Q}$ Lung"	$10 < \dot{V}_A/\dot{Q} < 100$
"Normal Lung Ventilation"	$0.10 \ \dot{V}_A/\dot{Q} < 10$
"Poorly Ventilated Lung"	$0.01 \ \dot{V}_A/\dot{Q} < 0.10$
"Intrapulmonary Shunt"	$\dot{V}_A/\dot{Q} < 0.01$

(#34)

Table **8.2** **Multiple inert gases dissolved in venous injectate**

Gas Species	Molec. Wt.	Blood:Gas Phase Partition
Sulfur hexafluoride	146.1	0.0063
Ethane	30.1	0.008
Cyclopropane	42.1	0.879
Enflurane	184.5	1.401
Diethyl Ether	74.1	8.932
Acetone	58.1	232.4

that ~1.5 L/min of $\dot{V}_A$ went to alveoli with $\dot{V}_A/\dot{Q}$ ratios of slightly more than 1.0; blood flow going to this same population of alveoli also was about 1.5 L/min. As is apparent from the super imposable curves, $\dot{V}_A/\dot{Q}$ and $\dot{Q}$ were well matched in this lung, and result in a highly efficient pattern of arterial oxygenation.

Pulmonary embolism (PE) provides a useful example of how the multiple inert gas technique detects $\dot{V}_A/\dot{Q}$ abnormalities (Fig. 8.5). Whereas normal lungs show well-matched $\dot{V}_A/\dot{Q}$ curves centered over 1.0, within minutes of PE a substantial fraction of $\dot{V}_A/\dot{Q}$ is ventilating alveoli whose microvasculature is occluded by blood clots, fat, or even the N_2 in air. For those units in this example, $\dot{V}_A/\dot{Q}$ is ~8 while the remaining $\dot{V}_A$ is ventilating relatively over-perfused alveoli. Overall, the PE has increased $\dot{V}_A$ and $\dot{Q}$ (see total area under those curves); hypoxemia and acidosis caused by these mismatches have stimulated breathing and increased **dead space ventilation** ($\dot{V}_D$, L/min).

The technique can distinguish between two forms of emphysema whose pathology and clinical presentations will be detailed in Chaps. 20 and 22. Patients with inherited **α1-antiprotease deficiency** exhibit the **type A** ("pink puffer") form of emphysema by the third or fourth decade of life, and present with rapid breathing **(tachypnea)**, moderate airflow obstruction, and mild hypoxemia. Their autopsied lungs show widespread loss of distal respiratory bronchioles and alveolar septa, presumably secondary to the unchecked activity of elastase and other proteases released by resident alveolar macrophages and recruited neutrophils (Chap. 10). Patients with smoking-related **type B** ("blue bloater") emphysema usually have more respiratory distress **(dyspnea)**, mucus production, bronchitis, severe **airflow** obstruction, and persistent hypoxemia. Their symptoms tend to worsen with a patient's **pack-year history of smoking**, perhaps evident only after 40-60 such units of time (one pack-year equals one pack of cigarettes smoked/day for one year). Their lungs show centrilobular loss of intermediate airways and terminal bronchioles due to deposition there of tobacco ash and other particulates and resulting proteolysis by recruited leukocytes. Alveolar architecture in such patients is often spared, since the organic and inorganic burden from tobacco is cleared upstream and does not penetrate the distal parenchyma.

Inert gas results for type A emphysema show that most $\dot{Q}$ goes to alveoli with $\dot{V}_A/\dot{Q}$ slightly less than 1.0, while $\dot{V}_A$ serves both alveoli with adequate $\dot{V}_A/\dot{Q}$ (~1.0) and those with little flow ($\dot{V}_A/\dot{Q} >5.0$) (Fig. 8.6). Such patients may maintain a normal P_aO_2, but their $\dot{V}_E$ is high due to increased physiological dead space. Type B patients have little wasted $\dot{V}_A$ since most gas ventilates intact alveoli, but they often deoxygenate because a large part of $\dot{Q}$ is wasted perfusing alveoli where $\dot{V}_A/\dot{Q} <0.1$ due to increased physiological shunt. Structurally these results make sense. Patients with type B disease lack intermediate airways that guide ventilation toward intact peripheral alveoli. Their airway resistance is high and **cyanosis** occurs due to physiological shunt. Persons with type A disease lack delicate structures that comprise terminal acini. Their airways provide adequate ventilation to distal lung

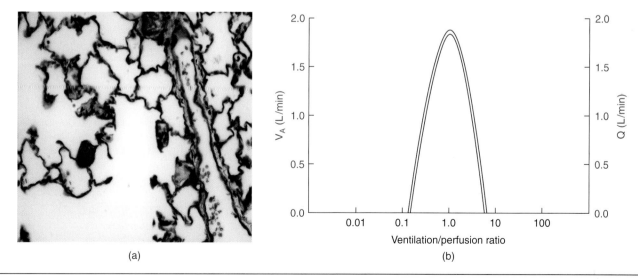

(a)   (b)

FIGURE 8.4 Normal lung tissue (a) yields well-matched $\dot{V}_A/\dot{Q}$ curves (b) by the multiple inert gas technique.

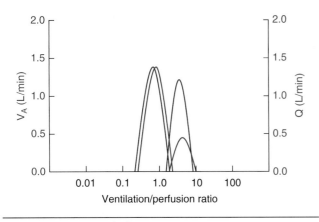

FIGURE 8.5 Defective $\dot{V}_A/\dot{Q}$ matching caused by pulmonary embolism. Note the bimodal distribution of both curves, and the vastly increased areas under those for alveolar ventilation compared to those for cardiac output.

regions that may be devoid of alveolar capillaries and so their volume adds to physiological dead space.

Alveolar Ventilation Equation

Given the preceding discussion, the importance of distinguishing $\dot{V}_A$ from $\dot{V}_D$ is clear and has led to several complementary approaches to estimating them from available patient data. In Chap. 4, $\dot{V}_A$ was introduced by stating that each tidal breath V_T is the sum of its dead space volume V_D plus its alveolar parenchymal volume V_A:

$$V_T = V_D + V_A \quad \text{(each in mL or L)}$$
$$V_T \cdot f = (V_D + V_A) \cdot f \quad \text{(where } f = \text{breaths/min)}$$
$$\dot{V}_E = \dot{V}_D + \dot{V}_A \quad \text{(each in L/min)}$$

Unlike $\dot{V}_E$, the $\dot{V}_D$ is difficult to measure directly in living subjects and so $\dot{V}_A$ cannot be determined by this equation alone. An indirect measure of $\dot{V}_A$ can be derived with two assumptions. First, since V_D equals that portion of V_T that cannot participate in diffusive gas exchange, **all expired CO_2 must originate in V_A**. Second, alveolar $F_A co_2 = F_E co_2$, measured as expiration approaches RV and exhaled gas is no longer diluted by dead space with its low $[CO_2]$ (Fig. 8.7). From these assumptions, a measured $\dot{V} co_2$ must equal the product of an unknown $\dot{V}_A$ (L/min) multiplied by estimated $F_A co_2$:

$$\dot{V} co_2 \text{ (L of } CO_2\text{/min)} = \dot{V}_A \text{ (L of air/min)} \cdot F_A co_2 \text{ (L of } CO_2\text{/L of air)}$$
$$V_A = \dot{V} co_2 / F_A co_2$$

This alveolar ventilation equation provides an accurate estimate of $\dot{V}_A$ using just spirometric testing and not requiring a blood sample. However $\dot{V} co_2$ is most often calculated under STPD conditions while $\dot{V}_A$ is usually reported in BTPS. Thus, a complete solution for $\dot{V}_A$ may necessitate converting between these volume measurements using the procedure outlined in Chap. 1: $(P_1 \cdot V_1)/T_1 = (P_2 \cdot V_2)/T_2$.

Physiological Dead Space Equation

An alternative approach to calculating $\dot{V}_A$ relies upon first estimating $\dot{V}_D$ and subtracting it from $\dot{V}_D$. Recall that anatomical and physiological dead space are assumed to contain no appreciable CO_2 as expiration begins. By that assumption, all CO_2 expired in one breath must equal the V_A for that breath multiplied by its $F_A co_2$:

$$\text{Total } CO_2\text{/breath} = V_A \cdot F_A co_2$$

At the same time, all CO_2 expired in one breath must equal the V_T for that breath multiplied by the average CO_2 of that V_T, its $F_E co_2$:

Total CO_2/breath $= V_T \cdot F_E co_2$
And thus: $V_T \cdot F_E co_2 = V_A \cdot F_A co_2$
Substituting: $V_T \cdot F_E co_2 = (V_T - V_D) \cdot F_A co_2$
Rearranging terms: $V_D/V_T = (F_A co_2 - F_E co_2)/F_A co_2$
By Dalton's law: $V_D/V_T = (P_A co_2 - P_E co_2)/P_A co_2$

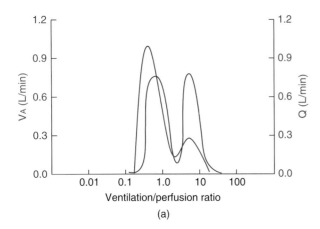

(a)

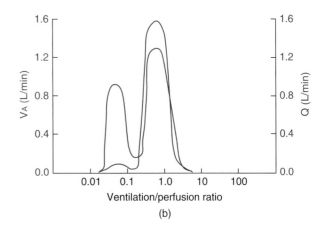

(b)

FIGURE 8.6 Multiple inert gas data for patients with the Type A "pink puffer" (a) and Type B "blue bloater" (b) forms of emphysema. See text for additional details regarding the most common etiologies of each.

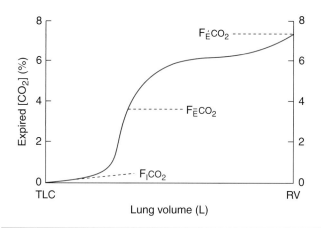

FIGURE 8.7 At the start of a complete exhalation from TLC, expired $[CO_2]$ is low, reflecting V_D gas resembling the low F_ICO_2. As exhalation continues, $[CO_2]$ increases to reflect levels in the alveolar parenchyma. As lung volume approaches RV, expired gas consists entirely of undiluted alveolar gas, and thus $F_ECO_2 = F_ACO_2$. A subject's F_ECO_2 is calculated by dividing the integrated area under the $[CO_2]$ curve by the volume of the full expiration.

Due to the high solubility of CO_2 in blood and tissues (Chap. 3), it is generally presumed that full equilibration occurs rapidly between levels in pulmonary arterial blood entering the alveolar parenchyma and gas within those alveolar airspaces. Thus, since $P_ACO_2 \cong P_aCO_2$, these two terms can be substituted for each other:

$$V_D/V_T = (P_aCO_2 - P_{\bar{E}}CO_2)/P_aCO_2$$
$$\text{Solving for } V_D \text{ yields: } V_D = [(P_aCO_2 - P_{\bar{E}}CO_2)/P_aCO_2] \cdot V_T$$

This physiological dead space equation yields a very similar estimate of V_D and $\dot{V}_D$ as deduced from the alveolar ventilation equation. The two mathematical approaches differ mostly by the assumptions made and the types of patient data needed to make the calculations: spirometric estimate of end-tidal CO_2 versus access to arterial blood gases. One is a non-invasive technique only requiring awake subjects who can respond to instructions to expire completely, etc. The other can be done at the bedside of intubated, catheterized patients irrespective of their cognitive status.

Anatomical V_D is ~2 mL/kg of predicted body weight (Chap. 4), with physiological V_D equal to or only slightly larger than anatomical V_D in healthy lungs. The ratio of physiological V_D/V_T is 0.2-0.4 at rest, decreasing with increases in V_T in healthy adults who breathe more deeply during exercise. A person's V_D/V_T increases with age, presumably due to progressive respiratory muscle weakness, loss of alveolar surface area, or fibrosis and may exceed 0.60 in individuals with cardiopulmonary disease. This increased V_D/V_T reflects worsening ventilation-perfusion mismatching or right-to-left shunt (Table 8.1). As V_D/V_T increases, the work of breathing becomes excessive as patients struggle to overcome such wasteful dead space ventilation (Chap. 6).

Alveolar Gas Equation

The alveolar gas equation estimates P_AO_2, and so provides a critical context for any P_aO_2 to assess whether the lungs are properly transferring O_2 into the blood (Chap. 9). Is a P_aO_2 of 38 mm Hg abnormal? What of $P_aO_2 = 55$ mm Hg, or 95 mm Hg? This equation also allows calculation of an important reference value, the partial pressure difference for O_2 between alveolar air (P_AO_2) and arterial blood (P_aO_2), the **(A – a) Po$_2$**. The equation requires just P_B plus the patient's F_IO_2 and arterial blood gases. Recall that as inhaled gas enters the airways, it is warmed to 37°C and saturated with water vapor to 100% relative humidity. Thus, by Dalton's law:

$$P_x = F_x \cdot (P_B - PH_2O)$$
$$P_IO_2 = 0.2093 \cdot (P_B - 47)$$
$$P_IO_2 = 149 \text{ mm Hg}$$

This P_IO_2 is further reduced as inhaled gas mixes with alveolar contents (as will its P_IN_2) and is diluted by CO_2 in the alveoli, that is, the P_ACO_2. A simplified equation estimates P_AO_2 with sufficient accuracy for routine use (while ignoring concurrent changes in P_IN_2):

$$P_AO_2 = P_IO_2 - (P_ACO_2/R)$$

where $R = \dot{V}CO_2/\dot{V}O_2$ (Chap. 3) and ranges from 0.7 to 1.0 depending on substrates being metabolized. If R is not measured directly, a value of 0.80 is often assumed based on one-third of calories being obtained from carbohydrates and two thirds from fat. If it is assumed again that $P_aCO_2 = P_ACO_2$, this expression becomes:

$$P_AO_2 = P_IO_2 - (P_aCO_2/R)$$

If arterial blood gases for a hypothetical patient breathing room air are presumed to be $P_aO_2 = 90$ mm Hg and $P_aCO_2 = 40$ mm Hg, it follows that:

$$P_AO_2 = 149 \text{ mm Hg} - (40 \text{ mm Hg}/0.8)$$
$$P_AO_2 = 99 \text{ mm Hg}$$

In this hypothetical patient, $P_AO_2 - P_aO_2 = 9$ mm Hg, well within a normal range of 5-19 mm Hg among healthy adults. If another patient also breathing room air at sea level has a $P_aO_2 = 53$ mm Hg and $P_aCO_2 = 48$ mm Hg, the calculated P_AO_2 would be 89 mm Hg and the (A – a) Po$_2$ = 36 mm Hg. Such a large (A – a) Po$_2$ would suggest that $\dot{V}_A$ is satisfactory because P_AO_2 is nearly normal, but diffusional impairment or intrapulmonary shunt defect is responsible for the abnormally low P_aO_2 (Chap. 9).

If P_IO_2 is constant but P_aCO_2 is elevated, perhaps due to hypoventilation, then both P_AO_2 and P_aO_2 must necessarily decrease by Dalton's law. Since P_AO_2 is calculated using known or assumed factors about the environment or patient, any change is generally predictable. In contrast, P_aO_2 is a measured value whose theoretical maximum is defined by P_AO_2 but whose minimum is determined by $\dot{V}_A/\dot{Q}$ mismatch, pulmonary diffusing capacity (Chaps. 9 and 17), and the O_2 content of mixed venous blood, $C_{\bar{v}}O_2$. Greater $\dot{V}_A/\dot{Q}$ mismatch inevitably creates larger (A – a) Po$_2$ differences.

Suggested Readings

1. Wagner PD. Ventilation-perfusion relationships. *Ann Rev Physiol.* 1980;42:235-247. *An authoritative early review by one of the principal developers of the multiple inert gas technique and its application to diagnosing a variety of pulmonary disorders.*

2. Cutaia M, Rounds S. Hypoxic pulmonary vasoconstriction: physiologic significance, mechanism, and clinical relevance. *Chest.* 1990;97:706-718. *In an evolving field, this remains one of the best summaries of experimental evidence supporting the local mediation of changing PVR by alveolar hypoxia.*

3. Putensen C, Rasanen J, Lopez FA. Improvement in $\dot{V}_A/\dot{Q}$ distributions during inhalation of nitric oxide in pigs with methacholine-induced bronchoconstriction. *Am J Respir Crit Care Med.* 1995;151:116-122. *A useful update on the preferred mix of infused gases to use when deciphering complicated ventilation/perfusion mismatch.*

CASE STUDIES AND PRACTICE PROBLEMS

CASE 8.1 Pre-employment pulmonary function test (PFT) data for a 37-year-old male smoker include the following results: $T_B = 38.1°C$; $P_B = 720$ mm Hg; $\dot{V}_{O_2} = \dot{V}_{CO_2} = 0.255$ L/min (STPD); $f = 15$/min; $F_{\bar{E}}CO_2 = 0.035$; $F_aCO_2 = 0.071$. What is his alveolar ventilation, $\dot{V}_A$ (L/min, BTPS)?

CASE 8.2 A 71-year-old female patient residing in a hospice with terminal metastatic disease has an estimated R = 0.70 at 5 days after refusing further parenteral feeding. While confined to bed she is receiving 3 L/min of intranasal oxygen that provide an estimated $F_{I}O_2 = 0.35$ at an ambient $P_B = 705$ mm Hg. Her most recent arterial blood gases are $P_aO_2 = 144$ mm Hg, $P_aCO_2 = 56$ mm Hg and $pH_a = 7.33$. What is her $(A - a)$ P_{O_2}?

CASE 8.3 A 28-year-old male medical student visits his hospital's PFT lab, where he learns that his $\dot{V}_E = 5.46$ L/min and his $\dot{V}_A = 3.77$ L/min, at an $f = 14$ breaths/min (BTPS units). What is his calculated dead space ventilation, $\dot{V}_D$ (L/min) and his dead space, V_D (L)?

CASE 8.4 An ICU patient is mechanically ventilated with $V_T = 450$ mL on air ($P_B = 740$ mm Hg) to maintain her $F_{\bar{E}}CO_2 = 0.040$. Current $T_B = 37°C$ and most recent ABGs are: $P_aO_2 = 92$ mm Hg; $P_aCO_2 = 39$ mm Hg. What is her current dead space volume, V_D (mL)?

CASE 8.5 A 55-year-old woman evaluated in the PFT lab gave the following results (all in BTPS): $T_B = 38.1°C$; $P_B = 725$ mm Hg; $\dot{V}_{O_2} = 0.282$ L/min; $\dot{V}_{CO_2} = 0.248$ L/min; $\dot{V}_E = 7.84$ L/min; $f = 19$/min; $F_{\bar{E}}CO_2 = 0.032$; $F_aCO_2 = 0.053$. What is her estimated physiological dead space ventilation, $\dot{V}_D$ (L/min, BTPS)?

Solutions to Case Studies and Practice Problems

CASE 8.1 To solve, choose a suitable equation for the available data:

$$\dot{V}_A = \dot{V}_{CO_2}/F_{\bar{E}}CO_2 = (0.255 \text{ L/min})/(0.071)$$
$$\dot{V}_A = 3.59 \text{ L/min (STPD)}$$

To convert the STPD answer to BTPS units, recall from Chap. 1 that:

$$V_2 = (P_1 \cdot V_1 \cdot T_2)/(P_2 \cdot T_1) = (760 \cdot 3.59 \cdot 311.1)/[(720 - 47) \cdot 273]$$
$$\dot{V}_A = 4.62 \text{ L/min (BTPS)}$$

Comment: The $F_{\bar{E}}CO_2$ in this subject is abnormally high, suggesting significant CO_2 retention and predicting a high V_D/V_T.

CASE 8.2 Using the ambient conditions given and Dalton's law, this woman's computed data include $P_IO_2 = 230$ mm Hg, $P_AO_2 = 150$ mm Hg, and $(P_AO_2 - P_aO_2) = 6$ mm Hg. Given this normal $(A - a)$ P_{O_2}, she has no diffusional impairment between alveolar gas and their capillaries (Chap. 9). However she is hypoventilating, indicated by her high P_aCO_2 and wide gap between P_IO_2 and P_AO_2.

Her declining condition and cachexia cannot sustain inspiratory efforts, although her pH_a suggests partial compensation for chronic respiratory acidosis (Chap. 17).

CASE 8.3 To solve for dead space ventilation $\dot{V}_D$, recall that:

$$\dot{V}_E = \dot{V}_D + \dot{V}_A$$
$$\dot{V}_D = \dot{V}_E + \dot{V}_A = (5.46 - 3.77) \text{ L/min} = 1.69 \text{ L/min}$$

To solve for dead space volume, V_D:

$$V_D = \dot{V}_D/f = (1.69 \text{ L/min})/14 = 0.121 \text{ L}$$

Comment: This student's $V_D/V_T = 0.31$, a normal value at rest.

CASE 8.4 To solve, first choose an equation suitable for the available data:

$$V_D/V_T = (P_aCO_2 - P_{\bar{E}}CO_2)/P_aCO_2$$

Note that $P_{\bar{E}}CO_2$ is needed but not given. However, Dalton's law will convert decimal gas fractions like $F_{\bar{E}}CO_2$ to their partial pressures:

$$P_{\bar{E}}CO_2 = F_{\bar{E}}CO_2 \cdot (P_B - P_{H_2O}) = 0.040 \cdot (740 - 47)$$

$$P_{\bar{E}}CO_2 = 28 \text{ mm Hg}$$

Then solve for the dimensionless ratio, V_D/V_T:

$$V_D/V_T = (39 - 28)/39 = 0.28$$

$$V_D = 0.28 \cdot (450 \text{ mL}) = 127 \text{ mL}$$

Comment: This patient appears to be well managed, with these nearly normal values for arterial blood gases (ABGs) and V_D/V_T.

CASE 8.5 To solve, choose the right equation; two in this chapter will eventually yield an estimate of V_D, but one requires ABG data. So choose:

$$\dot{V}_A = \dot{V}CO_2/F_{\bar{E}}CO_2 = (0.248 \text{ L/min})/(0.053)$$
$$\dot{V}_A = 4.68 \text{ L/min}$$

Then use this $\dot{V}_A$ and the given $\dot{V}_E$ to solve for V_D:

$$\dot{V}_D = \dot{V}_E - \dot{V}_A = 7.84 \text{ L/min} - 4.68 \text{ L/min} = 3.16 \text{ L/min}$$

Comment: Only 60% of this patient's V_T reaches her alveoli.

Chapter 9

Alveolar O_2 and CO_2 Exchange, Physiological Shunt, and Acid-Base Balance

ANDREW J. LECHNER, PhD

Learning Objectives

- The student will be able to define the terms governing alveolar O_2 diffusion, and the circumstances when O_2 uptake is limited by perfusion or diffusion.

- The student will be able to calculate the percentage of $\dot{Q}$ comprising physiological shunt by using appropriate patient data and knowledge of HbO_2 interactions in blood.

- The student will be able to summarize processes in CO_2 excretion and the manner by which blood CO_2 acts to maintain normal blood pH.

- The student will be able to use patient data to distinguish among respiratory acidosis, metabolic acidosis, respiratory alkalosis, and metabolic alkalosis.

Introduction to Alveolar Gas Diffusion

Once gases reach the alveolar parenchyma by ventilation, absorption into the blood or excretion from it occurs not by **convection,** but by molecular **diffusion** according to a physiological restatement of Ohm's law (Fig. 9.1). Diffusion of any gas through the septal barrier and into the blood is proportional to the **alveolar epithelial surface area** (S_A) and the **alveolar capillary endothelial surface area** (S_C) comprising the membrane available for such exchange. Quantitative measurements on electron photomicrographs of normal lung have estimated S_A and S_C to each be 50-70 m². This symmetry of S_A and S_C dimensions is perhaps not surprising, given the importance placed earlier on good $\dot{V}_A/\dot{Q}$ matching. Alveolar diffusion of any gas is inversely proportional to septal barrier thickness, estimated as its **harmonic mean** (τ_S) to emphasize statistically the thinnest regions where diffusion is presumably favored.

Given these lung anatomical features that affect all gases, other factors will determine whether diffusional equilibrium is achieved between an alveolar airspace and the blood flowing through its capillaries. Again by analogy to Ohm's law, each gas diffuses proportionally to the pressure gradient between its "source" (P_1, the higher value) and its "sink" (P_2, the lower value). For O_2, $P_1 = P_Ao_2$ (Chap. 8) and $P_2 = P_{\bar{v}}o_2$ as measured by a pulmonary artery catheter, yielding a normal inwardly directed gradient of ~60 mm Hg on room air. That gradient is dramatically affected by both F_Io_2 and P_B insofar as those affect P_Io_2 and thus P_Ao_2. For CO_2, $P_1 = P_{\bar{v}}co_2$, and $P_2 = P_Aco_2$ (= P_aco_2), for a normal outwardly directed gradient of 5-6 mm Hg and one that is less sensitive to F_Io_2 or P_B than that for Po_2. Indeed, data in Table 3.2 were used to make this point earlier of a tenfold larger gradient for O_2 despite that the flow of CO_2 outward and O_2 inward are nearly the same. How can

(#35)

this occur? Gases will diffuse at different rates, despite equal values for S_A, S_C, τ_S, and (P_1-P_2), because of differing **coefficients of diffusivity (D)**, defined as the solubility of a gas in aqueous media divided by its mass-dependent rate of gaseous-free diffusion. The value of D for CO_2 is ~20 times that of O_2 in biological systems, implying that lung disorders will present more often with **hypoxemia** (low blood O_2 content) than with **hypercarbia** (high blood CO_2 content). One can also appreciate that alveolar diffusion of all gases will diminish in a disease like emphysema where S_A and S_C are decreased (Fig. 9.2). Likewise, alveolar diffusion decreases in those diseases for which τ_S is increased, for example during the edema of acute lung injury (Chap. 28) or after the development of fibrosis in some interstitial lung diseases that show a restrictive pattern by pulmonary function test (PFT) (Chap. 24).

Distinguishing Diffusional and Perfusional Limits to Gas Exchange

Given this discussion, what time constraints exist on gas diffusion in the lung? This question can be answered by considering **capillary transit times** of erythrocytes in the lung in relation to the equilibration rate of alveolar gases with the interiors of those red blood cells (RBCs) (Fig. 9.3). An RBC spends ~0.8 seconds in an alveolar capillary at a resting $\dot{Q}$ but less than 0.3 seconds when $\dot{Q}$ approaches maximal values. The long RBC transit time at low $\dot{Q}$ is usually sufficient for N_2O (an anesthetic gas), CO, CO_2, and O_2 to equilibrate across the alveolar-capillary barrier, that is, $P_1 \cong P_2$ for

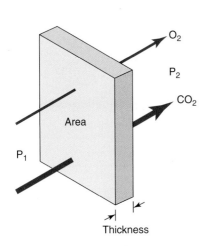

By Ohm's law:

$$V = (P_1 - P_2)/R$$

If conductance = $1/R$ then

$$V = C \cdot (P_1 - P_2)$$

where:

$$C = [D \cdot (S_A + S_C)]/(2 \cdot \tau s)$$

and where:

$$D_{gas\ x} = solubility_x / \sqrt{MW_x}$$

$D_{gas\ x}$ is its

coefficient of diffusivity

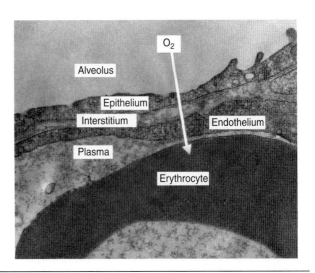

FIGURE 9.1 Alveolar diffusion as described by a physiological version of Ohm's law: Flow = $(P_1 - P_2)/R$, where P_1 and P_2 are the "source" and "sink" gas partial pressures in two adjacent compartments. Conductance (C) is the inverse of resistance R, and thus Flow = $C \cdot (P_1 - P_2)$. C is proportional to the average of all alveolar and capillary surface areas $[(S_A + S_C)/2]$ in the septa available for diffusion, and inversely proportional to the harmonic mean thickness of those septal barriers (τ_s). C is also proportional to Krogh's coefficient of diffusivity (D) for each gas, which is in turn the ratio of its solubility in saline divided by the molecular weight (MW) of each gas.

these gases near the venular end of alveolar capillaries. By example, N_2O is very soluble in blood but does not bind to Hb. Thus, it equilibrates across the barrier regardless of the original $(P_A N_2O - P_c N_2O)$ or transit time, so that its absorption is **perfusion limited** only by $\dot{Q}$. If $\dot{Q}$ increases, then N_2O uptake increases because more RBCs pass through the alveolar capillaries in the same interval of time. In contrast, CO binds to Hb in such large amounts that no RBC spends enough time in an alveolar capillary to equilibrate $P_A CO$ with $P_c CO$. Thus, the absorption of CO is **diffusion limited**, and simply increasing $\dot{Q}$ will not necessarily increase CO uptake. Rather, the alveolar uptake of

CO and other diffusion limited gases will more likely increase if S_A and S_C increase, or if τ_s decreases.

Normally O_2 has an intermediate equilibration rate to those of N_2O or CO. In healthy individuals, O_2 is a perfusion-limited gas over a wide range of $\dot{Q}$ (Fig. 9.3), and at sea level alveolar O_2 uptake usually is not considered to be the rate-limiting step to **maximal O_2 consumption**, $\dot{V}o_{2max}$ (Chap. 12). However, in diseased lungs with destroyed or fibrotic alveolar septa, O_2 becomes diffusion limited during moderate exercise, and potentially at rest despite long RBC transit times. Even in healthy individuals, O_2 becomes a diffusion-limited gas when

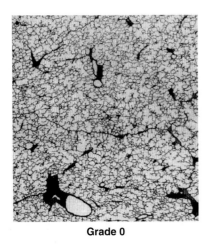
Grade 0

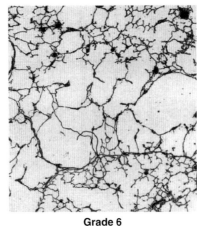
Grade 6

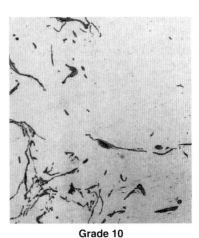
Grade 10

FIGURE 9.2 S_A is a key determinant of diffusion, and any decrease reduces maximal O_2 uptake and CO_2 excretion. Three images of lung tissue (all at the same magnification) are shown with their **Emphysema Severity Scores** assigned by the American Thoracic Society. A score of 0–2 would be normal for urban adults. *From Nagai et al. Am Rev Respir Dis. 1989;139:313-319.*

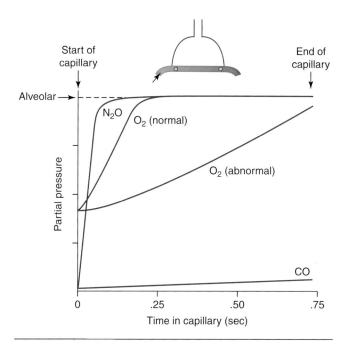

FIGURE 9.3 Equilibration rates of CO, nitrous oxide (N₂O), and O₂ along the alveolar capillary. P_cN_2O equilibrates rapidly with alveolar P_AN_2O, well before the capillary ends, and so N₂O is **perfusion limited**. In contrast, $P_{\bar{c}}CO$ in capillary blood is nearly unchanged during one capillary transit, and thus CO transfer is **diffusion limited**. O₂ transfer into alveolar blood can be perfusion limited or diffusion limited, depending upon conditions. *From West*, Respiratory Physiology; *2005.*

P_AO_2 is reduced by a low F_IO_2 or by the reduced P_B at high altitude (Chap. 13).

Based on its greater aqueous solubility, CO₂ diffuses into and out of tissues ~20 times faster than O₂ per mm Hg of pressure gradient. Consequently, there is usually ample capillary transit time for CO₂ to achieve equilibrium despite its much smaller partial pressure gradient versus O₂. However, under conditions of reduced RBC transit time or with thickening of the alveolar septal membranes, CO₂ transfer may be incomplete and result in hypercarbia.

Estimating Maximal Pulmonary Diffusing Capacity

The long equilibration time of inhaled CO is used clinically to estimate the single-breath **lung diffusing capacity for CO** (**DL$_{CO}$**). As detailed in Chap. 16, this pulmonary function test is most often conducted on patients who are suspected of having reduced S_A or S_C, or increased τ_s. Subjects begin the maneuver at their RV and inhale gas with a low F_ICO (usually ~0.003) up to their TLC. Once at TLC, the breath is held for 10 seconds and then exhaled completely. Concentrations of CO in the exhaled gas are measured to establish $F_{\bar{E}}CO$ and F_ECO (= F_ACO), and thus P_ACO by Dalton's law. These data yield the **CO uptake rate** (**$\dot{V}CO$**) plus the "P_1" from the equation in Fig. 9.1 that drove its absorption. "P_2" in that same equation, being the subject's $P_{\bar{c}}CO$, is considered zero since inhaled CO

never equilibrates with blood in the capillaries. The diffusivity coefficient D_{CO} is constant because the aqueous solubility and mass of CO are known. DL_{CO} is computed then as:

$$\dot{V}CO = C_{CO} \cdot (P_ACO - P_{\bar{c}}CO)$$
$$C_{CO} = \dot{V}CO/(P_ACO - P_{\bar{c}}CO)$$

where carbon monoxide conductance, $C_{CO} = [D_{CO} \cdot (S_A + S_C)]/(2 \cdot \tau_s)$. Thus, the working equation for the DL_{CO} test becomes:

$$(S_A + S_C)]/(2 \cdot \tau_s) = [\dot{V}CO/(P_ACO - P_{\bar{c}}CO)]/D_{CO}$$

Since all terms on the right side of this equation are measured by the single-breath DL_{CO} procedure, the test yields a robust "lump sum" or aggregate estimate of a subject's alveolar and capillary surface areas available for diffusion, as well as their alveolar barrier's thickness as an impediment to that diffusion. The subject's measured value for DL_{CO} then can be compared with expected normative values like other spirometric data to assess the severity of emphysema, edema, interstitial fibrosis, or other disease processes that impact S_A, S_C, or τ_S.

It should be emphasized that despite crossing the alveolar-capillary membrane, O₂ has yet to oxygenate the RBCs. Therefore, the lung's overall diffusing capacity for O₂ consists of two linked components: its membrane diffusing capacity for O₂, DM_O_2 representing the distance from alveolar airspace through the surfactant liquid, tissue, and plasma layers; and its erythrocytic diffusing capacity. As will be described in Chap. 16, this latter component depends on the **blood transfer conductance coefficient for oxygen** (Θ_{O_2}) between Hb and O₂, and on total pulmonary capillary blood volume, V_c. Perhaps surprisingly, the diffusive resistance of the membrane barrier ($1/DM_O_2$) accounts for only about half of overall resistance to O₂ uptake in the lung, with the balance of that resistance being due to the erythrocytes themselves.

Estimating Oxygen Delivery and Physiological Shunt

To this point, the P_{O_2} gradient in the body has encountered only one unavoidable reduction from the inspired P_IO_2, that occurring in conducting airways by Dalton's law, as O₂ is displaced by CO₂ and H₂O vapor. Thus P_AO_2 always is less than P_IO_2. The preceding discussion also implies that if O₂ is a perfusion-limited gas under most conditions, then the $P_{\bar{c}}O_2$ of blood draining alveoli should equal P_AO_2. However, as was seen in Chap. 8, a subject's actual P_aO_2 as reported from blood gas analyses is always at least slightly less than P_AO_2. Indeed, this (A – a) P_{O_2} difference can be quite large in some patients, implying that the higher $P_{\bar{c}}O_2$ of blood draining their alveolar capillaries is diluted downstream with blood with a P_{O_2} nearer to that of mixed venous blood. This **venous admixture**, or contamination of well-oxygenated blood draining the alveoli by less oxygenated blood, comprises the essence of **physiological shunt**.

By analogy to comments regarding anatomical and physiological dead space (Chap. 8), there can exist anatomical and physiological shunts in the pulmonary or systemic circulations. As for dead space, physiological shunt always includes anatomical shunt, that is, blood flow through pulmonary arteries that never enters the respiratory parenchyma to permit alveolar gas exchange. Examples of anatomical shunts include a **patent ductus arteriosus** (**PDA**) and **patent foramen ovale** (**PFO**) that allow systemic venous blood to bypass the lungs entirely (Chap. 7). Importantly, physiological shunt includes that blood flow plus any mixed venous blood that passes through the septal capillaries in the respiratory parenchyma without gaining access to ventilated alveoli. Such physiological shunt was noted earlier in the low $\dot{V}_A/\dot{Q}$ ratios of patients with type B emphysema, as documented with the multiple inert gas technique (Chap. 8). In simplified form, the development of physiological shunt is shown in Fig. 9.4.

A working version of the **shunt equation** can be derived from Fig. 9.4, where $\dot{Q}_T$ equals total cardiac output, and $\dot{Q}_S$ is that portion of $\dot{Q}_T$ being shunted around alveolar capillaries, either anatomically or due to low $\dot{V}_A/\dot{Q}$ ratios. The blood O_2 concentrations needed to solve the shunt equation for $\dot{Q}_S$ include that of blood in alveolar capillaries ($C_{\acute{c}}O_2$) with very high O_2 content, as well as blood in the systemic arteries (C_aO_2) and in the pulmonary artery ($C_{\bar{v}}O_2$). One can report a patient's physiological shunt ($\dot{Q}_S$) either in absolute terms (L/min) or as a percent of $\dot{Q}_T$. Deriving the shunt equation begins with the principle of mass balance for O_2 as expressed in the following equation:

$$\dot{Q}_T \cdot (C_aO_2) = [\dot{Q}_S \cdot (C_{\bar{v}}O_2)] + [(\dot{Q}_T - \dot{Q}_S) \cdot (C_{\acute{c}}O_2)]$$

Rearranging terms and making a sign change so that $\dot{Q}_S/\dot{Q}_T$ is a positive value, yields the working version of the shunt equation that is solvable using a patient's data:

$$\dot{Q}_S/\dot{Q}_T = (C_{\acute{c}}O_2 - C_aO_2)/(C_{\acute{c}}O_2) - (C_{\bar{v}}O_2)$$

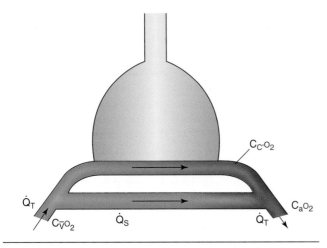

FIGURE 9.4 Measurement of **physiological shunt** $\dot{Q}_S$ assumes that the C_aO_2 of systemic arterial blood reflects the high $C_{\acute{c}}O_2$ of alveolar capillary blood diluted by shunted blood with its lower $C_{\bar{v}}O_2$. *From West*, Respiratory Physiology; *2005*.

In practice, shunt studies are done while subjects are breathing pure oxygen ($F_1O_2 = 1.00$). This minor intervention permits some simplifying assumptions about the amounts of HbO_2 versus dissolved O_2 needed in the calculation of total O_2 contents for each blood compartment. Shunt studies can be done on alert or sedated patients, provided that arterial and venous blood samples are available for determinations of P_aO_2 and $P_{\bar{v}}O_2$, blood [Hb], and **mixed venous % oxygenation or saturation, $S_{\bar{v}}O_2$** (%). The calculated $\dot{Q}_S/\dot{Q}_T$ is generally <10% in most healthy adults, but it may exceed 20% in disease conditions that are characterized by low $\dot{V}_A/\dot{Q}$ ratios as described in Chap. 8. Several examples of shunt calculation problems are included at the end of this chapter.

> ▶▶**CLINICAL CORRELATION 9.1**
>
> Shunt fractions approaching 50% are life-threatening and require aggressive management to restore at least some ventilation to lung regions where $\dot{V}_A/\dot{Q}$ ratios are extremely low. To do so often requires judicious application of mechanical ventilation with **positive end-expiratory pressure, PEEP** that attempts to provide an "air stent" to recruit alveoli that are consolidated into a nearly solid state by edema or are atelectatic due to excessive surface tension recoil (Chaps. 28 and 30).

Role of Alveoli in CO₂ Excretion and Acid-Base Balance

As detailed in Chap. 3, CO_2 is transported in blood as: dissolved CO_2 gas by Henry's law; as HCO_3^- from dissociated H_2CO_3 after CO_2 combines with H_2O (facilitated by carbonic anhydrase, CA); and as $HbCO_2$ from its reversible binding to Hb (Fig. 9.5). Recall that deoxy-Hb is a weaker acid than oxy-Hb and so binds H^+ more readily (the **Haldane effect**), particularly in active tissues where H_2CO_3 formation predominates.

If the relationship is plotted between P_{CO_2} and total [CO_2] in a blood sample at equilibrium, a **CO₂ dissociation curve** is obtained (Fig. 9.6) that is analogous to such graphs for the O_2 content of whole blood (Chap. 3). Because such plots of P_{CO_2} versus [CO_2] include all three forms of CO_2, the resulting curves are not linear, owing to the saturable $HbCO_2$ component and also to the exhaustible supply of donor H^+ from hemoglobin. Due to the Haldane effect, the [CO_2] for deoxygenated blood is higher than for oxygenated blood at all physiological values for P_{CO_2}.

As shown in the inset to Fig. 9.6, the physiological range for CO_2 exchange is normally between $P_aCO_2 = 40$ mm Hg and $P_{\bar{v}}CO_2 = 45$ mm Hg, which yields a net loss of about 5 mL CO_2/dL blood during each passage of blood through the lungs. Note that an essentially equivalent difference of 5 mL O_2/dL blood exists between arterial and venous bloods, although the required difference in P_aO_2 and $P_{\bar{v}}O_2$ is closer to

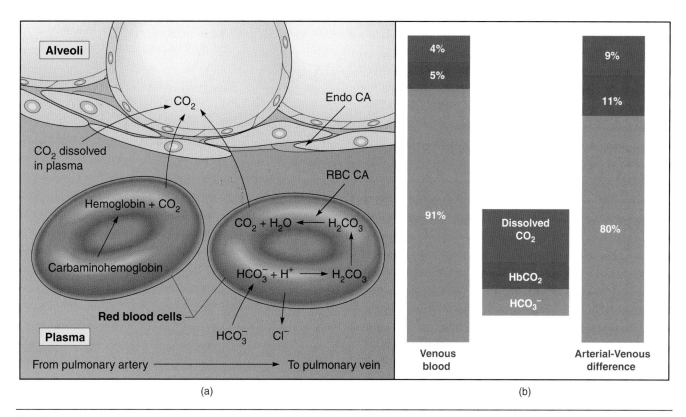

(a)   (b)

FIGURE 9.5 (a) Processes that absorb CO_2 in active tissues are reversed in pulmonary capillaries during excretion of CO_2 from mixed venous blood, even as oxygenation is occurring. Here, the roles of **carbonic anhydrase (CA)** within RBCs and on endothelial cells are emphasized. (b) About 91% of CO_2 in mixed venous blood exists as HCO_3^-, with 5% as $HbCO_2$ and 4% as dissolved CO_2 gas. Only ~7% of CO_2 in venous blood is excreted during one passage through the alveolar capillaries. Of that amount, ~80% is from HCO_3^- and ~9%-10% each from $HbCO_2$ and dissolved CO_2 pools. (a): *From Fox*, Human Physiology, *10th ed. 2008.*

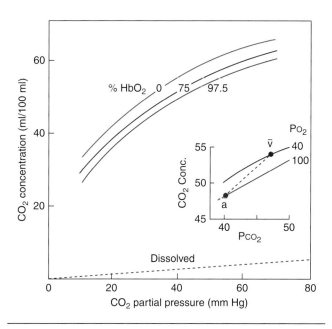

FIGURE 9.6 CO_2 dissociation curves for whole blood at different O_2 saturations. Oxygenated blood carries less CO_2 than deoxygenated blood at the same Pco_2, but both transport far more CO_2 than occurs as dissolved gas. The inset depicts differences between arterial and mixed venous blood. *Modified from West*, Respiratory Physiology; *2005.*

50-60 mm Hg to achieve this same amount of gas exchange, and that is normally occurring on the upper shoulder of the O_2 dissociation curve. The transport and release of CO_2 by the respiratory system have profound effects on the body's pH regulation and acid-base status. The following equation has been presented in the context of CO_2 transport, both for CO_2 uptake in metabolically active tissues, and for CO_2 excretion in the lungs:

$$CO_2 + H_2O \Rightarrow H_2CO_3 \Leftrightarrow H^+ + HCO_3^-$$

The equation as written represents events in the tissues, while the right-to-left direction would describe the reaction in the lungs. Importantly, mass action considerations apply in both directions: increasing the concentration of either substrates or products will shift the equilibrium points accordingly in response to those changed conditions. The equilibrium between the weak acid H_2CO_3 and its dissociated ions, H^+ and HCO_3^-, is described by the dissociation constant K_a:

$$K_a = [H^+] \cdot [HCO_3^-]/[H_2CO_3]$$

Taking logarithms of both sides and then substituting for H_2CO_3 based on Henry's law, yields the **Henderson-Hasselbalch equation** (see Chap. 17 for more detailed steps):

$$pH_a = pK_a + \log [HCO_3^-] - \log [H_2CO_3]$$

$$pH_a = pK_a + \log [HCO_3^-] - \log [(0.03) \cdot (P_aCO_2)]$$

where 0.03 represents the solubility coefficient to convert P_aCO_2 (in mm Hg) at 37°C into H_2CO_3 (in mM). In physiological systems, the value of pK_a for this first dissociation is 6.10 at 37°C, and an arterial pH of 7.40 is normally carefully regulated. Thus:

$$pH_a = 6.10 + \log ([HCO_3^-]/[(0.03) \cdot (P_aCO_2)])$$

$$7.40 = 6.10 + \log ([HCO_3^-]/[(0.03) \cdot (P_aCO_2)])$$

$$1.30 = \log ([HCO_3^-]/[(0.03) \cdot (P_aCO_2)])$$

$$20 = [HCO_3^-]/[(0.03) \cdot (P_aCO_2)]$$

Given a typical $P_aCO_2 = 40$ mm Hg, a normal resting $[HCO_3^-]$ is calculated to be:

$$20 = [HCO_3^-]/[(0.03) \cdot (40)]$$
$$[HCO_3^-] = (20) \cdot (1.2 \text{ mM}) = 24 \text{ mM}$$

Thus, to achieve a stable $pH_a = 7.40$ using the CO_2 buffer system requires maintaining an anion/acid ratio of approximately 20:1. Obviously, this 20:1 ratio can be satisfied by an infinite range of molarities for $[HCO_3^-]$ and $[H_2CO_3]$ (ie, P_aCO_2). Several decades ago it was presumed that all mammals operate at $P_aCO_2 = 40$ mm Hg. However smaller animals often function with a P_aCO_2 of 25-30 mm Hg, and have $[HCO_3^-]$ values that are appropriately lower, in the range of 18-20 mM. Nevertheless, at 37°C all mammals appear to protect a pH_a of ~7.40. Indeed, subsequent investigations confirmed that maintaining pH_a near 7.40 is far more important than is a particular value for total blood CO_2 content. Among healthy adults, total CO_2 is about 25.2 mM (= 24 mM HCO_3^- + 1.2 mM H_2CO_3). However this total can vary widely, such that the measured $[HCO_3^-]$ and total CO_2 content for individuals reflect either acute perturbations to their acid-base balance, or the chronic compensatory responses to such a perturbation (Chap. 17).

With the Henderson–Hasselbalch equation, knowing any two parameters among pH_a, P_aCO_2, and HCO_3^- fixes the third. Some years ago Davenport wrote *The ABC of Acid-Base Chemistry* that popularized the eponymous diagram in Fig. 9.7. It features an abscissa in pH units and an ordinate of $[HCO_3^-]$. Since knowing any pair of pH and $[HCO_3^-]$ values determines P_aCO_2, one can draw a family of PCO_2 **isobars** (lines of equal pressure) whose center point **A** shows that at 37°C, pHa = 7.40 if $P_aCO_2 = 40$ mm Hg and $[HCO_3^-] = 24$ mM. The line **CAB** here is the **CO_2 Blood Buffer Line** and describes the effects on pH and $[HCO_3^-]$ of blood titrated with acid in the form of H_2CO_3 and thus P_aCO_2. A similar **CO_2 Plasma Buffer Line** would have a shallower slope since plasma contains fewer proteins and is thus a weaker buffer than whole blood.

There are four principal ways to perturb acid-base homeostasis within the CO_2-based buffer system, namely raising or lowering either P_aCO_2 or $[HCO_3^-]$. Compensation usually involves altering the previously stable of the two

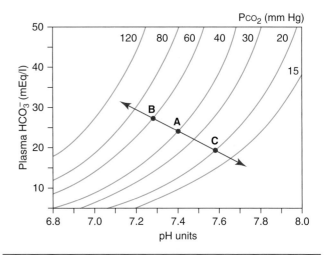

FIGURE 9.7 A Davenport diagram showing the basic relationships among blood HCO_3^-, pH_a, and P_aCO_2. Point **A** represents the normal values for healthy subjects at rest and with $P_aCO_2 = 40$ mm Hg; the center line **BAC** illustrates the normal buffering capacity for whole blood. *Modified from West,* Respiratory Physiology; *2005.*

(Fig. 9.8). Point **A** here and in Fig. 9.7 represents the normal, ideal balance among pH_a, P_aCO_2, and $[HCO_3^-]$. If P_aCO_2 abruptly increases toward a higher CO_2 isobar, this acute change in acid-base status to point **B** is termed **respiratory acidosis**. In the uncompensated phase of this response, P_aCO_2 is too high, pH_a is too low, and blood $[HCO_3^-]$ has not increased enough to reestablish a 20:1 ratio between $[HCO_3^-]$ and $[H_2CO_3]$. Remembering that homeostatic mechanisms will first and foremost attempt to restore a normal pH_a, one can easily predict the appropriate response. Since respiratory impairment already exists (P_aCO_2 is elevated), the appropriate compensation is to move along this new P_aCO_2 isobar toward point **D** by retaining $[HCO_3^-]$ in the kidneys and thereby regain a 20:1 ratio. Note that the uncompensated acidosis at point **B** does cause a slight increase in $[HCO_3^-]$ by simple mass action. However, this effect is not sufficient to correct the acidosis unless P_aCO_2 is allowed to increase very slowly from 40 to 60 mm Hg.

Acute respiratory acidosis may begin with food aspiration, heart attack, drug overdose, pneumothorax, head injury affecting ventilatory drive, etc. Chronic acidosis with some compensation via renal HCO_3^- retention is common with $\dot{V}_A/\dot{Q}$ abnormalities due to obstructive disease. As the term implies, respiratory acidosis is mainly a lung disorder, whether it is acute and uncompensated, or chronic and partially or fully compensated.

In the opposite direction, an individual may abruptly increase $\dot{V}_A$, causing P_aCO_2 to fall below 40 mm Hg. Such **respiratory alkalosis** is most often due to hyperventilation during pain or anxiety (or accidentally during mechanical ventilation), or as a direct result of exposure to environmental hypoxia, as occurs at high altitude. In Fig. 9.8, respiratory alkalosis is seen acutely as moving from point **A** to point **C** toward a

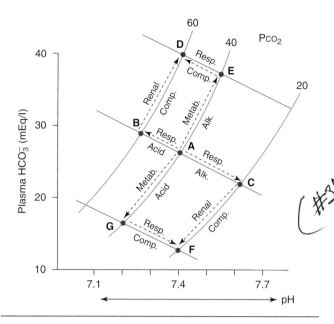

FIGURE 9.8   An expanded view of the physiological ranges encountered clinically for plasma HCO_3^-, pH_a, and P_aCO_2. Point **A** illustrates typical normal values at rest. The several paths to respiratory and metabolic disturbances are shown, and the typical compensatory responses to reestablish pH_a. *Modified from West,* Respiratory Physiology; *2005.*

lower P_aCO_2 isobar. Again in attempting to reestablish pH_a = 7.40, compensation will occur toward point **F** by promoting renal excretion of HCO_3^-. Again, such a respiratory disturbance could maintain the 20:1 ratio of $[HCO_3^-]/[H_2CO_3]$ if it occurred slowly, since HCO_3^- is eventually converted to H_2CO_3 by mass action. For example, ascent to altitude can be staged slowly enough to minimize such alkalotic increases in pH_a.

Numerous nonrespiratory diseases can affect pH_a, and their onset may be either acute or more chronic than respiratory acidosis and alkalosis. Excessive ingestion of antacids or prolonged vomiting can induce **metabolic alkalosis,** shown in Fig. 9.8 as moving from point **A** to point **E** along a constant P_aCO_2 isobar. Respiratory compensation occurs toward point **D** in the form of hypoventilation, again to restore the 20:1 ratio between anion and acid. This compensation increases total blood CO_2 content above that caused by the excessive $[HCO_3^-]$ in the acute, uncompensated phase. Assuming patients survive any immediate crisis caused by this elevated pH_a, their hypoventilation can be reversed later to excrete the additional CO_2 content that compensation induced.

Metabolic acidosis is a serious perturbation caused primarily by the excessive production of organic acids that overwhelm the body's supply of $[HCO_3^-]$. Diabetic ketoacidosis, septic shock, aspirin overdose, renal failure, and diarrhea are common causes. By observing movement from point **A** to point **G** in Fig. 9.8, the life-threatening nature of metabolic acidosis is apparent. Respiratory compensation from point **G** to point **F** requires lowering blood CO_2 content via hyperventilation, which consumes additional $[HCO_3^-]$. Thus, the 20:1 ratio for $[HCO_3^-]/[H_2CO_3]$ is restored in such a manner that if the underlying cause of acid generation is not corrected, blood $[HCO_3^-]$ stores are depleted, and irreversible acidosis and death ensue.

The numerous clinical variations of these acid-base disorders will be more extensively reviewed in Chap. 17, in the form of patient scenarios and their solutions.

▶▶ **CLINICAL CORRELATION 9.2**

Why is arriving at point **F** in Fig. 9.8 via point **G** more dangerous than getting to point **F** via point **C**, as occurs in respiratory alkalosis? The answer relates to the causes that lead to lost pH equilibrium. The hyperventilation of uncompensated respiratory alkalosis is more easily corrected (by descending from altitude or reducing anxiety with sedation) than is the ketoacidosis of diabetes or the ischemia and lactate acidemia of septic shock.

Suggested Readings

1. Davenport HW. *The ABC of Acid-Base Chemistry*, 6th ed. Chicago, IL: University of Chicago Press; 1974. *Many have tried and most have failed to teach as much about the fundamentals of acid-base balance in the lung as this author, whose contribution to the field continue in the diagrams bearing his name.*

2. Scheid P, Piiper J. Diffusion. In: Crystal RG & West JB, eds. *The Lung: Scientific Foundations.*. New York, NY: Raven Press; 1991. *Working predominantly at the Max Planck Institute in Gottingen, Germany, Drs. Piiper and Scheid pushed the experimental and mathematical boundaries of gas exchange to unprecedented heights, while influencing innumerable physiologists and clinicians with their insights and personalities.*

CASE STUDIES AND PRACTICE PROBLEMS

CASE 9.1 A 57-year-old female ICU patient with $T_B = 37°C$, $R = 1.0$, and $[Hb] = 16.0$ g/dL is ventilated with pure O_2 for 5 minutes at a $P_B = 750$ mm Hg before blood gas analyses show: $P_aO_2 = 400$ mm Hg, $P_aCO_2 = 40$ mm Hg, $P_{\bar{v}}O_2 = 85$ mm Hg, $S_aO_2 = 100\%$, $S_{\bar{v}}O_2 = 80\%$, and metHb = 3%. Is her physiological shunt fraction, $\dot{Q}_S/\dot{Q}_T$ (%) normal?

CASE 9.2 A 32-year-old male smoker breathes 100% O_2 at $P_B = 705$ mm Hg for 5 minutes before arterial and venous samples are drawn. Lab results indicate: $[Hb] = 15.5$ g/dL, metHb = 10%, $P_aO_2 = 390$ mm Hg, $P_aCO_2 = 52$ mm Hg, $P_{\bar{v}}O_2 = 68$ mm Hg, and $S_{\bar{v}}O_2 = 76\%$. Assuming $T_B = 37°C$, $\dot{Q} = 5.40$ L/min (by Swan-Ganz thermodilution catheter), $R = 0.80$, and 1.39 mL O_2/g Hb, what is his physiological shunt (L/min)?

CASE 9.3 A 38-year-old man is brought to the ER after being found near his home and apparently unable to stand upright. Physical examination reveals lethargy and mid-epigastric abdominal tenderness; skin turgor is poor and his mucous membranes are dry. Blood pressure is 85/60 mmHg while supine. Laboratory studies indicate serum $[Na^+] = 143$ mM, $[K^+] = 3.2$ mM, $[Cl^-] = 101$ mM, and total $[CO_2] = 11$ mM; arterial blood gases while on room air are $P_aO_2 = 80$ mm Hg, $P_aCO_2 = 23$ mm Hg, and $pH_a = 7.28$. Which of the following best describes his current acid-base status?

a. Uncompensated metabolic acidosis

b. Acute metabolic alkalosis

c. Chronic respiratory acidosis

d. Mixed respiratory acidosis and metabolic alkalosis

CASE 9.4 A 27-year-old woman with acute respiratory failure is ventilated with 100% O_2 ($P_B = 750$ mm Hg $T_B = 37°C$) for 5 minutes before arterial and venous samples are drawn. Lab results indicate: $[Hb] = 13.0$ g/dL, metHb = 0%, $P_aO_2 = 330$ mm Hg, $P_aCO_2 = 59$ mm Hg, $P_{\bar{v}}O_2 = 80$ mm Hg, and $S_{\bar{v}}O_2 = 90\%$. Assuming $\dot{Q} = 4.10$ L/min, $R = 0.90$, and 1.39 mL O_2/g Hb, what is her physiological shunt (L/min)?

CASE 9.5 A 14-year-old girl is taken to the emergency room by her teacher after the student succumbs to sulfuric acid fumes released by an accident in chemistry class. The student is unconscious but normothermic, and her respirations are shallow and rapid. She is immediately intubated and ventilated with room air while an initial arterial blood gas is obtained. Several minutes later, the laboratory reports the following: $pH_a = 7.30$, $P_aO_2 = 54$ mm Hg, $P_aCO_2 = 32$ mm Hg, $[HCO_3^-] = 15.2$ mM. Assuming a barometric pressure of 760 mm Hg and a respiratory quotient of 0.80, what is the $(A - a)$ Po_2 difference in this patient? What interventions might be useful in her emergent state?

Solutions to Case Studies and Practice Problems

CASE 9.1 *Recall the shunt equation:*

$$\dot{Q}_S/\dot{Q}_T = (C_{\acute{c}}O_2 - C_aO_2)/(C_{\acute{c}}O_2 - C_{\bar{v}}O_2)$$

Step 1. Compute $C_{\acute{c}}O_2$ using HbO_2 binding coefficient and Henry's law:

Hb-bound O_2 = (16.0 g Hb/dL) · (1.39 mL O_2/g Hb)
· (100%-3%)*
Hb-bound O_2 = 21.57 mL O_2/dL

(**accounts for presence of 3% metHb that does not bind O_2*)

Dissolved O_2 = (0.003 mL O_2/dL/mm Hg) · (750 – 47 – 40)†
Dissolved O_2 = 1.99 mL O_2/dL

(*use alveolar gas equation to solve for P_AO_2, which = $P_{\acute{c}}O_2$*)

Total $C_{\acute{c}}O_2$ = 21.57 + 1.99 = 23.56 mL O_2/dL

Step 2. Compute C_aO_2 for this patient, using P_aO_2 when needed:

Hb-bound O_2 = 21.57 mL O_2/dL *(same as for $C_{\acute{c}}O_2$)*
Dissolved O_2 = (0.003 mL O_2/dL/mm Hg) · (400)
= 1.20 mL O_2/dL

Total C_aO_2 = 21.57 + 1.20 = 22.77 mL O_2/dL

Step 3. Compute $C_{\bar{v}}O_2$ for this patient, using $P_{\bar{v}}O_2$ and $S_{\bar{v}}O_2$ when needed:

Hb-bound O_2 = (21.57 mL O_2/dL) · (0.80)   *(0.80 = venous oxygenation)*
Hb-bound O_2 = 17.26 mL O_2/dL

Dissolved O_2 = (0.003 mL O_2/dL/mm Hg) · (85) = 0.26 mL O_2/dL
Total $C_{\bar{v}}O_2$ = 17.26 + 0.26 = 17.52 mL O_2/dL

Step 4. Calculate the patient's shunt fraction:

$$\dot{Q}_S/\dot{Q}_T = (23.56 - 22.77)/(23.56 - 17.52)$$
$$\dot{Q}_S/\dot{Q}_T = 0.79/6.04 = 13\% \text{ (value is slightly above normal)}$$

CASE 9.2 *Step 1. Compute $C_{\acute{c}}O_2$, remembering to correct for 10% metHb:*

Hb-bound O_2 = (15.5) · (1.39) · (0.9) = 19.39 mL O_2/dL
Dissolved O_2 = (0.003) · [705 – 47 – (52/0.8)] = 1.78 mL O_2/dL
Total $C_{\acute{c}}O_2$ = 19.39 + 1.78 = 21.17 mL O_2/dL

Step 2. Compute C_aO_2, using P_aO_2 as given:

Hb-bound O_2 = 19.39 mL O_2/dL *(same as $C_{\acute{c}}O_2$)*
Dissolved O_2 = (0.003) · (390) = 1.17 mL O_2/dL
Total C_aO_2 = 20.56 mL O_2/dL

Step 3. Compute $C_{\bar{v}}O_2$, using $P_{\bar{v}}O_2$ and $S_{\bar{v}}O_2$ as given:

Hb-bound O_2 = (19.39) · (0.76) = 14.74 mL O_2/dL
Dissolved O_2 = (0.003) · (68) = 0.20 mL O_2/dL
Total $C_{\bar{v}}O_2$ = 14.94 mL O_2/dL

Step 4. Calculate the patient's shunt (in L/min):

$$\dot{Q}_S/\dot{Q}_T = (21.17 - 20.56)/(21.17 - 14.94) = 0.61/6.23 = 9.8\%$$
$$\dot{Q}_S = (5.40) · (0.098) = 0.53 \text{ L/min}$$

Comment: Considering the high [metHb], this percent shunt is within the normal range.

CASE 9.3 The most correct answer is a.

The patient's arterial pH of 7.28 is clearly not alkalotic (*answer b*), and his P$_a$CO$_2$ of 23 mm Hg is inconsistent with a respiratory cause for the reduced pH, either acute or chronic (*answers c, d*). The total [CO$_2$] of just 11 mM (normal range = 22-26) supports a metabolic cause of distress, perhaps a perforated ulcer or ruptured appendix that has initiated peritonitis. Given his low blood pressure and pallor, one cannot rule out septic shock at this point (Chap. 28).

CASE 9.4 *Using the same steps as in Cases 9.1 and 9.2, calculate that:*

For C$_{\bar{c}}$O$_2$: HbO$_2$ = (13.0) · (1.39) · (1.00) = 18.07 mL O$_2$/dL

Dissolved O$_2$ = (0.003) · [750 − 47 − (59/0.9)] = 1.91 mL O$_2$/dL

Total C$_{\bar{c}}$O$_2$ = 18.07 + 1.91 = 19.98 mL O$_2$/dL

For C$_a$O$_2$: HbO$_2$ = 18.07 mL O$_2$/dL *(same as C$_{\bar{c}}$O$_2$)*

Dissolved O$_2$ = (0.003) · (330) = 0.99 mL O$_2$/dL

Total C$_a$O$_2$ = 19.06 mL O$_2$/dL

For C$_{\bar{v}}$O$_2$: HbO$_2$ = (18.07) · (0.90) = 16.26 mL O$_2$/dL

Dissolved O$_2$ = (0.003) · (80) = 0.24 mL O$_2$/dL

Total C$_{\bar{v}}$O$_2$ = 16.50 mL O$_2$/dL

and thus: $\dot{Q}_S/\dot{Q}_T$ = (19.98 − 19.06)/(19.98 − 16.50)

= 0.92/3.48 = 26.4%

$\dot{Q}_S$ = (4.10) · (0.264) = 1.08 L/min

Comment: Concerns that this patient has ARDS are warranted, as her large shunt fraction demonstrates. Clinically, at least one fourth of her right ventricular cardiac output is perfusing alveolar units with $\dot{V}_A/\dot{Q}$ <0.01 (Chap. 8).

CASE 9.5 Using the ambient conditions and Dalton's law, the girl's computed data include P$_I$O$_2$ = 149 mm Hg, P$_A$O$_2$ = 109 mm Hg, and (P$_A$O$_2$ − P$_a$O$_2$) = 55 mm Hg. This very abnormal gradient (see Case 8.2, Chap. 8) indicates significant diffusional impairment and physiological shunt. As this case illustrates, inhaled acid fumes are a potent inducer of **acute lung injury, ALI** (Chap. 28), and the patient needs supplemental O$_2$ to raise her F$_I$O$_2$ and P$_A$O$_2$ plus ventilation with positive end-expiratory pressure (PEEP) to recruit edematous and atelectatic alveoli (Chap. 30).

Chapter 10

Airway and Parenchymal Defense Mechanisms

ANDREW J. LECHNER, PhD AND
GEORGE M. MATUSCHAK, MD

Learning Objectives

- The student will be able to define the general contributions of airway design, receptors, reflexes, and secretions in lung defense against microbes and other respiratory particulates.

- The student will be able to explain how impaction, sedimentation, Brownian motion, and mucociliary transport act to clear inhaled particles of various sizes.

- The student will be able to identify key leukocytes of airways and parenchyma, their roles in recognizing pathogens in proximal and distal airspaces, and their secretions of cytokines, chemokines, and other host defense molecules.

Introduction

Ventilation of the lung requires the daily inhalation of many thousands of liters of ambient air (Chap. 4), none of which can be presumed to be free of suspended microbes, inorganic particulates, organic fumes, or other noxious gases. Nevertheless, the delicate alveolar parenchyma remains remarkably intact and sterile in most individuals, unless **airway defense mechanisms** are disturbed. Those mechanisms include physical processes such as sedimentation, as well as biological barriers composed of resident leukocytes that begin in the nares and extend in various forms to, and even through the septal barrier.

Nasal Cavity and Sinus Defense Mechanisms

As described in Chap. 2, the nasal cavities are lined with **vibrissae** that are interspersed over the distal nasal turbinates, starting at the keratinized epithelial layers that exist inside the nares even before transition to the ciliated respiratory epithelium (Fig. 10.1). With their large size and scattered spacing, these hairs are sufficiently strong to ensnare larger objects that might be inhaled accidentally, such as small insects and large particles of ash. Tactile stimulation of these hairs is often sufficient to induce sneeze, cough, or glandular secretions that collectively act to consolidate and expel such foreign materials. However, they filter few objects that are smaller than the size that can be resolved with the unassisted human eye (~100 µm).

Less obvious are the delicate sensory nerve endings also present throughout the upper nasal passages. Collectively, these afferent fibers serve as **irritant receptors** capable of responding to both physical deformations, such as inhalation of a gnat, and physico-chemical stimuli like smoke, mineral dust, cold air, capsaicin, and ammonia vapors. Several classes of receptors present in this region send myelinated or unmyelinated fibers to the CNS via the vagus, trigeminal, and perhaps other cranial nerves. Additional details are presented in Chap. 11 about their sensitivity thresholds and their relative rapidity of adaptations to continued stimulation. Activating these receptors can induce bronchoconstriction, coughs, or sneezes that physically propel foreign debris out of the nasal passages. Receptor activation also stimulates serous or mucous glandular secretions, hypo- or hyperventilation, **apnea**, and potentially a full **diving reflex** that is particularly prominent in newborn infants and very young children (Chap. 39).

This combination of invoked responses in the nasal cavities to foreign objects or noxious stimuli is typical of reflexes that are present throughout the respiratory system. Virtually every child and adult has experienced the consequences of these responses, such as watery eyes, seasonal rhinitis, sinus congestion, and even emesis that may occur within minutes or hours of exposure to pollen, sawdust, animal dander, and foul odors. Interestingly, natural or pathological variations in the size and patency of the nasal vestibules will make individuals more or less susceptible to these stimuli. For example, deviations in the nasal turbinates or altered sinus drainage can confound the abilities of these defensive reactions to clear the offending stimuli, or drain the secretions they induce. Likewise, there is enormous range in innate or acquired responsiveness among otherwise healthy adults to the **antigenicity** of certain biological materials such as tree pollens, soil microbes, cats and other pets, or insect feces (see Chap. 21).

Defense Mechanisms of the Oropharynx and Upper Airways

Air streams inhaled through the nose or mouth eventually converge in the oropharynx. This makes the ventrolateral location there of the **tonsils** particularly important, often providing the

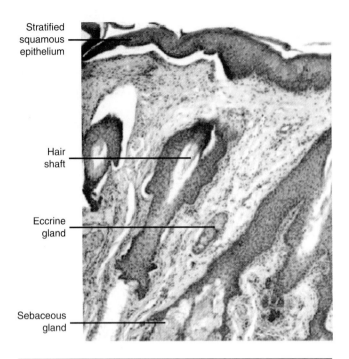

FIGURE 10.1 As presented in Chap. 2, nasal vestibules contain vibrissal hair follicles interspersed among eccrine and sebaceous glands that originate in the dermis and beneath the stratified squamous epithelium. The vestibule is keratinized distally but not proximally.

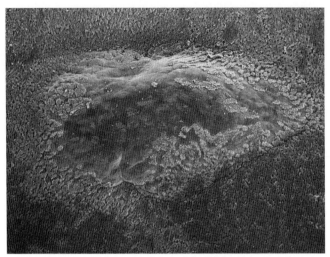

FIGURE 10.2 Scanning electron microscopic (SEM) view of the domed surface of a subepidermal lymphoid nodule, here surrounded by stratified squamous epithelium. Such foci are typical of respiratory **MALT**. *Souma T:* The distribution and surface ultrastructure of airway epithelial cells in the rat lung: a scanning electron microscopic study, Arch Histol Japon Oct; *50(4):419-436, 1987.*

respiratory system a first opportunity to commence **innate immunity** or the transition to **adaptive immunity**. These large, bilateral depots of predominantly lymphoid cells are ideally situated to sample all inspired gases. The tonsils are also continuously exposed to the mixture of normal mouth flora, exogenous microbes, and even refluxed gastrointestinal fluids that bathe the oropharyngeal surfaces. Less conspicuous than the tonsils are the lymphoid aggregates of variable sizes scattered in the lamina propria beneath the oropharyngeal epithelium and along the proximal and some distal airways (Fig. 10.2). These lymphoid aggregates were introduced in Chap. 2 as the **mucosa-associated lymphoid tissues** (**MALT**).

▶▶ CLINICAL CORRELATION 10.1

The importance of such lymphoid tissues in normal host defense can be illustrated by the example in AIDS patients. Particularly in the early days of the epidemic, virtually all HIV-infected individuals developed **oral thrush** from oropharyngeal colonization with *Candida albicans*, due to their impaired mucosal immunity. A much smaller percentage of these AIDS patients ever developed fungal pneumonia, candidemia, or disseminated candidiasis unless they also developed **neutropenia** for another reason. The pivotal role of **polymorphonuclear neutrophils** (**PMNs**) in maintaining sterility of the lung parenchyma is discussed in more detail below.

Inhaled gas or oropharyngeal aspirates that traverse the epiglottis at the larynx and enter the trachea encounter a more elaborate and comprehensive array of host defense barriers. In conventional terms, these include purely physical processes like **impaction** and **sedimentation**, as well as cell-mediated **mucociliary clearance**, **phagocytosis**, and **antigen presentation**. Each of these is summarized here in turn.

Impaction reflects the tendency for particles suspended in flight to remain on linear trajectories until an obstacle is encountered. Not surprisingly, the constantly bifurcating airways present such a barrier to deep lung penetration by larger airborne objects that are being inspired at relatively high velocities. Such inhaled particles collide with the apposing airway wall of each Y-shaped branch point, becoming entrapped there in the mucus layer that lines these airways (Fig. 10.3). Modeling studies and experimental evidence suggest that impaction is particularly effective at clearing inhaled particles >5 μm diameter. The subsequent fate of impacted particles is discussed below.

Smaller airborne particles (alive or inert) tend to remain suspended during rapid flight, despite the obstacles posed by approaching airway walls. However, these particles still have mass and respond to the effects of gravity, particularly as air speed diminishes with deeper penetrations into the conducting airways. For particles with diameters of 0.5-5 μm, **sedimentation** is an important clearance mechanism that resembles the way in which fine suspended particulates settle out of slowly moving water (Fig. 10.3). Once smaller particles sediment out and become entrapped in mucus, they also are expelled from the lungs so that the alveolar parenchyma is spared their effects.

Particles <0.5 μm in diameter are not effectively cleared by impaction or sedimentation. However, many of these become

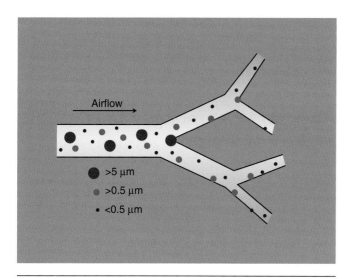

FIGURE 10.3 Clearance of airborne particles from inhaled air by impaction (red circles) and sedimentation (green circles). Very small particles (purple circles) may be cleared by collisions with airway walls, due to their random Brownian motion. These combined effects essentially sterilize inspired gas by the time it reaches the respiratory bronchioles.

embedded in epithelial mucus by random **Brownian motion** (termed "diffusion" by some authors), notably as airspeed slows even more due to the high resistance to flow in the smallest bronchioles. The net effects of impaction, sedimentation, and such random Brownian collisions are to sterilize the inhaled air of most objects down to the size of bacteria well before this gas enters respiratory bronchioles. Nevertheless viruses, aerosolized molecules like bacterial endotoxins, and organic vapors may persist within the inspired airstream that challenge respiratory system defensive functions within the alveolar parenchyma.

The consequences of these defensive processes can be dramatic. A commonly cited "clinical pearl" is that a pneumothorax caused by rupture of the visceral pleura covering the lungs creates a sterile wound. This is because the ambient air that entered the intrapleural space first passed through distal airways like respiratory bronchioles. Examples include spontaneous pneumothoraces that occur due to the rupture of a **congenital emphysematous bulla** (Chap. 37) or result from using excessive positive airway pressures during **mechanical ventilation** (Chaps. 28 and 30).

Mucociliary Clearance in the Proximal and Distal Airways

Most inhaled particulates become embedded in mucus secreted by respiratory mucosa. However, adhesion does not in itself protect the lung until this hazardous material is degraded or expelled. A second cleansing process depends upon the ciliated pseudo-stratified epithelium (Fig. 10.4), by which mucus-entrapped material is expelled by the synchronized and retrograde movement of cilia. The importance of ciliary function to host defense is underscored by the autosomal recessive disorder of **primary ciliary dyskinesia (immotile-cilia syndrome)** found in one of 10,000-30,000 persons. Subjects with impaired mucociliary clearance are prone to chronic cough, rhinosinusitis, and recurrent infections of the lower respiratory tract culminating in abnormal bronchial inflammatory dilatation termed **bronchiectasis**. Even under normal conditions, the viscosity of normal mucus makes ciliary expulsion challenging, if

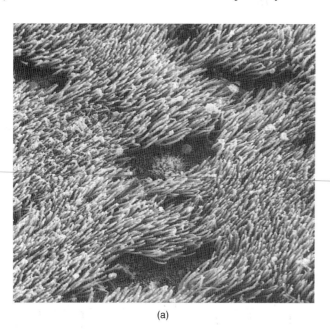 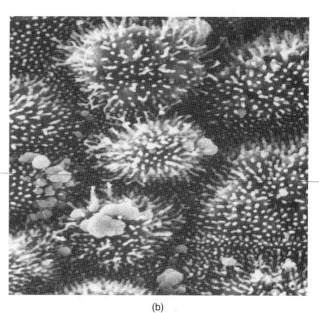

(a) (b)

FIGURE 10.4 In the trachea and upper airways, contiguous regions of ciliated cells (a) are intermingled with patches of goblet cells (b) that produce uninterrupted sheets of secreted mucus. Under normal conditions, these sheets of mucus are propelled by the cilia in a retrograde direction through the larynx to be expectorated or swallowed. *Souma T*: The distribution and surface ultrastructure of airway epithelial cells in the rat lung: a scanning electron microscopic study, Arch Histol Japon Oct; *50(4):419-436, 1987*.

not for the tearlike serous secretions of other epithelial cells creating an aqueous or "sol" phase beneath the mucus. As will be discussed in Chap. 38, the inability to secrete this serous subphase results in the tenacious, airway-plugging mucus of patients with **cystic fibrosis (CF)**.

As described in Chap. 2, the height and complexity of the respiratory mucosa decrease as airway branching forms progressively smaller bronchioles (Fig. 10.5). As this transition occurs, epithelial cells shorten and their cilia also become reduced in length and numbers. By the level of the deepest bronchioles and terminal bronchioles, ciliated cells are rare, seemingly replaced by shorter pear-shaped **brush cells**, each with a tuft of 120-140 nonmotile microvilli on its narrowed apex (Fig. 10.6). Little is known about the function of brush cells, despite their intriguing appearance and consistent presence in the smaller bronchioles of all mammalian lungs examined to date. Some experts favor the view that they function as chemosensory or sentinel cells, but further investigation is needed to provide a definitive answer.

At about the same airway depth, goblet cells become less numerous and are eventually replaced by apically domed **Clara cells** that appear to have multiple phenotypes and functions (Fig. 10.6). Many Clara cells are involved in production of **Clara cell secretory protein** and lysozyme; together these proteins comprise a major part of bronchiolar lining fluid. Clara cells also synthesize and recycle surfactant-associated proteins A and D, whose carbohydrate recognition domains bind to bacteria or viruses to promote phagocytosis by alveolar macrophages (see below). Some subsets of Clara cells are critical to host detoxification of inhaled xenobiotics like **lipopolysaccharide (LPS) endotoxin** through their unique **cytochrome P-450 mono-oxygenase, CYP4B1**. Clara cells also play poorly defined roles in innate immunity and cytokine production.

Alveolar Macrophages and Defense of the Respiratory Parenchyma

To this point, discussion of lung defensive strategies has emphasized physical processes like impaction and the roles of fixed or sedentary cell populations in creating or propelling airway lining liquids. However, the lungs contain one of the largest depots of tissue-based mononuclear phagocytes. These include **alveolar macrophages** that can be found patrolling the lumens of airways, inspecting the alveolar surfaces, migrating through septal interstitia, and adhering to the walls of blood and lymphatic vessels (Fig. 10.7). Some scientists divide these lung cells into specific subpopulations based upon their intrapulmonary locations. In any case, they appear phenotypically similar: large, aggressive, and highly mobile phagocytes that probably are a self-replicating population within the lung.

Alveolar macrophages function as initiators of inflammation and innate immunity by their abilities as professional phagocytes. Through their secretion of key proinflammatory cytokines including TNF-α, IL-1β, and IL-8, these macrophages also initiate the recruitment and activation of additional leukocytes to the lung. Such recruited cells include circulating monocytes and polymorphonuclear neutrophils (PMNs) that

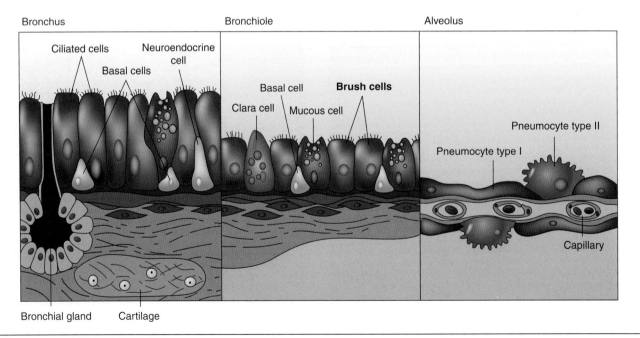

FIGURE 10.5 With decreasing airway diameter, the respiratory mucosa becomes thinner and less elaborate, although it retains the ability to produce and expel sheets of mucus. In particular, ciliated cells give way to brush cells with apical microvilli and Clara cells that secrete mucus but appear to have additional immunomodulatory roles.

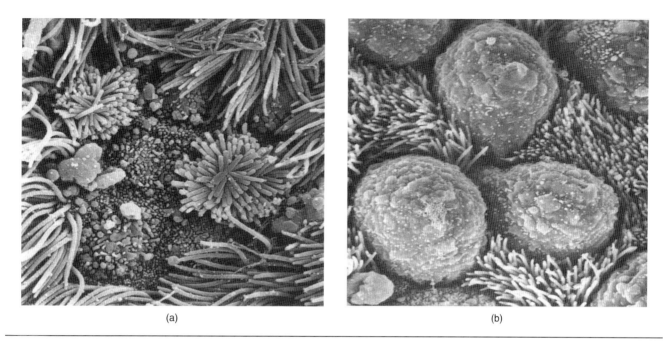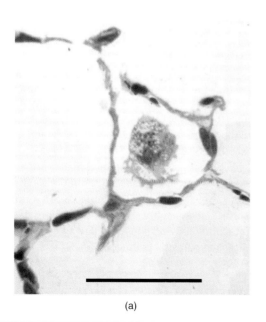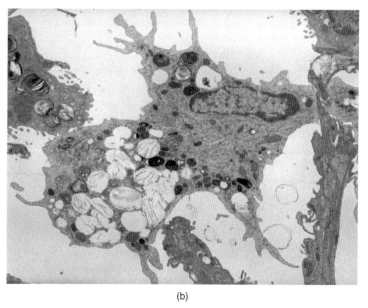

(a)

(b)

FIGURE 10.6 By the level of the smallest bronchioles and terminal bronchioles, the epithelium of the respiratory mucosa consists of: cuboidal brush cells with apical microvilli (a), interspersed with squamous epithelial cells that become more numerous by the level of respiratory bronchioles; and Clara cells that have prominent apical domes suggestive of their prominent secretory capacity (b). *Souma T:* The distribution and surface ultrastructure of airway epithelial cells in the rat lung: a scanning electron microscopic study, Arch Histol Japon Oct; *50(4):419-436, 1987.*

respond to chemotactic gradients by migrating from the blood through tissue barriers into the airspaces (Fig. 10.8).

Lung macrophage functions have been studied extensively since the development of **diagnostic bronchoscopy** as performed clinically using flexible bronchoscopes. During such a procedure, a small volume (100-150 mL) of sterile saline is sequentially instilled and then withdrawn yielding a suitable sample of **bronchoalveolar lavage fluid** (**BALF**) that represents alveolar epithelial cell lining fluid (Chap. 18). The BALF recovered from patients with pneumonia differs strikingly in its cell counts and cytokine concentrations versus fluid lavaged from healthy subjects.

(a)

(b)

FIGURE 10.7 Macrophages can occur virtually anywhere within airways, blood vessels, the adventitia of their walls, and within alveolar septa and the airspaces above them. Shown here are two examples; note their enormous size, highly ruffled borders and numerous phagocytic inclusions. (a) A macrophage nearly fills the entire alveolar airspace (thin plastic section, toluidine blue stain; bar = 100 μm). (b) An alveolar macrophage passing through a pore of Kohn bordered by the surfactant-secreting type 2 cell at center left and a squamous type 1 cell at bottom right.

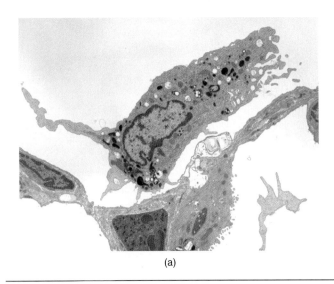

(a)

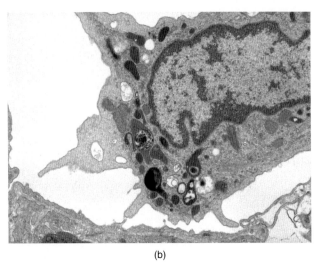

(b)

FIGURE 10.8 Lungs of a rat experimentally infected intratracheally with *Yersinia pestis* illustrate the pivotal role of alveolar macrophages in lung host defense. (a) Within 30 minutes of instilling live bacteria into the trachea, a macrophage internalized several into prominent vacuoles. Its rapid synthesis and release of TNF-α and CINC-1 (rat homolog of IL-8) recruit circulating PMNs like the one identifiable by its multilobed nucleus in an alveolar capillary at center bottom. Within 90 minutes, PMNs (mean diameter ~12 μm) leave blood vessels and enter airspaces by margination and diapedesis. (b) Higher magnification of the macrophage's phagocytic vacuoles and points of contact with the underlying septal wall.

Role of Surfactant-Associated Proteins in Defense of the Parenchyma

Epithelial type 2 cells and bronchiolar Clara cells constitutively express surfactant-associated proteins SP-A and SP-D within the distal airways. Both are pattern-recognition molecules of the collectin (collagenous Ca^{2+}-dependent lectins) family that opsonize pathogens with their C-terminal carbohydrate recognition domains (**CRD**). Thus, SP-A and SP-D are thought to be the lung's innate immune equivalents of multivalent IgG and IgM antibodies of adaptive immunity. SP-A monomers (~34 kDa) trimerize along their linear central and N-terminal domains with their clustered globular CRDs displayed outwardly; six such trimers join into octadecameric (6 × trimers) super molecules whose shape has been compared to a bouquet of tulips (Fig. 10.9). The CRD of SP-A is considered sufficiently hydrophobic to bind lipophilic membranes including the lipid A component of gram-negative bacteria. The CRDs of SP-D are more hydrophilic and bind surface glycoconjugates, including those on pathogens and the mannose receptors of host leukocytes. Secreted SP-D monomers (~43 kDa) also form axial trimers along their N-termini that organize into multimers, with dodecamers most common (4 × trimers) (Fig. 10.9). The CRDs of SP-D extend outward like wheel rims, maximizing their display and binding of simple and complex carbohydrates. Thus they promote binding of microbes by macrophages. In mice, deletion of SP-A primarily affects surfactant assembly, but SP-D deletions lead to ineffectual intrapulmonary responses to airway challenges of respiratory viral and bacterial pathogens.

Recruitment of Circulating Leukocytes into the Parenchyma

Circulating monocytes are normally present in the lungs only as they occur in pulmonary capillary blood. However, their numbers can increase greatly within minutes or hours of an

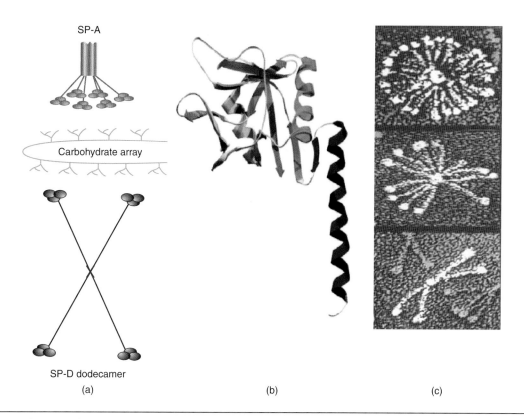

FIGURE 10.9 (a) Schematics of the multimeric forms of SP-A and SP-D as they likely exist in bronchiolar and alveolar lining fluids, with carbohydrate binding domains oriented toward the glycosylated surface of a bacterium. (b) The ribbon structure of SP-A monomer. (c) A single SP-D dodecamer (top) and two examples of variously sized SP-D multimeric "astral bodies". See Suggested Readings.[3]

inhaled or bloodborne threat to lung function. Once activated by chemotactic stimuli such as IL-1β or gram-negative bacterial LPS, they adhere to endothelial surfaces in large numbers, termed **margination** due to their alignment along vessel walls as seen histologically (Fig. 10.10). Within hours they move through blood vessel walls by **diapedesis**, presumably finding or making passageways that are not readily apparent in a quiescent lung. It is unresolved whether these

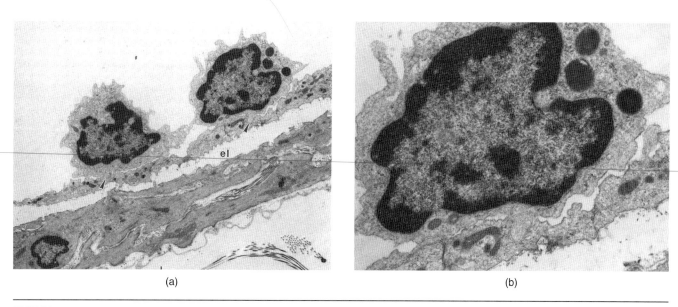

FIGURE 10.10 Two circulating monocytes adhering to a pulmonary arteriole within hours of onset of gram-negative bacteria caused by *E. coli*. Note the impressive thickness of the vessel wall, including its subendothelial elastin (**el**) above several layers of smooth muscle intertwined with ropelike collagen fibers. Arrowheads indicate the monocytes' points of adhesion, with that for the monocyte on the right in (a) shown at higher magnification in (b). *From Lechner et al:* Acute lung injury during bacterial or fungal sepsis, Micro Res Tech Dec 1; *26(5):444-456, 1993.*

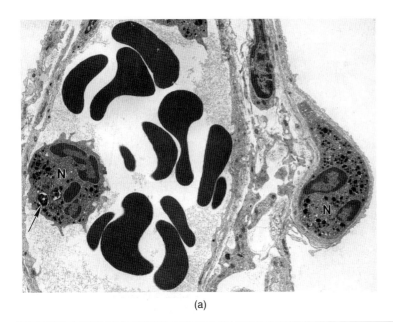
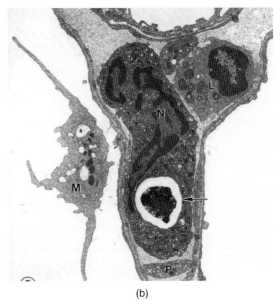

(a)   (b)

FIGURE 10.11 (a) Within 30 minutes of intravenous infusion of live *E. coli* into a rat, its circulating neutrophils (N) have begun adhering to pulmonary arteriolar walls and occluding alveolar capillaries; one contains a phagocytized bacterium (arrow). (b)Similarly, within 30 minutes of IV challenge with yeast-phase *Candida albicans*, a neutrophil containing a fungal blastospore (arrow) is surrounded by a lymphocyte (L) and two platelets (P) within the blood vessel. The proximity of the yeast or perhaps cytokine secretions from the neutrophil have apparently attracted the attention of an alveolar macrophage (M), whose larger size is not readily evident because the eccentric plane of section does not include a portion of its large central nucleus. *From Lechner et al:* Acute lung injury during bacterial or fungal sepsis, Micro Res Tech Dec 1; *26(5):444-456, 1993.*

recruited monocytes mature into **antigen-presenting dendritic cells** that are found in the lung during inflammation, since the dendritic phenotype is not particularly abundant in the healthy lung. Blood monocytes probably also replenish the alveolar macrophage population, since both cell types share developmental affinities to the same myeloid precursor stem cells.

Recruited PMNs follow a similar path and time course of migration into the alveolar zone during inflammatory situations, and they can quickly become the numerically dominant cell type recovered in BALF during severe pneumonia (Fig. 10.11).

Once within the alveoli, PMNs rapidly attack most biological substrates, which they phagocytize whole or can degrade extracellularly with secreted proteases. Like macrophages, PMNs interact with substrates that have been opsonized by SP-A, SP-D, and respiratory mucosal antibodies like IgG and IgA. Also like macrophages, these activated PMNs utilize **NADPH oxidase** and **myeloperoxidase** to produce **reactive oxygen species** (**ROS**). During such a **respiratory burst**, PMNs release ROS including **superoxide anion** ($\cdot O_2^-$), **hydroxyl radical** ($\cdot OH$), and **hypochlorite ion** (OCl^-). During inflammation, PMNs and macrophages upregulate their expression of **inducible nitric oxide synthase** (**iNOS**) that catalyzes formation of **nitric oxide** (**NO**), the predominant **reactive nitrogen species** (**RNS**). In addition to its role as a neuromodulator, NO is potently microbicidal. Furthermore, NO and $\cdot O_2^-$ combine spontaneously in vivo to produce **peroxynitrite anion** ($ONOO^-$), arguably the most active oxidant in terms of the damage it causes to cells and their macromolecules.

Unlike macrophages, mature PMNs do not replicate and can be relatively short-lived at sights of active infection like pneumonia. In patients with advanced forms of acute lung injury and ARDS, the PMNs that are recovered in BALF frequently show signs of apoptosis. PMNs are frequently seen in lung tissues within alveolar macrophages that have phagocytized these now exhausted leukocytes (Fig. 10.12).

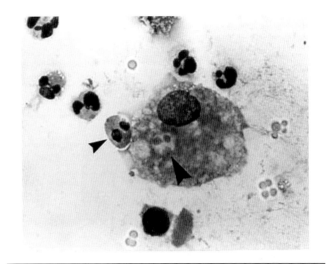

FIGURE 10.12 Cytospin of cells in BALF of a patient with ARDS. The large central cell is an alveolar macrophage. Arrowheads denote apoptotic PMNs. The outline of a phagocytized apoptotic PMN is visible within the macrophage itself. *From Matute-Bello et al.* Neutrophil apoptosis in the acute respiratory distress syndrome, Am J Respir Crit Care Med Dec; *156(6):1969-77, 1997.*

Fixed or circulating lymphocytes in the lung, such as the MALT mentioned above, offer multiple opportunities for inflammation and innate immunity to progress toward adaptive immunity. While usually rarer than macrophages, such luminal and MALT lymphocytes secrete pathogen-specific IgG and IgA into the serous phase of airway and alveolar fluids. Experimental studies indicate that activated alveolar macrophages and probably most other leukocytes routinely utilize the lymphatic drainage of the lungs and thorax to access axial lymph nodes and spleen. There, they encounter the full array of effector and helper cells to which they can present antigen and other pathogen-generated substrates to initiate antibody production, memory, and suppression as when exposures to foreign antigen occur in the GI tract, skin, and blood. Interested students should consult the review by Geissmann and colleagues for a detailed introduction to this field.

The Dilemma of Nondegradable Materials in the Lung

Many natural and synthetic materials can be suspended in air as a dust, aerosol, or fume. These may enter the airways in large amounts and challenge mechanisms that have evolved to protect the lungs. Some, like chlorine and cyanide gases and even distilled water, are injurious to the alveolar epithelium but have short half-lives. Thus patients either succumb to acute lung injury (ALI) abruptly, or survive with scarring or loss of functional parenchyma. At least as common are the many sources of organic and inorganic solids for which there is no biological degradative pathway. Among these are ground minerals containing silica, talc, coal, and asbestos, and paint aerosols containing titanium, lead, or cadmium (Fig. 10.13). Even a casual observer of mills, mines, construction sites, and road repair knows that many workers are exposed with insufficient respiratory protection. The accumulated burden in the lungs of unprotected workers is measured in the tens of grams, particularly if they engaged in such professions for several decades.

Regrettably, there is little available therapy to eliminate this foreign material. Innovative approaches like sequential single-lung lavage to clear paint aerosols have achieved mixed success. Much of the inhaled burden becomes inaccessible even to this strategy, once walled off by leukocytes and fibroblasts into granulomas, fibrotic plaque, and the like. Thus, an appropriate closing note for this chapter is to remind physicians-in-training that often the only treatment for such patients is prevention. A complete patient history documenting exposure to such risks often provides the best opportunity to intervene. Advice from a physician that includes suggestions for modifying personal behavior and improving workplace safety standards can prevent an existing threat from worsening.

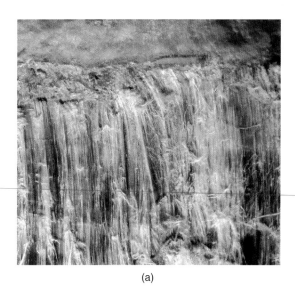
(a)

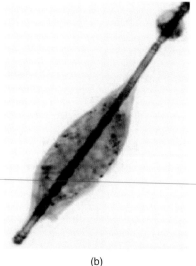
(b)

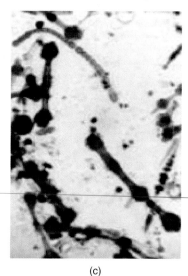
(c)

FIGURE 10.13 The mineral asbestos (a) offers a useful lesson in the challenge posed to lung defenses dusts containing inert particulates of pulverized rock, coal, talc, and ash. Despite aggressive attempts by macrophages to degrade amphibole asbestos fibers (b), virtually all persist indefinitely within the lung for decades following exposure (c), and lead to a large family of restrictive lung diseases (Chaps. 23 and 24).

Suggested Readings

1. Geissmann F, Manz MG, Jung S, et al. Development of monocytes, macrophages, and dendritic cells. *Science.* 2010;327:656-661. *A concise and readable overview of the most recent developments in the field, with excellent color images and supplemental data that will please even the most discerning reader.*

2. Lechner AJ, Ryerse JS, Matuschak GM. Acute lung injury during bacterial or fungal sepsis. *Microsc Res Tech.* 1993;26:444-456. *Several of the transmission electron microscopic images in this chapter were first presented in this article, reflecting our longstanding interest in the cellular players during lung infection and inflammation.*

3. Crouch E, Persson A, Chang D, Heuser J. Molecular structure of pulmonary surfactant protein. *D J Biol Chem.* 1994;269:17311-17319; Head JF, Mealy TR, McCormack FX, Seaton BA. Crystal structure of trimeric carbohydrate recognition and neck domains of surfactant protein. *A J Biol Chem.* 2003;278:43254-43260; *and:* Palaniyar N. Antibody equivalent molecules of the innate immune system: parallels between innate and adaptive immunity. *Innate Immun.* 2010;16:131-137. *These three articles provided key images used in Fig. 10.9 and offer the interested reader suitable chronological "bookends" to the fascinating field of collectin proteins as it continues to evolve.*

CASE STUDIES AND PRACTICE PROBLEMS

CASE 10.1 A 55-year-old woman presents with recent fever and weight loss. She has a cough that is productive of large amounts of sputum, but denies chest pain or shortness of breath. She has smoked a pack of cigarettes per day for 38 years, and admits to heavy alcohol usage, currently at least one pint of vodka per day. Her housemate states that the patient often drinks until she "falls asleep". Her chest radiograph (shown bleow) is read as positive for right middle lobe pneumonia. What pulmonary defense mechanisms are most likely compromised in this patient?

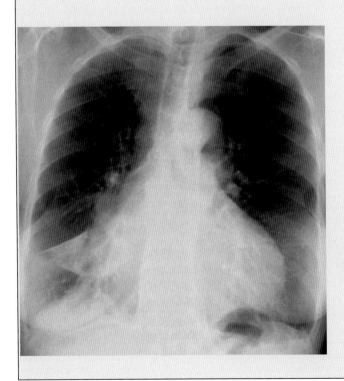

CASE 10.2 A 27-year-old woman is brought to the ER after she fell into a waste receptacle containing fine sawdust. Her vital signs are stable with respirations of 16/min. Physical exam shows a healthy woman who remains concerned about the prospect of subsequent inhalation-induced lung injury. The aspirated material from the patient's clothing shows particles all approximately 3 μm in diameter. The attending physician reassures the patient that the dust she aspirated is normally cleared rapidly from her airways by which of the following mechanisms (more than one may be correct)?

   a. Impaction

   b. Sedimentation

   c. Mucociliary transport

   d. Macrophage phagocytosis

   e. Neutrophil-derived ROS

CASE 10.3 A firefighter enters a room filled with smoke and airborne particles. Her mask is knocked off and she experiences shortness of breath and starts to wheeze. Her bronchospasm may be a good thing because it improves which of the following lung defensive strategies?

   a. Antigen presentation

   b. Cough

   c. Neutrophil recruitment

   d. Mucus clearance

   e. Sedimentation

Solutions to Case Studies and Practice Problems

CASE 10.1 This patient's lengthy history of smoking and daily alcohol consumption are both warning signs for serious lung disease, including lobar pneumonia. Nicotine powerfully suppresses mucociliary transport by its suppressive effects on both ciliary movements and secretion of a suitable "sol" phase under the mucus. Her airways that are narrowed by inflammation and unexpelled mucus will reduce airflow speeds more abruptly than normal. Thus for this woman, impaction and sedimentation will deposit ever larger ash burdens into her intermediate airways, where they are potent attractants of leukocytes secreting proteases. Lapsing into frequent alcohol-induced unconsciousness also increases manyfold the likelihood of aspirating stomach contents and oropharyngeal organisms into the trachea. Even if such aspirates were sterile, the gastric HCl they contain is a commonly noted initiator of acute lung injury that can denude the respiratory mucosa and permanently scar the alveolar parenchyma.

CASE 10.2 All answers are potentially correct.

The size of wood particle inhaled is most likely to be cleared by either impaction or sedimentation, and probably both will work to deposit the sawdust in her nasal vestibules, upper and middle airways. There sinus secretions and mucociliary transport will begin the usual process of expulsion, aided by the presence of resident macrophages that can phagocytize plant materials and use ROS (reactive oxygen species—like neutrophils) to assist in their degradation. The presumption in this case is that the type of wood involved is irrelevant, although many persons have allergic sensitizations to specific types such as cedar and oak.

CASE 10.3 Answer "e" is most correct.

Sedimentation will begin sooner in airways narrowed by bronchoconstriction, as this woman's acute wheeze suggests has occurred. Although cough, mucus clearance, and PMN recruitment (*answers b, c,* and *d*) will also help to clear her inhaled burden of ash, they are not necessarily initiated or enhanced by bronchoconstriction. Antigen presentation (*answer a*) in such a patient would occur only over the subsequent days of her convalescence, primarily in response to whatever smoke residue remains, its antigenicity, and the recovering strength of her adaptive immune system.

Chapter 11

Central and Peripheral Neural Controls of Respiration

W. MICHAEL PANNETON, PhD AND
ANDREW J. LECHNER, PhD

Introduction to the Control of Respiration

As demonstrated in earlier chapters, ventilation is simple in concept but complex in execution. The brain controls the basic pattern of breathing, integrating multiple influences within lower motor neurons of the brainstem and spinal cord to drive pharyngeal, laryngeal, diaphragmatic, intercostal, and other respiratory muscles. Recall that $\dot{V}_E$ (L/min) $= V_T \cdot f$. The central nervous system regulates respiration by controlling the rhythm and pattern of its output to respiratory muscles, adjusting f, V_T or both, depending on overall ventilatory needs for a greater or lesser $\dot{V}_E$ (Fig. 11.1).

The Central Rhythm Generator (#4)

The frequency of respiration, or its **rhythm**, is intrinsic to the brainstem. All vertebrates that use tidal oscillations for the exchange of O_2 and CO_2 in their lungs have such movements generated in their **medulla oblongata**. Indeed surgically isolated brainstem preparations, lacking afferent inputs from chemoreceptors and mechanoreceptors, still produce rhythmic outputs along the same cranial nerves as during normal respiration. One critical rhythm generator within a small area of the medulla and rostral to the obex is called the **pre-Bötzinger complex**. Bilateral lesions in this portion of the medulla induce complete respiratory arrest in humans. Whether this rhythmic discharge initiates within individual pacemaker cells, or from a network of such cells, remains a matter of debate. At this point, it is important to understand that a rhythm is constantly generated by the medulla, a rhythm that is modifiable by afferent input from sensory receptors.

The Central Pattern Generator

The **central pattern generator**, or the brainstem output controlling all muscles involved in respiration, is much more complex. This pattern generator algebraically sums all the afferent inputs to produce well-coordinated activations of the diaphragm, intercostal muscles, and abdominal muscles, and if needed, the accessory muscles of respiration. Like respiratory rhythm, the goal of such pattern generation is maintenance of normal P_aO_2, P_aCO_2, and pH_a. Extreme examples of modulating both the rhythm and pattern of respiration are seen during rigorous exercise and ascents to high altitude. The pattern of respiration is also modulated by events like coughing, speech, sleep, vomiting, micturition, and defecation, particularly as the latter may mimic a **Valsalva maneuver**. Although some of these events are episodic or relatively infrequent, they can affect the normal respiratory pattern in dramatic ways.

Defined Patterns of Respiration

Eupnea: is normal, quiet breathing at rest. Individuals are usually unaware of it.

Tachypnea or **polypnea**: is an increase in f without an increase in V_T. Tachypnea is not a normal stress response, unless hyperthermia or other factor has induced **panting**.

Hyperpnea or **hyperventilation**: denotes an increase in pulmonary ventilation involving both V_T and f, but without the subjectively stressful sensations of dyspnea (Fig. 11.2).

Dyspnea: is the sensation of inadequate or stressful respiration, with exaggerated awareness of one's need for increased respiratory effort. Dyspnea implies labored breathing, often involving accessory respiratory muscles. Many stimuli induce dyspnea.

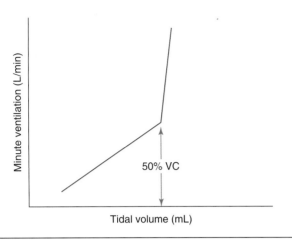

FIGURE 11.1 Relationship between $\dot{V}_E$ and V_T in normal awake subjects. With stimuli such as hypercapnia, $\dot{V}_E$ increases linearly with V_T up to about 50% of vital capacity (VC). Above that volume, $\dot{V}_E$ increases primarily by increasing f with little change in V_T.

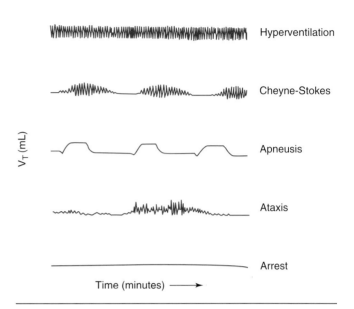

FIGURE 11.2 Characteristic waveforms of frequently encountered respiratory patterns. Both duration and amplitude of specific patterns vary widely among patients, and are affected by both central and peripheral processes. In each trace shown here, upward deflections represent inspiratory efforts.

Cheyne-Stokes respiration: is the most common form of abnormal breathing, with weak respiratory efforts that decrease to an apnea and then increase to hyperpnea. The "**crescendo-decrescendo**" oscillations of Cheyne-Stokes are most often caused by hypoxemia and are a frequently encountered symptom (see Chap. 25) (Fig. 11.2).

Apneusis: is an abnormally patterned breathing with prolonged inspirations that alternate with short expiratory movements (Fig. 11.2). **Apneustic breathing** is commonly noted after lesions in the **pontine pneumotaxic center** discussed below.

Ataxis or **ataxic respiration**: is an abnormal pattern with completely irregular breathing and increasing periods of apnea. As the pattern deteriorates, it may merge with agonal respiration. It is caused by damage to the medulla oblongata by stroke or trauma.

Apnea: is the absence of breathing. As generally used, apnea implies that the cessation is temporary. A prolonged apnea for any cause is considered **respiratory arrest**.

Respiratory Motor Neurons of the Spinal Cord and Medulla
The Spinal Cord

Spinal cord neurons are organized into **ventral horn** (motor), **dorsal horn** (sensory), and **lateral horn** (autonomic) regions. Those in the ventral horn are most critical to respiration, since they include **lower motor neurons** innervating somatic striated muscles (Fig. 11.3). Major somatic striated muscles involved in respiration include:

Diaphragm: its innervating motoneurons exit at C3-C5 as the phrenic nerve.
Intercostal muscles: innervated by motoneurons within the thoracic ventral horn with axons that exit the spinal cord and distribute via the intercostal nerves.
Abdominal muscles: their motoneurons have axons that track within the lower thoracic and upper lumbar cord regions.

Cervical spinal cord

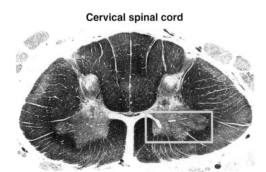

Thoracic spinal cord

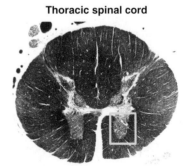

FIGURE 11.3 Cross sections of the cervical and thoracic spinal cords, with ventral horn regions in each indicated by the yellow boxes.

Accessory muscles: include all muscles that elevate and splay the ribs, notably the **levator costalis**, **scalene**, **transverse thoracic**, and **sternocleidomastoid**.

The Medulla

In addition to its role as the principal area of sensorimotor integration for respiration, the medulla contains lower motor neurons with fibers that exit via cranial nerves to innervate striated muscles in the head and neck (Fig 11.4). Motor neurons innervating the tongue muscles are found in the hypoglossal nucleus, while those innervating laryngeal, pharyngeal and facial muscles are found in the ventrolateral medulla. All of these muscles receive rhythmic central nervous system (CNS) motor input during every breath. Major cranial striated muscles that are involved during normal respiration includes

Laryngeal muscles: both laryngeal abductors and adductors are innervated by motoneurons in the **nucleus ambiguus**, whose axons travel with the vagus nerve.
Pharyngeal muscles: also receive motor input from the nucleus ambiguus by neurons whose axons exit via the glossopharyngeal and vagus nerves.
Facial muscles: most notably the **m. nasalis**, by motoneurons within the facial motor nucleus whose axons exit via the facial nerve.
Tongue muscles: principally the **genioglossus muscle** by motoneurons in the hypoglossal nucleus whose axons exit via the hypoglossal nerve.

Within the medulla are two recognized groups of neurons involved in the integration and coordination of breathing, whose functions continue to be intensively investigated. The first of these, the **ventral respiratory column**, is a longitudinal array of **respiratory-related neurons** that fire synchronously

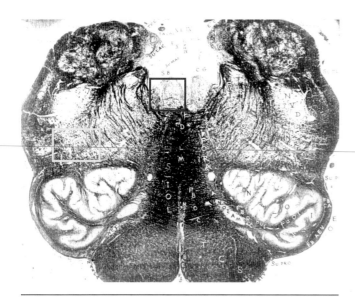

FIGURE 11.4 Cross section of the medulla with the **ventrolateral medulla** highlighted by the yellow box, and the **hypoglossal nucleus** by the red box.

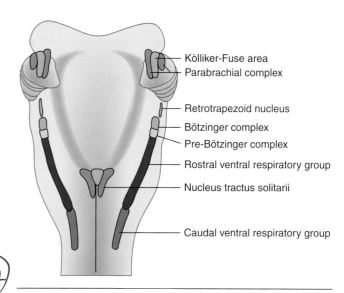

FIGURE 11.5 Schematic of principal respiratory areas in the mammalian brainstem.

with each phrenic nerve discharge. These neurons are found in the ventrolateral reticular formation of the medulla, generally just ventral to the nucleus ambiguus. A subject's basic respiratory rhythm persists if only these brainstem neurons are intact, albeit poorly controlled. Four main components of the ventral respiratory column have been identified (Fig. 11.5):

Caudal ventral respiratory group (cVRG): an expiratory area running from the spino-medullary junction to the obex;
Rostral ventral respiratory group (rVRG): the area of mixed inspiratory and expiratory respiratory neurons just rostral to the obex;
Pre-Bötzinger Complex: an area of neurons that is rostral to the rVRG and considered of central importance for rhythm generation;
Bötzinger Complex: an expiratory area just caudal to the facial nucleus.

In addition to the ventral respiratory column, a second brainstem area of importance to respiratory control contains the **dorsal respiratory group (DRG)**, being inspiratory neurons in the ventrolateral part of the **nucleus tractus solitarii** (**NTS**) (Fig 11.5).

The Pons

Situated rostral to the VRG and DRG neurons of the brainstem, the **pons** contains the **parabrachial nucleus** and the **Kölliker-Fuse area**, a neurophil surrounding the **brachium conjunctivum** (Fig. 11.6). These two regions contain neurons considered important as the main "off-switch" for spontaneous inspiration, and have been called the **pontine pneumotaxic center** because lesions here result in apneustic respiration.

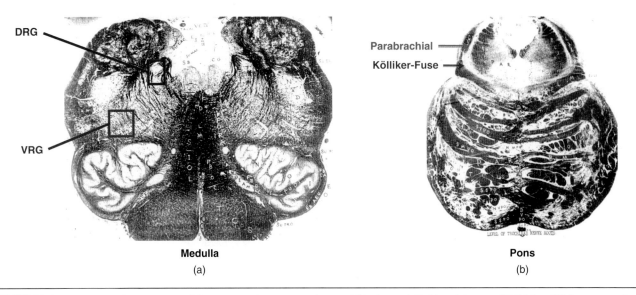

Medulla
(a)

Pons
(b)

FIGURE 11.6 Cross-sectional comparisons of the major respiratory control areas within the medulla (a) and the pons (b). DRG and VRG represent the dorsal and ventral respiratory groups of neurons, respectively.

Brainstem Integration of Respiration

Pontine and medullary respiratory neurons are quite interconnected, making it difficult to assign unambiguous functions to any particular group of neurons. Investigations of respiratory control usually are conducted while eliminating variables that are known to affect the rhythm or pattern of respiration. This usually means maintaining constant P_aO_2 or P_aCO_2 levels in animals that are anesthetized, vagotomized, and sometimes spinalized. Despite such limitations, it is clear that afferent inputs from higher brain areas, as well as from chemoreceptors and mechanoreceptors, converge on this network of brainstem respiratory neurons (Fig. 11.5). There they produce a pattern of muscle contractions and thus ventilation that are appropriate for metabolic needs.

> ▶▶ **CLINICAL CORRELATION 11.1**
>
> Respiratory pattern is a key indicator of improper brain functioning in a comatose patient. During diffuse forebrain depression, as in **metabolic encephalopathy** with liver failure, breathing may assume the crescendo-decrescendo pattern of Cheyne-Stokes respiration, with variable periods of apnea. Midbrain injury can cause hyperventilation, while injury to the rostral pons may produce apneusis (Fig. 11.2). Injury to the lower pons or upper medulla frequently induces ataxic breathing that often heralds complete respiratory arrest.

Sensory Modulation of Respiration

Respiratory rhythm generation is intrinsic to the medulla and proceeds even without additional sensory input. However, central respiratory neurons are modulated by afferent inputs affecting the depth, rate, and pattern of respiration. **Chemoreceptors** respond to changes in the composition of blood or other fluids around them. Major groups of chemoreceptors are located in the peripheral and central nervous systems.

Peripheral chemoreceptors are located in parenchymal lobules termed the **carotid bodies** above the bifurcations of the common carotid arteries (Fig. 11.7), and the **aortic bodies** located along the superior aspect of the aortic arch. Although the lobules are organized similarly at each location, the carotid bodies send afferent impulses via the carotid sinus nerve branch of cranial nerve IX, while the aortic bodies send signals via cranial nerve X to the NTS in the CNS. In general terms, these peripheral chemoreceptors respond quickly to decreasing P_aO_2 and pH_a, and increasing P_aCO_2, with discharge rates alterable during a single respiratory cycle. Importantly, they cause all increased ventilation in response to arterial hypoxemia, although their effect is not appreciable until P_aO_2 declines to ~40 mm Hg. Thus, their role in regulating eupneic breathing is small. It is also thought that their response to increased P_aCO_2 is less important than that of central chemoreceptors.

The major populations of **central chemoreceptors** are located near the ventral surface of the medulla, many near levels of the exiting hypoglossal nerve (Fig. 11.8). They are bathed in brain **extracellular fluid** (**ECF**) that rapidly equilibrates with gaseous CO_2 diffusing from blood vessels into **cerebrospinal fluid** (**CSF**). This local rise in PCO_2 acidifies CSF and thus stimulates the chemoreceptors, even though $[H^+]$ and $[HCO_3^-]$ do not readily cross the blood-brain barrier. In this manner, a reduction in pH_a stimulates ventilation centrally while an increased pH_a is inhibitory (Fig. 11.8).

Systemically the body seldom experiences isolated hypoxia, hypercapnia, or acidemia. Moreover, the ventilatory response to a set of variables is greater than the response to each component, due to integration of these modulatory influences within the CNS.

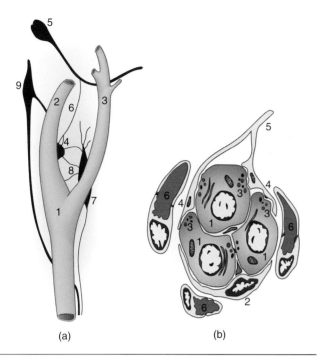

Receptors of the Lower Airways

There are several important types of sensory receptors associated with afferent fibers in the vagus nerve that respond to either mechanical or chemical stimulation of the tracheobronchial tree, including its respiratory mucosa (Table 11.1).

Important subtypes of receptors within the lower airways and/or the lung parenchyma include three main groups:

Slowly adapting pulmonary stretch receptors (SARs): Myelinated SARs are situated among airway smooth muscle cells and send afferent fibers centrally via the vagus nerve. They discharge in response to distension of the lung, and show little adaptation over time to sustained lung inflation. Activation of SARs reduces respiratory frequency by increasing the expiratory time interval, the so-called **Hering-Breuer reflex**. These SARs are inactive in awake subjects unless V_T is large (>1 L), but they may be prominent in anesthetized animal preparations.

Rapidly adapting pulmonary receptors (RARs), also termed by some authors as **irritant receptors**: Myelinated RARs lie between airway epithelial cells and also send afferent fibers centrally via cranial nerve X (vagus). Some RARs are mechanoreceptors that fire during hyperinflation or forced deflation of the lungs. Most are chemoreceptive RARs activated by exogenous agents (eg, noxious gases, cigarette smoke, and cold air) and endogenous chemicals (eg, histamine, prostaglandins, and serotonin). Their reflex effects include bronchoconstriction, hyperpnea, and

FIGURE 11.7 (a) The common carotid artery (1) bifurcates into internal (2) and external (3) branches, with the carotid body (4) near the bifurcation. Sensory fibers from cranial nerve IX (5) reach the carotid body via the carotid sinus nerve (6). The superior cervical ganglion (7) innervates the carotid body via the ganglioglomerular nerves (8), as does the inferior or nodose ganglion of CN X (9). (b) A carotid body or aortic arch lobule contains chemoreceptor cells (1) supported by sustentacular cells (2). Chemoreceptors have a heterogeneous population of synaptic vesicles (3), some near sensory nerve endings (4) of the carotid sinus nerve (5). Each lobule is surrounded by a dense network of capillaries (6).

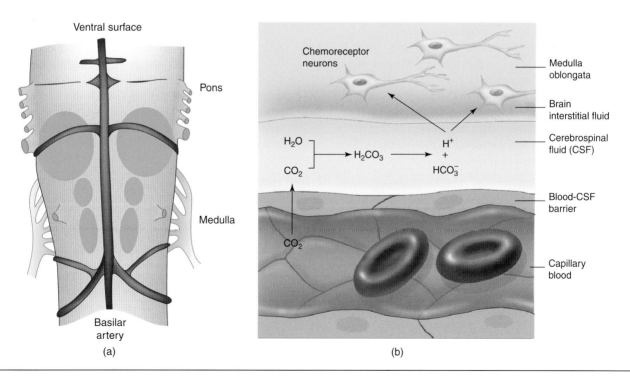

FIGURE 11.8 (a) General locations of central chemoreceptors along the ventral surface of the medulla are shown as three pairs of blue circles. (b) Mechanism by which increases in P_aco_2 and thus pH_a are transduced by central chemoreceptors located across the blood-brain barrier that is considered normally impermeable to charged molecules like H^+ and HCO_3^-. (b): *From Fox,* Human Physiology, *10th ed. 2008.*

Table **11.1** **Tracheobronchial receptor properties**

Receptor Type	Location	Stimulus	Reflexes
Myelinated vagal fibers			
Slowly adapting receptors (SAR)	among airway smooth muscle	lung inflation	Hering-Breuer reflexes, tachycardia, bronchodilation
Rapidly adapting receptors (RAR)	among airway epithelial cells	lung hyperinflation, noxious gases, smoke histamine, prostaglandins	hyperpnea cough, mucus secretion bronchoconstriction
Unmyelinated vagal fibers			
C-fiber free nerve endings	lung interstitium; close to pulmonary and bronchial circulations	large hyperinflation smoke, capsaicin, gases histamine, serotonin prostaglandins, bradykinin	apnea, then tachypnea cough, mucus secretion bronchoconstriction bradycardia, hypotension

cough. Indeed, a presumptive cough receptor has been discovered recently. It is not clear whether RARs function during eupneic respiration. However, their responsiveness to inflammatory mediators and other endogenous chemicals indicate they may be important in disease (Chap. 10).

Tracheobronchial C-fibers: Unmyelinated C-fibers comprise >75% of afferent fibers emerging from the lungs. Their nerve endings generally function as chemoreceptors that are sensitive to histamine, prostaglandins, bradykinin, and serotonin, as well as cigarette smoke, noxious gases, and capsaicin. Thus they probably play a prominent role in asthma, allergic bronchoconstriction, pulmonary vascular congestion, and pulmonary embolism. Although C-fibers are relatively inactive during eupneic breathing, they respond to lung hyperinflation and can induce reflex apnea (followed by tachypnea), bronchoconstriction, hypotension, bradycardia, and mucus secretion.

Other Peripheral Sensory Receptors

Receptors of the upper airways: There are un-encapsulated (free) nerve endings arrayed within the respiratory mucosa from the nasal cavity to the larynx (Chap. 2). Their afferent fibers travel via the trigeminal, glossopharyngeal, and vagus nerves and respond to chemical and mechanical stimuli. Induced respiratory responses caused by their stimulation include sneezing, coughing, bronchoconstriction, and apnea, depending on stimulus nature and the region within the upper respiratory tract being stimulated.

Such sensory innervations of the larynx via the superior laryngeal nerve are of considerable clinical importance, since these receptors monitor airflow, laryngeal temperature, and other mechanical and chemical stimuli (Fig. 11.9).

Receptors in muscle: Dynamic or static contractions of limb muscles induce many autonomic effects including hyperpnea, although P_aCO_2, P_aO_2, and pH_a change little during moderate exercise. Moreover, experimental data indicate that neither the carotid chemoreceptors nor respiratory muscle afferent fibers provide the primary stimulus for such hypernea. Rather, most evidence suggests that the small myelinated and unmyelinated fibers of sensory nerves (Groups III and IV) that innervate striated muscle initiate this response. It also has been proposed that a **central command mechanism** may initiate hypernea during exercise. This topic is addressed further in Chap. 13.

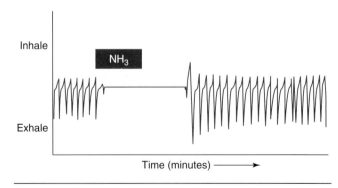

FIGURE 11.9 Applying ammonia vapor (NH_3) to the nasal mucosa induces an abrupt apnea. Many substances induce similar responses when applied to either the nasal or laryngeal mucosa. *From Panneton, recording in an anesthetized rat.*

Respiratory Control during Sleep

Sleep is a complex diurnal rhythm having a different time scale that is superimposed on the normal respiratory rhythm. Although sleep consists of various stages, it is often simplified to be either rapid eye movement (REM) sleep or non-REM sleep. Respiration slows and chemoreception is blunted during sleep, such that prolonged apnea and marked CO_2 retention may occur. From a cardiovascular perspective, sleep also induces bradycardia and mild hypotension. These autonomic effects are especially evident during REM sleep, during which there is **atonia** or **hypotonia** of skeletal muscles. This hypotonia increases upper airway resistance by relaxing pharyngeal muscles. It is thought that snoring, as well as **obstructive sleep apneas** (**OSA**) is the result of this atonia (Chap. 25). Perhaps the most important effect of sleep on respiration is loss of what some researchers refer to as the **wakefulness stimulus**, an overriding controller or integrator of all other respiratory inputs and functions.

Higher Neural Controls of Respiratory Function

Eliminating suprapontine inputs to brainstem respiratory centers has only minor effects on resting respiration, suggesting that such areas modulate but do not control basal respiratory patterns and rhythms. Suprapontine areas are active in volitionally altered respiration associated with speech, singing, and similar activities (Fig. 11.10). Thus, cortical areas are capable of affecting the pattern generator and of activating different muscle groups of respiration. Although little is known currently about the anatomy and physiology of cerebral cortical areas that modulate respiration, new imaging methods using functional MRI and/or PET scans are beginning to identify important regions.

Pathological Breathing Patterns

Respiratory rhythm is usually regular and continues throughout life without conscious effort. Indeed, consciousness of one's breathing often signifies the presence of extreme environmental conditions or pathological states. When respirations become arrhythmic, the term **periodic breathing** is applied, while **apnea** refers to an absence of breathing that is usually temporary. Apneas are **obstructive** when caused by upper-airway blockage despite efferent impulses to breathe, or **central** when without respiratory movements, or may be of **mixed** type. However other apneas exist, including **obstructive expiratory apnea**, **obstructive hypoventilation**, and **central hypoventilation syndrome** ("**Ondine's curse**"); these will be discussed in Chap. 25.

The term **dyspnea** was introduced earlier to describe a patient's sensation of inadequate or stressful respiration, or an

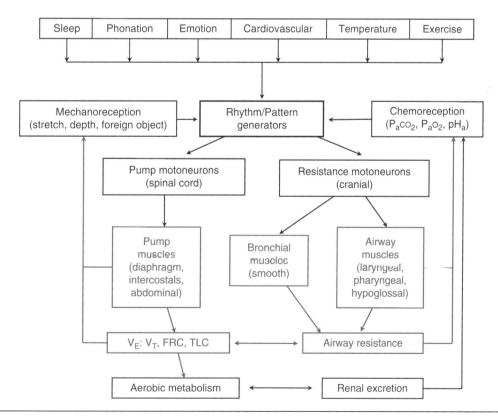

FIGURE 11.10 An integrated perspective showing the interactions among central and peripheral control mechanisms of respiration residing within the autonomic domains, and the known or putative inputs from cerebrocortical brain regions and other organ systems such as skeletal muscles, the heart, and kidneys. FRC and TLC represent functional residual capacity and total lung capacity, respectively.

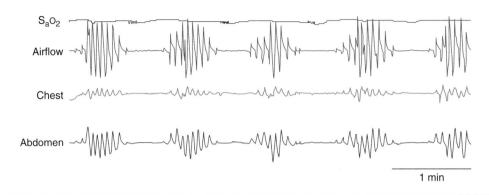

FIGURE 11.11 Cheyne-Stokes breathing in a patient with congestive heart failure. Shown from top to bottom are the patient's arterial saturation by pulse oximetry (S_aO_2), airflow rate measured at the mouth, chest movements by thoracic tension belt, and abdominal wall movements by a similar device. Note the reproducible periodicity, with the complete cycle repeated every 70-90 seconds.

exaggerated consciousness of a need for increased respiratory effort. Clinically, dyspnea usually implies labored respiration and the use of some or all accessory respiratory muscles, as in many patients with acute lung injury and the acute respiratory distress syndrome (Chap. 28). Many factors induce dyspnea, but it is important to remember that it is a sensation that may not have an underlying pathophysiological explanation in every case.

Periodic Breathing

Periodic breathing is characterized as clusters of breaths separated by intervals of apnea or near-apnea. A clinically useful definition of such periodic breathing might be when at least three respiratory pauses, each lasting 3 seconds or longer, are separated by periods of normal breathing, each lasting less than 20 seconds. **Cheyne-Stokes breathing** as commonly seen in congestive heart failure is an example of such periodic breathing (Fig. 11.11). Periodic breathing usually occurs during sleep and can occur in healthy individuals,

and the apnea there is usually of central rather than obstructive origin.

Periodic breathing is a normal respiratory pattern in premature infants during active REM-sleep and non-REM sleep. It persists in infants, but decreases as a percentage of the population as children mature. Among term infants, periodic breathing usually is confined to REM sleep. Persistence of periodic breathing during longer portions of sleep may be abnormal, and reflect immaturity or an abnormality of brainstem respiratory control (Chap. 39). Sleep apnea occurs in 2%-3% of children, 3%-7% of middle-aged adults, and 10%-15% of otherwise healthy adults who are > 65 years old. Periodic breathing is generally considered to be a consequence of chemoreceptor function. When P_aCO_2 or P_ACO_2 is far below normal eupneic values, or when P_aO_2 or P_AO_2 is far above, then at least transient apnea will almost certainly ensue. Thus, there are **apneic thresholds** for both **hypocapnia** and **hyperoxia** that may differ strikingly among healthy individuals. Whether their periodic breathing is more, the result of activation of central versus peripheral chemoreceptors remains unresolved to date.

Suggested Readings

1. Feldman JL, Mitchell GS, Nattie EE. Breathing: rhythmicity, plasticity, chemosensitivity. *Ann Rev Neurosci.* 2003;26:239-266. *Reviews the rhythm generator in the ventral medulla, as well as central chemoreceptors; also a good source of other literature.*

2. Chamberlain N. Functional organization of the parabrachial complex and intertrigeminal region in the control of breathing. *Respir Physiol Neurobiol.* 2004;143:115-125. *Summarizes the function of neurons in the parabrachial complex (parabrachial and Kölliker-Fuse nuclei). Also reviews the neuroanatomical connections of the dorsolateral pons with laryngeal, hypoglossal, and facial motor neurons.*

3. Canning BJ, Mori N, Mazzone SB. Vagal afferent fibers regulating the cough reflex. *Respir Physiol Neurobiol.* 2006;152:223-242. *These authors review potential neural pathways regulating cough, particularly fibers innervating the tracheobronchial tree.*

4. Horn EM, Waldrop TG. Suprapontine control of respiration. *Respir Physiol.* 1998;114:201-211. *Despite a sparse literature, this is an excellent summary of areas of the cortex, hypothalamus, basal ganglia, and midbrain that may be important for volitional and suprabulbar reflexive respiratory control (defense reaction and locomotion).*

5. Jordan D. Central nervous pathways and control of the airways. *Respir Physiol.* 2001;125: 67-81. *Reviews CNS integration of airway receptors, the nucleus tractus solitarii, and activation of somatic and autonomic motoneurons, details that clinicians should know before prescribing drugs.*

CASE STUDIES AND PRACTICE PROBLEMS

CASE 11.1 A semi-comatose 80-year-old male is brought to the ER on a respirator. Tests show he has developed bilateral hemorrhagic infarcts of his lateral medulla. He has no noticeable respiratory efforts. This effect is best explained by necrosis of which of the following structures?

a. Neurons generating the "wakefulness stimulus"

b. Lower motor neurons in nucleus ambiguus innervating the diaphragm

c. Central chemoreceptors in the ventral medulla

d. Lower motor neurons of the major respiratory pump muscles

e. The central locus for controlling the rhythm of respiration

CASE 11.2 A 57-year-old woman enters the emergency room displaying 'bluish' lips and complaining of difficulty in catching her breath walking up stairs. The attending physician admits the woman for observation. Several hours later the resident places the patient on $F_IO_2 = 1.00$ at 4.0 L/min via a nasal cannula hoping to rectify her cyanotic lips, but within two minutes the patient stops breathing. What is the most likely explanation for this patient's apnea?

a. The patient crossed her hyperoxia apnea threshold.

b. The nasal cannula has accidentally obstructed the patient's pharynx.

c. An infarct in the lateral medulla has destroyed her pre-Bötzinger complex.

d. The patient has attempted suicide by holding her breath until she dies.

e. Central chemoreceptors have been stimulated by her high P_aCO_2.

CASE 11.3 A 54-year-old woman presents with a chief complaint that her spouse noticed an irregular feature of her breathing, particularly if he awoke before the patient did in the morning. Physical exam shows a female with normal color and skin tone and a moderately increased body mass index; results of an office chest x-ray are pending. She cannot recall the names of current medications. An overnight sleep study indicates the patient exhibits a crescendo-decrescendo pattern of breathing. Which of the following best characterizes this form of abnormal respiration?

a. Obstructions of the upper airways are usually evident.

b. It is usually caused by weakness of respiratory pump muscles.

c. It is common in sleeping patients with congestive heart failure.

d. Prolonged inspirations are followed by periods of apnea.

e. The pattern is common among obese patients who snore.

Solutions to Case Studies and Practice Problems

CASE 11.1 The most correct answer is e.

The central locus for controlling the rhythm of respiration; bilateral lesions of the ventrolateral medulla induce respiratory arrest, most probably by disrupting the central rhythm generator. The "wakefulness stimulus" dominates respiratory behavior when awake, but respiration is maintained without it during sleep and coma (*answer a*). Motor neurons for the diaphragm originate in the ventral horn of cervical levels 3-5 (*answer b*). Stimulation of central chemoreceptors induces hyperpnea; their distribution is widespread and total ablation would be very rare (*answer c*). Motor neurons for the diaphragm, intercostal and abdominal muscles, and accessory muscles of respiration are in the spinal cord, while those innervating the pharyngeal and laryngeal muscles are in the nucleus ambiguus (*answer d*).

CASE 11.2 The most correct answer is a.

The patient was cyanotic with an unknown $\%S_aO_2$; placing her on $F_IO_2 = 1.00$ exceeded her hyperoxic threshold and induced an apnea. Even if the nasal cannula became obstructed (*answer b*), she could have breathed through her mouth, and a sudden bilateral infarct of her medulla is improbable given her history and presentation (*answer c*). Suicides by such a means have never

been documented (*answer d*) and all available scientific evidence indicates that once consciousness is lost, chemoreceptor activation would override the loss of a wakefulness stimulus and restore breathing. Stimulation of central chemoreceptors would cause hypernea, not apnea (*answer e*).

CASE 11.3 The most correct answer is c.

It is common in sleeping patients with congestive heart failure; the crescendo-decrescendo breathing pattern is indicative of Cheyne-Stokes breathing, which is highly correlated with the diagnosis of congestive heart failure (CHF). Obstruction of the upper airways, particularly the pharynx, occurs in obstructive sleep apnea and is commonly seen in obese patients. When such patients awaken, pharyngeal muscle tone strengthens and alleviates the obstruction and they may become hyperpneic due to chemoreceptor activation (*answers a, e*). Muscle weakness typically occurs during both sleep and wakefulness and usually does not alter normal respiratory rhythms (*answer b*). This patient does not have an apneustic breathing pattern (*answer d*) which is uncommon and carries a poor prognosis; it is most usually associated with infarcts and lesions of the dorsolateral pons.

Chapter 12

Importance and Derivation of Aerobic Capacity

GERALD S. ZAVORSKY, PhD AND
ANDREW J. LECHNER, PhD

Introduction

A subject's **aerobic capacity** is an important assessment in respiratory physiology because the lungs may comprise a primary limitation on O_2 transport and $\dot{V}O_2$ (Chap. 1). Furthermore, abundant scientific evidence supports the contention that aerobic capacity is a very powerful predictor of both life expectancy and **mortality** from many diseases. Aerobic capacity has several synonyms in the literature, including exercise capacity, aerobic fitness, maximal or peak oxygen consumption ($\dot{V}O_{2max}$ and $\dot{V}O_{2peak}$, respectively), metabolic equivalent of the task (MET) capacity (see below), and cardiovascular fitness. For consistency, the terms aerobic capacity and $\dot{V}O_{2max}$ will be used throughout this chapter.

Definition and Calculation of Aerobic Capacity

Aerobic capacity is defined by the **American College of Sports Medicine (ACSM)** as "The ability to perform dynamic exercise that involves large muscle groups at a moderate to high intensity for prolonged periods." $\dot{V}O_{2max}$ is the most widely accepted measure of such aerobic capacity. Recall that $\dot{V}O_2$ always is equal to the product of the amount of blood delivered to all body tissue, that is, the cardiac output, multiplied by the amount of oxygen extracted from the blood during each passage through the tissues, that is, its arterial-venous oxygen content difference. Mathematically this relationship is expressed by the **Fick equation**:

$$\dot{V}O_2 = \dot{Q} \cdot (C_aO_2 - C_{\bar{v}}O_2)$$

And thus: $\dot{V}O_{2max} = \dot{Q}_{max} \cdot (C_aO_2 - C_{\bar{v}}O_2)_{max}$

Clearly an individual's $\dot{V}O_{2max}$ may be limited by any factor that constrains either cardiac output or the (arterial-venous) O_2 content difference. Each of these components will be discussed in this chapter. One general comment is worth noting at this point. When evaluating aerobic capacity using weight-bearing exercises like running, walking, or climbing stairs,

the $\dot{V}O_{2max}$ is expressed in mL/kg/min or L/kg/min to correct for differences in a subject's body weight (and from which can be calculated their **body mass index, BMI**). When evaluating aerobic capacity using non-weight-bearing exercises like swimming, rowing, or biking, then $\dot{V}O_{2max}$ is expressed in mL/min or L/min to exclude influences of a subject's body weight.

A useful alternative is to express $\dot{V}O_{2max}$ in **METs**, with one MET being the average for a subject's resting $\dot{V}O_2$. Historically, **1 MET = 3.5 mL/kg/min**, although recent research indicates that a truer estimate over a wider range of body weights is 2.6 mL/kg/min. Thus, a subject with $\dot{V}O_{2max}$ of 8 METs has an aerobic capacity approximately seven-fold above their resting metabolic rate. This subject would also be described as having a **metabolic reserve** of 7 METs. Tables 12.1 and 12.2 provide normative data for weight-adjusted aerobic capacity (mL/kg/min) for subjects sorted by age and sex. The verbal classification rankings in each table are useful in distinguishing among patients from a range of lifestyles, and have been validated using the *ACSM Guidelines Handbook*.

Influence of Aerobic Capacity on Mortality

Aerobic capacity is a more powerful predictor of mortality than any other established risk factor for cardiovascular disease. Indeed, as reported in the *New England Journal of Medicine* in 2002 by Myers and colleagues, a high aerobic capacity is protective even in the presence of other known risk factors (Fig. 12.1). When subjects are defined according to other known risk factors like diabetes, the risk of death from any cause in subjects whose exercise capacity is <5 METs is nearly double that of subjects whose exercise capacity is >8 METs.

Because physical fitness is a modifiable risk factor, improving it enhances patient prognoses: Each MET of

Table **12.1** ACSM percentiles for aerobic capacity in males (mL/kg/min)

Age (y)	20-29	30-39	40-49	50-59	60-69	70-79	Classification
95%	56.2	54.3	52.9	49.7	46.1	42.4	Superior
80%	51.1	47.5	46.8	43.3	39.5	36.0	Excellent
60%	45.7	44.4	42.4	38.3	35.0	30.9	Good
50%	43.9	42.4	40.4	36.7	33.1	29.1	Fair
40%	42.2	41.0	38.4	35.2	31.4	28.0	Fair
20%	38.1	36.7	34.6	31.1	27.4	23.7	Poor
1%	26.6	26.6	25.1	21.3	18.6	17.9	Very poor

increased aerobic capacity yields ~12% improvement in survival. As shown in Fig. 12.2, mortality rates differ strikingly just between the least-fit **quintile** (lowest 20% of the population) and the next-least fit quintile (the second-lowest 20% of the population). Regardless of whether patients have cardiovascular disease, survival declines as aerobic capacity decreases. In this multicenter study, fewer than 50% of patients with an aerobic capacity <5 METs survived 14 years from the study's inception versus >75% of patients with an aerobic capacity >8 METs.

Using the Fick Equation to Estimate $\dot{V}o_2$ and $\dot{V}o_{2max}$

In 1870, the German physician and physiologist **Adolf Eugen Fick** developed the eponymous equation that was introduced above to estimate $\dot{Q}$ when the O_2 concentrations of arterial and venous blood and of the exhaled gas are known or can be measured. Thus, the Fick equation demonstrates the combined efficacies of the heart, lungs, and peripheral muscles to achieve a maximal effect systemically:

$$\dot{V}o_{2max} = \dot{Q}_{max} \cdot (C_aO_2 - C_{\bar{v}}O_2)_{max}$$

As introduced in Chap. 1, **O_2 delivery** is defined from this equation as the product of $\dot{Q}$ and C_aO_2, while **O_2 extraction** is similarly defined as the difference between C_aO_2 and $C_{\bar{v}}O_2$.

Therefore, $\dot{V}o_2$ equals the product of $\dot{Q}$ and O_2 extraction, and $\dot{V}o_{2max}$ is the physiological optimization of all three terms by the heart ($\dot{Q}$), the lungs (C_aO_2), and the working muscles ($C_{\bar{v}}O_2$). In determining $\dot{V}o_{2max}$ for a healthy subject or a particular patient, the physician is often simultaneously assessing which of these three terms is rate-limiting under the clinical and environmental conditions present during assessment.

As established in Chaps. 3 and 9, the C_aO_2 depends on four variables: blood [Hb]; the binding capacity of Hb for O_2 (1.39 mL O_2/g Hb); the effective P_AO_2; and the amount of dissolved O_2, also dependent on P_aO_2 (Chap. 3). Mathematically this becomes:

$$C_aO_2 = \text{Hb-bound } O_2 + \text{Dissolved } O_2$$
$$C_aO_2 \text{ (mL } O_2/\text{L blood)} = \{S_aO_2 \cdot [\text{Hb}] \cdot 1.39\} + \{23.3 \text{ mL/L/atm} \cdot (P_aO_2/P_B)\}$$

In a healthy nonsmoking man with [Hb] = 15.6 g/dL breathing air at sea level, this yields:

$$C_aO_2 \text{ (mL } O_2/\text{L)} = \{0.98 \cdot 156 \text{ g/L} \cdot 1.39\} + \{23.3 \cdot (100/760)\}$$
$$C_aO_2 \cong 215.6 \text{ mL } O_2/\text{L blood}$$

Anemia and methemoglobinemia reduce the effective arterial [Hb] and thus the maximal C_aO_2, while high altitude, hypoventilation, and pulmonary fibrosis reduce C_aO_2 by their

Table **12.2** ACSM percentiles for aerobic capacity in females (mL/kg/min)

Age (y)	20-29	30-39	40-49	50-59	60-69	70-79	Classification
95%	50.2	46.9	45.2	39.9	36.9	36.7	Superior
80%	44.0	41.0	38.9	35.2	32.3	30.2	Excellent
60%	39.5	36.7	35.1	31.4	29.1	26.6	Good
50%	37.4	35.2	33.3	30.2	27.5	25.1	Fair
40%	35.5	33.8	31.6	28.7	26.6	23.8	Fair
20%	31.6	29.9	28.0	25.5	23.7	21.2	Poor
1%	22.6	22.7	20.8	19.3	18.1	16.4	Very poor

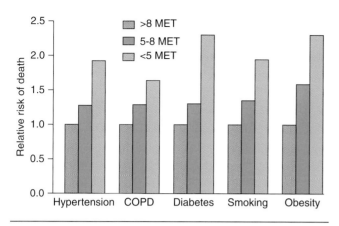

FIGURE 12.1 Relative risk of death by any cause in subjects with various risk factors who achieved aerobic capacities of <5 METs, 5-8 METs, or >8 METs. Data are based on 6213 patients of mean age = 59 years. *From Myers et al:* Exercise capacity and mortality among men referred for exercise testing, N Eng J Med Mar 14; *346(11):793-801, 2002.*

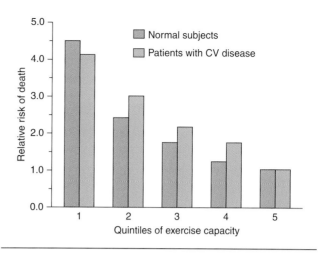

FIGURE 12.2 Age-adjusted risk of death from any cause by quintiles of exercise capacity in normal subjects or patients with cardiovascular disease. Subgroups with the highest exercise capacity (quintile #5) are the reference cohort in each. *From Myers et al:* Exercise capacity and mortality among men referred for exercise testing, N Eng J Med Mar 14; *346(11): 793-801, 2002.*

effects on $P_{A}O_2$. Not surprisingly, physicians as well as many professional athletes are personally aware of training approaches and pharmaceutical agents that affect aerobic capacity by their impact on C_aO_2 (see Chap. 13). It is important for both clinical and lay audiences to remember that increasing C_aO_2 may not in itself increase aerobic capacity. For example, the polycythemia from administering erythropoietin may increase blood viscosity to the point where $\dot{Q}_{max}$ decreases by Ohm's law. On the other hand, one benefit of consistent and prolonged aerobic training is the strengthening of respiratory muscles that collectively may improve P_AO_2 and/or P_aO_2 at any P_IO_2.

When considering factors that optimize $\dot{V}o_{2max}$ by lowering $C_{\bar{v}}O_2$, the primary variable governing maximal O_2 extraction is how low tissue Po_2 and pH can fall and thus how much $S_{\bar{v}}O_2$ can decrease. Generally $S_{\bar{v}}O_2$ is ~75% in resting subjects, but may decrease to 25% during heavy exercise, corresponding to $P_{\bar{v}}O_2$'s of ~40 mm Hg at rest and ~15 mm Hg during heavy exercise. It remains unclear why some athletes are able to sustain their tissues at a lower Po_2 and thereby achieve a

larger maximal $(C_aO_2 - C_{\bar{v}}O_2)$ difference. Some studies suggest that aerobic training enhances tissue capillarity, [myoglobin], the density or proximity of mitochondria to blood vessels, and even tissue tolerance to the acidemia that occurs with accumulation of lactate, which would permit a larger Bohr effect to occur precisely at the point of O_2 delivery.

Table 12.3 summarizes mean values for the key measured variables in the Fick equation during maximal exercise, including several beyond the scope of this book relating to $\dot{Q}_{max}$. As Table 12.3 shows, the decreases in maximal heart rate, stroke volume, and O_2 extraction all contribute to the age-related decline in $\dot{V}o_{2max}$, irrespective of changing body weight and fat content. When calculated in mL/kg/min, just being 30-40 years older is itself associated with a 40%-45% reduction in $\dot{V}o_{2max}$ among sedentary subjects, and a 25%-32% reduction in $\dot{V}o_{2max}$ among trained individuals. As illustrated in Fig. 12.3, a substantial portion of this decline relates directly to $\dot{Q}_{max}$.

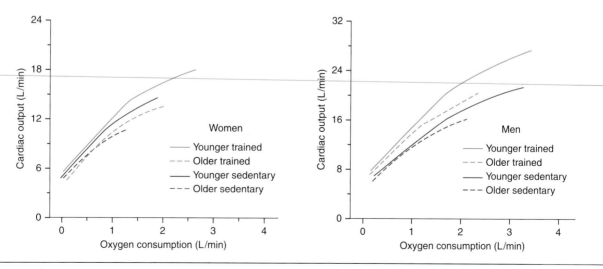

FIGURE 12.3 $\dot{Q}_{max}$ increases with aerobic training but decreases with age in both men and women. *Modified from the study by Ogawa et al:* Effects of aging, sex, and physical training on cardiovascular responses to exercise, Circulation Aug; *86(2):494-503, 1992.*

Table **12.3** Age, gender, and training effects on the Fick equation in maximal exercise

Parameter	Sedentary men		Trained men		Sedentary women		Trained women	
Age Group (yrs)	23-31	58-68	21-31	59-72	20-27	60-72	18-30	51-63
Height (cm)	177 (8)	177 (6)	180 (5)	173 (6)	165 (7)[b]	165 (8)[b]	167 (6)	165 (6)
Weight (kg)	75 (12)	83 (12)	68 (12)	66 (7)	58 (9)[b]	67 (15)[b]	55 (7)	59 (6)
Body fat (%)	17 (7)	29 (6)[a]	9 (3)	18 (4)[a]	22 (7)	36 (6)[ab]	17 (5)	25 (6)
$\dot{V}O_{2}max$ (L/min)	3.4 (.4)	2.2 (.3)[a]	4.4 (.5)	3.1 (.4)[a]	2.1 (.4)	1.5 (.2)	2.9 (.4)[b]	2.1 (.2)[ab]
$\dot{V}O_{2}max$ (mL/kg/min)	46 (6)	27 (5)[a]	64 (4)	48 (4)[a]	37 (4)	22 (3)[ab]	52 (3)[b]	35 (4)[ab]
$\dot{V}O_{2}max$ (mL/kg fat-free mass/min)	55 (6)	38 (5)[a]	70 (5)	58 (6)[a]	47 (5)[b]	35 (3)[a]	63 (5)[b]	49 (4)[b]
$\dot{Q}max$ (L/min)	21 (2)	16 (3)[a]	27 (3)	21 (2)[a]	15 (3)	12 (2)[ab]	18 (2)[b]	14 (2)[ab]
HRmax (beats/min)	185 (9)	163 (15)[a]	178 (6)	165 (9)[a]	189 (5)	162 (10)[a]	181 (9)	167 (9)[a]
SVmax (mL/beat)	115 (16)	101 (19)	154 (20)	124 (14)[a]	80 (12)	74 (8)[b]	102 (12)[b]	85 (9)[#]
$C_{a}O_{2} - C_{\bar{v}}O_{2}$ (mL/dL)	15 (1)	14 (1)a	16 (1)	15 (1)	14 (1)	12 (2)[b]	15 (1)	14 (1)

[a] $P <.05$ versus younger subjects of same sex and training.
[b] $P <.05$ versus men of same age and training status. Trained individuals exercised aerobically ≥3 times/week for ≥30 min/event during the preceding 3 years.

Values are means (± SD) for 110 subjects studied by Ogawa et al: Effects of aging, sex, and physical training on cardiovascular responses to exercise, Circulation Aug; 86(2):494-503, 1992.

A declining **stroke volume (SV)** accounts for nearly 50% of the age-related decreases in $\dot{V}O_{2max}$ and $\dot{Q}_{max}$, while increases in SV form a very substantial fraction of the increases in $\dot{Q}_{max}$ that occur with aerobic training (Fig. 12.4). Indeed as this figure shows, the increase in SV with aerobic training is just as impressive among the old as it is among the young. During a **stepwise exercise stress test** in which work intensity is increased every several minutes by adjusting treadmill speed and/or elevation, SV_{max} is achieved well before most subjects reach their $\dot{V}O_{2max}$.

The remaining age-related decreases in $\dot{Q}_{max}$ evident in Fig. 12.3 are best explained by reductions in a subject's **maximal heart rate, HR_{max}**. The often-applied formula to estimate this value in an aging population involves this simple calculation:

$$HR_{max} = 220 - (\text{subject's age in years})$$

By this rubric, a 70-year-old woman should expect her HR_{max} to be ~150 beats/min. What are the effects of aerobic training on HR and HR_{max}? First, the HR that is required to

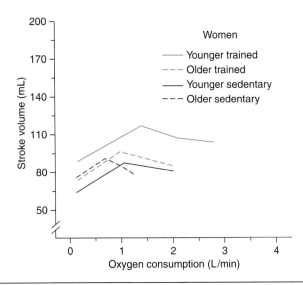
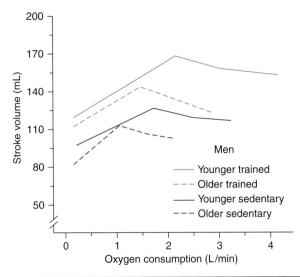

FIGURE 12.4 Changes in stroke volume account for most of the increases in $\dot{Q}_{max}$ that occur with aerobic training, as well as the decreases in $\dot{Q}_{max}$ that occur with normal aging. *Modified from the study by Ogawa et al: Effects of aging, sex, and physical training on cardiovascular responses to exercise, Circulation Aug; 86(2):494-503, 1992.*

sustain any submaximal level of $\dot{Q}$ decreases with training, due to the increase in SV that occurs (Fig. 12.4). This effect of aerobic training on HR should lead to an expanded aerobic capacity proportional to the increase in $\dot{Q}_{max}$ that the greater training-induced SV_{max} allows. Interestingly however, several studies have indicated that a subject's HR_{max} may actually decrease slightly with such aerobic training, perhaps by ~8-12 beats/ min between an elite-trained athlete and a sedentary subject of the same age. Postulated mechanisms for this reduction in HR_{max} with increasing aerobic fitness include both factors intrinsic to the heart (reduced β-adrenergic receptor density; altered sinoatrial node electrophysiology) and extrinsic to it (expanded plasma volume; altered baroreceptor sensitivity). Most experts in the field consider the matter unresolved at this time. In any case, this apparent depression in HR_{max} by endurance training is rapidly reversed when a person experiences detraining or extended bed rest.

When $\dot{V}o_{2max}$ and $\dot{Q}_{max}$ are normalized to fat-free mass, many of these age and training-related differences are reduced by 24%-47% (Table 12.3). However, these effects of age and training on $\dot{V}o_{2max}$, $\dot{Q}_{max}$, and SV_{max} at the peak of aerobic tolerance are not fully explained by differences in body composition alone. This conclusion indicates that there are probably a number of small, incremental improvements occurring at multiple points in the O_2 transport cascade (Chap. 1).

Given the focus of this book, to what extent does the respiratory system participate in training-induced increases in $\dot{V}o_{2max}$ or in its age-related declines? As Fig. 12.5 shows, O_2 extraction as estimated by the quantity $(C_aO_2 - C_{\bar{v}}O_2)$ continues to increase almost linearly with the intensity of a subject's aerobic work output. Furthermore, there are clear training and age-related effects on $(C_aO_2 - C_{\bar{v}}O_2)$ present for both men and women. However, such results do not in themselves indicate whether endurance training improves O_2 extraction by

increasing a subject's C_aO_2 or by decreasing $C_{\bar{v}}O_2$, or perhaps by affecting both.

As an earlier section of this chapter indicated, there are many clinical scenarios in which C_aO_2 or $C_{\bar{v}}O_2$ are affected. Some of these, like muscle [myoglobin], fiber type, oxidative capacity, and capillary geometry show training-induced effects that collectively allow $C_{\bar{v}}O_2$ to drift lower during peak aerobic activity among elite endurance athletes than the lowest $C_{\bar{v}}O_2$ reported from exercise testing of sedentary subjects.

As summarized above, the absolute value of C_aO_2 depends upon both hematological parameters like [Hb] and %Met-Hb (methemoglobin), and the lungs themselves. Among the key factors that determine P_AO_2 and P_aO_2 and thus C_aO_2 are: the ambient F_IO_2 and P_IO_2; the amount of physiological dead space ventilation $\dot{V}_D$; the severity of any $\dot{V}A/\dot{Q}$ mismatch and/or physiological shunt $\dot{Q}_S/\dot{Q}_T$; and the success of alveolar diffusion as dictated by alveolar surface area S_A and septal barrier thickness τ_s. Several studies have demonstrated that raising the F_IO_2 which elite athletes are breathing using a hyperoxic gas mixture increases their $\dot{V}o_{2max}$, whereas lowering their F_IO_2 with a hypoxic gas or altitude ascent decreases the $\dot{V}o_{2max}$ in such subjects (Fig. 12.6). However, sedentary individuals or subjects who exercise less do not show appreciable changes in their $\dot{V}o_{2max}$ over a similar range of inspired F_IO_2's, particularly if the exercise testing that is being used fails to increase their cardiac output toward a true maximal value.

Most significant for this discussion, there is no persuasive evidence that the alveolar parenchyma of the adult lung increases its area, or diminishes its barrier thickness, or otherwise responds directly to aerobic training. Indeed, neither absolute lung volumes nor respiratory muscle oxidative capacities are appreciably altered by endurance exercise. This finding is not particularly surprising for several reasons. First, anatomical constraints on thoracic dimensions in humans are

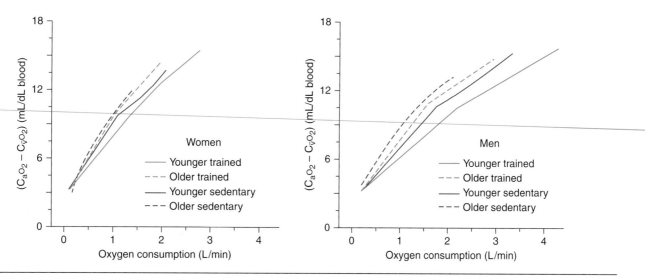

FIGURE 12.5 O_2 extraction defined as $(C_AO_2 - C_{\bar{v}}O_2)$ shows both training and age-related effects during progressively greater $\dot{V}o_2$'s. What cannot be deduced from these graphs alone is whether extraction increases due to higher values for C_aO_2 or lower values for $C_{\bar{v}}O_2$. *Modified from the study by Ogawa et al*: Effects of aging, sex, and physical training on cardiovascular responses to exercise, Circulation Aug; 86(2):494-503, 1992.

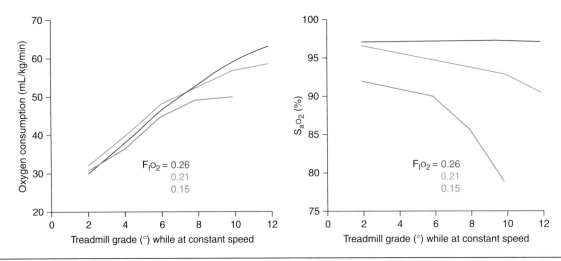

FIGURE 12.6 The ambient F_IO_2 to which elite athletes are exposed can dramatically affect their maximal O_2 consumption (left), here achieved by increasing treadmill grade stepwise every 2.5 minutes. Particularly when breathing hypoxic gas mixtures ($F_IO_2 = 0.15$), many such athletes will experience arterial deoxygenation (right) as the intensity of work increases. Sedentary individuals exposed to the same stepwise exercise test may fail to show such arterial deoxygenation if there are nonpulmonary limits to their performance. *Modified from the study by Ogawa et al: effects of aging, sex, and physical training on cardiovascular responses to exercise, Circulation Aug; 86(2):494-503, 1992.*

genetically determined, and will limit chest expansion by the second decade of life due to epiphyseal closure of the related skeletal elements that surround the lungs. Second, for the vast majority of sedentary or lightly trained individuals, whether non-obese or obese, the lung is already "overbuilt" for the usual aerobic demands of most whole-body exercises, even at what is their $\dot{V}O_{2max}$.

However, the lungs may be the limiting factor in very fit and perhaps genetically gifted endurance athletes whose $\dot{Q}_{max}$ is double that of sedentary individuals of the same age, and whose skeletal muscles optimize O_2 extraction. In several studies, 40%-50% of male and female endurance athletes develop **arterial deoxygenation** ($\downarrow \%S_aO_2$) with heavy exercise at sea level, termed **exercise-induced arterial hypoxemia (EIAH)**. During such EIAH, the $(A - a)P_O_2$ difference also increases, with values exceeding 25 mm Hg. Thus, as exercising athletes approach their $\dot{V}O_{2max}$, any previously unremarkable amounts of anatomical or physiological shunt, dead space ventilation, diffusional defect, or other limiting factor can emerge within their respiratory systems.

▶▶ CLINICAL CORRELATION 12.1

Mild EIAH at sea level is defined as $S_aO_2 = 93.0\%$-94.9%, moderate EIAH = 88.0%-92.9%, and severe EIAH as <88.0%. P_aO_2 is also an excellent marker for EIAH, with a value $\leq$80 mm Hg during sea level exercise defining EIAH, using a radial or brachial arterial sample. Pulse oximetry alone should not define EIAH due to excessive motion artifacts and the large error range. Blood temperature or T_B must be measured simultaneously since a 1°C rise in T_B increases the measured P_aO_2 and P_aCO_2 by 5-7 mm Hg, decreasing the estimated $(A - a)$ P_O_2 difference by 20%-30%. In other words, failing to correct data for the hyperthermia that often accompanies exercise will underestimate the true P_aO_2 and thus overestimate the true $(A - a)P_O_2$.

Effect of Detraining on Aerobic Capacity

Detraining reduces aerobic capacity through its effect on several components of the Fick equation (Fig. 12.7). The decline is noticeable within 12 days of ceasing aerobic exercise, and is predominantly attributable to decreases in SV_{max} and thus $\dot{Q}_{max}$. The reduction in SV_{max} is in turn due primarily to the reduction in total blood volume within 2 weeks of inactivity, most of that being the contraction of total plasma volume.

Effects of Prescribed Bed Rest on Aerobic Capacity

As Table 12.3 documents, cardiovascular capacity decreases with aging and thus leads to a decline in $\dot{V}O_{2max}$. Longitudinal data in Table 12.4 collected in the same patients over a span of 30 years shows that prolonged inactivity is as detrimental as aging itself to the cardiovascular system and $\dot{V}O_{2max}$. Here, 3 weeks of bed rest in men 20 years old caused a more profound deterioration of $\dot{V}O_{2max}$ than 30 years of aging. Thus, even the simple immobility of a postsurgical convalescence in a hospital ward can be quite detrimental to aerobic capacity. Therefore, physicians increasingly instruct their patients to resume exercise therapy as soon after surgery as practical. Note that this study clearly showed that aging affects maximal O_2 extraction (ie, $C_aO_2 - C_{\bar{v}}O_2$) more than $\dot{Q}_{max}$.

Effect of Genetics on Aerobic Trainability

While vigorous exercise training can enhance aerobic fitness regardless of genetic background, the limits on improving aerobic capacity are linked closely to natural endowment. When two similarly active individuals engage in the same exercise

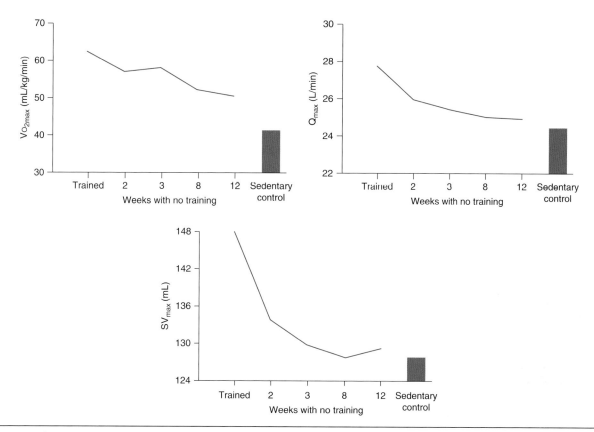

FIGURE 12.7 $\dot{V}O_{2max}$ declines significantly within 2-3 weeks of ceasing aerobic training, mostly due to reduced plasma volume, which decreases preload and so SV_{max}. *With permission from Coyle EF, et al: Time course of loss of adaptations after stopping prolonged intense endurance training, J Appl Phy. Dec 1;57(6):1857-1864, 1984.*

program, it is possible that one might show a tenfold greater improvement than the other. Research has indicated a genotypic dependency for much of this responsiveness to training. Identical twins generally show a very similar response to equivalent intensities of training (Fig. 12.8). When one identical twin is a low responder to an aerobic exercise training program, it is likely that the other twin will also be a low responder to the same training program.

Exercise Prescriptions to Improve Aerobic Capacity (#46)

To encourage physical fitness and reduce rising rates of mortality and morbidity, the ACSM and the **US Centers for Disease Control and Prevention (CDC)** have jointly issued public health recommendations stating that, "Every US adult should accumulate 30 minutes or more of moderate intensity physical

Table **12.4** **Effect of bed rest and aging using the Fick equation at maximal exercise**

Study Date	1966 (subjects 20 years old)		1996 (subjects 50 years old)
Variable at maximal exercise	*Baseline*	*After 3 wks bed rest*	*Baseline*
$\dot{V}O_{2max}$ (L/min)	3.3	2.4	2.9
METs	14.2	10.7	12.3
$\dot{Q}_{max}$ (L/min)	20	14.8	21.4
HR_{max} (beats/min)	193	197	181
SV_{max} (mL)	104	75	121
$C_aO_2 - C_vO_2$ (mL/dL)	16.2	16.4	13.8

Data from the cited study by McGuire et al. Circulation 104:1350-1357, 2001.

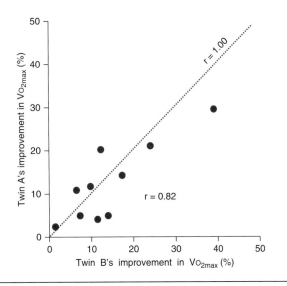

FIGURE 12.8 Effect of training on $\dot{V}o_{2max}$ among ten pairs of identical twins. In this study, 67% of the total variance in their percentage improvements in $\dot{V}o_{2max}$ can be attributed to genetic heritability $[(0.82)^2 = 0.67]$. *Adapted from Bouchard C et al: Aerobic performance in brothers, dizygotic and monozygotic twins, Med Sci Sports Exer Dec; 18(6): 639-646, 1986.*

activity on most, preferably all, days of the week" (Table 12.5, also modified from the **ACSM Guidelines Handbook**).

Recently, there has been considerable interest in whether aerobic capacity is improved by **interval training** that consists of brief, repeated, very intense bursts of exercise that are separated by recovery periods lasting several minutes. The acknowledged benefits of interval training include that it is a very potent stimulus for skeletal muscles to increase their oxidative capacity, and is highly time efficient for the subject versus more ponderous training at lower intensities. Interval training increases muscle carbohydrate stores, mitochondrial enzymes, muscle buffering capacity, and the percentage of highly oxidative **type IIa** muscle fibers. The disadvantage of interval training is that such workouts require high motivation and cause extreme fatigue. There is no convincing evidence that interval training has any greater impact on respiratory system components beyond their limited responsiveness to training as discussed above.

Table **12.5** CDC/ACSM aerobic training and muscular strength guidelines

Aerobic Activities	Muscle Strengthening Activities
For adults 18-65 years old: ≥30 min moderate intensity 5 days/week or ≥20 min vigorous intensity 3 days/week moderate = 3-6 METs; vigorous = >6 METs	8-10 strength exercises, 8-12 repetitions, at least 2 nonconsecutive days/week, using all major muscle groups
For adults >65 years old: Same duration/frequency as above but with moderate = 5-6 on a 10-point subjective scale vigorous = 7-8 on a 10-point subjective scale	8-10 strength exercises, 10-15 repetitions, at least 2 nonconsecutive days/week, with effort = 6-8 on a 10-point subjective scale

Suggested Readings

1. Thompson WR, Gordon NF, Pescatello LS, eds. *American College of Sports Medicine. Guidelines for Exercise Testing and Prescription*, 8th ed. Baltimore, MD: Lippincott Williams & Wilkins; 2009. *The gold standard of exercise testing and prescription for healthy and clinical populations.*

2. Myers J, Prakash M, Froelicher V, Do D, Partington S, Atwood JE. Exercise capacity and mortality among men referred for exercise testing. *N Engl J Med.* 2002;346:793-801. *A classic study demonstrating that aerobic capacity is more powerful in predicting mortality than other established risk factors for cardiovascular disease.*

3. Ogawa T, Spina RJ, Martin WH, et al. Effects of aging, sex, and physical training on cardiovascular responses to exercise.

Circulation. 1992;86:494-503. *As the graphs and table in this chapter emphasize, this was a definitive study in its day.*

4. McGuire DK, Levine BD, Williamson JW, et al. A 30-year follow-up of the Dallas bed rest and training study: I. Effect of age on the cardiovascular response to exercise. *Circulation.* 2001;104:1350-1357. *One of the few truly meaningful longitudinal studies on a cohort of aging athletes.*

5. Bouchard C, Lesage R, Lortie G, et al. Aerobic performance in brothers, dizygotic, and monozygotic twins. *Med Sci Sports Exer.* 1986;18:639-646. *Important reading for those interested in the "nature vs. nurture" argument as it pertains to aerobic fitness.*

CASE STUDIES AND PRACTICE PROBLEMS

CASE 12.1 A 23-year-old male college runner (weight = 70 kg) wishes to know his aerobic capacity. He does an exercise test to exhaustion in a lab on a treadmill. Calculate his O_2 delivery in L/min, his O_2 extraction in mL O_2/L, and his $\dot{V}O_{2max}$ in L/min and mL/kg/min, given the following data at the point of maximum exercise: HR = 190 beats/min; SV = 150 mL/beat; [Hb] = 145 g/L; % S_aO_2 = 96%; $S_{\bar{v}}O_2$ = 20%; O_2 binding capacity = 1.39 mL of O_2/g Hb; P_aO_2 = 90 mm Hg; $P_{\bar{v}}O_2$ = 20 mm Hg; P_B = 760 mm Hg.

CASE 12.2 A 45-year-old male patient (82 kg) has a peak exercise capacity of 10 METs. He breaks both femurs in a motor vehicle accident, and two leg casts are placed on him for 8 weeks. After the leg casts are removed, he begins rehabilitation therapy. Two weeks later, his $\dot{V}O_{2max}$ is again 8 METs. Which variable in the Fick equation is most responsible for the patient's decreased aerobic fitness?

a. Decreased stroke volume at maximal exercise
b. Increased heart rate at maximal exercise
c. Decreased O_2 extraction at maximal exercise
d. Increased O_2 extraction at maximal exercise
e. Decreased heart rate at maximal exercise

CASE 12.3 A sedentary 37-year-old man who is morbidly obese (BMI = 50 kg/m^2) wishes to understand the benefits of physical activity and exercise training on his health. Which of the following is the most relevant advice for this patient?

a. Aerobic capacity correlates with the relative risk of death.
b. Aerobic capacity does not influence the relative risk of death in patients with cardiovascular disease.
c. Aerobic exercise in morbidly obese patients causes exercise-induced arterial hypoxemia, and therefore is not recommended in these patients.
d. Aerobic capacity in an obese patient (mL/kg/min) is greatly reduced versus an age-matched, nonobese individual.

Solutions to Case Studies and Practice Problems

CASE 12.1

First, calculate the subject's **maximal cardiac output**:

$$\dot{Q}_{max} = HR_{max} \cdot SV_{max}$$
$$\dot{Q}_{max} = 190 \text{ beats/min} \cdot 150 \text{ mL/beat} = \textbf{28.5 L blood/min}$$

Second, calculate the subject's **maximal arterial blood O_2 concentration**:

$$[C_aO_2]_{max} = \{S_aO_2 \cdot [Hb] \cdot 1.39 \text{ mL } O_2/g \text{ Hb}\} + \{23.3 \text{ mL/L/atm} \cdot (P_aO_2/P_B)\}$$
$$[C_aO_2]_{max} = \{0.96 \cdot 145 \text{ g/L} \cdot 1.39\} + \{23.3 \cdot (90/760)\}$$
$$[C_aO_2]_{max} = (193.5 \text{ mL } O_2/L) + 2.8 \text{ mL } O_2/L = \textbf{196.3 mL } O_2\textbf{/L blood}$$

Third, calculate this subject's **maximal O_2 delivery**:

$$[O_2 \text{ delivery}]_{max} = Q_{max} \cdot C_aO_{2max}$$
$$[O_2 \text{ delivery}]_{max} = 28.5 \text{ L/min} \cdot 196.3 \text{ mL/L} = \textbf{5.59 L } O_2\textbf{/min}$$

Fourth, calculate the subject's **maximal mixed venous O_2 concentration**:

$$[C_{\bar{v}}O_2]_{max} = (S_{\bar{v}}O_2 \cdot [Hb] \cdot 1.39) + \{23.3 \text{ mL/L/atm} \cdot (P_{\bar{v}}O_2/P_B)\}$$
$$[C_{\bar{v}}O_2]_{max} = (0.20 \cdot 145 \text{ g/L} \cdot 1.39) + \{23.3 \cdot (20/760)\} = \textbf{40.9 mL } O_2\textbf{/L blood}$$

Fifth, calculate the subject's **maximal O_2 extraction**:

$$[C_aO_2 - C_{\bar{v}}O_2]_{max} = 196.3 - 40.9 = \textbf{155.4 mL } O_2\textbf{/L blood}$$

Sixth, calculate this subject's **aerobic capacity**:

$$\dot{V}O_{2max} = \dot{Q}_{max} \cdot (C_aO_2 - C_{\bar{v}}O_2)_{max}$$
$$\dot{V}O_{2max} = 28.5 \text{ L/min} \cdot (155.4 \text{ mL } O_2/L \text{ blood}) = \textbf{4.43 L } O_2\textbf{/min}$$
$$\dot{V}O_{2max} = 4.43/70 \text{ kg} = \textbf{63.3 mL } O_2\textbf{/kg/min}$$

CASE 12.2 The most correct answer is b.

A decrease in stroke volume at maximal exercise is the most consistent finding during bed rest and other forms of detraining. Consult Table 12.3 and Figs. 12.3 and 12.4 for more specifics based upon age and gender.

CASE 12.3 The most correct answer is d.

Aerobic capacity in the obese patient expressed in mL/kg/min is greatly reduced compared to the aerobic capacity of an age-matched individual who is not obese. *Answer a* is its opposite, and *answer b* is also incorrect because a higher aerobic capacity is protective with or without coexistent cardiovascular disease. *Answer c* is incorrect in that most morbidly obese patients have a normal P_aO_2 and S_aO_2 during exercise.

Chapter 13

Respiratory Responses to Extreme Environments

GERALD S. ZAVORSKY, PhD AND
ANDREW J. LECHNER, PhD

Learning Objectives

- The student will be able to describe the effects of cold, hot, and humid environments on the patterns of ventilation.

- The student will be able to define cardiovascular drift and the experimental approach that is used to measure it.

- The student will be able to enumerate changes in lung function after acute exposures to particulates, ozone, and other constituents of smog.

- The student will be able to identify the changes in arterial blood gases, hyperventilation, and red cell mass with acute or chronic high altitude exposure.

- The student will be able to explain the pulmonary physiology associated with breath-hold diving and deeper submersions using scuba gear.

Introduction to the Nomenclature of Biological Change

Lung tissues and the processes of respiration are stressed when exposed to the extreme environments that humans inhabit. Although detailed discussions of each such environment are beyond the scope of this book, there are general respiratory responses that reflect the system's adaptability over time, age, and level of aerobic capacity (Chap. 12). Situations that induce the most relevant adaptations include: cold, hot, and humid environments; regions with significant and persistent air pollution; short and long-term life at high altitude; and submersion under water using breath-holding or compressed air such as scuba diving gear. Each of these will be discussed here.

For clarity, this chapter recognizes three levels of organismal response to changing environmental conditions. **Acclimation** is a suite of responses induced in an organism by a single changed factor (like temperature, water supply, or light/dark cycle), usually in a laboratory setting where all other known variables are controlled. Periods of acclimation rarely last more than 2 months and involve individual organisms. For example, after spending a year living next to the airport you may barely hear its noise, but friends do not like to sleep over. Once you have moved away for a year, you will not sleep well at your old place either. Acclimations are transient and reversible.

Acclimatization is a more complex suite of responses by an organism to natural, multifactorial changes in the environment, perhaps encountered seasonally or when migrating across biomes. To achieve its full potential in the organism, acclimatization must optimize rapidly enough to yield benefits within one lifetime; fur density and lipid deposition only improve survival in the winter if they are in place by fall. Acclimatization usually involves at least a familial bloodline or other closely aligned group. Importantly too, larger groups undergoing acclimatization simultaneously have a higher likelihood of their changes enduring in the population. For example,

(#47)

families that bicycle or run regularly together often have similar body phenotypes. They are manipulating common pressure points within their similar genotypic backgrounds to affect more durable change within their own lifetimes. Any reader who owns animals in a temperate climate is familiar with their seasonal changes in girth, fur length, and breeding behaviors.

Knowing this, **adaptation** in a physiological sense is a durable response that has begun to integrate into the genome. Adaptation necessarily involves a population of organisms large enough to offer genotypic diversity to the selective pressures applied by an environment. In this sense of the word, adaptation is always at least partially genetic and inheritable. There are human groups that have lived at high altitudes (>3,500 m above sea level) in relative isolation for millennia. They share common physiques that differ from groups at sea level, such as greater chest circumference/height ratios, which their children show even if born and raised at sea level. Their erythropoietic responses to severe hypoxia differ from those of sea level natives. Indeed, hemoglobin diversity teaches some of the most interesting lessons in adaptive evolution for this reason.

Cardiopulmonary Function in Cold Environments

The severity of cold stress is determined by both ambient temperature and wind speed—what everyone appreciates as the "wind chill factor" in a weather report. Most heat is lost from the body while in the cold by **conduction**, that is, direct physical contact with colder substrates, and by **convection**, that is, heat transfer to colder substrates through the intervening air. Clearly, insulated clothing can limit most heat loss except from body surfaces like the face that are difficult to cover completely. Insufficient insulation while in the cold elevates $\dot{V}o_2$, a physiological response involving isometric contraction of voluntary muscles (**shivering thermogenesis**) and adrenergic stimulation of organs like brown adipose tissue (**non-shivering thermogenesis**). Thus $\dot{V}_E$ must increase.

Interestingly, simply inhaling cold air to meet an increased $\dot{V}o_2$ has few effects on whole-body heat exchange, until metabolism significantly increases $\dot{V}_E$. Pharyngeal and upper airway temperatures decrease, particularly when breathing extremely cold air, through the mouth. However, temperatures in the lower respiratory tract remain normal. Thus most pulmonary functions are unaffected by breathing cold air during exercise, although asthmatics may experience **bronchospasms** when doing so (Chap. 21). Individuals who experience bronchospasm from cold air can show a >15% reduction in FEV_1. The trigger for this hyperreactive airway response is unresolved. Older data implicated progressive water loss from the lower respiratory tract, but a 1999 study found that the amount of evaporative water loss did not correlate with severity of the obstructive response. Thus, dehydration of the lower respiratory tract does not appear to be the primary cause of cold-induced asthma.

If ambient cold reduces T_B, **aerobic capacity** also declines versus at 37°C. Most of the decline reflects the dependence of tissue metabolism on T_B, an effect more commonly observed in poikilothermic organisms with a labile T_B. Lower tissue temperatures reduce the maximal force achieved by muscle contractions, thus restraining both $\dot{Q}$ and power generated by voluntary muscles during exercise. Such **hypothermia** also increases HbO_2 affinity (Chap. 3), causing a leftward shift of the HbO_2 dissociation curve that promotes O_2 uptake in the lung but decreases O_2 release in the peripheral tissues. C_aO_2 is unaffected by cold stress or can increase slightly, while resting O_2 delivery ($= \dot{Q} \cdot C_aO_2$) increases to meet the needs of skeletal muscles that are shivering in the cold.

Such increases in resting $\dot{Q}$ and muscle metabolism during cold stress may reduce the work capacity of remaining body elements, proportionally to the metabolic cost of maintaining thermal equilibrium in the cold. As example, envision a male runner wearing only a singlet and shorts while doing hill repeats when ambient conditions are −5°C and 30 km/h wind. Heat lost from his exposed body parts (head, upper torso, arms, hands) stimulates shivering thermogenesis in those muscles, although they do little to propel him up the hill. The demand for additional blood flow to these non-running muscles reduces the amount of $\dot{Q}$ available to serve running muscles of the pelvis and legs. This runner is not likely to achieve his best times going up the hill because his leg power output is lower, although his $\dot{Q}_{max}$, aerobic capacity, and $\dot{V}_{Emax}$ are essentially the same as the day he ran last month when ambient conditions were 15°C and 5 km/h wind.

Repeated exposure to breathing cold air during a season of exercising outdoors will result in only limited acclimation, because individuals rarely spend more than a few hours per day in harsh ambient conditions before retreating to milder thermal conditions indoors. There is no persuasive evidence that the lungs acclimatize or adapt to prolonged life in the cold versus the substantial changes that take place in the integument, skeletal muscles, and adipose tissues during chronic cold exposure. In animals like rodents that are continuously exposed to the cold, the non-pulmonary organ responses can seasonally increase $\dot{V}o_{2max}$, as by non-shivering thermogenesis due to increased brown fat deposition. As discussed in Chap. 12, the lungs of such acclimatized animals are still less likely than the heart to be the rate-limiting step of aerobic capacity.

Cardiopulmonary Function in Hot and Humid Environments

When resting in hot, humid environments [$T_A \geq 30$°C; relative humidity (RH) $\geq 70\%$] for less than an hour, lung function in healthy individuals is not appreciably altered versus spirometric volumes and FEV_1 under more hospitable conditions (10°C $\leq$ $T_A \leq 25$°C; RH $\leq 50\%$). As noted for cold exposure however, hot and humid environments do affect key components of the **Fick equation** (see Chap. 12). Sub-maximal exercise in the heat for more than 15 minutes causes significant water loss by sweating and by fluid shifts from plasma to tissues. Any rise in T_B due to exercise or ambient thermal stress also redistributes blood flow away from working muscles to the skin for evaporative cooling. The progressive fall in plasma volume decreases ventricular preload and thus stroke volume (SV). This reduction in SV by thermal stress requires a compensatory rise in HR if $\dot{Q}_{max}$ is to be maintained (see Fig. 13.1). This increase in HR to compensate for the decreased SV that ensues during long-term heavy exercise is termed **cardiovascular drift**.

Not surprisingly, cardiovascular drift can be pronounced in the heat. Consider the runner again, now doing hill repeats when $T_A = 36$°C and RH = 75% with no breeze. He cannot expect to achieve a personal best time today either, not because of lost aerobic capacity. Rather, there is again reduced work output by his running muscles, whose blood flow is being diverted to skin for evaporative cooling. Recent studies suggest a dramatic effect on cardiovascular drift and aerobic capacity of exercising during extreme elevations of T_A. In a study by Lafrenz and colleagues (Fig. 13.1), the participants' HR, SV, and $\dot{Q}$ were measured after 45 minutes of strenuous cycling (60% of aerobic capacity) in either 22°C or in 35°C (RH = 40% in both). Despite adequate hydration in all athletes, T_B increased by 1°C in the 35°C group versus 0.5°C in the 22°C group by 45 minutes, and showed cardiovascular drifts of 11% versus 2%, respectively. A stepwise exercise stress test (Chap. 12) conducted immediately after cycling found that aerobic capacity fell 15% in the 35°C group versus 5% in the 22°C cohort (Fig. 13.1).

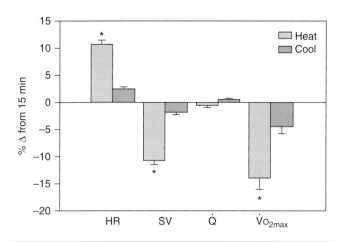

FIGURE 13.1 Changes in metabolic performance during 45 minutes of cycling exercise when ambient temperature was 22°C (cool) or 36°C (heat). Data are means ± standard deviations. *From LaFrenz AJ et al:* Effect of ambient temperature on cardiovascular drift and maximal oxygen uptake, Med Sci Sports Exer Jun; *40(6):1065-1071, 2008.*

Repetitive daily thermal stress induces heat acclimation, including an expansion of plasma volume by 5%-30% after prolonged intervals of heat exposure. When healthy persons were exposed to hot and dry conditions ($T_A = 50°C$, RH ≤20%) for 2 hours per day for up to 2 weeks, their onset of sweating began at a lower T_B versus their own pre-acclimated state, and their maximal sweat production ($mg/m^2/s$) was threefold higher. Indeed their resting T_B was 0.4°C lower after heat acclimation than before. As a result of this heat acclimation, their V_T, f, and $\dot{V}_E$ increased by 0.5 L/breath, 2 breaths/min, and 10 L/min, respectively, at an equivalent T_B. These acclimation-induced changes in respiratory dynamics were associated with a $P_{A}O_2$ increase of about 4-5 mm Hg. Thus, repetitively performing exercise in the heat leads to an increase in $\dot{V}_E$ commensurate with the enhanced rate of sweating when controlling for metabolic rate.

Respiratory Function and Environmental Pollutants

Periodic exposure to even low concentrations of **ozone** (0.2 ppm for 4 h/d × 2 d) can cause airway inflammation, leading to decreased FEV_1 and FVC because of increased airway resistance. However, there is apparently natural variability in this responsiveness to ozone and to other constituents of smog. In more reactive individuals, ozone appears to directly activate airway irritant receptors (Chap. 11), leading to bronchoconstriction and contraction of distal smooth muscle within alveolar ducts. Such reactions decrease spirometric volumes and may or may not be reversible. Acclimatization to breathing in an environment with chronically poor air quality is conceivable. However, it has not been systematically observed in human populations or adequately modeled in animal studies.

Lung function is also affected by airborne debris, even ultrafine particles <0.5 μm in diameter (Chap. 10). Fine particulates are generated by machinery such as sand blasters and

diesel engines, and can remain suspended for long periods of time. The amount deposited in upper and middle airways reflects the average $\dot{V}_E$ during exposure, and thus increases with even brief periods of exercise. In healthy adults, abruptly breathing moderately clean air containing just 20,000 particles/cm^3 can decrease FEV_1 by 11 mL and FEF_{25-75} by 50 mL/s. The **Environmental Protection Agency (EPA)** reported that air collected within 20-50 m of major highways contained 300,000 particles/cm^3. This was an amount 30-40 times higher than the EPA measured in parks or on lightly driven streets just a kilometer away. Thus, acute exposure to a large particulate burden can decrease a healthy person's FEV_1 by ~150 mL and FEF_{25-75} by 500 mL/s. In asthmatics, the risk of an adverse event from such exposure is greatly increased due to their hyper-reactive airways and enhanced susceptibility. Chronic exposure to air containing large particulate burdens causes lung injury similar to that noted with tobacco smoke and some occupational hazards. Whether human respiratory systems adapt over generations to poor air quality is an experiment in progress.

Lung Function at High Altitude

Hypobaric hypoxia (altitude) directly affects many parameters within the respiratory system. As discussed in Chap. 1, dry air contains 20.93% O_2, 0.03% CO_2, traces of helium (He) and argon (Ar), and 79.02% N_2. Partial pressures of these gases are proportional to their fractional concentrations by Dalton's law (Chap. 1). Because P_B decreases by half for every 5,500 m of elevation, the partial pressures of all atmospheric gases also diminish with altitude, leading to predictable reductions in both $P_{A}O_2$ and $P_{a}O_2$ (Table 13.1).

These unavoidable reductions in P_IO_2 at altitude eventually reduce Po_2 in the alveoli, arterial blood, and systemic capillaries. Decreasing P_B with altitude reduces $P_{A}O_2$ until O_2 becomes **diffusion-limited** rather than perfusion-limited (Chap. 9). Native populations in the Andes and Himalayas at the highest permanent habitations of about 5,000 m show physiological adaptations to altitude, both genetic and developmental. Mountaineering above this elevation, particularly by sea level natives, is usually possible only for short durations and carries with it considerable risk (Fig. 13.2).

Acute altitude exposure stimulates chemoreceptors in the aortic arch and carotid bodies within seconds of a reduced $P_{a}O_2$. Over the ensuing hours and days, $\dot{V}_E$ acclimatizes to a sustained higher level whose magnitude depends on elevation and P_IO_2. At the same time, the **acute hypoxic pressor response (AHPR)** quickly responds across the ventilated lung (Chap. 8) in an effort to maximize $P_{a}O_2$. However, the results of such AHPR activation will further decrease $P_{a}CO_2$ and increase pH_a, resulting in progressive **respiratory alkalosis** (pH >7.44; $P_{a}CO_2$ <40 mm Hg) (Table 13.2). Alkalosis causes an abrupt leftward shift in HbO_2 affinity that favors O_2 binding in the lung. However, the persistent tissue hypoxia that develops at moderate altitudes usually stimulates the increased synthesis of 2,3-DPG by erythrocytes that reverse

Table **13.1** **Expected arterial blood gases at various altitudes above sea level**[a]

Elevation		P_B	$P_{I_{O_2}}$	$P_{a_{O_2}}$	$P_{a_{CO_2}}$	$S_{a_{O_2}}$
(m)	(ft)	(mm Hg)	(mm Hg)	(mm Hg)	(mm Hg)	(%)
0	0	760	149	95	40	98
1,500	5,000	630	123	67	39	93
2,500	8,000	565	109	60	37	89
3,000	10,000	524	100	54	36	85
3,600	12,000	484	92	52	35	82
4,600	15,000	413	76	44	32	75
5,500	18,000	379	69	40	29	70
6,100	20,000	348	63	38	21	65
7,300	24,000	280	52	34	16	50
8,848	28,028[b]	253	43	28	8	70[b]

[a]For subjects at rest, most without acclimatization.
[b]The extreme alkalosis of climbers on the summit of Mt. Everest causes a large leftward shift of their HbO_2 dissociation curves in vivo.

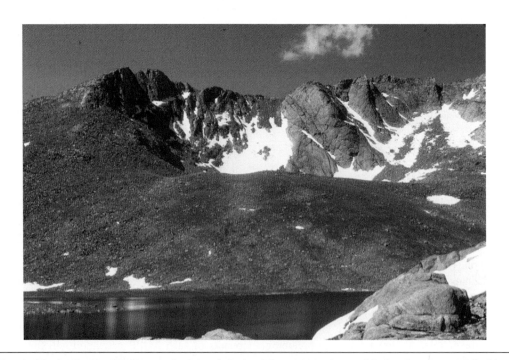

FIGURE 13.2 View looking southwest at **Mt. Evans** in the Colorado Rockies [elev. = 4,347 m (14,264 ft)] taken from Summit Lake [elev. 3,910 m (12,830 ft)]. Cars can use what is called the "World's highest paved road" to reach the peak, or passengers can join a select group of runners each summer who begin a 23-km road race to the summit from Echo Lake [elev. 3,230 m (10,600 ft)]. The current record pace for male finishers is 6:42/mile (6 minutes, 42 seconds per mile) set in 2008 by Matt Carpenter (a 10-time winner of the Pikes Peak Marathon), and for women is 8:24/mile, set in 2010 by Kim Dobson. To put these times in proper perspective, the previous women's pace record was 8:42/mile, set in 2008 by Naoko Takahasha, the gold-medal marathoner at the 2000 Sydney Olympics in 2:23:14 (it is still the women's Olympic record) and the first woman to break the 2:20 barrier for 26.2 miles, at the Berlin Marathon in 2001, setting a blistering pace of 5:20/mile. The take-home lesson is that even the fittest aerobic athletes can look slow at altitude.

Table **13.2** Respiration in a sea level resident exposed to 4,300 m for 2 weeks

Parameter	Sea Level	Day 1	Day 7	Day 14
$P_{A_{O_2}}$ (mm Hg)	105	46	51	55
$P_{A_{CO_2}}$ (mm Hg)	41	37	32	28
$\dot{V}_E$ (range, L/min)	8-10	9-11	11-12	12-13
pH_a	7.40	7.45	7.49	7.45
$S_{a_{O_2}}$ (%)	97	80	86	88

this left shift (Chap. 3). At even higher altitudes, the leftward shift predominates due to persistent alkalosis almost irrespectively of aerobic metabolism (Table 13.2).

Within several days of continuous high altitude exposure, this alkalotic pHa begins to normalize through compensatory renal HCO_3^- excretion (Chap. 9). There is evidence that the chemoreceptor sensitivity to hypoxia among sea level natives increases during acclimatization, making hyperventilation more likely even with moderate exertion. In contrast, populations of individuals who are born at altitude often have a **blunted ventilatory response** to hypoxia that may persist or be slowly normalized by prolonged residence at sea level. Mammals that are native to high altitude tend to have lower P_{50}'s than their sea level counterparts, good examples being the llamas and alpacas of the Andes, whose low P_{50}'s contrast with higher P_{50} values among other members of the Camelidae. These findings strongly suggest that a left-shifted HbO_2 dissociation curve is the favored evolutionary adaptation to persistent hypobaric hypoxia.

Another common feature of altitude acclimatization among sojourners from sea level is an increased hematocrit. Initially this finding reflects **hemoconcentration** of red cells by plasma extravasation through vessel walls, but it is followed within days by authentic **erythropoiesis** to increase total red blood cell mass. These responses appear to be driven by the initial drop in P_aO_2 that reduces renal oxygenation and thereby stimulates release of **erythropoietin (EPO)** by the kidneys. Elevations in plasma EPO are potent stimuli to myeloid tissues throughout the body, and the peripheral blood soon reflects increased reticulocyte counts as evidence of this erythropoiesis. The resulting **polycythemia** increases the O_2 carrying capacity of blood, usually by 3-6 g Hb/dL. However, actual O_2 delivery to systemic tissues at altitude may be confounded by both reduced oxygenation in the lungs, witnessed as a fall in S_aO_2 (Table 13.2), and by the increased blood viscosity that accompanies the rise in blood [Hb].

There is little persuasive evidence that polycythemia is a true adaptation to high altitude, since few animal species native to high altitude or long-standing human populations show it unless they are transported experimentally to even higher elevations. Stated differently, Sherpas of the Himalayas who routinely guide sojourners to the summit of Everest

(elev. 8,848 m) are rarely polycythemic at their native elevations of ~4,500 m, but even their hematocrit begins to increase by the time they reach South Base Camp I at the foot of the Khumbu Icefall (elev. 5,500 m).

Due to both the AHPR-induced pulmonary vasoconstriction and the effects of increased blood viscosity due to polycythemia, **pulmonary arterial hypertension** is a nearly invariant finding among sea level sojourners at altitude that dramatically increases the work requirements of the right heart. As was surveyed in Chap. 7 and will be discussed in Chap. 27, pulmonary hypertension in this setting can quickly lead to **high altitude pulmonary edema (HAPE)**, as well as hypertrophic remodeling of pulmonary blood vessel walls, and ultimately right heart failure (**cor pulmonale**).

▶▶CLINICAL CORRELATION 13.1

The mild to moderate interstitial edema that occurs at altitude resembles a low-grade permeability defect that has been noted during some forms of high intensity, maximal effort exercise. Fortunately perhaps, combining the stresses of heavy exercise and altitude does not consistently lead to a worse edema. In one study of elite athletes exercising while exposed to a P_IO_2 = 106 mm Hg for 4 hours, their 60%-70% prevalence of mild interstitial edema matched the rate in elite athletes doing maximal effort exercise at sea level [Zavorsky (2007)]. Although mild forms of pulmonary edema caused by intense exercise do not adversely affect pulmonary gas exchange or arterial blood gases [Zavorsky (2006)], which is usually not the case in HAPE.

Unless there is severe HAPE, pulmonary DL_{CO} increases at altitude because there are fewer O_2 molecules competing for binding sites on Hb. Typically carbon monoxide diffusion in the lung (DL_{CO}) increases by about 0.31% per mm Hg of decrease in P_IO_2: at 4,600 m of elevation (15,000 ft), the measured DL_{CO} is about 23% higher compared to values found in the same subjects at sea level. During continued exposure to high altitude, the DL_{CO} further increases due to the onset and persistence of polycythemia that expands the red cell conductance term detailed in the derivation of DL_{CO} pertaining to alveolar capillaries (Chap. 16).

Some spirometric indices are also directly affected at altitude. In one study, subjects were studied twice daily during an ascent from 2,800 m (mean $P_B = 551$ mm Hg) to 5,300 m (mean $P_B = 404$ mm Hg) during a period of 10-16 days. Measurements of their FVC, FEV_1, **peak expiratory flow rate (PEF)**, S_aO_2 by pulse oximetry, and **acute mountain sickness (AMS)** assessment scores were analyzed. When averaged for all climbers, FVC decreased by 4% at 2,800 m versus each subject's sea level values, and by 9% at 5,300 m, although their FEV_1 did not change with increasing altitude. Over the same interval, PEF increased with altitude by a mean of 9% at 2,800 m, and 16% at 5,300 m, both being smaller than the increases predicted from the change in atmospheric density. These declines in FVC may be due to reduced inspiratory force generation that effectively reduces TLC. Alternatively, subclinical pulmonary edema, or an increase in pulmonary capillary blood volume, or premature airway closure could also explain this reversible loss of FVC. The absence of correlation between severity of spirometric volume loss and either S_aO_2 or AMS may reflect that these measurements of pulmonary function are not sufficiently sensitive indicators of altitude-related disease.

Lung Function during Breath-hold Dives and When Using Scuba

Breath-hold diving allows many recreational swimmers to explore shallow areas of clear water. Even in a swimming pool the duration of a dive depends on the elapsed time until P_aCO_2 reaches a level that stimulates inhalation (Chap. 11). Duration also depends on a diver's TLC and RV. Trained breath-hold divers typically hyperventilate before submerging, employing a V_T that is nearly equal to vital capacity. After 10 seconds of such deep hyperventilation, P_aCO_2 can decline by 15-20 mm Hg while putting perhaps a liter of O_2 within the alveoli. With practice, as much as 650 mL of this O_2 can be consumed before P_aO_2 declines and P_aCO_2 rises sufficiently to stimulate breathing. There are risks to such hyperventilation before a breath-hold dive. First, reducing P_aCO_2 by hyperventilation causes alkalosis with unpredictable systemic consequences. Second, a rapid decline in P_aCO_2 reduces cerebral blood flow and can elicit vertigo or loss of consciousness even before the dive begins. With practice, breath-hold diving probably adjusts chemoreceptor sensitivity to tolerate alkalosis as well as a higher P_aCO_2, a lower pH_a and P_aO_2, or a higher [lactate] before breathing is stimulated.

Such respiratory system adaptations are common among marine mammals, and are augmented by a fully developed diving reflex (Chap. 39) that induces not just apnea but an abrupt bradycardia and profound vasoconstriction to all tissues except heart and brain. Some have suggested that respiration among Japan's **Ama pearl divers** has acclimatized or adapted to the daily repetitive dives that this population has performed over many centuries. However, more objective evidence indicates that these individuals rely instead on accrued cultural knowledge of how to economize energy expenditures during such dives. From a very young age, the Ama are taught to grasp a heavy rock to descend with less effort, to plug their nares and ear canals hands-free with balls of waxed fibers, and to coat their skin with animal fat that retards heat loss. The Ama also employ mostly shallow water dives, rarely to depths of more than 20 m and never approaching the impressively deep and prolonged dives of seals and whales.

Snorkeling with face mask and breathing tube facilitates diving farther from shore, but physiologically it resembles breath-hold diving. Some inventive practitioners of the sport have attempted to use a longer snorkeling tube, reasoning that they could submerge to greater depths for longer times. Unfortunately this logic fails for several reasons. First, inflating the lungs is more difficult at greater depth because of the increased trans-thoracic pressure exerted on the chest wall by the water (Table 13.3). The lungs, airways, and even the snorkel tube are prone to collapse as water depth increases. Second, adding airway resistance in the form of a longer "trachea" increases the work of breathing (Chap. 6). Third, a tube increases "anatomical" dead space, remembering that V_D is already ~2 mL/kg at the surface (Chap. 4). Thus, insufficient fresh air would enter the lungs through a long snorkel tube unless a subject's V_T is very large, and that would require enormous effort to expand the chest against the water pressure.

During submersion, gas pressures within any body cavities must continually equalize with the surrounding external hydrostatic pressure to prevent barotrauma. Air trapped within a nasal sinus or the middle ear by inflammation and mucus can create tissue injury and pain when compressed, even at shallow depths. Indeed, patients afflicted with poorly drained sinuses experience pain even with small changes in ambient pressure, like those felt in an airplane or elevator, or with approaching weather fronts. Fortunately for swimmers, the normally compliant chest wall allows for at least partial equilibration during submersion, compressing the air that is within the lungs when the dive begins (Table 13.3). Then as the breath-holding diver ascends toward the surface, air within lung spaces re-expands to its original volume, minus O_2 that was absorbed and displaced only with highly soluble CO_2. Not unexpectedly, many marine mammals tolerate extremely long and deep dives precisely because their entire respiratory system (including the trachea) readily accommodates compression by external water pressure.

A **self-contained underwater breathing apparatus (scuba)** permits much longer submersions and to greater water depths, but such gear creates new problems for the lungs and chest. As reviewed in Chap. 1, **Boyle's law** specifies that the volume of a gas varies inversely with its pressure. Water exerts one atmosphere of pressure (1 atm = 760 mm Hg $\cong$ 14.2 lbs/inch^2) for every 10 m of depth. The effects of these laws on actual lung volume during deep breath-hold diving are impressive (Table 13.3). For example, the lungs of a diver who inhales 5 L at the surface contain only 2.5 L of gas at a depth of 10 m, as lungs and trachea are compressed by water surrounding the thorax.

The challenges faced by the lungs of a scuba diver are complex. First, as they prepare for descent, air from their

Table **13.3** **Effect of water depth on pressure exerted on adjacent gas volumes**

Water Depth		Barometric Pressure		$P_{I_{O_2}}$	$P_{I_{N_2}}$	Lung Volume
(m)	(ft)	(atm)	(mm Hg)	(mm Hg)	(mm Hg)	(mL)
0	0	1	760	150	600	6,000
10	33	2	1,520	300	1,200	3,000
20	66	3	2,280	450	1,800	2,000
30	99	4	3,040	600	2,400	1,500
40	132	5	3,800	750	3,000	1,200
50	165	6	4,560	900	3,600	1,000
60	198	7	5,320	1,050	4,200	857
180	594	19	14,440	2,850	11,400	316

storage tank enters the face mask at a regulated manifold "head" pressure that only slightly exceeds the 1 atm of P_B at sea level. With descent this regulated manifold pressure must increase to prevent collapse of the mask against the face by the same water weight that would collapse the diver's chest, trachea, and lungs. Breathing in this manner resembles the use of **continuous positive airway pressure** (**CPAP**) masks to treat obstructive sleep apnea (Chap. 25) or intubation to apply **positive end-expiratory pressure** (**PEEP**) during mechanical ventilation (Chap. 30). Both strategies provide an **air stent** that maintains airway patency, albeit at much lower values of P_{AW} than would develop during scuba diving. The student should also recall the negative effect that high airway pressures have on alveolar blood flow (Chap. 7). At a moderate diving depth of 40 m (132 ft), the regulated manifold pressure must be at least 5 atm in order to stent the mask, airways, and thorax open (Table 13.3).

The manifold pressure at this dive depth presents the lungs with an effective $P_{I_{O_2}}$ of 750 mm Hg, equivalent to breathing pure O_2 at the surface. Prolonged exposure to such a high $P_{I_{O_2}}$ causes hyperoxic lung injury of the type that critical care physicians try to avoid by reducing a patient's $F_{I_{O_2}}$ in the ICU to the lowest value consistent with good oxygenation (Chap. 28). During ascent, a scuba diver who has maintained nearly sea-level lung volumes while under water by breathing pressurized air must stop inhaling and continuously exhale to expel the expanding gas in their lungs. Surfacing too quickly to allow pressure equilibration through the mouth and nose may rupture lung tissues and airways due to the force of gas re-expansion.

More subtle than this effect of scuba breathing on the gas-containing spaces within the lungs is the dissolution during the dive of inhaled air into body tissues, notably as O_2 and N_2 diffuse down their potentially enormous partial pressure gradients (Table 13.3). Because of its relatively low aqueous solubility, N_2 may continue to dissolve in tissues throughout a dive's duration. Thus, ascent after prolonged dives can cause **decompression sickness** (or the **bends**), as

dissolved tissue N_2 coalesces into bubbles throughout the body. Such bubbles continue to merge and enlarge as they enter the vascular system, where the risks of air emboli and tissue infarctions are high (Chap. 27). Decompression sickness is most commonly reported today among inexperienced divers. However, it also can occur in persons working underwater beneath an inverted bell (**caisson**) that is continuously ventilated with sufficient amounts of pressurized air to exclude water (Fig. 13.3). Indeed, decompression sickness was first identified in the medical literature as **caisson disease** for this reason.

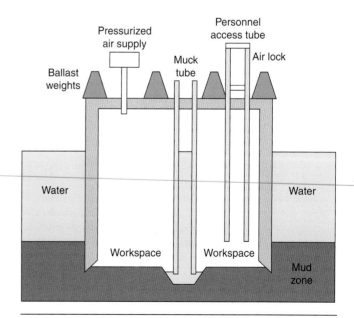

FIGURE 13.3 Schematic of a pneumatic caisson as used for underwater ship repair or construction of a bridge pier or dam. The internal air pressure needed to exclude water and keep a dry environment depends upon its working depth.

The potential severity of decompression sickness is such that scuba divers use depth tables and dive computers to limit both their time under pressure and their ascent speed. The effects of too rapid decompression range from joint pain and rashes to paralysis and death. When feasible, decompression sickness is treated by **hyperbaric oxygen therapy** in a **hyperbaric chamber** to maximize the partial pressure gradient that favors N_2 excretion. If treated early, there is a significantly greater likelihood of minimizing permanent injury. Mild interstitial edema is common in the respiratory parenchyma of decompression victims but it usually resolves within 2-3 hours of surfacing. Spirometric lung volumes and DL_{CO} have been reported to be normal within the same recovery period after dives to 65 m in depth that lasted 60-80 minutes.

▶▶CLINICAL CORRELATION 13.2

Nitrogen narcosis (also termed **inert gas narcosis**, **raptures of the deep**, **Martini effect**) is a reversible alteration in mental status that occurs while scuba diving at depth. This narcosis resembles alcohol intoxication or nitrous oxide inhalation, but impairment is not usually noticeable above 30 m (100 ft). The most dangerous aspects of nitrogen narcosis are impaired decision-making ability, loss of focus, poor judgment, failure at multi-tasking, and reduced musculoskeletal coordination. Affected divers complain of vertigo, exhaustion, and tingling or numbness of the lips, mouth and fingers, while their dive companions note exhilaration, giddiness, extreme anxiety, depression, or paranoia. While narcosis affects all divers, predicting the depth when impairment becomes serious is difficult; susceptibility varies from dive to dive and among individuals. The condition is reversed by ascent and appears to have no long-term effects.

Diving beyond 40 m (130 ft) is considered non-recreational, and carries very substantial risks for nitrogen narcosis, oxygen toxicity, and decompression sickness. Such deep dives require specialized gas manifold regulators, advanced conditioning and training, and comprehensive dive management by a medically qualified team at the surface. One important aspect of such specialist training is the use of various gas mixtures such as **heliox** that consist of O_2 blended with inert gases like helium instead of N_2 to reduce the total amount of dissolved gases in the tissues.

Suggested Readings

1. Gomes EC, Stone V, Florida-James G. Investigating performance and lung function in a hot, humid and ozone-polluted environment. *Eur J Appl Physiol.* 2010;110:199-205. *This paper describes acute effects of ozone and humidity on patient spirometry pre and post exercise.*

2. Lafrenz AJ, Wingo JE, Ganio MS, et al. Effect of ambient temperature on cardiovascular drift and maximal oxygen uptake. *Med Sci Sports Exer.* 2008;40:1065-1071. *As described in the text, these authors established a direct effect of exercise in the heat on aerobic capacity measured at the conclusion of submaximal cycling.*

3. Rundell KW, Slee JB, Caviston R, Hollenbach AM. Decreased lung function after inhalation of ultrafine and fine particulate matter during exercise is related to decreased total nitrate in exhaled breath condensate. *Inhal Toxicol.* 2008;20:1-9.

These authors demonstrated the importance of particulate concentrations on spirometric parameters.

4. McArdle WD, Katch FI, Katch VL. *Exercise Physiology: Energy, Nutrition and Human Performance*, 7th ed. Baltimore, MD: Lippincott Williams and Wilkins; 2010. *The text has excellent chapters on altitude, sport diving, thermal stress, and microgravity.*

5. Zavorsky GS. Evidence of pulmonary edema triggered by exercise in healthy humans and detected with various imaging techniques. *Acta Physiol Scand.* 2007;189:305-317.

6. Zavorsky GS, Saul L, Murias JM, et al. Pulmonary gas exchange does not worsen during repeat exercise in women. *Respir Physiol Neurobiol.* 2006;153:226-236.

CASE STUDIES AND PRACTICE PROBLEMS

CASE 13.1 One morning in mid-July around 8 am PDT, participants in the Badwater Ultramarathon start running at Badwater CA on the floor of Death Valley [elev. 86 m (260 ft) below sea level, the lowest point in North America]. The raceday high temperature at Badwater averages 45°C (113°F) with RH ≤3%. Registrants have 60 hours to traverse 217 km (135 miles) of open, unsheltered terrain before ending at Whitney Portal [elev. 2,548 m (8,300 ft)], the trailhead to Mt. Whitney where the average daytime high is 21°C (70°F) and RH ≅ 30%. A few participants continue up trail several more kilometers to the summit of Mt. Whitney, at 4,421 m (14,505 ft) the highest point in the 48 contiguous United States. Some of this group even turn around at the summit and run back to Badwater!

Contrast these runners' likeliest respiratory pattern 30 minutes before the race begins with their pattern at the race midpoint near Panamint Springs (115 km marker, elev. 585 m) and as they approach the finish at Portal.

CASE 13.2 A 20-year-old female vacationing in the Bahamas joins a charter boat of snorkelers and scuba enthusiasts to explore nearby coral reefs. She is a competent swimmer but has never swum in the ocean, worn a face mask, or used a breathing tube. What specific advice might the dive director on board provide to this woman to ensure that she has a safe and enjoyable experience?

Solutions to Case Studies and Practice Problems

CASE 13.1 Resting quietly, although expectantly, at the starting line exposes these race participants only to warm, dry air that should not affect their breathing aside from drying their nasal mucosa. As the race begins, they have their maximal available cardiac output devoted to running rather than cooling or shivering, and their deep, regular breaths should provide excellent arterial oxygenation.

Over the 115 km to Panamint Springs (72 miles) they will lose many liters of water as sweat and by evaporation from the lungs as they pant with rapid, shallow breaths. This water loss and contraction of their plasma volume will collectively result in a moderate increase in hematocrit but a reduced circulating blood volume, potentially compromising pulmonary diffusing capacity. Their T_B will have been elevated for hours, although many participants will hit this mark in the early morning of the following day.

Approaching Whitney Portal, their T_B should normalize but P_aO_2 will be approaching 60 mm Hg. At this level of arterial hypoxemia, S_aO_2 will be poised to plunge off the plateau of the HbO_2 dissociation curve if they are unable to sustain sufficient ventilatory effort. If they have maintained adequate hydration, they should have a nearly normal cardiac output devoted to their running muscles. Their ventilation/perfusion matching should be optimal, since at this elevation a mild hypoxic pressor response will provide enough hypertension to ensure perfusion of all available alveoli, even those apical regions that are presumptively in Zone 1.

CASE 13.2 The dive director must assess both swimming ability and sound judgment in a novice, and so would probably insist upon a series of observed performance tasks in this approximate order. Dive directors must always reserve the right to stop advancement if the participant fails a step, refuses to follow instructions, or appears disoriented for any reason. One possible sequence might be as shown below. **Self-Test: What is the director's key objective in each instruction?**

a. "Show me that you can swim on the surface and briefly below it."

b. "Show me that you can take a small mouthful of saltwater and expel it without getting nauseous or vomiting."

c. "Submerge your entire body no more than 1 m (3.28 ft) and hold your breath for as long as is comfortable; I will time you." Repeat until times stabilize.

d. "Submerge to 2 m if you can; I will time you." Repeat until times stabilize.

e. "Put on just your face mask and submerge again to 1 m. I will hold a message board under water; read it and repeat its content to me when you surface."

f. "Put the tube on your snorkel mask and swim shallowly while breathing through it. I will again ask you to repeat to me the message on this board."

g. "Submerge to 1 m with the face mask and tube on. Do not attempt breathing while the tube is below the surface. Repeat the message when you surface."

h. "Find a competent partner, practice for 10 minutes beside the boat, and then report back to me. Do not dive more deeply than 2 m."

i. "Good job. Have fun today but stay with your dive partner."

j. "Come back after a week of practice and we'll try the scuba tanks!"

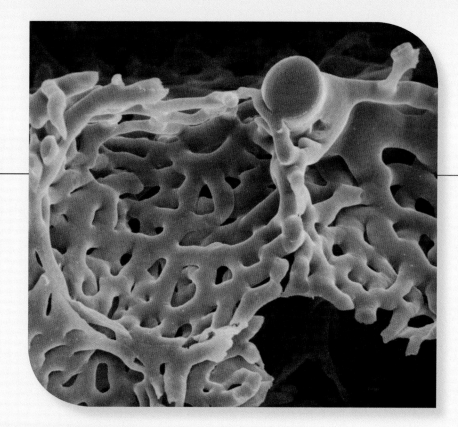

EVALUATING PATIENTS WITH RESPIRATORY DISEASES

Conduct and Interpretation of the Basic Chest Exam

WILLIAM C. MOOTZ, MD AND
GEORGE M. MATUSCHAK, MD

Introduction

Physical examination of the patient's chest adds valuable information to direct clinicians toward a correct diagnosis when symptoms suggest a lung disease or disorder. This chapter summarizes first the key elements of a basic chest exam, using the four modalities of **inspection, palpation, percussion,** and **auscultation.** It then gives guidance on interpreting those findings, using estimates of the discriminatory power of certain results, or their absence, by means of **positive likelihood ratios (+LR)** or **negative likelihood ratios (−LR).** It is important to note that students must practice the chest exam on standardized patients and real patients. Such practice should be augmented with breath sound simulators, a valuable way to become familiar with abnormal lung and adventitious sounds that standardized patients usually do not have.

General Considerations

Although this chapter focuses on the basic chest exam, assessing all vital signs is crucial in patients who present with symptoms that suggest a lung disease or disorder. Here, four modalities are discussed in succession. In practice, most physicians first evaluate the patient for any signs of respiratory distress including use of accessory muscles of respiration, then examine the posterior chest and lung fields using all four modalities, and finally examine the anterior chest wall and lung fields using all modalities. The posterior chest wall is best examined with the patient sitting erect on an exam table or hospital bed. Even frail, bedridden patients can generally be safely held in a sitting position by assistants, while the physician examines the posterior chest and lung fields. Some experts recommend examining the anterior chest wall with the patient sitting, while others prefer that the patient be supine for the anterior chest exam, so that a female patient's breasts may be gently displaced.

The lungs are nearly symmetrical structures, and except for the lower anterior chest wall where the heart intervenes, each side serves as a natural control to the other. Indeed, a proper chest exam carefully evaluates any side-to-side asymmetries. The exam should not be made through a hospital gown, since this can alter the findings of all four modalities. Physicians can learn to respect patient modesty while completing a thorough exam.

Inspection

There are four questions to be answered during the inspection phase of the chest exam:

1. Is the patient using the accessory muscles of respiration?

2. Is the trachea deviated from a midline position?

3. Are there any chest wall structural abnormalities such as kyphosis or scoliosis?

4. Is chest expansion of the two hemithoraces symmetric, or asymmetric?

Inspection of the Accessory Muscles
Method

Observe the patient's neck during several breathing cycles, especially the sternocleidomastoid and scalene muscles, noting whether these muscle groups are participating in inspiration. Under normal circumstances, patients do not manifest inspiratory contraction of the accessory muscles.

Interpretation

Use of accessory muscles is a sign of acute respiratory distress and/or significantly reduced pulmonary reserve, correlating with an FEV_1 <70% of predicted values. Hence, accessory muscle use is usually accompanied by an increased respiratory rate (ie, tachypnea). Even so, accessory muscle use is not specific to the type of underlying respiratory system disorder.

Inspection of Tracheal Position

Method

Using a ruler and the medial ends of the clavicles as reference points, determine whether the trachea is equidistant between the ends. If it is not midline, observe whether there is a visible neck mass.

Interpretation

Normal tracheal position is from exact midline up to 4 mm to the right of midline. A trachea even 1 mm to the left of the midline is left-deviated. A trachea that is more than 4 mm to the right of midline is right-deviated. Tracheal deviation is due to a neck mass, a superior mediastinal mass, or significant unilateral chest pathology. This differential diagnosis is resolved as follows. If there is no visible neck mass, proceed with completing the chest exam. If further exam demonstrates no major unilateral abnormality, then imaging studies of the superior mediastinum are indicated to confirm and delineate the process.

Inspection of Chest Expansion

Method #1

While standing behind the patient, the physician's hands are placed at the level of the patient's 10th ribs, with fingers pointed laterally and parallel to the ribs, and thumbs placed medially (Fig. 14.1). Then the physician's hands are slid medially to raise a small amount of loose skin between them, while keeping the thumbs 2-4 cm apart on the respective hemithoraces. The patient is instructed to take several deep breaths as the physician's thumbs are noted for symmetric or asymmetric movement.

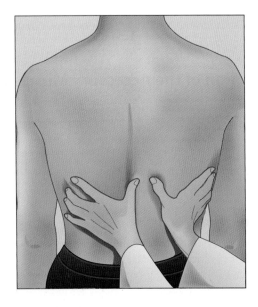

FIGURE 14.1 Proper hand placement to evaluate chest expansion when viewed posteriorly.

Method #2

While standing behind the patient who is looking straight ahead, the physician places her left and right hand on the patient's left and right lateral chest walls. The patient is instructed to take several deep breaths, while the physician observes both the motion of her hands and the force exerted on them by the patient's chest wall. Asymmetry in either the extent of hand movement, or the force exerted upon them, is an abnormal finding.

Interpretation

Asymmetric movement indicates a unilateral pathology on the side with less movement. Symmetric expansion has no diagnostic value, since it occurs in normal persons, patients with diffuse lung diseases, and many with unilateral pathologies. Thus this test is specific for unilateral pulmonary pathology, but it lacks sensitivity.

Palpation

There is one question being asked during palpation of the chest: Is **fremitus** in this patient symmetric?

Method

Fremitus, also called **tactile fremitus** or **vocal fremitus**, refers to vibrations produced by the patient's speech that are detected when the physician's hands are placed on the patient's chest wall. The examiner instructs the patient to repeat a brief expression, such as "ninety-nine", or "toy boat". As the patient complies, the examiner systematically surveys the chest wall for vibrations, always comparing one side to the other for evidence of asymmetry. For optimal detection of vibrations, some physicians use the ulnar surface of their hand or fifth digit, while others employ the palmer surface that overlies the distal end of metacarpal bones 2-5. Some clinicians test for fremitus using both hands simultaneously to compare the two sides, whereas others prefer a systematic survey of the chest wall with one hand. If using the one-handed technique, a sequential ladder pattern (Fig. 14.2) ensures that comparisons at each site are immediately preceded or followed by their mirror images from the opposite hemithorax.

Interpretation

There is considerable variation in the prominence of detected fremitus among healthy subjects and patients, and thus it is not a useful modality when comparing individuals. The method is more sensitive to lower-frequency vibrations than to those of higher frequency, and so fremitus tends to be more prominent in men than women. Diagnostically, physicians expect fremitus to be symmetric in an individual patient, and any detected asymmetry is an abnormal finding. An area of asymmetry is then evaluated to determine whether its fremitus is increased or decreased relative to a presumptively normal area

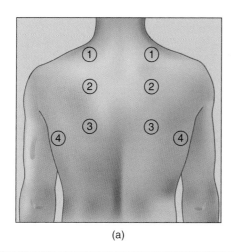 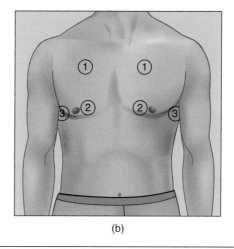

(a)   (b)

FIGURE 14.2 Posterior (a) and anterior (b) views of the single or paired hand positions to be completed in ascending numerical order when conducting palpation.

on the patient's other side. This distinction is best made by comparing the asymmetric regions to other adjoining regions. Decreased fremitus can occur in any disease that places a material other than normal lung against the inner chest wall, thus decreasing transmission of vibrations to the physician's hands. Thus, decreased fremitus is associated with an ipsilateral (same-side) **pneumothorax**, **pleural effusion**, pleural scarring, or tumor mass adjacent to the chest wall. Increased fremitus, in most cases, indicates the presence of the consolidation of **pneumonia**.

Percussion (#51)

Three questions need to be answered during the percussion phase of the chest exam:

1. Do all areas of the lung fields yield a resonant note?

2. Are the two hemidiaphragms at the same level?

3. Do both hemidiaphragms descend during inspiration?

Percussion of the Lung Fields

Method

There are two basic chest percussion techniques. The **direct method** of Auenbrugger, in 1761, was the first report of percussion as part of the physical exam. In this method, blows are struck directly on the surface of the patient's body. Most physicians today prefer the **indirect method** in which the examiner places a finger at the site to be percussed and then strikes that finger. The finger placed on the patient is the **pleximeter**, usually the third digit of the physician's nondominant hand, although some use the second digit. The palmar surface of the pleximeter finger is placed firmly and horizontally in the intercostal space, keeping the other four digits and hand off the patient. The pleximeter is struck at its distal interphalangeal (DIP) joint, using the third digit, or the second and third digits,

of the physician's dominant hand. The metacarpo-phalangeal (MCP) joints, the proximal interphalangeal (PIP) joints, and the DIP joints of the striking finger(s) are flexed to allow the fingertip(s) to strike the pleximeter. Nails on the striking fingers should be trimmed to avoid damaging the pleximeter finger.

It is critical that the physician use a consistent percussion technique to ensure reliable detection of unilateral abnormalities. Consistency includes the placement and pressure applied by the pleximeter finger, and the force used to strike the pleximeter once it is positioned. Students learning the percussion technique often fail to produce a resonant note that would be the normal finding over healthy lung fields. Rather than increasing the force of the strike, more consistent results are found by increasing the pressure being applied by the pleximeter before striking it. Only when this approach fails to produce a resonant note, should the force of the strike be increased.

To systematically percuss the posterior chest wall, the examiner stands to one side of the patient to facilitate placing the pleximeter finger in a consistently horizontal position relative to the intercostal spaces. While percussing the posterior chest, the patient's arms should be folded anteriorly to shift the scapulae laterally. As was recommended for palpation, the posterior wall of the thorax should be sequentially percussed using a ladder pattern (Fig. 14.3) to assure that attention is focused on comparing the two sides for symmetry of the notes produced. While examining the anterior chest wall, the patient's arms should be at their sides as the examiner again uses a ladder pattern.

Interpretation

Textbooks differ on the number of different types of percussion notes that may be encountered. Some authors distinguish only three types of note: tympany, resonance, and dullness; others add one or two notes to these, hyperresonance and/or flatness. **Tympany** is the normal note sound over the abdomen, especially the left upper quadrant. It is usually found in Traube's space, the most inferior region of the lower anterior chest wall, and represents the proximity of the stomach.

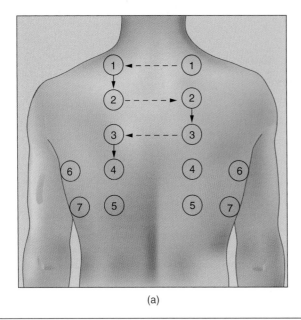
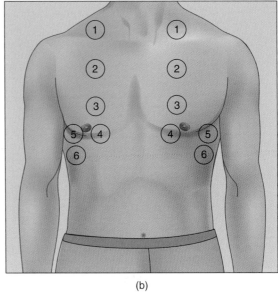

(a)   (b)

FIGURE 14.3 A recommended "ladder" sequence to be used for percussion of the posterior wall of the thorax (a) and anterior chest (b). Circles indicate approximate positions of the examiner's pleximeter finger.

Resonance is the normal note sound over the lung fields. **Dullness** is the normal note sound over the liver. Focal dullness in a lung field suggests one or both of two conditions: an underlying area of lung consolidation, that is, pneumonia (Chap. 35); or the presence of a pleural effusion (Chap. 29). For clinicians who include **flatness** as a percussion note type, it is the normal note over the anterior thigh. **Hyperresonance** generally is not considered a normal note sound over any part of the chest in health, but can be encountered in patients with COPD or a pneumothorax. Students will need experience before they develop confidence in distinguishing hyperresonance from resonance.

Percussion to Assess Position of the Hemidiaphragms

Method

The level of the hemidiaphragm for each side of the posterior chest wall is estimated as the position where a resonant note is replaced by a dull note while proceeding downward. Patients are asked to breathe normally to keep diaphragmatic excursions small, as the chest wall is being percussed at this stage to identify the level where note transition occurs. Those levels should be symmetric, or be no more than one intercostal space higher on the right side.

Interpretation

If the right hemidiaphragm is more than one intercostal space higher, or if the left hemidiaphragm is higher than the right, an explanation should be pursued. The two most likely causes for such an asymmetric finding are a unilateral pleural effusion and hemidiaphragmatic paralysis.

Percussion to Assess Respiratory Excursion of the Hemidiaphragms

Method

The pleximeter finger should be positioned at the highest level on each side at which a dull note has been produced. The patient is then instructed to take a deep breath and hold it, as percussion is repeated to identify the new highest level that produces a dull note and that difference is measured.

Interpretation

The new position for the transition between resonance and dullness is 5-6 cm lower in healthy adults as their diaphragms descend with deeper breaths. Patients with significant obstructive airway diseases and presumed resting hyperinflation may be expected to show minimal if any additional descent of their hemidiaphragms. However, this expectation is not consistently reflected by a significant LR, either positive or negative.

Auscultation

There are four questions to be asked during the auscultation phase of the chest exam:

1. Which type of breath sound is heard at this site?

2. What is the intensity of the breath sounds at this site?

3. Are there any adventitious (added) breath sounds present at this site?

4. Are there any sites manifesting abnormal voice transmission?

Method: Breath Sounds

In a quiet room, the patient is asked to breathe deeply, but with an open mouth, as the stethoscope diaphragm is pressed firmly against the skin to survey the anterior and posterior chest walls systematically with the sequential ladder pattern approach. At each site being auscultated, the physician should determine the type of breath sound present, its intensity, and whether there are any extra **adventitious breath sounds**. After completing auscultation of a patient's normal breath sounds, auscultation during vocalization is done if clinically warranted (see below).

Interpretation of Breath Sound Type

While three types of breath sounds have been described (vesicular, bronchovesicular, and bronchial) new students should learn two: vesicular and bronchial. **Vesicular breath sounds** are the normal breath sound heard over healthy lung fields. They are muted, low-pitched, and characterized by an inspiratory:expiratory (I:E) duration of about 3:1. This ratio occurs because expiratory sounds normally end well before the actual expiratory phase of respiration has ceased. **Bronchial breath sounds** are a normal finding only over the sternal manubrium. They are louder than bronchovesicular breath sounds, have a higher pitch, and their I:E is <1. Bronchial breath sounds also tend to be harsher than vesicular sounds, and are occasionally called tubular breath sounds by clinicians who consider their sound to resemble that of air passing through a tube.

Interpretation of Breath Sound Intensity

With practice, students can expand beyond a beginner's simple intensity dichotomy of "presence or absence" of sound to a standardized breath sound scoring system having five tiers. The most common scoring system applied to breath sounds is: absent (0 points); barely audible (1 point); faint but definitely heard (2 points); normal (3 points); and louder than normal (4 points). This five-tiered system is applied at six defined points on the patient's thorax: bilaterally on the upper anterior chest wall, bilaterally in the mid-axillary line, and bilaterally on the lower posterior chest wall. Thus, an aggregate score generated for the entire chest ranges from 0 points (breath sounds absent at all sites) to 24 points (breath sounds louder than normal at all sites), with normal being defined here as 18 points.

Interpretation of Adventitious Sounds

The abnormal breath sound most usually termed **crackles** (or **rales**) is a series of short (5-30 msec), discontinuous notes that have been likened to the sound produced by the pulling apart of strips of Velcro®, or the sound of longer hair strands being rubbed together. Some physicians distinguish two categories of such sounds: **fine crackles** that are more muted and higher-pitched than **coarse crackles**, which are louder, lower-pitched, and fewer per breath. Independent

evidence that these two levels of crackles differentially assist in the diagnosis of specific diseases is lacking. A different characteristic of crackles that does have diagnostic utility in certain situations is their inspiratory timing. **Early inspiratory crackles** do not persist into the second half of inspiration, and are more typical of obstructive airway diseases (Chap. 22). **Late inspiratory crackles** continue throughout the inspiratory phase and often suggest diseases of the lung parenchyma such as alveolar edema in heart failure or ARDS (Chap. 28).

A **wheeze** is a continuous adventitious sound that lasts much longer (~250 msec) than an individual crackle, is musical in quality, and often is high-pitched. Wheezes usually occur during expiration, but are sometimes present during both inspiration and expiration. They are a manifestation of narrowing in the smaller airways of the lung causing increased airflow resistance, signifying that a patient most likely has an obstructive airway disease such as COPD or **asthma**. However, absence of wheezing does not exclude either COPD or asthma, because most of these patients do not wheeze when their disease is well-controlled, or conversely when their airway obstruction is so severe such that little air movement is occurring.

The term rhonchus (plural: rhonchi) presents students with the challenge of interpreting an adventitious breath sound with a name that is not used consistently within the profession. As defined by the **American Thoracic Society**, rhonchi are continuous adventitious sounds lasting ~250 msec and are low-pitched in tone. Despite this definition, the term rhonchi is applied inconsistently even by experienced clinicians. It is therefore recommended that new students avoid the term, and instead classify all continuous sounds as either a high-pitch wheeze or a low-pitch wheeze.

Stridor is a continuous, loud, adventitious sound of constant pitch that is acoustically similar to a wheeze. Stridor is distinguished from wheeze by two criteria: (1) stridor is louder over the neck, while wheezes are louder over the chest wall; and (2) stridor occurs during inspiration while wheezes can occur throughout the respiratory cycle. Stridor is caused by high-grade obstruction of the upper airway, and represents a medical crisis. Physicians-in-training hearing what they believe is stridor should seek immediate assistance since the patient's airway may need to be secured emergently.

A **pleural rub** is a sound of variable intensity that suggests grating of the visceral and parietal pleural surfaces that normally slide silently against one another. Although some pleural rubs have phonic components that sound like crackles, the creaking or crackling of a rub is more often heard during inspiration than expiration. The presence of a pleural rub indicates the patient has a disease that involves inflammation of the pleurae.

Method: Voice Sound Transmission

When auscultating over normal lung fields, a patient's voice is muffled and unintelligible. Several terms have been introduced to signify abnormal voice transmission. **Bronchophony** indicates that voice sounds are louder than normal, whether or not they are intelligible. **Pectoriloquy** is used to indicate that words are intelligible by auscultation, and **whispered pectoriloquy** if intelligible even at very low spoken sound volume. **Egophony** is a change in the timbre of the vowel sound "EE", giving it a nasal quality that sounds more like "AA" or "AH". In the United States, egophony is often called an "E to A Change".

Interpretation

Abnormal voice transmission suggests that the patient has either pneumonic consolidation or a large-volume pleural effusion with compressive atelectasis. These two possibilities can be distinguished because consolidation increases tactile fremitus while a pleural effusion decreases fremitus except at the top of a large effusion where there may be a zone of increased fremitus. In many cases, altered voice sound transmission is accompanied by bronchial breath sounds, as both are caused by enhanced transmission of sounds from the central airways to the chest wall through consolidated lung.

Use of Likelihood Ratios in the Chest Exam

Likelihood ratios (LRs) that are calculated from a test's sensitivity and specificity allow the physician to quickly estimate to what extent, if any, the presence or absence of a particular clinical finding changes the probability that the patient suffers from a particular disease. A **positive likelihood ratio** (**+LR**) is equal to the proportion of patients known to have disease "XY" and exam result "AB" divided by the proportion of patients known not to have disease "XY" but who also have result "AB". A **negative likelihood ratio** (**−LR**) is equal to the proportion of patients known to have disease "XY" who lack result "AB", divided by the proportion of patients known not to have disease "XY" who also lack result "AB". LRs can range from zero (disease is excluded absolutely) to infinity (disease is confirmed absolutely). An LR value of 1 indicates that the result lacks any discriminatory power whatsoever to confirm or refute a particular diagnosis.

The LR system offers several advantages over test sensitivities and specificities alone, including ease of use (Fig. 14.4). With the nomogram shown, a physician applies a patient's exam result to strengthen or weaken the likelihood of a specific pretest diagnosis, by drawing a line that starts at the patient's pretest probability through the result's LR to establish the posttest probability. If such a nomogram is unavailable, acceptable approximations are that a +LR of 2, 5, or 10 for a result increases a pretest probability by 15%, 30%, or 45%, respectively. Conversely, a −LR of 0.5, 0.2, or 0.1 for a

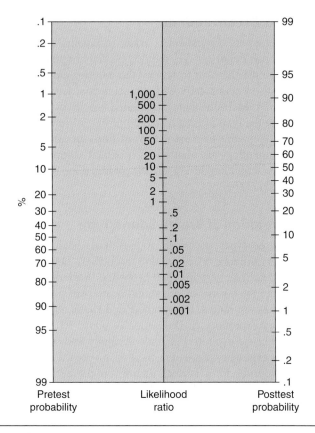

FIGURE 14.4 A standard nomogram of likelihood ratios (LR). The physician draws a straight line that begins with an estimated pretest probability of a patient diagnosis (left axis) through the LR ratio for the exam finding that is being conducted on the patient (center axis) to determine the posttest probability that the pretest diagnosis is correct. *Adapted from Haynes RB, Sackett DL, et al:* Clinical epidemiology: How to do clinical practice research, 3rd edition. *Philadelphia, PA: Lippincott Williams & Wilkins, 2005.*

result decreases a pretest probability by 15%, 30%, or 45%, respectively.

A second advantage is that an LR can be determined for exam results with graded outcomes, such as the scoring system for intensity of breath sounds that ranges from 0 to 24 and in which 18 is normal (as described above). When this sound intensity scoring system was studied for its suitability as a test for COPD, intensity scores ≤9 had a +LR = 10.2, scores of 10-12 had a +LR = 3.6, scores of 13-15 had a +LR not different from 1.0, and scores ≥16 had a + LR = 0.1. One important caveat is that the LRs for two different exam findings that may be associated with the same disease cannot necessarily be combined, since those two findings may not be independent of one another. For example, it might be tempting when evaluating a patient who has bronchial breath sounds and increased fremitus to use the posttest probability of one finding as the pretest probability for the second. This could mislead diagnosis because both findings have similar underlying pathophysiological causes. The only time it is completely safe to combine LRs is when they have been studied as a combination.

In the next section of this chapter, LR values of chest exam findings of use in certain clinical scenarios are presented.

Possible Findings in Patients with Specific Diseases

Community-Acquired Pneumonia in Adults

Several abnormalities may be noted in the chest exam of adults with community-acquired pneumonia (CAP), including increased fremitus, dullness to percussion, decreased breath sounds, bronchial breath sounds, crackles, and egophony (Chap. 35). However, none of these findings has high sensitivity, and thus their absence does not refute a provisional diagnosis of CAP. Three of these findings, when present, have useful positive likelihood ratios: dullness to percussion (+LR = 3.0), bronchial breath sounds (+LR = 3.3), and egophony (+LR = 4.1). To help clinicians improve the accuracy of bedside diagnosis of CAP, several scoring systems have been developed. A system developed by Heckerling and colleagues assigns one point for each of five possible findings: T_B >37.8°C; heart rate >100 beats/min; diminished breath sounds; crackles; and absence of asthma. A score of 4 or 5 in this system has a +LR = 8.2 for pneumonia, while a score of 0 or 1 has a +LR of 0.3. When diagnostic certainty is essential for a particular patient, such as a nurse stricken with CAP who wants to resume work among the elderly, the physician should order a chest x-ray for confirmation when the Heckerling score is ambiguous.

Chronic Obstructive Pulmonary Disease

Possible abnormal findings from the physical exam in patients with chronic obstructive pulmonary disease (COPD) include barrel chest from longstanding pulmonary hyperinflation, pursed lip breathing, use of accessory muscles, hyperresonance on percussion, decreased breath sound intensity, early inspiratory crackles, and wheezing. The clinical literature may confuse diagnosis, in part because of differences in patient populations and the presence or absence of superimposed acute exacerbations of COPD. However, certain points are consistent across

studies. First, the most useful information comes not from the chest exam, but the medical history. In patients without previously known airflow limitation, a smoking history of >40-pack-years has a +LR = 12 for COPD, while lifelong nonsmokers have a –LR = 0.16. Second, studies that focused specifically on the presence or absence of early inspiratory crackles found a +LR = 14.6 for that finding, while absence of early inspiratory crackles showed an unhelpful –LR not different from 1. Third, an auscultatory finding of decreased breath sounds is associated with high +LRs that can be conclusive, as summarized above. Given this challenging literature, it is worthwhile to remember that the definitive test for diseases with airflow limitation, namely spirometry, is safe, non-invasive, and readily available (Chap. 16).

Pulmonary Embolism

Experienced clinicians appreciate the difficulty in confirming or refuting a diagnosis of **pulmonary embolism** based only on patient history and physical exam. This is because no one finding or combination of findings from the chest exam makes the diagnosis with sufficient certainty to treat an often fatal disease with an effective, but potentially dangerous and lifelong course of anticoagulation (Chap 27). Thus, several structured scoring systems have been validated to estimate bedside pretest probability of PE. In the **Wells Pulmonary Embolism Score**, seven factors from the bedside evaluation are used to produce a numerical sum from 0 to 12.5, including current signs/symptoms of **deep venous thrombosis (DVT)** of the leg (3.0), no alternate diagnosis more likely (3.0), heart rate >100 beats/min (1.5), immobilization or surgery in past 4 weeks (1.5), past history of PE or DVT (1.5), hemoptysis (1.0), cancer treated in past 6 months (1.0). A Wells score places a patient into one of three pretest probability groups: low (0-1), moderate (2-6), or high (≥7). Clinicians often combine a Wells PE score with results of a D-dimer assay to decide whether the diagnosis of embolism may be safely rejected, or whether further testing is necessary.

Pleural Effusion

Physicians-in-training should remember that pleural effusion is not a final diagnosis, but the manifestation of many different diseases (Chaps. 19 and 29). While additional diagnostic work may identify the underlying pathophysiology, it remains valuable to assess quickly the presence and size of a pleural effusion. Abnormalities in the chest exam of patients with pleural effusions may include asymmetric chest expansion, decreased fremitus (but large effusions may have a narrow band of increased fremitus at the top of the effusion), dullness to percussion, decreased breath sounds, crackles, and pleural friction rubs. When present, two of these findings make the diagnosis very likely: dullness to percussion (+LR = 8.7); and asymmetric chest expansion (+LR = 8.1). The finding during a routine chest exam that most reduces the probability of a diagnosis of pleural effusion is the absence of decreased tactile fremitus, for which the –LR = 0.21.

Suggested Readings

1. Bickley LS, Szilagyi PG. *Bates' Guide to Physical Examination and History Taking,* 10th ed. Philadelphia, PA: Wolters Kluwer Health/Lippincott Williams & Wilkins; 2009. *A well illustrated student favorite. All students need such a guide to help them learn physical examination.*

2. McGee SR. *Evidence-based Physical Diagnosis,* 2nd ed. St. Louis: Saunders; 2007. *Brings the evidence together in one book.*

3. Simel DL, Rennie D, Keitz SA. *The Rational Clinical Examination-Evidence Based Clinical Diagnosis.* New York, NY: McGraw-Hill; 2009. *The application of likelihood ratios to the standard chest exam has been essential to managing health care and its costs/benefits analysis throughout contemporary medicine.*

CASE STUDIES AND PRACTICE PROBLEMS

CASE 14.1   A 67-year-old male presents to an acute care clinic complaining of 5 days of cough. He is a lifelong nonsmoker with no history of asthma, but worries that he has pneumonia. Physical exam reveals $T_B = 37.6°C$, HR = 88 beats/min, f = 20 breaths/min, and systemic BP = 136/84 mm Hg. The trachea is midline. Chest exam findings are the following: the trachea is midline; there is a normal chest wall and symmetric chest expansion; there is symmetric fremitus and resonance to percussion throughout the lung fields; vesicular breath sounds are present throughout the lung fields; no wheezes, crackles, or rubs are heard. The pretest probability for pneumonia in patients presenting with the complaint of cough is ~5%. Using the scoring system of Heckerling and colleagues, what is the probability that this patient has pneumonia?

   a. 3.5%

   b. 2.1%

   c. 1.3%

   d. 0.8%

   e. 0.2%

CASE 14.2   A 27-year-old male presents to the emergency room after the sudden onset of right-sided chest pain 1 hour ago. His pain is accompanied by acute, but not severe, dyspnea. He has had no cough with this illness and is on no medications. The pain is described as sharp, and is worse with each chest excursion. He has never been hospitalized, never had surgery, and has no history of cancer, deep venous thrombosis, pulmonary embolus, or current leg pain. He has smoked one pack of cigarettes per day for 12 years. His vital signs are: $T_B = 37.0°C$, HR = 96 beats/min, f = 28 breaths/min, and systemic BP = 142/86 mm Hg. His chest wall is normal to inspection but chest expansion is decreased on the right side. His trachea is deviated 2 mm to the left. Fremitus is symmetric except for the right upper anterior chest wall, where it is decreased. Percussion yields a resonant note throughout the lung fields. Vesicular breath sounds are heard throughout the lung fields, but are of decreased intensity at the right upper anterior chest wall. There are no crackles, wheezes, rubs, or stridor. Which of the following is the most likely diagnosis?

   a. Consolidation

   b. Pleural effusion

   c. Pleural scarring

   d. Pneumothorax

   e. Pulmonary embolism

Solutions to Case Studies and Practice Problems

CASE 14.1   The most correct answer is b, 2.1%.

This patient's Heckerling score is 1 (see Community-Acquired Pneumonia in Adults earlier in the chapter). In this scoring system, a score of 0-1 has a +LR = 0.3. While students may think that this should be considered a –LR because it is < 1, the use of a multitiered scoring system dictates that all LRs are expressed as positive numbers. Using the nomogram in Fig. 14.4, the posttest probability is read as ~2.1%.

CASE 14.2   The most correct answer is d, pneumothorax.

Significant findings in this case include decreased right side chest expansion, tracheal deviation to the left, and decreased fremitus and decreased breath sounds on the right upper anterior chest wall.

Importantly, the percussion note at that site is resonant. Consolidation does not usually cause tracheal deviation and it would be expected to yield a dull percussion note, rather than a resonant one, as would pleural effusion and pleural scarring. Pneumothorax causes decreased fremitus and decreased breath sounds, while yielding a percussion note that is resonant, or hyper-resonant. Tracheal deviation to the contralateral side is also a feature of pneumothorax, even in those who have not developed intrathoracic tension. Primary spontaneous pneumothorax is typically a condition noted in young male smokers, as is this patient. While sudden onset of chest pain and dyspnea should always cause a clinician to consider pulmonary embolism, this patient has a Wells Pulmonary Embolism Score of 0 (see Pulmonary Embolism earlier in the chapter).

Chapter 15

Interpreting Chest X-Rays, CT Scans, and MRIs

ASHUTOSH SACHDEVA, MD AND
GEORGE M. MATUSCHAK, MD

Learning Objectives

- The student will be able to describe basic chest radiographic patterns and identify normal contours created by the boundary of intrathoracic structures with aerated lung tissue.

- The student will be able to recognize common abnormal radiographic patterns and be able to localize lung pathology and gather clinical information from the radiographs.

- The student will be able to identify the basic anatomical unit of lung structure and how different diseases variably affect these structures on chest CT scans.

- The student will be able to apply knowledge of chest x-rays and CT scans to assist in the diagnostic interpretation of clinical cases.

Introduction

Imaging the chest with radiographs (x-rays) and computed tomography (CT) is an integral part of the diagnostic work-up of patients with symptoms of respiratory disease. The natural contrast of aerated pulmonary tissue provides a window into the body allowing for x-ray and CT evaluation of diseases involving the lungs, tracheobronchial tree, and pleura, as well as the thoracic lymph nodes, thoracic skeleton and chest wall, heart, esophagus, and upper abdomen. For chest x-rays in particular, it is important to understand fundamental aspects of image acquisition and the technical factors that can limit the utility of the resulting studies and interpretation of their findings. Simplistically, radiography uses ionizing x-ray radiation to generate a film image. Interactions of the x-rays with the targeted matter and the subsequent fate of x-ray photons collectively determine the generation of an image, whose characteristics will vary according to whether the radiation is completely absorbed, transmitted unchanged through the patient, or scattered within the body (Fig. 15.1).

Normal anatomical features of the respiratory system, as well as pathologies of the lungs and cardiothoracic system are visualized by the interplay among seven different **radiographic densities** (Fig 15.1): air, fat, soft tissue (eg, muscle vs blood or fluid), calcium, x-ray contrast media, and metal ($\cong$ dense bone). Discrimination among these features is accomplished because of differential absorption of radiation by various normal or diseased tissues that ultimately results in the creation of radiographic images. Of note, an intra-thoracic structure is best rendered visible by the juxtaposition of two different radiographic densities. Moreover, it is necessary for the x-ray beam to tangentially strike the interface between tissues of different density in order to appear as a well-defined boundary line on chest radiographs. Because diseases of the respiratory system often result in differential x-ray absorption, both the absence of a normal **radiographic interface** and the presence of an unexpected interface are valuable clues to underlying pathological changes.

By convention, the routine frontal chest x-ray view is taken in the radiological suite with the patient upright and during full inspiration. In this view the x-ray beam is horizontal to the patient, and the x-ray tube is ~2 m from the film detector as the beam traverses the patient from a **posterior to anterior (PA)** direction or view. This distance used in acquiring the PA view reduces unnecessary magnification and enhances sharpness as does the close apposition of the chest and the film. In contrast, it is frequently necessary in hospitalized and critically ill patients to obtain portable chest x-ray images at the bedside, which are performed using an **anteroposterior (AP)** direction or view. Such AP films involve less powerful radiation energy and a shorter x-ray tube-to-film distance, resulting in greater magnification but reduced anatomical resolution.

Using only the PA view, it is often difficult to detect chest lesions located behind the heart, near the mediastinum, or near the hemidiaphragms because these are radiographically denser structures with poor interfaces. For this reason, the **lateral chest x-ray view** is also performed to pinpoint such lesions three-dimensionally and localize them within the lungs. The lateral view is routinely taken with the left side of the patient against the film cassette.

Interpretation of Chest X-Rays

A **systematic approach** is essential for evaluating the normal anatomy of the lungs and thorax, and for recognizing the basic patterns of respiratory diseases. Such an approach minimizes diagnostic errors while guiding additional studies to achieve the correct diagnosis in a given patient.

#53

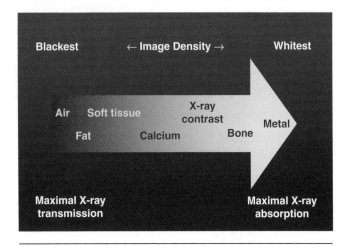

FIGURE 15.1 Schematic of the relative visual densities of biological structures visualized by standard x-ray imaging intensities.

In reviewing chest x-ray images, it is important to simultaneously assess the quality of the study with respect to technical aspects including film exposure, since overexposure will decrease and underexposure will increase radiographic densities. Attention should also be paid to the positioning of the patient and the degree of the inspiratory effort at the instant of image capture.

The keys to successful reading of chest x-rays well are a sound understanding of normal anatomy and an orderly search pattern. The following structures are easily recognized on a PA and lateral film and should be recognized on every examination. The arrows on Figs. 15.2 and 15.3 correspond to the numbered descriptions below, respectively.

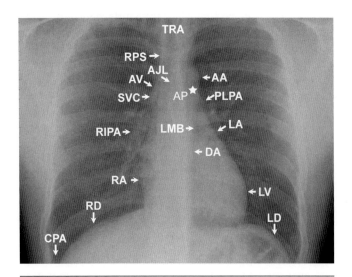

FIGURE 15.2 A standard AP x-ray film of the chest; see the text for the anatomical landmarks noted by their most common abbreviations here. Students should appreciate that not each structure will be readily identified in every film examined.

Common Landmarks on Frontal (PA or AP) Chest Radiographs

1. The **aortic arch** (**AA**) normally dominates the left superior cardiomediastinal contour of the patient, although it may form part of the right cardiomediastinal contour in older individuals.
2. The left lateral wall of the **descending aorta** (**DA**) is usually visible as it courses inferiorly through the thorax.
3. The **proximal left pulmonary artery** (**PLPA**) is visible in the left hilar region just inferior to the aortic arch. When visualized, the **left interlobar pulmonary artery** (**LIPA**) is noted to be inferior and lateral to PLPA.
4. The **aorto-pulmonary** window is the concavity created by the overlap of the aortic arch and the left pulmonary artery shadow.
5. The **left mainstem bronchus** (**LMB**) is often seen on frontal views just below the main pulmonary artery segment and the left pulmonary artery.
6. The appendage of the **left atrium** (**LA**) projects slightly inferior to the left mainstem bronchus and along the left cardiomediastinal contour. The **left ventricle** (**LV**) completes the rest of the left cardiomediastinal contour.
7. The **superior vena cava** (**SVC**) is seen in the most superior portion of the patient's right cardiomediastinal contour.
8. The **right paratracheal stripe** (**RPS**) is the soft tissue stripe created by the interface of the right lateral tracheal wall and right upper lobe. Near the inferior RPS in the right tracheobronchial angle the **azygos vein** (**AV**) may be seen.
9. The **right interlobar pulmonary artery** (**RIPA**) exits through the right hilum inferiorly and laterally and is the predominant shadow in this region.
10. The **right atrium** (**RA**) forms the right cardiac border, and occasionally coursing through the cardiophrenic angle between the heart and the right diaphragm is the shadow representing the **inferior vena cava** (**IVC**).
11. The **trachea** (**TRA**) is usually easily seen on PA or AP (frontal) radiographs.
12. The **right diaphragm** (**RD**) and **left diaphragm** (**LD**) contours are clearly visible.
13. The **costophrenic angle** (**CPA**) is visible in the lower left portion of the thorax.
14. The **anterior junction line** (**AJL**) may be seen as an obliquely oriented line overlying the mediastinum representing points of contact between the two lungs.

Role of the Lateral Chest Radiograph

The lateral radiograph complements frontal images. Here students should focus on recognizing the normal anatomical shadowing and understand structural relationships.

Common Landmarks on Lateral Chest Radiographs

1. The **retrosternal space (RS)** is the clear region anterior to, and just beneath, the sternum. This space is decreased with enlargement of the right ventricle during conditions that result in **pulmonary hypertension (PHT)**.
2. The **TRA** is again easily visualized as in the frontal view.
3. The bronchial orifice of the **right upper lobe (RUL)** appears as a circular lucency that projects over the continuation of the tracheal air column.
4. The posterior wall of the bronchus intermedius is represented by the soft tissue stripe just below the orifice of the right upper lobe bronchus.
5. The **left pulmonary artery (LPA)** appears as a structure having soft tissue density that courses over the bronchus of the **left upper lobe (LUL)**.
6. The **right pulmonary artery (RPA)** is visible as a rounded soft tissue density. It is anterior and inferior to the orifice of the RUL bronchus (#3 above).
7. The **infrahilar window (IH**, at the ✱ in Fig. 15.3) is seen just beneath the RPA; normally, this area is clear and contains only vessels and bronchi. Therefore, unexpected contouring may represent pathological adenopathy or a lung mass.
8. The **left atrium (LA)** is visible along the postero-superior aspect of the cardiac contour and just below the RPA. One or more **pulmonary veins (PVs)** may be seen as tubular or nodular soft tissue densities projecting over this region.
9. The **LV** forms the posteroinferior cardiac contour.
10. The **right ventricle (RV)** comprises the anterior and superior portions of the cardiac contour on lateral x-rays. The RV contour is rarely visible on AP x-rays.

11. One or both **posterior costophrenic angles (PCPA)** are visible inferiorly.
12. The RD and LD contours are visible inferiorly.

▶▶ CLINICAL CORRELATION 15.1

Additional radiographic projections may be used in the chest x-ray evaluation of patients with diseases of the respiratory system. For example, **lateral decubitus views** obtained with the patients lying on their right side, left side, or both sides in sequence are helpful in distinguishing **pleural effusions** from underlying lung consolidation. If effusions are present, such decubitus views help determine whether they are loculated or free-flowing, and thereby amenable to thoracentesis (Chaps. 19 and 29). Lateral decubitus views are also useful in evaluating the possible presence of a **pneumothorax**, as are frontal films taken in full expiration. Classically, frontal **lordotic x-rays** of the chest taken with the patient leaning backward were used in evaluating opacities in the apices of the lungs. However, the wide availability of chest CT scans has now largely supplanted this latter imaging strategy.

Lung Anatomy and the Localization of Pulmonary Disease   (#54)

Knowledge of lobar and segmental lung anatomy is indispensible for understanding patterns of lung disease and parenchymal collapse (**atelectasis**). Application of this knowledge during review of a chest radiograph is furthermore important in planning additional diagnostic and therapeutic procedures, such as bronchoscopy, surgery, or radiation therapy. In this context, one of the most commonly recognized and helpful radiological signs during review of chest x-rays is the **silhouette sign** (loss of normal interface). Under normal conditions a distinct boundary is seen when aerated lung contacts a structure of different radiographic density such as the heart, mediastinum, or diaphragm through the creation of an interface as defined above (Fig. 15.4).

However, diseases of the respiratory system often feature replacement of air in the alveolar spaces with inflammatory cells, pus, blood, or edema fluid that singly or combined, result in **consolidated lung** tissue. When such consolidated lung is adjacent to soft tissues that have similar soft tissue/water density such as that of the heart or mediastinum, the normal interface created by aerated lung is lost. This loss of normal air-water radiographic density interface is termed the **silhouette sign** (Fig.15.5).

Detecting Air in the Pleural Space—Pneumothorax

Abnormal presence of air in the pleural space, or **pneumothorax**, is generally manifested radiologically as unilateral, darker homogeneous shadowing outside the zone of vascular lung

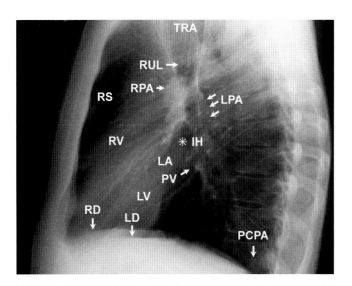

FIGURE 15.3 Typical lateral chest x-ray, taken from the patient's left side. See the text for anatomical landmarks noted by their common abbreviations here.

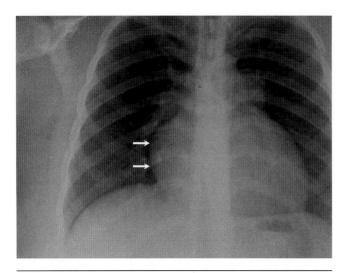

FIGURE 15.4   The normally prominent interface between the right atrium (arrows) and right middle lobe lung tissue is evident in this AP x-ray. Note the prominent acute angles formed by interfaces of aerated parenchyma with the left and right hemidiaphragms. Students will also learn to appreciate the prominent pulmonary vasculature with bulging right atrial shadow as seen in this patient with pulmonary hypertension.

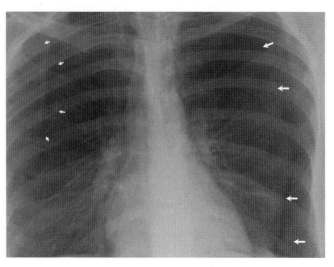

FIGURE 15.6   Left-side spontaneous pneumothorax (large white arrows) in a patient with preexisting bilateral bullae, seen here with sharply demarcated areas of emphysematous lung (small white arrows mar the fine whitish lines of the bullae edges). Note the continuity of the visceral pleural line on the left side in contrast to the irregular bullae.

markings on a frontal chest x-ray (Fig. 15.6). Pneumothorax can occur spontaneously after rupture of a visceral pleural bleb or following invasive procedures such as **thoracentesis** that puncture the visceral pleura and cause an air leak (Chaps. 19 and 37). Placing the patient in an erect position to obtain PA or AP frontal views is ideal to diagnose a pneumothorax, although this condition can also be detected by a lateral decubitus film when taken with the presumed affected side facing upward.

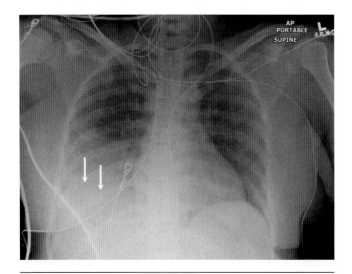

FIGURE 15.5   The white arrows in this AP x-ray indicate a right-sided silhouette sign caused by loss of visualization of the right diaphragmatic contour due to adjacent consolidated lung in the right lower lobe. Compare this interface with the prominent right costophrenic angle visible in Fig. 15.4.

▶▶ **CLINICAL CORRELATION 15.2**

It is critical to promptly recognize a pneumothorax on chest x-rays of hospitalized patients receiving positive-pressure ventilation, or in acutely traumatized patients requiring emergent operation for their injuries who are about to receive mechanical ventilatory assistance. Pneumothorax under these conditions of superimposed positive-pressure ventilation can rapidly progress to life-threatening **tension pneumothorax**, characterized by elevations in intrapleural pressure that progressively impede systemic venous return, reduce cardiac output, leading to arterial hypotension and **cardiovascular collapse**. Definitive treatment of pneumothorax consists of needle decompression followed by tube thoracostomy.

Detecting Air Outside the Chest— Subdiaphragmatic Gas Shadows

To extract maximal diagnostic information from chest x-rays, it is important to systematically look for shadowing that is indicative of abnormal air/gas collections, not just within the chest wall margins but outside the chest wall as well. Normally, the stomach gas "bubble" is visible just below the left diaphragmatic shadow (Fig. 15.2), unless there exists transposition of the intrathoracic and abdominal organs that is termed **situs inversus**. Any gas shadowing in the subdiaphragmatic region on the patient's right side, or the presence of double diaphragm shadowing is abnormal and suggests a high possibility of a **perforated viscus** (Fig. 15.7).

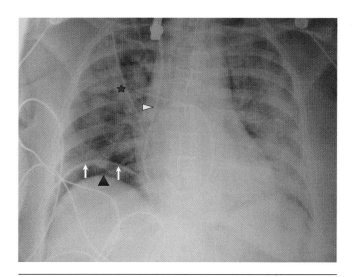

FIGURE 15.7 An abnormal right subdiaphragmatic gas collection (white arrows) above the liver (blue triangle) is seen, secondary to an esophageal tear caused by errant nasogastric tube placement. Also depicted are a right chest thoracostomy tube (red star), PA catheter (yellow arrowhead), and bilateral air-space opacities.

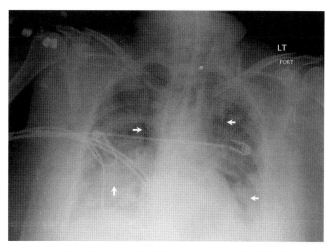

FIGURE 15.8 Bilateral air opacities of the type seen with acute lung injury. The lower two arrows indicate zones of lower lobe consolidation; air bronchograms are also visible (upper two arrows).

The Six Basic Patterns of Lung Disease Visualized by X-Rays

1. **Air-space opacities:** These appear as confluent, ill-defined opacities that obliterate the normal shadows created by pulmonary blood vessels, and often display a tendency to extend to the pleural surfaces. Air-space opacification occurs with the replacement of the air in the alveolar spaces of the lung parenchyma by an alternate substance such as inflammatory cells in acute respiratory distress syndrome (ARDS), pus in conditions of pneumonia, blood from pulmonary hemorrhage, water representing cardiogenic or noncardiogenic pulmonary edema fluid, or tumor cells. An **air bronchogram** is the characteristic manifestation of air-space opacity and may be seen when the alveoli surrounding a patent air-filled bronchus are rendered airless (Fig. 15.8). An air bronchogram is therefore a fundamental sign of consolidation and enables confident localization of the opacity within the lung parenchyma.

2. **Interstitial opacities:** These are described as linear or reticular, or as septal lines, peribronchovascular thickening, nodules, or as a generalized **miliary** pattern consisting of innumerable small opacities (miliary is defined medically as multiple small foci that resemble small millet seeds on an x-ray) (Fig. 15.9). Collectively, these radiographic findings suggest disease processes that are localized to the pulmonary interstitium; depending on the patient's clinical history, they may suggest specific diagnoses.

3. **Nodules and masses:** A nodule is a discrete opacity on a chest x-ray measuring <3 cm in diameter. Nodules are further characterized with respect to their numbers, size, border configurations, anatomic location, and the presence or absence of either internal calcification or cavitation (Fig. 15.10a). Nodules may manifest as airspace opacities or can appear predominantly as interstitial opacities. By convention, discrete opacities >3 cm on chest x-rays are referred to as masses (Fig. 15.10b).

4. **Lymphadenopathy:** Abnormal contouring of the mediastinal shadows in frontal PA or AP views may represent lymph node enlargement (Fig.15.11) or a mass. Characteristic locations of commonly observed intrathoracic lymphadenopathy on PA x-rays include the right paratracheal area, the hilar regions, the aortopulmonary window, the subcarinal region, and the superior mediastinum. Lymphadenopathy in the retrosternal area is best visualized using lateral radiographs, since lymph node enlargement fills the normally clear infrahilar window with an unexpected contour.

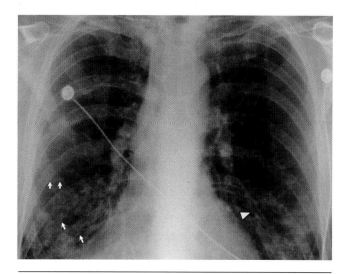

FIGURE 15.9 Linear (septal) interstitial opacities (upper arrow pair), reticular opacities (lower slanting arrow pair), and peribronchial thickening (yellow arrowhead) in a patient with interstitial lung disease due to scleroderma.

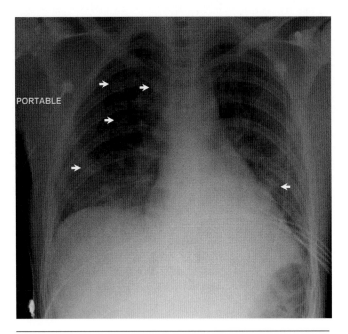

FIGURE 15.10 a. AP x-ray showing numerous small nodules (arrows) of varying densities and interfaces of greater or less contrast. This patient was diagnosed with methicillin-resistant *Staphylococcus aureus* bacteremia; the nodules represent septic pulmonary emboli.

5. **Cysts and cavities:** These abnormalities include areas of pulmonary parenchymal space that normally contain lung tissue but instead are filled with air, fluid, or both. Cysts usually have thin walls that may be composed of cellular elements. Cavities are usually created by tissue necrosis within a lung nodule or mass, and they evolve to become air-filled when the internal necrotic elements

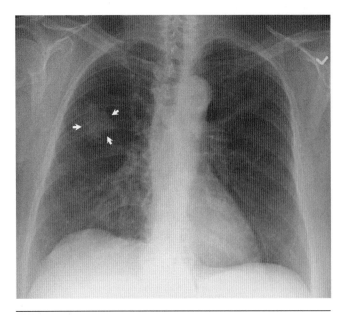

FIGURE 15.10 b. AP chest x-ray showing a mass (arrows) in a 60-year-old woman with a history of smoking who presented with persistent cough. Subsequent biopsy of this mass revealed a non-small cell lung cancer.

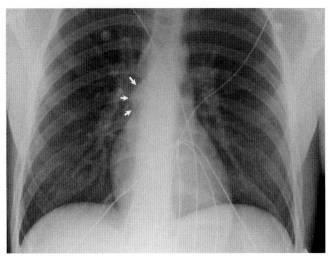

FIGURE 15.11 A rather subtle example of right mediastinal adenopathy with abnormal contouring (compare to Fig. 15.2), and density just below the carinal bifurcation of the right and left mainstem bronchi in a 19-year-old man diagnosed with mediastinal abscesses due to *Streptococcus intermedius* pneumonia.

are expelled into the tracheobronchial tree (Fig. 15.12). Pulmonary cysts and cavities are characterized on chest films by noting their distribution, number, any special characteristics of their inner lining, the thickness of their walls, and the nature of their contents.

6. **Pleural abnormalities:** Pleural disease has several manifestations, the commonest being **pleural effusions,** which when free-flowing characteristically blunt the costophrenic angle to form a meniscoid opacity. Large effusion volumes may show blunting or opacify an entire hemithorax (Fig. 15.13). In contrast to free-flowing effusions, **pleural thickening** reveals its nondependence on gravity and a nonlayered appearance on lateral decubitus x-rays. Nodular pleural thickening may

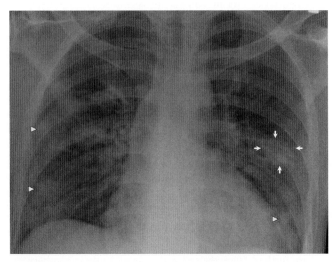

FIGURE 15.12 This is an example of a cavitary lesion (small arrows) arising from a necrotic lung nodule in a patient with HIV infection. Note also the fainter nodular opacities as marked bilaterally by the arrowheads.

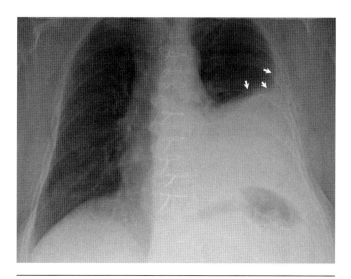

FIGURE 15.13 A large left-sided pleural effusion (arrows) that coincidentally results in a silhouette sign with the left hemidiaphragm.

suggest malignancy. **Pleural calcifications** are common in asbestos-related pleural disease, or as the sequelae of a prior hemothorax or tuberculous empyema.

Chest CT Scans

By itself, a chest x-ray often cannot clearly define disease processes, due to inherent limitations of resolution, imprecise segmental lung localization, and two-dimensional representation. In contrast, a chest CT scan provides **three-dimensional visualization** of intrathoracic anatomical structures including the lung parenchyma, making diagnostic interpretation easier and more accurate albeit at increased cost and radiation dose. For example, the radiation dose to the patient from a single chest x-ray is 10 mrem versus ~580 mrem for a standard chest CT scan, but the chest CT increases contrast resolution by a factor of 200. Such resolution is particularly useful for defining the segmental localization of parenchymal opacities, assessing mediastinal structures including lymphadenopathy, and evaluating pleural diseases. Importantly, **CT angiography** of the chest that is performed with intravenous injections of contrast media has become the primary method for detecting **pulmonary embolism** (Fig. 15.14) (Chap. 27).

High-Resolution CT Scans

High-resolution CT scans (HRCT) are most useful in evaluating patients with suspected interstitial lung disease, since their history and physical exam are frequently of limited diagnostic value. Optimal utilization of HRCT findings requires appreciation of the **secondary pulmonary lobule** as the lung's basic structural unit (Chap. 2) whose several components are normally visible on thin-section HRCTs of the lung. The **interlobular septal region** consists of peripheral interstitium containing interlobular septa and subpleural septa, pulmonary veins, and lymphatics. The **centrilobular region** contains the axial interstitium with its peribronchovascular structures including bronchiolar, pulmonary arterial, and lymphatic branches. The **lobular**

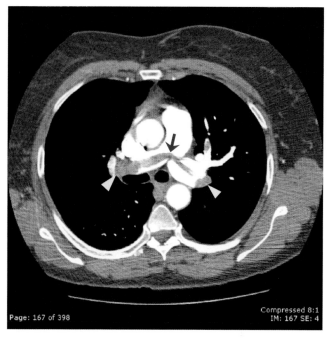

FIGURE 15.14 Contrast CT angiogram of the chest showing a "saddle" pulmonary embolism (red arrow) as well as filling defects in the left and right pulmonary artery branches (yellow arrowheads) secondary to obstruction by thromboembolic materials.

parenchyma region contains alveoli and their pulmonary capillaries as well as intralobular septal fibers (Fig. 15.15).

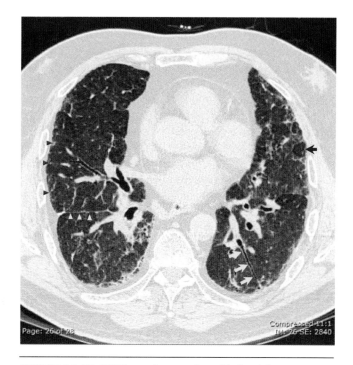

FIGURE 15.15 HRCT image from a patient with chronic hypersensitivity pneumonitis, a form of interstitial lung disease (ILD). Depicted are thickened interlobular septa (blue arrowheads), fissure prominence (yellow arrowheads) due to fibrosis, and traction bronchiectasis (yellow arrows) due to subpleural and intralobular fibrosis. Note also the **mosaic attenuation** of the left upper lobe (blue arrow) with darker and whiter shades in the same lung segment consistent with air-trapping.

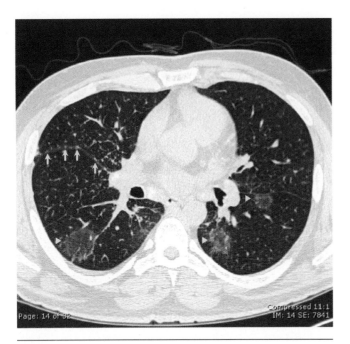

FIGURE 15.16 HRCT chest image from a patient with **sarcoidosis** showing nodular opacities (arrows) over the fissure consistent with lymphatic distribution of granulomatous inflammation. **Ground-glass opacities** (arrowheads) in this setting represent alveolar sarcoidosis.

HRCT Radiological Patterns of Diffuse Parenchymal Lung Disease

Recognizing abnormal structures of the secondary pulmonary lobule is fundamental to interpreting HRCT scans (Fig. 15.16). Pathological alterations visible on thin-section CT scans include interlobular septal thickening, diseases with peripheral lobular distribution, centrilobular abnormalities, and panlobular abnormalities. To simplify the approach with HRCT, the signs of diffuse lung disease can be grouped into four general patterns: (1) increased attenuation, referred to as "ground glass opacity" or consolidation; (2) reticulation with parenchymal distortion, typified by pulmonary fibrosis; (3) nodules, whether large or small, singular or multiple; and (4) mosaic patterns and cysts. These patterns of disease are combined with the distribution of disease to formulate a differential diagnosis.

Magnetic Resonance Imaging of the Chest

Magnetic resonance imaging (MRI) is a non-invasive diagnostic scanning technique to identify the distribution of water and other hydrogen-rich molecules in the body through the use of a powerful and highly uniform, static magnetic field but no ionizing radiation. MRI provides a comprehensive but non-invasive evaluation of the morphology and function of intrathoracic vessels, including the aorta and its branches, the pulmonary vasculature, and the central veins. This imaging

modality has several advantages including multiplanar images, intrinsic contrast between blood pool and vessel wall, and a wide range of soft tissue contrasts that delineate vascular and perivascular structures while avoiding the use of iodinated contrast media or radioisotopes.

Indications for performing an MRI study of the chest include: evaluation of mediastinal masses; investigation of suspected **Pancoast tumor** of the pulmonary apices especially when involvement of the brachial plexus is considered; diagnosis of the **superior vena cava syndrome** as an aid to lung cancer staging when invasion of great vessels, chest wall or diaphragm is suspected; and detection of congenital and acquired cardiac diseases. In this context, the principal utility of MRI studies of the chest is in evaluating cardiac function, including flow dynamics and major vessels and cardiac chambers or their constituent parts. The use of MRI is evolving for the evaluation and ongoing management of patients with **pulmonary arterial hypertension** (**PHT**), given the reproducibility of this technique and its accuracy for assessing right ventricular structure and function (Fig. 15.17). On the other hand, using MRI for lung imaging is currently limited by the longer time required to completion versus a CT scan, the greater cooperation required of a patient, and its unsuitability for very large or claustrophobic individuals. The proximity of an implant or any other metallic object in the vicinity of the chest may be a relative or absolute contraindication for MRI studies.

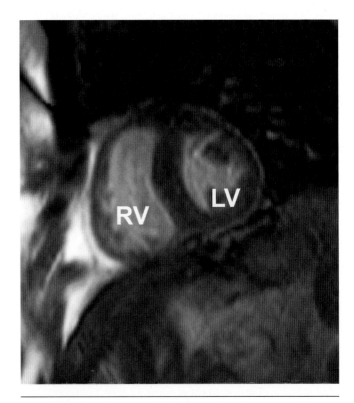

FIGURE 15.17 The cardiac MRI image from a patient with pulmonary hypertension reveals right ventricular enlargement. Note that the cross-sectional area of the RV exceeds that of the LV during end-systole.

Suggested Readings

1. Goodman LR. *Felson's Principles of Chest Roentgenology - A Programmed Text*, 2nd ed. Philadelphia, PA: Saunders; 1999. *This is a concise, case-based, conceptual text that teaches the "how" of radiographic interpretation.*

2. Chen MYM, Pope TL, Ott DJ. *Basic Radiology*, 2nd ed. New York, NY: McGraw-Hill; 2010. *The chapter on chest radiology provides a case-based approach with questions followed by discussion related to the case.*

3. Austin JH, Muller NL, Friedman PJ, et al. Glossary of terms for CT of the lungs: recommendations of the Nomenclature Committee of the Fleishner Society. *Radiology.* 1986;200:327-331. *An excellent resource for students building their vocabularies of diagnostic procedures.*

4. Webb WR. The 2004 Fleishner Lecture: Thin-section CT of the secondary pulmonary lobule: anatomy and the image. *Radiology.* 2006;239:322-338. *This review article provides a thorough understanding of the anatomy of secondary pulmonary lobules as it relates to interpreting thin-section CT scans of the chest for diffuse lung diseases.*

CASE STUDIES AND PRACTICE PROBLEMS

CASE 15.1 A 64-year-old man presents with persistent cough and a 9 kg (20 lb) weight loss over 6 months. He is a current smoker with a 50-pack-year history of tobacco use. Physical exam reveals stable vital signs with $f = 14$ breaths/min. There is no abnormality to percussion on chest exam; bronchovesicular breath sounds are auscultated without wheezes. His chest radiograph (shown below) is reported as being abnormal. Given the patient's history, what is the most accurate description of this radiological abnormality?

a. Consolidation of the left upper lobe
b. Left upper lobe atelectasis
c. Mediastinal mass
d. Left upper lobe mass
e. Aneurysmal dilatation of left pulmonary artery

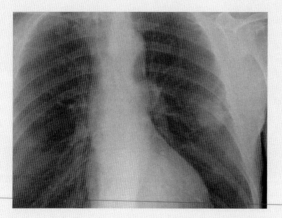

a. Diagnostic bronchoscopy
b. Thoracentesis with tube thoracostomy on the right side if diagnostic of empyema
c. Empiric antimicrobial therapy and discharge home
d. CT scan of the chest with contrast

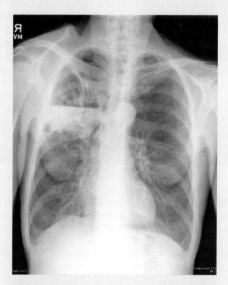

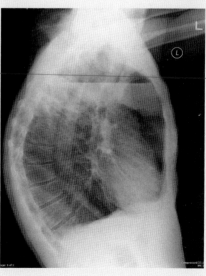

CASE 15.2 A 49-year-old man (current smoker) presents with progressive dyspnea, associated with right-sided chest discomfort, 12 kg (26 lb) weight loss, and whitish productive phlegm of two weeks' duration. Over the past 48 hours, he has coughed up dark red blood in small amounts. Physical exam reveals stable vital signs but with increased $f = 22$ breaths/min. An oral cavity exam reveals poor dentition with multiple caries of his teeth. There are decreased breath sounds on the right side by auscultation. His chest x-rays (shown at right) are reported as being abnormal. Given this patient's history and chest x-ray findings, what is the most appropriate next step in his diagnosis and/or treatment?

Solutions to Case Studies and Practice Problems

CASE 15.1 The most correct answer is d, a left upper lobe mass.

The chest radiograph shows a round opacity projecting just laterally and cephalad to the left hilum. Because the medial margin of the opacity is seen, a mediastinal mass is excluded (*answer c*). The left pulmonary artery can be seen easily in its normal location (*answer e*). The opacity is smaller than the left upper lobe, and no air bronchograms are present, excluding consolidation (*answer a*). The inferior margin of the opacity is not a long straight or gently curving line, as is the major fissure, and therefore left upper lobe atelectasis is also not evident (*answer b*). The chest CT scan for this patient is shown below as confirmation.

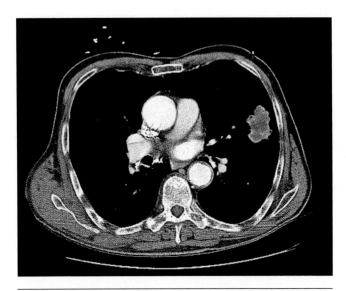

CASE 15.1. CT scan of chest confirming presence of a left upper lobe mass. Students should remember to visualize such CT slices as if they were standing at the foot of the patient's bed as the man lies supine. Thus, like x-rays, the patient's left is on the right.

CASE 15.2 The most correct answer is d, obtain a CT of chest with contrast.

The chest radiograph shows a large round opacity with incomplete margins and a right-sided air-fluid level suggestive of a lung abscess. The lateral view confirms these findings and suggests that the fluid-filled cavity is rather large, spanning the entire anterior to posterior aspect of the right upper lobe. Diagnostic bronchoscopy is recommended to exclude an endobronchial lesion (*answer a*), but not before doing a further diagnostic test to exclude possible accompanying pleural infection, and to define the segmental anatomy. Thoracentesis would be appropriate if a pleural fluid collection is confirmed (*answer b*). Initiation of antimicrobial therapy after obtaining blood and sputum cultures is important, especially with the patient's history and physical findings, but discharging him home without the appropriate workup is not recommended (*answer c*). A CT scan of the chest with contrast (shown below) defines segmental anatomy to achieve the best possible bronchoscopy samples, and may exclude pleural fluid collection and other complications of infection. The IV contrast agent will help to delineate mediastinal structures and also assess for lymphadenopathy; if present such enlarged lymph nodes can be easily sampled during bronchoscopy.

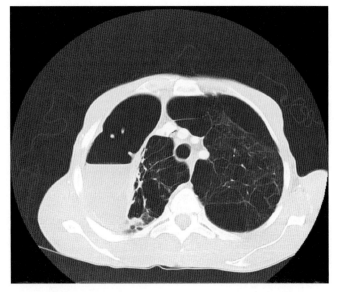

CASE 15.2 CT scan image with contrast of the chest in the 49-year-old patient reveals a fluid-filled right lung abscess. An infected emphysematous bulla is in the differential diagnosis.

Chapter 16

Pulmonary Function Testing, Plethysmography, and Pulmonary Diffusing Capacity

GERALD S. ZAVORSKY, PhD AND
ANDREW J. LECHNER, PhD

Learning Objectives

- The student will be able to identify the static and dynamic pulmonary function tests (PFTs) commonly performed to establish obstructive and/or restrictive patterns.

- The student will be able to describe the operating principle of a whole-body plethysmograph and the measurements obtained from such an apparatus.

- The student will be able to explain the use of carbon monoxide to estimate pulmonary diffusing capacity and diseases in which diffusion is altered.

Introduction

This chapter examines the many practical applications of **pulmonary function testing (PFT)** for evaluating lung function and disease progression in individual patients, as well as identifying broader public health concerns across populations. The full range of PFT procedures can assess airway resistance, functional residual capacity (FRC) and residual volume, pulmonary diffusing capacity, arterial blood gases (ABGs), exercise capacity, and even energy expenditure. While spirometry was introduced in Chaps. 4 and 6, the more detailed descriptions here include specific diagnostic criteria for grading the severities of obstructive and restrictive lung disease types, as developed by the **American Thoracic Society** and **European Respiratory Society (ATS/ERS)** (Table 16.1).

Spirometry as the Entry Point to Pulmonary Function Testing

Spirometry is non-invasive, dynamic pulmonary function testing that indirectly assesses airway resistance, notably in medium-sized bronchi. Among the lung volumes estimated by spirometry to distinguish obstructive and restrictive disorders are: **vital capacity (VC), forced vital capacity (FVC), forced expiratory volume in one second (FEV$_1$), peak expiratory flow (PEF) rate**, and **forced expiratory volume over the middle half of expiration (FEF$_{25-75}$)**. There are three distinct steps to obtaining a reliable FVC. First, maximal inspiration is measured by the subject inhaling as deeply as possible toward TLC before pausing for 1 second at that volume. Second, the subject exhales maximally as quickly as possible toward RV, continuing for at least 6 seconds, yielding an **expiratory flow volume curve** or **loop** [Fig. 16.1 (a)]. Third, the subject immediately inhales again toward TLC to obtain an **inspiratory flow volume loop**. At least three such efforts, but not more than eight, are performed in a given PFT session, with brief resting intervals using a normal V$_T$ between efforts if needed.

With these data, the subject's largest FVC and FEV$_1$ from any of the attempts are recorded, even if the highest values for FVC and FEV$_1$ do not occur in the same expiratory effort. However, the highest two estimates of FVC and FEV$_1$ should not differ by more than 150 mL to assure an appropriate degree of **repeatability**. If the patient's best results differ by more than 150 mL, it is usually recommended that another full test be conducted. Similarly, once the expiratory flow-volume loops have been plotted, the patient's PEF results should be evaluated to ensure that peak rates (usually near the start of expiration) do not vary by more than 5% between the highest two values. If patient variance exceeds this benchmark, another full test should be completed.

The shape of the flow-volume loop during expiration [Fig. 16.1 (b)] is modified by dynamic airway compression that is effort-independent during expiration (Chap. 6). A "choke point" may exist throughout expiratory flow, so that whenever P$_{IP}$ exceeds P$_{AW}$, airway collapse can occur (Fig. 16.2), making expiratory flow-volume loops concave. Dynamic compression of airways does not occur during inspiration because P$_{IP}$ < P$_{AW}$ throughout that phase of breathing, stenting the airways and alveoli open.

Comparing a subject's measured spirometry results and subsequent PFT data (eg, lung volumes and DL$_{CO}$ described below) to appropriate reference values is essential to proper interpretation. Reference values are derived from studies of large, well-defined healthy populations of children and non-smoking adults, expressed as normal intervals or frequency distributions representing 95% of the sample population. The most common method of analysis is to compare the observed

Table **16.1** **Primary reasons for pulmonary function testing**

Confirming a Diagnosis of Primary or Secondary Lung Disease	
To evaluate:	New signs of diminished breath sounds, crackles, clubbing, hyperinflation; Symptoms of dyspnea, wheezing, orthopnea, cough, sputum production, chest pain; Abnormal imaging studies and arterial blood gases (hypoxemia, hypercapnia).
To measure:	Effects of new systemic diseases on pulmonary function.
To screen:	Past and present smokers, and those exposed to second-hand smoke; Individuals with occupational, domestic, or social risk factors.
To assess:	Preoperative risk and/or prognosis for lung transplantation, cystic fibrosis (CF), etc.
Sequential Monitoring during Management of Known Lung Disease	
To assess:	Therapeutic interventions for asthma with bronchodilators, corticosteroids, etc; Complications from systemic disorders (congestive heart failure, sarcoidosis, etc); Adequacy of antibiotics for CF, antiarrhythmics that affect DL_{CO}, etc.
To define:	Pulmonary complications from cardiovascular and neuromuscular diseases.
To monitor:	Adverse drug reactions when pulmonary toxicity is known or suspected; Mitigation efficacy against occupational or domestic risk factors for lung disease.
Evaluating Known or Suspected Disabilities and Impairments	
To assess:	Patient suitability for medical, industrial, or vocational rehabilitation programs.
To confirm:	Eligibility for insurance or worker's compensation, and personal injury lawsuits; Compliance with behavioral, pharmacological, or other prescribed activities.
Establishing Public Health Policies, Regional Action Plans, and Legislative Agendas	
To survey:	Identified or suspected populations at risk for pulmonary disease.
To validate:	Subjective complaints of occupational, environmental, or industrial risk or injury; Reference equations derived to predict any related feature of lung function.

data to the mean reference value, with results expressed both as absolute numeric values and as the percent of predicted value. The **lower limit of normal** (LLN) describes the lowest 5th percentile according to reference equations based on age, gender, and height, and sometimes ethnicity. Any value below the LLN is deemed clinically abnormal. To determine the severity of obstruction, the FEV_1 expressed as percentage predicted is often used (Table 16.2).

▶▶**CLINICAL CORRELATION 16.1**

An FEV_1/FVC ratio that is less than normal when FEV_1 and FVC are both within normal ranges may be observed in healthy subjects, including athletes. Whether it is a true airflow obstruction depends on prior probability of obstructive disease and should be pursued with additional tests such as response to bronchodilator challenge, DL_{CO}, respiratory muscle strength, or exercise tolerance.

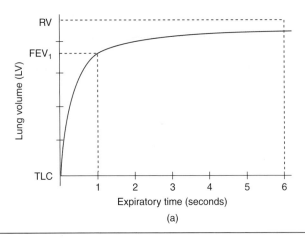

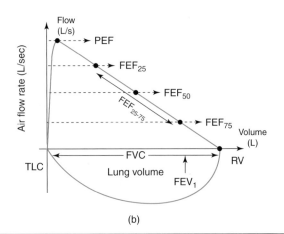

FIGURE 16.1 (a) A typical expiratory volume curve plotted against time since starting exhalation. (b) A normal complete flow-volume loop, plotted with flow rate as a function of lung volume from TLC to RV. Note that the **expiratory flow-volume curve** is plotted above the x-axis and the **inspiratory flow-volume loop** plotted below it.

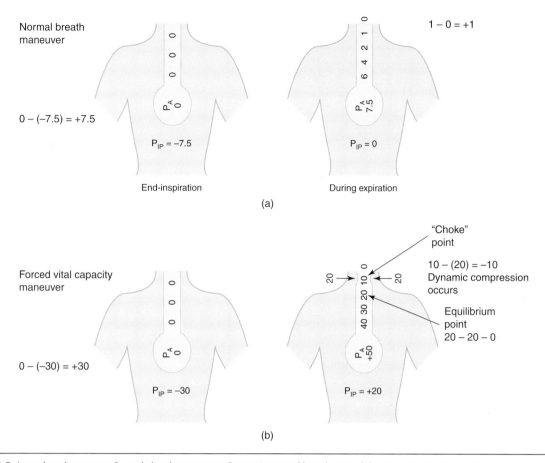

FIGURE 16.2 Intrapleural pressures, P_{IP} and alveolar pressures, P_A vary in normal breathing and during a spirometry test. Dynamic airway compression is most likely during the expiratory phase of an FVC maneuver. At the end of normal or forced inspiration, $P_A = P_{ATM}$ because no airflow occurs.

Some additional ATS/ERS guidelines for the use and interpretation of basic spirometry data include the following points:

1. Interpretation of spirometric results should include FVC, FEV_1, and FEV_1/FVC as well as PEF, FEF_{25-75}, and TLC to reduce the number of **false positives** (false alarms) in healthy adult or pediatric populations.
2. Spirometric results vary with time and testing conditions, but ≥15% yearly changes in FEV_1 or FVC are generally considered clinically significant. Regularly monitoring a patient's FVC may provide the most

useful data for following the course of a restrictive chest disease (Chap. 24).
3. Low lung function levels by spirometry predict poor prognoses in patients with heart and lung disease, even among never-smokers. In patients with cystic fibrosis (CF) (Chap. 38), an FEV_1 <30% of predicted has been associated with a two-year mortality rate of 50%. Nevertheless, symptom severity or mortality risk for an individual patient cannot be predicted by FEV_1 alone.
4. Lack of acute improvement in a patient's FEV_1 with bronchodilators does not preclude a clinical response to long-term bronchodilator therapy, and the patient's reported volumes may change with medication due to reduction in dynamic gas trapping and chest hyperinflation. More on this subject is presented in later discussions of chronic obstructive lung disease and asthma (Chaps. 21 and 22) in the context of irreversible airway remodeling.

Determining the Need for Advanced Pulmonary Function Testing

With these basic spirometric results in hand, clinicians then can decide whether follow-up procedures are warranted. The assessment and treatment algorithm (Fig. 16.3) developed by

Table **16.2** **Airflow obstruction by ATS/ERS* criteria**

Degree of Severity	FEV₁ (% of Predicted)
Mild	>70%
Moderate	60%-69%
Moderately severe	50%-59%
Severe	35%-49%
Very severe	<35%

*ATS/ERS = American Thoracic Society/European Respiratory Society

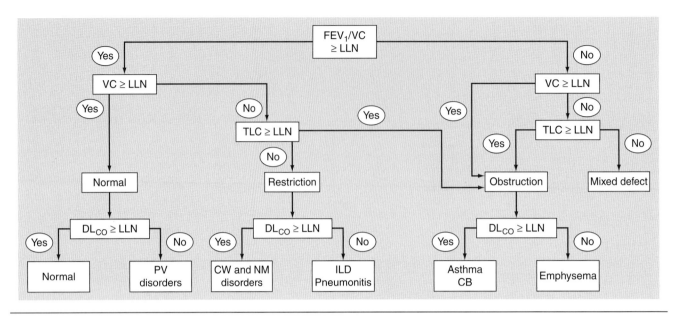

FIGURE 16.3 An assessment algorithm for lung function using ATS/ERS guidelines. Patients may not present with a classic pattern, if, for example, their VC is outside the lower limit of normal (LLN). Clinical decisions of how far to follow this algorithm depend on the need for additional intervention, but FEV$_1$/VC is a good starting point. Data for TLC confirm or exclude a restrictive defect. Other abbreviations are: PV = pulmonary vascular; CW = chest wall; NM = neuromuscular; ILD = interstitial lung diseases; CB = chronic bronchitis.

the ATS/ERS is a useful guide. However, patients may not present with every feature of a classic obstructive or restrictive pattern, depending on how immediate their illness is and its severity are affected by baseline lung function that existed before the onset of new symptoms or an acute exacerbation of preexisting disease.

Measurement of Absolute Lung Volumes *(# 56)*

Direct measurement of TLC is necessary to confirm a restrictive disease that may be suggested by a low spirometric estimate of VC. Gas dilution techniques (Chap. 4) and plethysmography can directly measure FRC and thus TLC, core PFT values not obtainable by spirometry alone. Unlike the helium (He) dilution and N$_2$ washout techniques described in Chap. 4, however, **whole-body plethysmography** estimates all intra-thoracic air volume, even gas-filled spaces that may be isolated from the major airways. Such noncommunicating air spaces are common in the form of the subpleural **blebs** or **bullae** in diseases like cystic fibrosis or **congenital bullous emphysema** (Chaps. 37 and 38). Thus, the use of plethysmography to measure FRC (and thus TLC) is preferred over gas dilution techniques in those patients with obstructive conditions where air trapping may occur, or in patients suspected of having coexistent restrictive and obstructive diseases.

Plethysmography is based on the physics of Boyle's law (Chap. 1), which states that isothermally changing the volume of a known amount of gas changes the gas pressure inversely, so that: $P_1 \cdot V_1 = P_2 \cdot V_2$. A whole-body plethysmograph is an airtight Plexiglas chamber (a "body box" in PFT lexicon)

about the size of a telephone booth. According to current ATS/ERS criteria, a subject should be sitting upright in the box while wearing nose clips and breathing through a mouthpiece fitted with a **pneumotachometer** to measure airflow (Fig. 16.4). The chamber should be large enough to accommodate the subject without having to bend or hyperextend the neck to reach the mouthpiece. Multiple transducers are

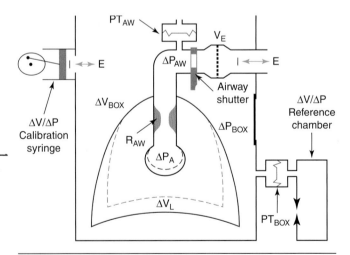

FIGURE 16.4 Diagram of a pressure-corrected integrated-flow plethysmograph. Green arrows show how a subject breathes by a mouthpiece through the chamber wall to room air (right), an action emulated by a calibration syringe (left). Pneumotachometers in the mouthpiece (PT$_{AW}$) and chamber wall (PT$_{BOX}$) deduce volume changes in the patient's chest (ΔV_L) and the box (ΔV_{BOX}) and their associated pressure changes (ΔV_{AW}, ΔV_{BOX}) during normal breathing, or when inspiration and expiration are attempted against a closed shutter in the airway that momentarily prevents actual lung ventilation.

arrayed within the chamber to measure pressures within the box, in the airway, and across the pneumotachometer itself.

A subject first breathes quietly in the plethysmograph for 8-10 breaths, as system temperatures stabilize and a reproducible end-expiratory volume (ie, FRC) is achieved. Then as the subject next pauses at FRC, a shutter closes to occlude the airway for perhaps 2-3 seconds. With the shutter closed, the subject is asked to perform mild panting ($f = 0.5\text{-}1$ Hz) with enough effort to create oscillations in their P_{AW} of about ± 8 mm Hg. Ideally, 3-5 technically correct panting maneuvers can be recorded before the shutter is released. Once the airway is reopened, the subject exhales completely to RV, then slowly inhales to TLC, and then slowly exhales back to RV. This sequence of steps is considered one complete FRC maneuver. The subject is then instructed to resume quiet normal respiration until the shutter is closed and another trial is attempted.

Although no air moves into the lungs during the attempted panting, PAW fluctuates by a measurable amount, ΔP_{AW}, while the fixed amount of gas in the lungs (= FRC) expands and contracts by an unknown amount, ΔV_L. During the same panting efforts, the volume of air surrounding the subject in the box also fluctuates by an unknown amount, ΔV_{BOX}, even as its pressure oscillates by a measurable amount, ΔP_{BOX}. Periodic air injections are made by a calibrated push-pull syringe operating at typical respiratory frequencies while the subject is in the box. These injections provide precise values for the ratio $\Delta V_{BOX}/\Delta P_{BOX}$ with the subject inside. Those ratios are then used in sequential iterations of Boyle's law to solve first for the unknown ΔV_{BOX} (while the subject pants), then the subject's unknown ΔV_L (while panting), and finally the subject's actual FRC. To achieve an appropriate level of repeatability, at least three such panting maneuvers should be performed that yield estimates of the subject's actual FRC within 5% of each other.

▶▶CLINICAL CORRELATION 16.2

This derived relationship between a subject's FRC and the chamber's nonsubject air volume under static shutter conditions is then extrapolated to dynamic events while the subject is breathing freely. In this manner, dynamic airway resistance (R_{AW}) is calculated by Ohm's law from the observed $\dot{V}_E$ and ΔP_A. Design innovations by manufacturers of these apparatus continue to provide additional information, better accuracy, and greater ease of operation, including some that no longer require a subject to be physically enclosed within an airtight chamber.

Measurement of Pulmonary Diffusing Capacity (#57)

The **pulmonary diffusing capacity for carbon monoxide** (**DL$_{CO}$**) is a standard lung function test that estimates alveolar-capillary diffusion for gases such as O_2 and CO_2. However,

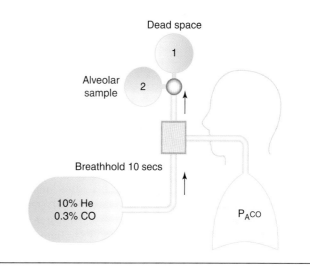

FIGURE 16.5 The single-breath method for determining DL$_{CO}$. A subject previously breathing air or O_2 is switched while at RV to inhaled gas containing known concentrations of He and CO that will be used to determine FRC and diffusive capacity, respectively.

measuring rate-limiting O_2 transfer across the alveolar membranes presents technical difficulties that are caused by high background levels of O_2. Consequently, CO has been used extensively as a surrogate index of O_2 transfer, due primarily to its high affinity for Hb that results in CO being considered a diffusion-limited gas (Chaps. 3 and 9).

The most widely used DL$_{CO}$ protocol is the **single-breath method** (Fig. 16.5). After a few normal breaths at rest, subjects exhale to RV and then inhale a standard mixture of gases ($F_ICO = 0.003$; $F_IHe = 0.100$; $F_IO_2 = 0.207$; $F_IN_2 = 0.690$) to TLC. To complete the single-breath test properly, >85% of a subject's VC should consist of this standard gas mixture just inhaled to TLC. While holding at TLC for 10 seconds, subjects should avoid every positive airway pressures that decrease pulmonary blood flow and capillary volume, V_c (see **Valsalva maneuver**) or extremely negative airway pressures that artifactually increase $\dot{Q}$ and V_c (see **Müller maneuver**). After the 10-second breathhold at TLC, the subject exhales completely to RV in a smooth, unforced, and uninterrupted manner. Owing to undiluted gases within the dead space volume, the first liter of exhaled air is discarded. The second liter of gas exhaled by the subject is collected and analyzed to compute both the equilibrated alveolar concentration of CO, F_ACO and its partial pressure, P_ACO (Chap. 8) at the end of the breathhold. DL$_{CO}$ is then calculated as the total amount of CO absorbed by the subject from the amount inspired ($F_ICO - F_ACO$) divided by the P_ACO that served as the driving pressure gradient into the patient's pulmonary capillary blood. Simultaneous measurement of the equilibrium [He] allows an accurate estimate of lung volume by the dilution principles discussed in Chap. 4.

The DL$_{CO}$ estimated for the entire lung by this test consists of the sequential diffusive capacities of the alveolar-capillary membrane and of pulmonary capillary blood (Chap. 9).

Indeed, DL_{CO} is calculated using the equation for resistors in series:

$$\frac{1}{DL_{CO}} = \frac{1}{DM_{CO}} + \frac{1}{\Theta_{CO} \cdot V_c}$$

where DM_{CO} = alveolar membrane diffusing capacity for CO, V_c = pulmonary capillary blood volume (Chap. 7), and Θ_{CO} is the **blood transfer conductance coefficient for CO**. The Θ_{CO} is the standard rate at which 1 mL of whole blood will take up CO in mL STPD per minute per milliliter of mercury of partial pressure. The unit for DL_{CO} is mL·(min^{-1}·mm Hg^{-1}) or mL·min^{-1}·mm Hg^{-1}, or it can be written as mL/(min·mm Hg). The units for DL_{CO} in most textbooks and research papers report DL_{CO} as mL/min/mmHg (mL/min/kPa in Europe). The most commonly used approximation for Θ_{CO} was derived by Roughton and Forster (1957) who showed that:

$$1/\Theta_{CO} = 0.73 + \{0.0058 \cdot (P_{A}O_2) \cdot 14.6/[Hb]\}$$

where [Hb] is expressed in g/dL of arterial or venous blood. **Membrane diffusive resistance, $1/DM_{CO}$** and red cell resistance, $1/(\Theta_{CO} \cdot V_c)$ usually contribute about equally to the overall diffusive resistance of the lung, $1/DL_{CO}$. To estimate the individual contributions made by DM_{CO} and V_c to DL_{CO}, the single-breath method is done twice, at an $F_IO_2 = 0.207$ and then at 0.897 to achieve two widely separated values for $P_{A}O_2$ of about 100 mm Hg and 600 mm Hg, respectively. Using the subject's $P_{A}O_2$ measured during each single-breath test, the value of $1/DL_{CO}$ is plotted on the y-axis and $1/\Theta_{CO}$ is plotted on the x-axis. A straight line drawn through these two points yields the y-intercept ($1/DM_{CO}$) and the slope ($1/V_c$) (Fig. 16.6). Sufficient accuracy can usually be achieved with just four to six single-breath tests, usually two to three at low $P_{A}O_2$ and two to three at high $P_{A}O_2$.

No more than five DL_{CO} tests should be performed per session to avoid accumulation of HbCO, since HbCO increases by ~0.7% per single-breath test. For each 1% increase in HbCO, there is an approximate 1% decrease in DL_{CO} due to the reduction in $1/\Theta_{CO}$ that is caused by such dysfunctional hemoglobins. Regular smokers may have an HbCO of 5%-10%, much higher than in nonsmokers, whose HbCO = 0.7%-1.0%. When two DL_{CO} tests fall within 3 mL·min^{-1}·mm Hg^{-1} of each other, the average of both tests is reported. Normal month-to-month variations in DL_{CO} are about 5 mL·min^{-1}·mm Hg^{-1}. Thus larger variations are clinically meaningful. A classification scheme for severity of a decrease in DL_{CO} compared to normative values is shown in Table 16.3.

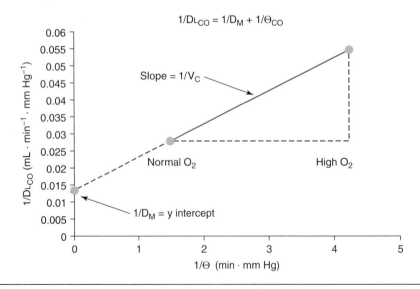

FIGURE 16.6 Schematic of Roughton and Forster's two-step method to compute DM_{CO} and pulmonary capillary blood volume (V_c) from a conventional single-breath DL_{CO} test. As described in the text, a subject inhales from RV to TLC a gas mixture of 0.3% CO/10.0% He/20.7% *or* 89.7% O_2/ balance N_2. When the results are plotted as shown, the inverse of the slope = V_c, and the inverse of the y-intercept = DM_{CO}.

Table 16.3 DL_{CO} severity assessment by ATS/ERS criteria

Degree of Severity	DL_{CO} as % of Predicted Value
Mild	>60%, but less than the LLN*
Moderate	40%-60%
Severe	<40%

*LLN = lower limit of normal range for age, gender, height, ethnicity

▶▶ CLINICAL CORRELATION 16.4

Only four contraindications have been established for any of the lung function tests that are described in this chapter: chest or abdominal pain; oral or facial pain; stress incontinence; and dementia. Neither pregnancy nor advanced age is considered a contraindication per se for measurement of pulmonary diffusing capacity using the single breath DL_{CO} technique.

Suggested Readings

1. Miller MR, Hankinson J, Brusasco V, et al. Standardisation of spirometry. *Europ Respir J*. 2005;26:319-338; and Miller MR, Crapo R, Hankinson J, et al. General considerations for lung function testing. *Europ Respir J*. 2005;26:153-161. *These two papers contain the 'gold standards' for routine spirometry testing and describe patient considerations and laboratory details as recently approved jointly by the American Thoracic Society and the European Respiratory Society (ATS/ERS).*

2. Wanger J, Clausen JL, Coates A, et al. Standardization of the measurement of lung volumes. *Europ Respir J*. 2005;26:511-552; and Macintyre N, Crapo RO, Viegi G, et al. Standardization of the single-breath determination of carbon monoxide uptake in the lung. *Europ Respir J*. 2005;26:720-735. *The first paper provides definitive guidelines for static lung volume assessment and the second for determining DL_{CO}, both approved policy statements jointly promulgated by the ATS/ERS.*

3. Pellegrino R, Viegi G, Brusasco V, et al. Interpretive strategies for lung function testing. *Europ Respir J*. 2005;26:948-968. *This paper describes references equations, consideration of ventilator defects and other obstacles for proper interpretation of PFT results, again approved jointly by the ATS/ERS.*

4. Roughton FJW, Forster RE. Relative importance of diffusion and chemical reaction rates in determining rate of exchange of gases in the human lung, with special reference to true diffusing capacity of pulmonary membrane and volume of blood in the lung capillaries. *J Appl Physiol*. 1957;11:290-302. *These authors were among the first to develop a conceptual model of DL_{CO} that included both the alveolar membrane and the erythrocytes as sequential resistances to gas flow.*

CASE STUDIES AND PRACTICE PROBLEMS

CASE 16.1 Describe the physiological pattern (eg, obstructive vs restrictive) that is most likely to be measured in a subject who is unable or unwilling to perform the expected expiratory spirometric maneuvers with maximal effort?

CASE 16.2 What results for FEV_1 and FVC are expected in a subject with a combined airflow limitation, as might occur with poorly controlled asthma plus an underlying restrictive process such as interstitial fibrosis? What additional pulmonary function testing might help resolve the situation in such a patient?

CASE 16.3 In addition to changes in the caliber of conducting airways and the elasticity of lung parenchyma, what other non-pulmonary, anatomical, or functional factors can influence a subject's measured FVC?

CASE 16.4 A 55-year-old man who has smoked 10 cigarettes in the preceding 90 minutes now has a measured HbCO of 10%. If his measured DL_{CO} on this same day is 21.4 mL·min⁻¹·mm Hg⁻¹, what is the best approximation of this patient's actual DL_{CO}?

a. 18.2 mL·min⁻¹·mm Hg⁻¹
b. 23.5 mL·min⁻¹·mm Hg⁻¹
c. 19.1 mL·min⁻¹·mm Hg⁻¹
d. 20.1 mL·min⁻¹·mm Hg⁻¹
e. 22.5 mL·min⁻¹·mm Hg⁻¹

Solutions to Case Studies and Practice Problems

CASE 16.1 The physiological pattern in such a patient most likely would be obstructive. Every effort should be made to perform spirometry to the best of a patient's ability. Premature termination of a spirometry test is not in itself a sufficient reason to eliminate results from evaluation. Often at least the estimated FEV_1 is useful, depending on the length of exhalation, and should be reported even for prematurely terminated maneuvers.

CASE 16.2 A patient with mixed pulmonary disorders may have an FEV_1 below that predicted for age, height, and gender, and also an FVC below the lower limit of normal, LLN. In such patients, the ratio FEV_1/FVC may be normal, or at least > LLN. To test for a restrictive pattern and confirm a low FVC result, the patient's TLC should be measured by whole-body plethysmography. If plethysmography confirms that TLC < LLN, then the patient has both obstructive and restrictive disorders. However, if TLC > LLN, then the patient has primarily an obstructive disorder and a DL_{CO} test is warranted. If DL_{CO} > LLN, the patient most likely has asthma and/or chronic bronchitis. If DL_{CO} < LLN, then emphysema is more likely (see Fig. 16.3, the lung function assessment algorithm).

CASE 16.3 Several nonpulmonary conditions can affect FVC. For example, fractured ribs may increase compliance of the thorax and thus estimates of both FVC and TLC. Obesity, abdominal trauma, hepatomegaly, and peritoneal ascites generally act to reduce FVC. During the prolonged submersions that scuba divers and snorkelers experience, the external pressure of water on thoracic elements usually decreases FVC and TLC. Restraint jackets or other restrictive clothing can also reduce FVC and TLC.

CASE 16.4 The most correct answer is b.

For every % of HbCO present, the measured DL_{CO} is decreased by about the same amount from the actual DL_{CO}. In this patient with HbCO = 10%, the measured DL_{CO} is 21.4 mL·min^{-1}·mm Hg^{-1}. Multiplying the measured value of 21.4 by 110% will correct upward toward the actual value of 23.5 mL·min^{-1}·mm Hg^{-1} that would have been found if this patient's HbCO had been 0%.

Chapter 17

Blood Gas Analyses and Their Interpretation

MARY M. MAYO, PhD AND ANDREW J. LECHNER, PhD

Learning Objectives

- The student will be able to identify primary acid/base disorders given patient laboratory results and the degree of compensation.

- The student will be able to distinguish between the roles of the lungs and kidneys in maintenance of acid/base homeostasis.

- The student will be able to identify common causes of metabolic acidosis and alkalosis, and of respiratory acidosis and alkalosis.

- The student will be able to use the calculation of the anion gap to identify causes of metabolic acidosis.

Introduction

Although the human diet is essentially neutral with respect to its pH, various aerobic and anaerobic metabolic processes create large amounts of acid daily from the catabolism of carbohydrates, fats, and proteins. The body maintains a constant $[H^+]$ such that blood and extracellular pH is near 7.4 and intracellular pH is about 7.1. The buffer most responsible for this is the HCO_3^-/H_2CO_3 system, regulated by the coordinated behavior of the lungs and kidneys. Aerobic metabolism yields gaseous CO_2 that combines with water to form volatile carbonic acid, H_2CO_3. The lungs are primarily responsible for elimination of CO_2. Anaerobic metabolism of glucose and fat, as well as some protein catabolism yield fixed or **nonvolatile acids** such as lactic acid, sulfuric acid, and phosphoric acid, most being excreted by the kidneys. In one 24-hour period, a 70-kg person produces 70-100 mmol of such nonvolatile acids versus 20 moles CO_2, all without appreciable change in plasma pH. An effective $\dot{V}_A$ controls CO_2 excretion, while the kidneys excrete nonvolatile acids and reabsorb or regenerate HCO_3^-. The lungs and kidneys maintain a balance of CO_2 and HCO_3^-, and thus pH_a near 7.4 (Fig. 17.1).

Basic Categories of Acidosis and Alkalosis

Acidosis and **alkalosis** are terms that describe primary processes modulating $[H^+]$ in patient populations. Each may be **metabolic** or **respiratory** in origin, based on whether the primary deviation is in arterial $[HCO_3^-]$ or P_aCO_2, respectively. Respiratory disorders are caused by inappropriate excretion of CO_2 that raises or lowers $[H_2CO_3]$ in body fluids. Metabolic disorders reflect primary changes in plasma $[HCO_3^-]$ due to excessive intake, production, or loss of HCO_3^- or inappropriate handling of H^+ and anions from dissociated nonvolatile acids. **Primary acid-base disorders** and the compensations that must follow to restore pH to normal are shown in Table 17.1.

In **respiratory acidosis**, excessive CO_2 raises blood P_{CO_2}, and produces by the mass action principle more H_2CO_3 which

then dissociates into H^+ and HCO_3^- to reduce pH_a (Fig. 17.2). Compensation for this drop in pH_a is attempted in the kidneys through reabsorption of filtered HCO_3^- to restore pH_a toward 7.4. In **respiratory alkalosis**, a reduced P_aCO_2 forces by mass action the resynthesis of H_2CO_3 from free H^+ and HCO_3^- and thereby raises pH_a (Fig. 17.2). Compensation for the rise in pH_a is attempted in the kidneys by excretion of more anion, including HCO_3^-. (#58)

In **metabolic acidosis**, excess H^+ from various nonvolatile acids causes pH_a to fall below 7.4, even as blood $[HCO_3^-]$ decreases due to its recombination with those protons (Fig. 17.3). Respiratory compensation requires hyperventilation to excrete the added acid burden and restore pH_a to 7.4, although this response simultaneously lowers P_aCO_2. In **metabolic alkalosis**, the blood $[HCO_3^-]$ is abnormally elevated, raising pH_a above 7.4. Respiratory compensation attempts to increase P_aCO_2 by hypoventilation, which then acts to restore pH_a downward toward 7.4 by forming more H_2CO_3.

Derivation of the Henderson–Hasselbalch Equation (#59)

Laboratory assessment of a patient's acid-base status involves quantifying components of this HCO_3^-/H_2CO_3 buffer system. **Arterial blood gas (ABG)** specimens are the most commonly submitted, and must be drawn directly into special syringes that contain heparin as an anticoagulant. Specimen integrity is extremely important. Each must be collected anaerobically, after which the needle is removed and the syringe capped, placed on ice or otherwise stored <4°C (<39.2°F) and then delivered immediately to the laboratory. Every effort is made to ensure that specimens are analyzed within 20-30 minutes of their

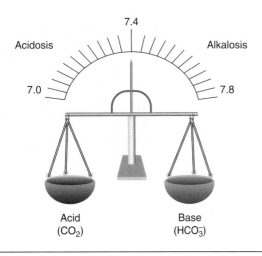

Table 17.1 Simple acid-base disorders and their compensations

Disorder	Primary Deviation	Compensatory Response
Metabolic acidosis	$\downarrow HCO_3^-$	$\downarrow P_aco_2$
Metabolic alkalosis	$\uparrow HCO_3^-$	$\uparrow P_aco_2$
Respiratory acidosis	$\uparrow P_aco_2$	$\uparrow HCO_3^-$
Respiratory alkalosis	$\downarrow P_aco_2$	$\downarrow HCO_3^-$

FIGURE 17.1 Acidosis and alkalosis refer to primary processes that increase or decrease blood [H⁺], respectively. Acidemia refers to a blood pH <7.36 and alkalemia to a blood pH >7.44. Compensation occurs as either the metabolic (renal) or respiratory response that attempts to restore blood pH when altered by some primary process.

collection to retard degradation by ongoing metabolism of blood-formed elements. The three measured parameters on each ABG include its pH_a, P_aco_2, and P_ao_2, with pH_a and P_aco_2 obviously being the parameters associated with assessing acid-base balance. The pH_a is measured by means of a H⁺-sensitive glass electrode. P_aco_2 is measured using a modified pH electrode whose tip is surrounded by a membrane selectively permeable to CO_2. Blood P_ao_2 is measured amperometrically with an oxygen-sensitive electrode. In practice, each of the three electrodes undergoes periodic automated recalibrations using

standard buffers (for pH) or custom gas mixtures (for Pco_2 and Po_2) that ensure at least a 2-point "slope and intercept" linearity over the expected biological range of measurements. The sample's [HCO_3^-] is a calculated parameter, determined by the **Henderson–Hasselbalch equation** (Chap. 9). Recall that a weak acid HA dissociates only partially into its constituent ions, H⁺ and A⁻, as described by its equilibrium constant, K_a:

$$K_a = [H^+] \cdot [A^-]/[HA]$$

Solving for [H⁺] yields:

$$[H^+] = K_a \cdot [HA]/[A^-]$$

Converting all terms to their negative $\log_{10}$ equivalents gives:

$$-\log [H^+] = -\log K_a - \log ([HA]/[A^-])$$

Substituting "p" for $-\log_{10}$ yields:

$$pH = pK_a + \log ([A^-]/[HA])$$

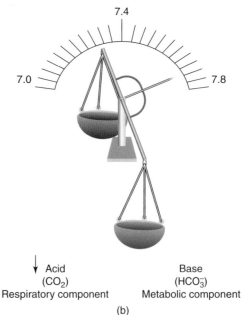

FIGURE 17.2 Respiratory acidosis (a) occurs when the acid component (CO_2) increases, promoting by mass balance the formation of more H_2CO_3 and thus free H⁺, decreasing pH. Respiratory alkalosis (b) occurs when this acid component represented by CO_2 decreases, thereby increasing pH_a.

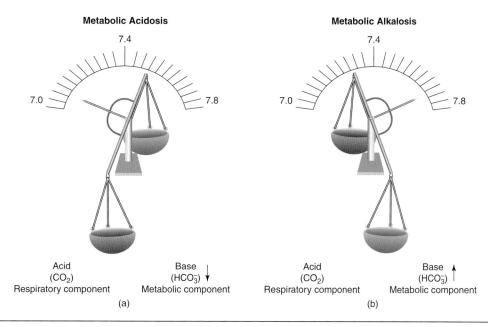

FIGURE 17.3 Metabolic acidosis (a) occurs when the base component (HCO_3^-) decreases, resulting in relatively more H_2CO_3, increasing [H^+], and decreasing blood pH. Metabolic alkalosis (b) occurs when the base component (HCO_3^-) increases, lowering H_2CO_3, decreasing [H^+], and increasing blood pH.

For the HCO_3^-/H_2CO_3 buffer system in blood, the most frequently cited value of pK_a is 6.1 for dissociation of the first H^+ from carbonic acid at 37°C. Thus, this generic equation for pH determination in arterial blood becomes:

$$pH_a = 6.1 + \log ([HCO_3^-]/[H_2CO_3])$$

The actual [H_2CO_3] cited here is not measurable directly but can be estimated from the sample's P_aco_2 and Henry's law (Chap. 1). By this approach, the solubility coefficient to estimate [H_2CO_3] in aqueous media is 0.03 mM/mm Hg P_aco_2. This substitution yields a working version of the **Henderson–Hasselbalch equation**. With the blood gas analyzer having directly measured two of the equation's three variables, its computer software solves for and reports an arterial [HCO_3^-] in mM using:

$$pH_a = 6.1 + \log ([HCO_3^-]/0.03 \cdot P_aco_2)$$

Reference ranges (or normal values) for these parameters are: pH_a = 7.36-7.44 or [H^+] = 40 nM; [HCO_3^-] = 22-28 mM; P_aco_2 = 35-45 mm Hg; and P_ao_2 = 85-100 mm Hg (when breathing room air, but higher when the F_Io_2 is increased). Their determinations allow assessment of a patient's current (A − a) Po_2 difference (Chap. 8) and acid/base status as well as the degree of compensation by the kidney or lungs for the primary abnormality. As stressed in Chap. 9, all disturbances in acid-base balance can be mathematically viewed as undesirable deviations from the 20:1 ratio of blood [HCO_3^-]/[H_2CO_3] that normally maintains pH_a at 7.4. This is so because the $\log_{10}$ of 20 = 1.3, which when added to the first dissociation constant pK_a for H_2CO_3 of 6.1 yields the protected pH_a of 7.4 at 37°C (98.6°F). Needless to say, there is an infinite number of paired values for [HCO_3^-] and [H_2CO_3] that can still satisfy this 20:1 ratio.

Determination and Interpretation of the Anion Gap

Most ABG measurements in patients are routinely accompanied by determination of the major serum electrolytes, notably [Na^+], [K^+], and [Cl^-]. Collectively these data provide estimates of all easily measured cations and anions in blood, whose charge totals must equal one another to achieve the electrochemical neutrality that exists in blood. However, routine serum assays do not measure the concentrations of other organic anions derived from dissociating weak acids in biological specimens, including lactate, pyruvate, and phosphates. The sum of all non-quantified anions is the **anion gap**, and must equal the difference between the sums of all measured cations and all measured anions. An accurate calculation of the most commonly reported **four-ion anion gap** is thus simply solved from:

$$\text{Anion gap (mM)} = ([Na^+] + [K^+]) - ([Cl^-] + [HCO_3^-])$$

For a calculated four-ion anion gap, the **normal reference range = 8-18 mM**. (At some institutions, serum [K^+] is excluded from anion gap calculations, lowering their normal reference range accordingly.) The anion gap distinguishes among the many causes of metabolic acidosis, notably those that induce elevated levels of lactate and other organic anions. As a general rule, the anion gap is increased proportionally to the aggregate concentration of these unmeasured anions. Consequently, a pure metabolic acidosis that is caused only by a direct reduction in [HCO_3^-] does not increase the calculated anion gap (Fig. 17.4).

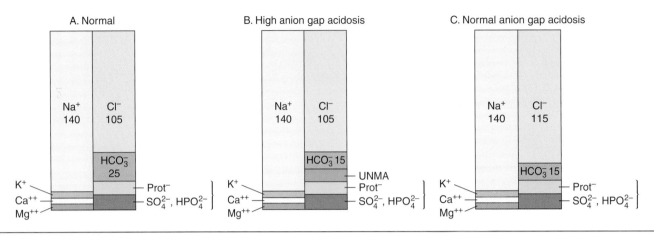

FIGURE 17.4 Histogram plots of measured cations and anions as well as all unmeasured anions (UNMA) in normal subjects and patients with metabolic acidosis with either elevated or normal anion gaps.

Clinical Algorithm to Assess Acid-Base Status

Using the theoretical constructs detailed above and patient data from the clinical laboratory, a simple stepwise method to assess acid-base balance can be applied:

Step 1: **Check arterial pH.**
  If pH_a <7.36, acidosis is present.
  If pH_a >7.44, alkalosis is present.

Step 2: **Check P_aCO_2.**
  For any acidotic pH_a:
  If P_aCO_2 <40 mm Hg, **metabolic acidosis** is present.
  If P_aCO_2 >40 mm Hg, **respiratory acidosis** is present.
  For any alkalotic pH_a:
  If P_aCO_2 <40 mm Hg, **respiratory alkalosis** is present
  If P_aCO_2 >40 mm Hg, **metabolic alkalosis** is present.

Step 3: **Calculate the anion gap.**
  This calculation is critical when Step 2 indicates metabolic acidosis.

Step 4: **Assess results and prepare differential diagnosis.**

Many chapters in this book combine these ABG results and anion gap determinations with other anatomical and physiological information to deduce likely disease states. Among the most problematic categories is metabolic acidosis, because it can be caused by many pathophysiological processes. Simplistically, these processes can be divided among those that increase circulating levels of nonvolatile acids and thus the anion gap, versus those that reduce blood [HCO_3^-] by any number of mechanisms. The principal causes of each category are listed in Table 17.2.

Pathophysiology of Metabolic Acidosis and Metabolic Alkalosis

The many causes of **anion gap metabolic acidosis** share several features in common. Methanol, paraldehyde, salicylate,

ethanol, ethylene glycol, and isoniazid can all result in elevated serum organic acids upon their metabolism. Virtually all of the anions created by dissociation of those organic acids are unmeasured, thereby increasing the reported anion gap. Uremia due to renal failure likewise elevates serum levels of weak nitrogenous acids. Diabetic ketoacidosis secondary to insulin insufficiency and hyperglycemia is a well-known development in which fatty acids and related compounds are oxidized to several ketoacids. Serum [lactate] most often increases during tissue hypoxia, when pyruvate is converted anaerobically to lactate instead of entering the tricarboxylic acid cycle for full oxidation to CO_2. **Nonanion gap metabolic acidosis** is usually the result of a direct loss of HCO_3^- or reduced ability of the kidneys to excrete acid. Serum [Cl^-] is often increased in these situations, so that the calculated anion gap remains within the reference range.

In both anion gap and nonanion gap metabolic acidosis, the expected respiratory response is hyperventilation that reduces P_aCO_2. This respiratory compensation can start within

Table **17.2** **Differential causes of metabolic acidosis**

Abnormal Anion Gap "MUDPILES"	Normal Anion Gap "HARDUP"
Methanol ingestion	Hypertonic saline infusion
Uremia	Acetazolamide administration
Diabetic ketoacidosis	Renal tubular acidosis
Paraldehyde poisoning	Diarrhea (most causes)
Isoniazid, Iron overload	Ureteral diversion
Lactic acidemia	Pancreatic fistula
Ethanol or ethylene glycol intoxication	
Salicylate overdose	

minutes and have an observable effect within 2 hours, such that maximal compensation is usually reached within 12-24 hours.

As indicated by the algorithm above, **metabolic alkalosis** is characterized by a significant elevation in pH_a that is accompanied by increased blood or serum $[HCO_3^-]$. The principal causes of metabolic alkalosis include:

- **Loss of nonvolatile acids** through vomiting or excessively acidic urine.
- **Hypochloridemia** (reduced serum $[Cl^-]$), which tends to enhance reabsorption of $[HCO_3^-]$ within the renal tubules.
- **Hypokalemia** (low serum $[K^+]$), which stimulates K^+ transport from the intracellular space in exchange for extracellular H^+ into cells. Hypokalemia also stimulates the reabsorption of HCO_3^- within the distal renal tubules.
- **Mineralocorticoid or corticosteroid excess**, which promotes an increase in renal Na^+ reabsorption in exchange for excretion of K^+ and H^+, resulting in hypokalemia and alkalosis, respectively.

The expected respiratory response to metabolic alkalosis is hypoventilation, causing an increasing in P_aCO_2. Compensation to correct the elevated pH_a by hypoventilation is expected within 2 hours, but may not be maximally effective for 12-24 hours. In general agreement with the concept of maintaining a constant 20:1 ratio of plasma $[HCO_3^-]/[H_2CO_3]$, respiratory compensation should increase P_aCO_2 by about 0.7 mm Hg for every 1 mM increase in plasma $[HCO_3^-]$.

Estimation of Base Excess

Base excess (**BE**) is a calculated term from a routine ABG assay that some clinicians use to determine if a patient's blood $[HCO_3^-]$ is above or below normal levels. If the BE is negative (= a **base deficit**) as in metabolic acidosis, the value is used to estimate how much IV HCO_3^- would correct the patient's pH or at least slow its descent. Thus, another definition of BE is the amount of acid or base that must be added to 1 liter of blood to return its pH to 7.4 when $P_aCO_2 = 40$ mm Hg. By this definition, for a blood sample whose pH = 7.40 and $P_aCO_2 = 40$ mm Hg at 37°C (98.6°F), and [Hb] = 15.0 g/dL, the BE = 0. Generally, the normal reference range for base excess is −2 mM to +2 mM.

Pathophysiology of Respiratory Acidosis and Respiratory Alkalosis

The measured P_aCO_2 reflects the balance between CO_2 production and its removal by ventilation of the lungs. Thus, the increased P_aCO_2 of respiratory acidosis usually represents hypoventilation in resting subjects, or an insufficient rise in ventilation when their $\dot{V}CO_2$ increases as during exertion. The principal causes of respiratory acidosis are many, with the most notable including:

- Obstructive lung diseases including asthma, emphysema, chronic bronchitis, acute bronchial pneumonia, allergic bronchoconstriction, and exacerbations of cystic fibrosis (see Chaps. 21, 22, and 38).
- Impaired function of central or peripheral receptors or control pathways, as with head or spinal trauma, sedation, anesthesia, certain sleep-related breathing disorders, and heart/lung transplantation (see Chaps. 11, 25, and 33).
- Mechanical hypoventilation, often done intentionally to create a temporary state of **permissive hypercapnia** when using the low tidal-volume protective strategy to ventilate intubated ALI and ARDS patients (see Chaps. 28 and 30).

Conversely, the decreased P_aCO_2 of respiratory alkalosis usually represents hyperventilation above the level that would normally be required to accommodate a subject's $\dot{V}O_2$ and $\dot{V}CO_2$. The principal causes of respiratory alkalosis include:

- Hypoxemia of any cause, including myocardial infarction, shock, pulmonary embolism, anemia, and high altitude hypoxia (see Chaps. 12, 13, 27, and 28).
- Anxiety, emotional distress, and related psychosomatic disorders that do not in themselves increase a subject's $\dot{V}O_2$ proportionally to the increase in $\dot{V}_E$.
- Hyperventilation during mechanical ventilation, generally considered to be caused by inappropriate management of V_T, f, or peak airway pressures, resulting in increased physiological dead space and thus $\dot{V}_A/\dot{Q}$ mismatch.
- Trauma, burns, and sepsis when accompanied by significant pain or insufficient pain management, particularly if such injuries involve those nonpulmonary organs that have the potential to powerfully stimulate nociceptive pathways.

Suggested Readings

1. Toffaletti JG. *Blood Gases and Electrolytes,* 2nd ed. AACC Press. *Authored by a clinical chemist, this book does an excellent job of explaining blood gases, acid-base balance, and various disorders of electrolytes.*

2. Sherwin AE. Acid-base control and acid-base disorders. In: *Clinical Chemistry: Theory, Analysis, Correlation,* 5th ed. St. Louis, MO: Mosby; 2010. *This is an excellent chapter that describes the various acid base disorders and the measurements to help diagnose causes of the disorders.*

CASE STUDIES AND PRACTICE PROBLEMS

CASE 17.1 Patients A and B present with the following arterial values:

	Patient A	Patient B	Reference range
pH_a	7.21	7.21	7.36-7.44
P_aCO_2	24 mm Hg	24 mm Hg	35-45 mm Hg
$[HCO_3^-]_a$	9 mM	9 mM	22-28 mM
$[Na^+]$	140 mM	140 mM	135-145 mM
$[K^+]$	5 mM	5 mM	3.5-5.0 mM
$[Cl^-]$	96 mM	121 mM	96-111 mM
[Glucose]	110 mg/dL	110 mg/dL	70-115 mg/dL

What is the most likely explanation for the lab findings of each patient?

	Patient A	Patient B
a. Diabetic ketoacidosis	_____	_____
b. Fever	_____	_____
c. Respiratory acidosis	_____	_____
d. Salicylate intoxication	_____	_____
e. Diarrhea	_____	_____

CASE 17.2 Arterial blood gases and serum chemistry data for a 71-year-old male patient show the following results: $[Na^+]$ = 139 mM; $[K^+]$ = 4.4 mM; $[Cl^-]$ = 85 mM; pH_a = 7.37; P_aCO_2 = 79 mm Hg; and $[HCO_3^-]$ = 43 mM. No other reliable history or physical exam information is available regarding this patient. Which of the following is the most likely explanation for these results?

a. Diabetic ketoacidosis
b. Excessive vomiting
c. Renal tubular acidosis
d. Emphysema
e. Septicemia

CASE 17.3 Which of the following situations would be most likely to cause a decrease in the P_aO_2 of a 5 mL arterial sample just drawn for blood gas analysis?

a. There is a 0.5 mL air bubble in the syringe.
b. The blood sits for 45 minutes at 27°C before delivery to the lab.
c. The blood sample is stored on ice for 30 minutes.
d. A needle is left on the syringe when delivered to the lab.

CASE 17.4 A 33-year-old woman with a history of anxiety and poor weight control presents to her primary care physician. She was referred by her dentist who noted erosion on the posterior surfaces of her central and lateral incisors. The physician orders arterial blood gas analysis. Which results are most consistent with this patient's clinical history?

a. pH_a = 7.40; P_aCO_2 = 40 mm Hg; $[HCO_3^-]_a$ = 24 mM
b. pH_a = 7.32; P_aCO_2 = 30 mm Hg; $[HCO_3^-]_a$ = 18 mM
c. pH_a = 7.35; P_aCO_2 = 55 mm Hg; $[HCO_3^-]_a$ = 32 mM
d. pH_a = 7.46; P_aCO_2 = 30 mm Hg; $[HCO_3^-]_a$ = 21 mM
e. pH_a = 7.49; P_aCO_2 = 46 mm Hg; $[HCO_3^-]_a$ = 33 mM

Solutions to Case Studies and Practice Problems

CASE 17.1 The most correct answer for Patient A is d, salicylate intoxication. The pH_a is <7.36 and P_{CO_2} is <40 mm Hg, indicating a metabolic acidosis (recall the simple series of steps to determine this). Calculation of the four-ion anion gap yields: $(140+5)-(9+96)=$ 40 mM, which is significantly elevated above normal range. Among the possible answers, only diabetic ketoacidosis and salicylate intoxication are part of the mnemonic **MUDPILES**. Since blood [glucose] is not elevated in Patient A, diabetic ketoacidosis is unlikely, leaving only salicylate intoxication in the differential diagnosis.

The most correct answer for Patient B is e, diarrhea. It has already been established that this is another case of metabolic acidosis. Calculation of the four-ion anion gap in this case yields: $(140 + 5) - (9 + 121) =$ 15 mM, which is within the reference range for a four-anion gap

calculation. The only choice in this offered differential diagnosis that produces metabolic acidosis without an increased anion gap is diarrhea.

CASE 17.2 The most correct answer is d.

With pH_a = 7.37, this is a mild acidosis within the reference range. However, $[HCO_3^-]$ and P_aCO_2 are clearly abnormal, suggesting a compensated acid-base abnormality; because P_aCO_2 >40 mm Hg, a respiratory acidosis is most likely. Among causes offered in the differential diagnosis, only emphysema would cause respiratory acidosis, probably of the type 2 variant associated with airway obstruction, reduced $\dot{V}_A$, and increased physiological shunt (Chap. 8). Thus the increased $[HCO_3^-]$ reflects its retention by the kidneys to offset the hypoventilation-induced elevation of P_aCO_2.

CASE 17.3 The most correct answer is b.

Of the four choices, only storage on ice for up to 30 minutes (*answer c*) is the appropriate way to hold and/or transfer such an ABG sample. However, leaving a needle on the syringe or introducing an air bubble (*answers a and d*) will raise the sample's apparent P_aO_2 and its pH_a, and lower its P_aCO_2 due to the higher ambient PO_2 in air with its low PCO_2 (Chap. 8). Storage of the sample at room temperature will not prevent ongoing aerobic metabolism by the sample's leukocytes and platelets, and thus a decrease in the sample's P_aO_2 will have occurred by the time it is measured 45 minutes later.

CASE 17.4 The most correct answer is e.

Presumably the woman's dentist is concerned that the patient's tooth enamel is being eroded by recurrent exposures to stomach acid during vomiting. Such persistent metabolic alkalosis (*answers d or e*) will lead to chronic elevations in plasma $[HCO_3^-]$. The appropriate compensation is at least moderate hypoventilation that elevates P_aCO_2 to reestablish the desired 20:1 ratio between bicarbonate and carbonic acid concentrations.

Chapter 18

Diagnostic Flexible Bronchoscopy

DAVID A. STOECKEL, MD AND
GEORGE M. MATUSCHAK, MD

Learning Objectives

- The student will be able to identify clinical indications and contraindications for flexible bronchoscopy for diagnostic evaluation of respiratory system diseases.

- The student will be able to describe the stepwise performance of a diagnostic flexible bronchoscopy, the equipment utilized, and possible complications.

- The student will be able to enumerate the types of diagnostic samples obtained by flexible bronchoscopy and their utility in establishing an etiologic diagnosis.

Introduction

Bronchoscopy adds light and color to the study of diseases of the respiratory system. As one of the most important diagnostic procedures in pulmonary medicine, it enables the physician to **visually inspect** the tracheobronchial tree and to **obtain samples** from the lungs, including distal air spaces, in a non-invasive fashion. Clinical bronchoscopic procedures date back to Gustav Killian, who in 1897 performed the first inspection and therapeutic intervention within the human tracheobronchial tree. Reports indicate that he used a rigid bronchoscope to successfully remove a foreign body lodged in the patient's right mainstem bronchus. During the early twentieth century, a **rigid bronchoscope** remained the only tool available to thoracic physicians to diagnose and treat diseases of the respiratory system. Such rigid bronchoscopes consisted of a hollow metal tube plus a light source that allowed for passage of suction catheters and various tools to extract aspirated foreign bodies. The rigid bronchoscope did not allow access to smaller lobar airways or to any airway segment that could not be linearly aligned with the oropharynx. In 1967, Ikeda of Japan developed the **flexible fiberoptic bronchoscope**, enabling procedures to be performed with greater ease and comfort for awake patients using minimal anesthesia, and giving access to segmental and even subsegmental airways.

Contemporary Bronchoscopy Equipment

(#10)

The modern flexible adult bronchoscope has a diameter of 5-6 mm and is 50-60 cm in length (Fig. 18.1). Most flexible bronchoscopes have a **fiberoptic light source** as well as a lens for viewing, and a hollow channel for suction that also permits the passage of instruments to and beyond the distal tip of the bronchoscope. Such bronchoscopes are maneuvered manually through the patient's airways by variably deflecting its distal end, using a lever mounted on the proximal portion of the instrument that is held by the physician. Images are generally displayed on a video screen in the bronchoscopy suite or at the bedside of critically ill patients. In addition to providing a means to aspirate tracheobronchial secretions, blood, or other airway debris via suction, the hollow working channel allows for the passage of a wide variety of specially designed tools into the airways. These include small sampling brushes, miniature forceps for obtaining tissue samples and needles for obtaining aspirates. The working channel can also be used to deliver medications such as **topical anesthetic** and to deliver saline to **lavage** the airways (see below).

The modern **bronchoscopy suite** (Fig. 18.2) usually is a room specifically equipped for, and dedicated to, these procedures. In some clinical settings, bronchoscopies may be performed in a common area used for multiple types of endoscopic procedures. Bronchoscopies are also routinely performed in operating rooms and intensive care units (ICUs). The bronchoscopy suite typically utilizes a bed or table that can accept a **portable fluoroscopy "C-arm" unit** for positioning over the chest region of interest. Radiological imaging using fluoroscopy increases patient safety when obtaining samples from the lung periphery through airways that are too small to permit direct visualization. Always present in the bronchoscopy suite is all equipment needed to automatically monitor a patient's vital signs including a continuous reading of S_aO_2, and to provide supplemental O_2, suction, and emergency resuscitation.

Indications and Contraindications for Bronchoscopy

The possible indications for flexible bronchoscopy are numerous and will vary with the unique circumstances of each individual patient. In general, indications can be divided into those involving known or suspected abnormalities of the **large**

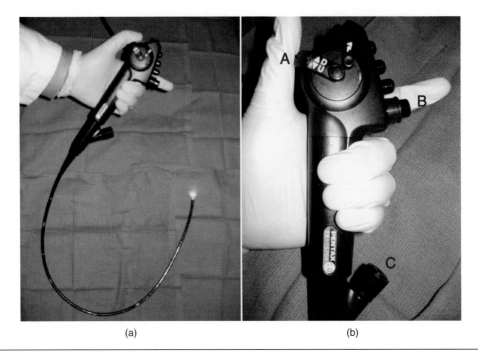

(a)   (b)

FIGURE 18.1 (a) Adult flexible fiberoptic video bronchoscope, with illumination evident at distal end. (b) Close-up view of bronchoscope handle showing directional lever used to flex or extend its distal tip (A), suction control button (B), and proximal port (C) for accessing the internal channel that extends to the distal tip.

airways, those involving the **lung parenchyma**, and abnormalities of **extrapulmonary** or **mediastinal structures** (Table 18.1). Indications where inspection and possible sampling of the large airways are the primary objectives include evaluation for suspected **tracheal stenosis** or excessive tracheal collapse during the respiratory cycles secondary to abnormal inflammatory softening of the tracheal walls known as **tracheomalacia** (Chap. 37). Likewise, bronchoscopy allows inspections

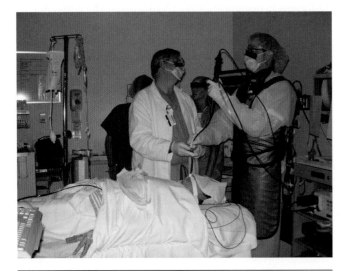

FIGURE 18.2 Performance of a diagnostic flexible fiberoptic procedure in the bronchoscopy suite. In this case, the bronchoscope is being passed via an electively placed endotracheal tube to permit simultaneous assisted ventilation when needed.

Table **18.1** **Possible indications for diagnostic flexible bronchoscopy**

Evaluation of Large Airway Abnormalities	Evaluation of Parenchymal Abnormalities
Tracheal stenosis	Pneumonia
Tracheomalacia	Pneumonitis
Upper airway obstruction	Diffuse alveolar hemorrhage (DAH)
Hemoptysis	Pulmonary nodules and masses
Chronic cough	Diffuse lung disease
Endobronchial tumors	Sarcoidosis
Tracheobronchitis	Organizing pneumonia
Tracheobronchial trauma	Lung transplant rejection
Inhalational injury	
Evaluation of Extrapulmonary or Mediastinal Abnormalities	
Hilar and/or mediastinal lymphadenopathy	
Mediastinal masses	

for tracheobronchial obstruction, endobronchial tumors in patients with a known or suspected malignancy (Chap. 31), persistent atelectasis on thoracic imaging studies (Chap. 15), and investigation of hemoptysis. In other conditions such as penetrating or nonpenetrating **thoracic trauma** or **inhalational injury**, bronchoscopy is useful to directly assess acute airway damage and altered anatomical integrity. Indications for diagnostic flexible bronchoscopy where the primary objective is to sample the lung parenchyma include evaluating unexplained, recurrent or severe **pneumonias**, investigating **diffuse alveolar hemorrhage (DAH)**, and sampling selected **pulmonary nodules** and **mass lesions**. Flexible bronchoscopy has a more limited role in diagnosing diffuse interstitial pulmonary processes (Chap. 24), although excluding infection and malignancy remain important. Indications where sampling of extrapulmonary or mediastinal structures is the goal include evaluating mediastinal or hilar **lymphadenopathy**, mediastinal masses and, increasingly, nodal involvement in patients with known or suspected lung cancer (Chaps. 31-33).

There are few absolute contraindications to diagnostic flexible bronchoscopy, and as for the indications, most contraindications vary with the unique circumstances of individual patients (Table 18.2). Impending hypoxic or hypercarbic respiratory failure without a **secured airway** (ie, an indwelling endotracheal tube to permit assisted ventilation and oxygenation) is a common contraindication. Likewise, nonsecured airways in patients with severe **OSA, mixed sleep apnea**, or **OHS** (Chap. 25) are contraindications, since sedating patients with these conditions for the procedure may worsen their reduced ventilatory drive and upper airway obstruction, culminating in progressively reduced $\dot{V}_A$, hypercapnea, and hypoxemia.

Marked large airway abnormalities, including partial tracheal obstruction, can be a contraindication despite the presence of an endotracheal tube or tracheostomy. High oxygen requirements and high airway pressures are also common contraindications. An untreated **pneumothorax** is a contraindication to flexible bronchoscopy, as are hemodynamic instability accompanying circulatory shock, unstable angina, recent myocardial infarction, coagulopathies, and platelet disorders. Recent oral intake or the inability to obtain adequate informed consent can be contraindications. Finally, lack of adequate trained personnel and lack of adequate equipment to perform the procedure is a contraindication. As with any procedure, the thoughtful and informed consideration of the risks and benefits of diagnostic bronchoscopy prior to performance of the procedure will allow for the safest environment and best overall outcome for the patient.

Performing the Procedure

Once informed consent is obtained and monitoring devices are in place, the patient's upper airway is typically anesthetized with a topical anesthetic such as 2% **xylocaine** delivered by nebulization. Most patients are provided with moderate or **conscious sedation** using intravenous **benzodiazepine** and **opiates**, with the level of sedation carefully maintained throughout a procedure. The bronchoscope is then advanced through the nose or mouth to a position just above the vocal chords. Additional local anesthetic (1% xylocaine) is usually administered to these structures at this point via the working channel of the bronchoscope. After observing the structure and function of the vocal chords and the appearance of the surrounding supraglottic structures, the bronchoscope is passed between the vocal chords as they open during inspiration. The tracheal column is then inspected for mucosal lesions (Fig. 18.3) and for its overall caliber (Chap. 37) until the carina is reached, representing division of the trachea into the right and left mainstem bronchi (Fig. 18.4).

Table **18.2** Possible contraindications to diagnostic flexible bronchoscopy

Severe hypoxemia or hypercarbia with impending respiratory failure
Severe obstructive sleep apnea syndrome without a secure airway
High grade tracheal obstruction
High inspired oxygen requirements
High airway pressures during mechanical ventilation
Untreated pneumothorax
Hemodynamic instability including shock
Unstable angina or recent myocardial infarction
Coagulopathy or platelet disorders
Recent oral intake
Inability to obtain informed consent
Lack of equipment or adequately trained personnel

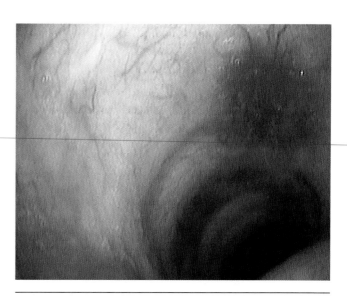

FIGURE 18.3 Bronchoscopic view of the tracheal wall demonstrating an erythematous lesion (upper right) consistent with a **Kaposi sarcoma**.

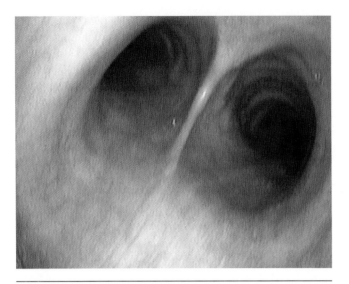

FIGURE 18.4 Bronchoscopic view of the normal sharply defined **carina** dividing the right and left mainstem bronchi. The posterior tracheal wall is at the bottom of the figure.

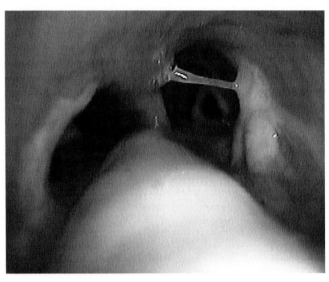

FIGURE 18.6 Purulent yellowish secretions associated with an underlying bacterial pneumonia involving the distal trachea and the bilateral mainstem bronchi.

Even at this proximal level of the tracheobronchial system, grossly abnormal findings including proximal neoplasms (Fig. 18.5; Chap. 31) and purulent secretions typifying bacterial pneumonia (Fig. 18.6; Chaps. 19 and 34) can be frequently encountered.

After inspection of the carina, the entire tracheobronchial tree is systematically evaluated according to a pre-procedural bronchoscopic plan. Thus, one side is selected first and the bronchoscope is passed from that mainstem bronchus into the lobar bronchi, segmental bronchi, and subsegmental bronchi in a systematic fashion until all lobes of a given lung have been examined. Assessment is specifically made for mucosal

irregularities, endobronchial obstructing lesions (Fig.18.7), and evidence of extrinsic airway compression by masses within the adjacent lung parenchyma or mediastinum (Fig. 18.8). Then the process is repeated to examine the opposite lung. To suppress the cough reflex, additional doses of topical anesthetic are given periodically throughout the exam via the working channel of the bronchoscope.

Next, specific areas of interest identified on any pre-procedure thoracic imaging studies or by the endobronchial exam become the focus of diagnostic sampling procedures. Knowledge of the endobronchial anatomy facilitates selective sampling of various sublobar pulmonary segments, or the

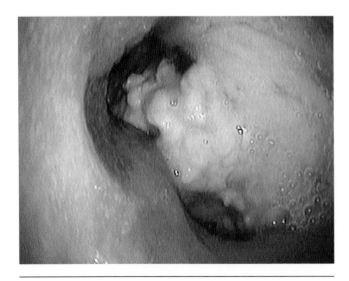

FIGURE 18.5 Squamous cell lung cancer that involves the carina and has extended into both mainstem bronchi.

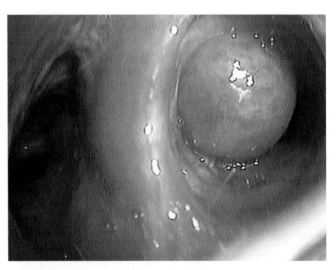

FIGURE 18.7 An endobronchial obstructing tumor (right side of field) that was subsequently diagnosed as a carcinoid tumor.

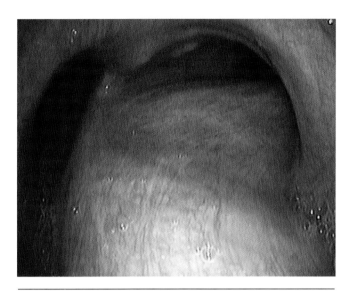

FIGURE 18.8 Extrinsic compression of the distal posterior tracheal wall and of the mainstem bronchus by a mediastinal mass.

transbronchial needle aspiration sampling of hilar and mediastinal lymph nodes and masses. Once sampling is complete and hemostasis is ensured, the bronchoscope is removed and the patient allowed to recover from sedation. Typical diagnostic bronchoscopies last from <15 minutes to >1 hour depending on complexity. Outpatients usually can return home safely after several hours' recovery.

Although it is common for patients to complain of a mild sore throat or even a low grade fever in the 24 hours following a procedure, major complications are rare. Asymptomatic or minimally symptomatic pneumothorax is likely to be the most common significant complication, especially following bronchoscopic lung biopsy procedures. Severe bleeding, respiratory failure, and cardiovascular events are less common, and mortality overall is less than 1 in 2,500 procedures.

Diagnostic Techniques

Bronchoalveolar lavage (BAL) is a very important sampling technique and has been referred to as a "liquid lung biopsy," since properly performed lavage is thought to sample the cells and other contents of approximately a million alveoli simultaneously. To obtain BAL fluid (BALF), the distal tip of the bronchoscope is carefully wedged into a subsegmental bronchus of interest. For diffuse pulmonary infiltrates, the right middle lobe or lingula is usually selected because BAL fluid return is maximized by gravity dependence. An aliquot of 50-60 mL of **normal sterile 0.9% NaCl (NS)** is then instilled through the working channel of the bronchoscope. After a few seconds, the NS is retrieved using gentle suction. These steps are usually repeated once or twice. BALF has special utility in the identification of pulmonary infections (see Chap. 19). A Gram stain and quantitative bacterial culture are usually performed on the BALF, with infection being suggested by the presence of polymorphonuclear neutrophils (PMNs, Chap. 10) that contain phagocytized microorganisms, confirmed by culture findings

of >10^4 colony-forming units (CFU)/mL of BALF. Such BALF samples are generally also sent for acid-fast smear and culture for *Mycobacterium* species as well as for fungal smear and culture (Chaps. 19, 35, and 36). Likewise, viral and *Legionella* cultures can be ordered on BALF, as can silver stains for *Pneumocystis jiroveci*.

▶▶CLINICAL CORRELATION 18.1

In addition to identifying specific infections of the lower respiratory tract, analysis of the **cell count** and **differential** of BALF may suggest specific pathological conditions. For example, the normal percentage of PMNs in BALF of healthy nonsmoking adults is 2%-3%, but increases to ~5%-7% in active smokers. By contrast, high percent of PMNs (ie, >20%) suggests **acute inflammation** within distal airspaces that frequently occurs during **infectious pneumonias**. Alternatively, an elevated percentage of eosinophils may indicate a **drug reaction** or **eosinophilic pneumonia**. A BALF sample that becomes progressively bloodier with sequential aspirations of instilled NS is compatible with the bleeding of **diffuse alveolar hemorrhage (DAH)**. Such DAH may accompany connective tissue disorders or drug reactions that cause bilateral pulmonary infiltrates, even in the absence of frank **hemoptysis**. Flow cytometric analysis of BALF is very useful in identifying a **pulmonary lymphoma** (Chap. 31) and to determine the $CD4^+/CD8^+$, that is, the T-cell helper to suppressor ratio in the fluid. This latter result may help identify a noninfectious diffuse lung disease such as **sarcoidosis** (a $CD4^+$ T-cell dominant pulmonary process) versus **hypersensitivity pneumonitis** (a $CD8^+$ T-cell dominant process) (Chaps. 23 and 24). Lastly, BALF can be sent for cytologic analysis in an attempt to identify particular malignancies (Table 18.3).

Table **18.3** Utility of bronchoalveolar lavage in diagnosing respiratory diseases

Diagnostic	Suggestive
Infectious pneumonias:	Sarcoidosis
Bacterial, *Legionella*, *Mycobacteriae*, fungi,	Hypersensitivity pneumonitis
Pneumocystis jiroveci, viral	Amiodarone pulmonary toxicity
Eosinophilic pneumonia	Pulmonary lymphoproliferative disorders
Lung cancer (lymphangitis carcinomatosa)	
Pulmonary alveolar proteinosis	
Diffuse alveolar injury, incl. hemorrhage	
Langerhans' cell histiocytosis	

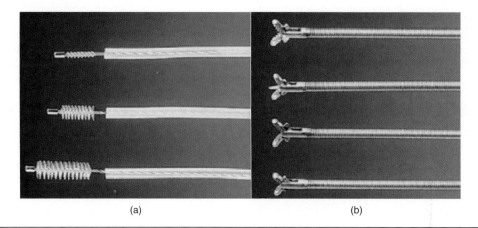

(a)   (b)

FIGURE 18.9 Shown are brushes of increasing sizes (a) and different types of biopsy forceps (b) that can be passed through the working channel of a flexible fiberoptic bronchoscope for diagnostic purposes. The brushes are shown protruding from their surrounding plastic sheaths and the forceps are splayed. *From Prakash U.* Bronchoscopy. In: Clinical Respiratory Medicine, 3rd ed., Albert R, Spiro S, Jett J., eds. *Philadelphia: Mosby, 2008.*

In addition to permitting performance of BAL, the working channel of the bronchoscope allows for the passage of various miniature devices into the airways (Fig. 18.9). One type of sampling device is a sterile brush, located at the end of a long wire that can be protruded from its protective plastic sheath, once the bronchoscope is properly located in an airway of interest. These brushes can be used to collect specimens for culture or cytologic analysis directly from a visualized endobronchial lesion, or from the walls of small distal airways. **Fluoroscopy** is instrumental in helping to guide these brushes to areas of specific interest in the peripheral lung regions.

The working channel of the bronchoscope also accommodates small biopsy forceps attached via a long wire to a handle that opens and closes their cutting or grasping jaws. Forceps are used to biopsy bronchial walls of interest identified by visual inspection, and may be passed into smaller airways under fluoroscopic guidance to biopsy more peripheral regions of interest. Using this technique of **transbronchial lung biopsy**, alveolated lung tissue is obtained for histological examination (Fig. 18.10).

Samples from a transbronchial lung biopsy can be sent for both histopathological and microbiological evaluations. Although very useful diagnostically (Table 18.4), specimens obtained by this technique are small, and may be insufficient in size to characterize many diffuse inflammatory and fibrotic parenchymal and interstitial lung conditions.

Finally, the working channel of the flexible bronchoscope can allow for the passage of various needle devices into the airways (Fig. 18.11). Such needles are used for **transbronchial needle aspiration** to obtain aspirates of visualized endobronchial lesions, or more distal parenchymal lesions with the assistance of fluoroscopy. The needles also permit sampling of mediastinal and hilar lymph nodes and masses by passing the needle through walls of the trachea or bronchi.

Careful review of imaging and a keen understanding of endobronchial, mediastinal, and thoracic anatomy allow performance of this procedure to be safe and rewarding. The aspirates are typically sent for cytologic analysis. In addition, larger needles can be used to obtain "core biopsies" that can be sent for histopathologic analysis.

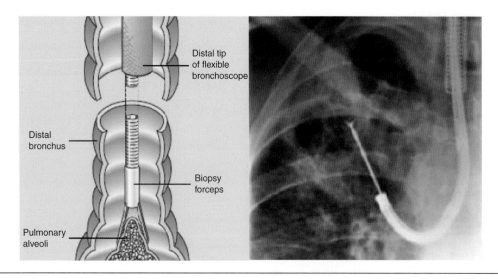

Distal tip of flexible bronchoscope

Distal bronchus

Biopsy forceps

Pulmonary alveoli

FIGURE 18.10 Performance of transbronchial lung biopsy with fluoroscopic guidance. *From Prakash U.* Bronchoscopy. In: Clinical Respiratory Medicine, 3rd ed., Albert R, Spiro S, Jett J., eds. *Philadelphia: Mosby, 2008.*

Table **18.4** **Respiratory conditions with high diagnostic yield by transbronchial biopsy**

Mycobacterial infections	Sarcoidosis
P jiroveci infection	Pulmonary alveolar proteinosis
Fungal infections	Primary or metastatic lung cancer
Cytomegalovirus infection	Allograft rejection following lung transplantation
Diffuse pulmonary lymphoma	Hypersensitivity pneumonitis
Eosinophilic pneumonia	Langerhans' cell histiocytosis

▶▶ **CLINICAL CORRELATION 18.2**

In general, diagnostic yields from flexible fiberoptic bronchoscopy for specific respiratory system diseases are amplified by acquisition of multiple types of specimens during the same procedure. For example, in the case of **visible endobronchial tumors**, combining bronchial washings and brushings for cytological analysis with at least three endobronchial biopsies for histopathological evaluation maximizes the likelihood of establishing the diagnosis.

The Future of Diagnostic Flexible Bronchoscopy

If the past decade is a reliable indication, clinicians can expect rapid innovations in the field of diagnostic flexible bronchoscopy. Ultrasound-tipped flexible bronchoscopes have recently been introduced that allow for accurate identification and sampling of mediastinal lymph nodes and masses once inaccessible via standard flexible fiberoptic bronchoscopy (Fig. 18.12). In addition,

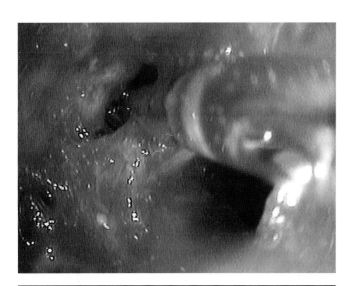

FIGURE 18.11 Transbronchial needle aspiration from the wall of a narrowed right middle lobe bronchus. Note the splayed jaws of the enclosing forceps (the dark bar in upper left center of image) that shield the needle prior to use.

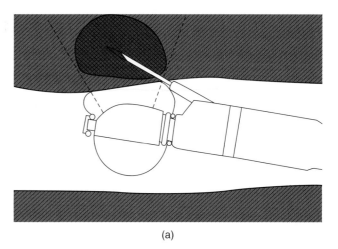

(a)

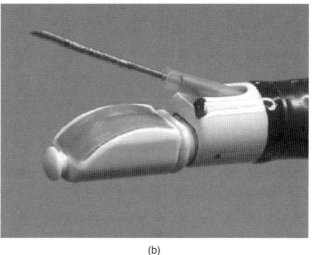

(b)

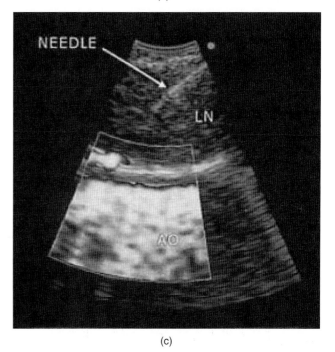

(c)

FIGURE 18.12 Schematic (a) and photograph (b) of an endobronchial ultrasound bronchoscope. An ultrasound image (c) shows a fine needle aspiration of a lymph node near a large blood vessel. *From Sheski F, Mathur P: endotracheal Ultrasound, Chest. Jan;133(1):264-70, 2008.*

small ultrasound probes can be passed through a standard bronchoscope to help locate nodules and masses in the distal lung.

Advances in CT imaging and computerized reconstruction have fostered development of three-dimensional **virtual bronchoscopy** by which endobronchial anatomy is analyzed prior to the bronchoscopic procedure and aides in localization of lesions. Taking this approach a step further, virtual bronchoscopy can be fused with the actual procedure in real time to provide **electromagnetic navigational bronchoscopy** to enhance the precision of finding and sampling peripheral lung lesions.

Finally, replacing the conventional light source of a flexible bronchoscope with light of a different wavelength or with highly restricted wavelengths is being investigated to detect premalignant or small malignant lesions involving the endobronchial mucosa. These are known respectively as **autofluorescence bronchoscopy** and **narrow band imaging bronchoscopy**. These exciting new technologies will expand the roles of diagnostic flexible bronchoscopy toward more accurate and minimally invasive procedures than previously have been required.

Suggested Readings

1. Prakash U. Bronchoscopy. In: Albert R, Spiro S, Jett J., eds. *Clinical Respiratory Medicine*, 2nd ed. Philadelphia, PA: Mosby; 2004. *A concise review of bronchoscopy with many helpful tables, illustrations and photographs.*

2. Ernst A. *Introduction to Bronchoscopy*. New York, NY: Cambridge Univ. Press; 2009. *An in-depth and very readable review of basic bronchoscopy. Contains many fine color photographs and illustrations.*

CASE STUDIES AND PRACTICE PROBLEMS

CASE 18.1 Which of the following would benefit most from a diagnostic flexible bronchoscopy?

a. A 34-year-old man with HIV and low CD4$^+$ count who developed fever and nonproductive cough over the past week; his chest x-ray reveals diffuse opacities.

b. A 60-year-old woman with hypertension who developed fever, cough productive of "rusty" sputum, and right-sided pleuritic chest pain over the past 4 days; her chest x-ray reveals an infiltrate in the right lower lobe.

c. A 28-year-old woman just admitted to the ICU with ARDS after nearly drowning in salt water; she is intubated and being ventilated at $F_IO_2 = 1.00$ and $P_{PEAK} = 30$ cm H_2O to maintain her S_aO_2 at 88%.

d. A 70-year-old diabetic man with worsening cough, frothy sputum and shortness of breath over the past 2 days; his chest x-ray reveals bilateral pleural effusions and bilateral perihilar infiltrates, and he is tachycardic with an irregular heart rhythm.

CASE 18.2 Which of the following is the most serious contraindication to performing diagnostic flexible bronchoscopy?

a. Arterial [Hb] = 7.5 g/dL

b. Implanted cardiac pacemaker and defibrillator

c. Intubated patient with severe obstructive sleep apnea

d. Hypercarbic respiratory failure requiring non-invasive mechanical ventilation

CASE 18.3 Which of the following techniques would be most helpful in confirming a diagnosis of diffuse alveolar hemorrhage?

a. Transbronchial lung biopsy

b. Transbronchial fine needle aspiration of mediastinal lymph nodes

c. Bronchoalveolar lavage

d. Visual evaluation of the endobronchial tree to the level of the subsegmental airways

Solutions to Case Studies and Practice Problems

CASE 18.1 The most correct answer is a.

The 34-year-old man with HIV and a low CD4 count may have a typical community acquired pneumonia, but is at risk for a wide range of opportunistic infections. A diagnostic flexible bronchoscopy with BAL will help to determine the pathogen and most appropriate therapy. The 60-year-old woman likely has typical community acquired pneumonia and would not require a diagnostic bronchoscopy

unless her sputum studies were not diagnostic and she failed to improve with appropriate therapy (*answer b*). The 28-year-old woman with ARDS after a near drowning will require appropriate ventilator therapy for her lung injury. Bronchoscopy may actually be contraindicated given her high F_IO_2 requirements and high airway pressures (*answer c*). The 70-year-old diabetic man likely has congestive heart failure and does not require bronchoscopy (*answer d*).

CASE 18.2 The most correct answer is d.

Hypercarbic respiratory failure would preclude a safe diagnostic bronchoscopy without the presence of a secured airway via endotracheal intubation. Moderate anemia (*answer a*), cardiac pacemakers and defibrillators (*answer b*), or severe obstructive sleep apnea in a patient with a secure airway via endotracheal intubation (*answer c*) are not typically contraindications to flexible diagnostic bronchoscopy.

CASE 18.3 The most correct answer is c.

The presence of progressively bloody serial bronchoalveolar lavages is very suggestive of diffuse alveolar hemorrhage. Visual evaluation (*answer d*) may or may not reveal blood in the visible larger airways in patients with diffuse alveolar damage (DAD), but it is not sensitive or specific for that diagnosis. Similarly, transbronchial lung biopsy (*answer a*) or fine needle aspiration of mediastinal lymph nodes (*answer b*) would not be the test of choice for diffuse alveolar hemorrhage.

Chapter 19

Evaluating Sputum and Pleural Effusions

MARY M. MAYO, PhD AND
ANDREW J. LECHNER, PhD

Introduction to Laboratory Analysis of Sputum

Pneumonia is an infectious process affecting the parenchyma of the lungs. Infectious agents that are potentially responsible for such pneumonia include bacteria, fungi, viruses, and rarely parasites. The goal when evaluating sputum in the laboratory is to confirm the diagnosis of pneumonia, identify the etiologic agent(s) responsible for producing the present disease, and guide selection of appropriate antibiotic therapy.

Sputum Collection and Gram Staining

Expectorated sputum is the most common lower respiratory tract specimen received in the clinical microbiology laboratory. Sputum can be collected either by **spontaneous expectoration** or after **sputum induction**, which is collected following instillation or inhalation of an irritating aerosol such as hypertonic saline. Sputum induction is performed when the patient cannot produce sputum. Generally, the first morning sputum samples are the best specimens; a volume of 5-10 mL is usually adequate. Because many received specimens consist mostly of pharyngeal secretions and upper airway cells rather than sputum, the first step in evaluating a specimen's suitability uses a **Gram stain** (Fig. 19.1). Use of such a Gram stain assesses specimen acceptability for further processing, and aids interpretation by identifying the morphology of any likely etiologic agents of pneumonia in a specimen that is acceptably **purulent**.

Ideally, a sputum sample examined microscopically should contain <10 epithelial cells per low power field (LPF), or from 10-25 epithelial cells and >25 leukocytes/LPF. Sputum specimens containing >25 squamous epithelial cells are rejected because these represent oropharyngeal secretions that will be heavily contaminated with normal throat flora. Likewise, a sputum specimen containing no epithelial cells, leukocytes, or bacteria is rejected because the specimen is an inadequate representation of conditions in the intermediate airways. Most hospital laboratories have well-established guidelines of this type, including stipulations as to the handling of such potentially dangerous biological specimens. These guidelines can be adjusted when a particular patient's needs are communicated to the laboratory personnel.

The Gram stain report on a sputum sample includes the types of organism seen, whether they are gram-positive or -negative, and the architecture of the organism, whether cocci or bacilli. Such information gives important clues as to possible identifications of organisms found. For example, gram-positive cocci that appear as grape-like clusters raise suspicion for *Staphylococcus* spp., while gram-positive lancet-shaped diplococci suggest *Streptococcus pneumoniae*. The presence of gram-negative coccobacilli often indicates *Haemophilus influenzae*. In the same sputum report, the number of organisms present is usually estimated as **many**, **moderate**, **few**, or **rare**. In most laboratories, these terms pertain to the number of similar organisms present per high power field (HPF) using oil immersion: **many** >10 organisms/HPF; **moderate** = 5-10 organisms/HPF, **few** = 1-5 organisms/HPF, and **rare** <1 organism/HPF.

Sputum Culture

A sputum sample can be cultured as indicated, both for routine bacterial pathogens, as well as for a variety of other microorganisms including *Mycobacteriae* and fungi (Fig. 19.2).

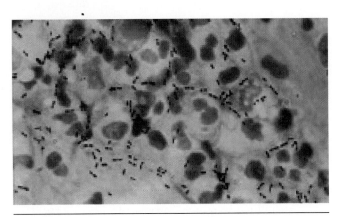

FIGURE 19.1 A typical sputum sample that has been Gram-stained to show neutrophils, epithelial cells, and gram-positive bacteria, in this case diplococci. *Courtesy of C. Sinave, MD.*

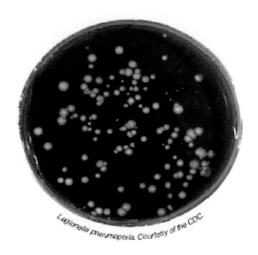

FIGURE 19.3 Cultures of *Legionella pneumophila* growing on charcoal yeast extract agar. *Image courtesy* of the Centers for Disease Control and Prevention (CDC).

Some culture results are available within days while others, particularly for fungi and *Mycobacteriae*, may require several weeks to yield definitive results. Sputum smears and cultures for fungi and/or *Mycobacteriae* must be ordered separately in most laboratory settings, since special culture media are needed for many of the atypical bacterial infections, such as *Mycobacterium* and *Legionella* (Fig. 19.3).

Some organisms are best discovered using serology, notably *Chlamydia* and *Mycoplasma*. These organisms will not grow on routine microbiological culture media. Urine antigens also can be assessed for *Legionella* and *S. pneumoniae*.

Sputum for Cytology

Sputum specimens may also be submitted for cytological exam of individual cells, usually when looking for neoplasms (Chap. 31). For such purposes, the sputum specimen is collected into a cup with a special mucolytic fluid that improves visualization

of the cells contained therein (Fig. 19.4). These specimens are sent to surgical pathology and not to the microbiology section of a hospital laboratory. As with other sputum specimens, these should be delivered to the laboratory as soon as possible.

Introduction to Analysis of Pleural Effusions

The pleural space often is described as a **potential space** that exists between the juxtaposed **visceral pleura** covering the outer surface of the lung and **parietal pleura** lining the inner surface of the chest wall. As such, the pleural space normally contains just a few milliliters of fluid (Fig. 19.5). Laboratory characteristics of **normal pleural fluid** include: pH = 7.6, [protein] = 1-2 g/dL (vs plasma [protein] $\cong$ 7 g/dL), [glucose] $\cong$ plasma [glucose], and [lactate dehydrogenase] <50% of

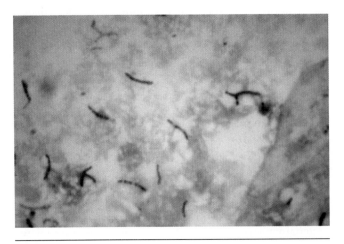

FIGURE 19.2 Use of the Ziehl-Neelsen stain to visualize *Mycobacteria* in a sputum sample. *Mycobacteria* are acid-fast and retain the red color of the carbolfuchsin.

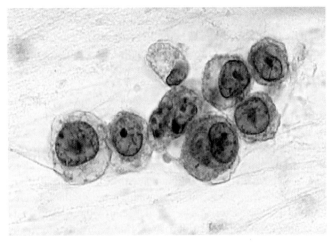

FIGURE 19.4 View of non-small cell carcinoma in a mucolytically processed sputum sample. See Chap. 31 for additional information.

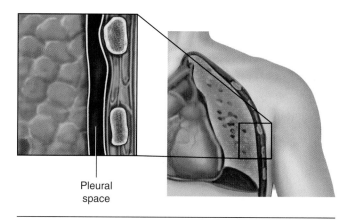

Pleural
space

FIGURE 19.5 Diagram of the pleural space created by close apposition of the visceral and parietal pleura. *Adapted from A.D.A.M. Interactive Anatomy* http://adameducation.com/aionline_student.aspx.

plasma [LDH]. The number of WBC in pleural fluid is normally <1,000/mL and consists predominantly of mononuclear cells with a few erythrocytes and mesothelial cells. Normally there are <10 mL of pleural fluid in the entire thoracic space of a healthy adult.

Physiology of the Pleural Space

A detailed description of the physical forces that create pleural fluid is presented in Chap. 29. In brief, pleural fluid is formed by the same forces that generate edema elsewhere, according to Starling's law of the capillary (Chap. 7). The normal hydrostatic pressure of ~30 mm Hg in systemic capillaries of the parietal pleura drives extravasation of ultrafiltrate into the pleural space. This occurs because this hydrostatic pressure exceeds the net colloid osmotic pressure gradient of ~24 mm Hg between those systemic capillaries and the few proteins in normal pleural space fluid.

At the same time, the normally low hydrostatic pressure of ~12 mm Hg within pulmonary capillaries lying beneath the visceral pleura is considerably less than this same colloid osmotic pressure gradient of 24 mm Hg between the plasma and normal pleural fluid. This osmotic gradient thus normally drives pleural fluids into the lung tissue, adding to pulmonary lymph created within all of the alveoli (Chap. 7). By this mechanism, as long as the protein concentration within the pleural space remains low and/or pulmonary capillary pressure is normal, virtually all of the fluid being lost from systemic capillaries into the pleural space is rapidly removed into the lungs across the visceral pleural membrane to form lymph.

Conversely, such extravasated fluids accumulate into a **pleural effusion** if increased capillary hydrostatic pressures overwhelm the osmotic pressure gradient, as in systemic or pulmonary hypertension. A pleural effusion created by such altered hydrostatic forces would be considered a **transudate**. Pleural fluid also accumulates if the colloid osmotic pressure

within the pleural space becomes elevated, as by neoplasm or infectious agent. Such an increase in pleural fluid osmotic pressure reduces the normally large osmotic gradient between plasma proteins and proteins within the pleural space. A pleural effusion created under such conditions would be classified as an **exudate**, and as discussed below may become **empyemic**. Effusions of either type will accumulate when lymphatic obstruction or other defect prevents their timely drainage or reabsorption. Additional sources of pleural fluid include excessive drainage of lymph from the interstitial spaces of the lung into the visceral pleura, or **ascites** fluid from the peritoneal cavity that enters the thoracic space via small holes in the diaphragm.

Laboratory Analysis of Pleural Fluids

Thoracentesis is the intentional and guided collection of pleural fluid from the otherwise closed chest, a procedure that may yield several liters depending on the cause of a patient's effusion (Fig. 19.6). Not surprisingly, thoracentesis can have both diagnostic and therapeutic values, since evacuating effusions may remove infectious material and permit re-expansion of lung lobes that develop atelectasis by fluid compression.

Proper technique for handling pleural effusions includes sending all fluid obtained, even if consisting of several liters. Samples are refrigerated if analyses will be delayed, but no fixative is needed. Separate specimens are needed for studies in microbiology, hematology, and chemistry. In practice, these are processed by most laboratories "24/7". Specimens are sent to flow cytometry when lymphoma or leukemia is suspected.

Once a sample of pleural effusion is obtained, the first step in its evaluation is to determine whether the fluid is a transudate or an exudate. Often the physician will have a strong suspicion regarding its type in a patient with known underlying disease.

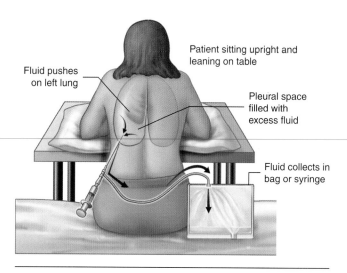

Patient sitting upright and leaning on table

Fluid pushes on left lung

Pleural space filled with excess fluid

Fluid collects in bag or syringe

FIGURE 19.6 Diagram of a patient undergoing thoracentesis to clear a left-sided pleural effusion. Note the use of gravity to facilitate drainage into a container that is suitable for volume measurement and subsequent laboratory analysis.

For example, a transudate is far more common when other signs suggest a patient with worsening **congestive heart failure (CHF)**. In addition to CHF, transudates may be present in any of the following conditions: cirrhosis with ascites; **nephrotic syndrome** when resulting in hypoproteinemia; recent peritoneal dialysis; myxedema in patients with **hypothyroidism**; acute lobar atelectasis due to multiple causes; **constrictive** pericarditis; superior vena caval obstruction; and pulmonary embolism.

Exudates are caused by local factors that create abnormal pleural fluids or obstruct their reabsorption, often in the presence of free or adherent cells. Normal leukocytes that are commonly found in exudates include resident lung macrophages and lymphocytes, as well as neutrophils recruited by chemokines and microbial secretions (Chap. 10). Their intrapleural release of cytokines and other inflammatory mediators augments the local concentration of high molecular weight proteins. This increase in intrapleural colloid osmotic pressure retards fluid reabsorption into the lung lymphatics, in addition to whatever primary immunomodulatory effects these mediators induce. Abnormal host cells that are commonly associated with exudates include many neoplastic forms that represent primary thoracic tumors or metastases to the pleural compartment. Although many neoplastic cells will exist as large aggregates (Chap. 31), there are sufficient numbers of free cells to be retrieved during thoracentesis. Of course, almost any combination of microbial pathogens can be identified in exudates, with those found free within the fluid phase representing potentially massive abscesses.

Exudates may need extensive testing to establish their etiologies, given that the list is long of diseases in which they may develop:

- Pneumonias of nearly all types
- Neoplasms, either primary or secondary
- Pulmonary embolism
- Sarcoidosis and other connective tissue diseases
- Hematogenously spread systemic infections
- **Chylothorax**
- **Postmyocardial infarct syndrome**
- **Asbestosis**
- **Meigs syndrome** (a benign ovarian tumor producing ascites)
- Pancreatic disease
- Uremia
- Chronic atelectasis
- Adverse drug reaction

Distinguishing between Transudates and Exudates

The two most useful criteria for identifying an effusion as an exudate or transudate are its [LDH] and total [protein]. Acknowledging the role of [protein] on pleural colloid osmotic

pressure, an exudate is defined by at least one of the three following criteria:

- Pleural fluid [protein]/serum [protein] >0.5
- Pleural fluid [LDH]/serum [LDH] >0.6
- Pleural fluid [LDH] >200 IU/L, or >2/3 normal upper limit for serum

Depending upon the outcomes of these initial evaluations, other useful testing includes:

- Pleural fluid specific gravity, >1.016 in exudates
- Pleural fluid [cholesterol], >60 mg/dL in exudates
- Pleural fluid fibrinogen, seen in exudates and potentially indicating a clot
- Pleural fluid number of WBCs, >1,000/μL in exudates
- Pleural fluid number of RBCs, > 100,000/μL in exudates (including malignancy, pulmonary embolism/infarction, or trauma)
- Pleural fluid [bilirubin]/serum [bilirubin], >0.6 g/dL in exudates
- Pleural fluid [amylase] or its activity, elevated in some types of exudates

Figure 19.7 is a flow diagram that summarizes a useful sequence of laboratory studies to systematically identify an effusion as an exudate or transudate.

Macroscopic and Microscopic Evaluation of Effusions

In terms of gross appearance, transudates are clear and **straw-colored**, rarely turbid (Fig. 19.8). In contrast, there are many described types of exudates, all of which are translucent at best and opaque more often. An effusion that is **red-tinged** or obviously bloody can be due to trauma, malignancy, or a pulmonary infarct. A **green-white, turbid** effusion is often indicative of **rheumatoid pleuritis**, while a **milky white** color indicates a pseudochylous or **chylous effusion** (Fig. 19.8). An effusion that is **cloudy and purulent** usually indicates an infection (Fig. 19.9).

The standard laboratory examination of exudative pleural fluids should include their gross description, assays for [glucose] and [amylase], a differential cell count, microbiological cultures, and cytology. The [glucose] of an exudate is usually less than 60 mg/dL in rheumatoid arthritis, malignancy, or purulent infection, while [amylase] is elevated above normal range in esophageal rupture, pancreatitis, or malignancy. Exudate values for [triglycerides] are elevated above normal serum ranges in **chylothorax**, and occasionally in patients with **pseudochylous** effusions.

To perform a differential cell count, an effusion sample is spun in a **cytocentrifuge** to sediment its cells onto a microscope slide that is then examined as a thin Wright-stained smear or pellet. Cells that are routinely identified on such a cytospin

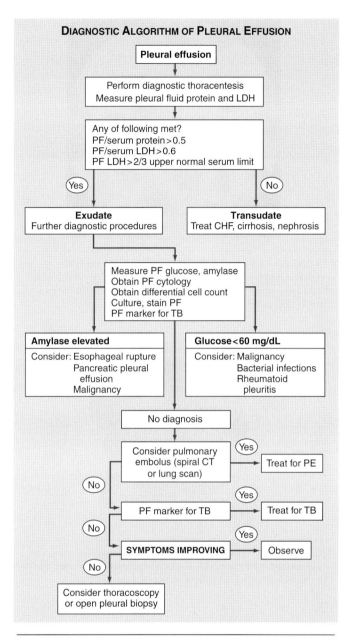

DIAGNOSTIC ALGORITHM OF PLEURAL EFFUSION

FIGURE 19.7 Diagnostic algorithm for determining the etiology of pleural effusions. *From* Harrison's Principles of Medicine, *17th ed. New York, NY: McGraw-Hill.*

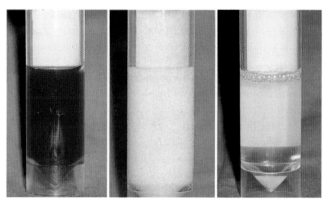

FIGURE 19.8 Visual comparison of three pleural effusions obtained by thoracentesis. At left is a blood-stained exudate from a patient with pleural metastases from breast carcinoma. At center is a milky white chylous exudate from a patient with bronchial carcinoma that invaded and obstructed the thoracic duct. At right is a clear transudate typical of those found in patients with heart failure or other causes of generalized edema. *From Forbes CD, Jackson WF,* Color Atlas and Text of Clinical Medicine, *3rd ed. London, UK: Mosby; 2003.*

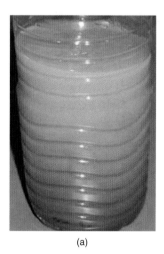

(a)

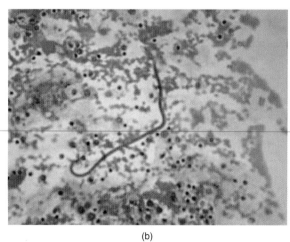

(b)

FIGURE 19.9 (a) A cloudy, purulent exudative effusion obtained from a patient with **lymphatic filariasis** caused by *Wuchereria bancrofti,* a common disease spread by mosquitoes in tropical and subtropical climes. The intact nematode parasite is seen in (b) in a microscopic view of such an effusion.

slide include erythrocytes, lymphocytes, macrophages, and mesothelial cells; a few eosinophils and plasma cells may also be present. The leukocyte count for a normal pleural fluid is <1,000/µL, and erythrocytes are normally <10,000/µL. Increased numbers of neutrophils are among the most common findings in effusions caused by bacterial infections, and are indicative of **empyema**. Lymphocyte counts are increased in exudates from patients with active tuberculosis, malignancy, and viral infections. Eosinophilia (>10% counted cells) most often occurs in patients with pneumothorax, empyema, parasitic infections, malignancies, or in some idiopathic effusions.

(#65)

Microbiological testing should include at least a Gram stain, fungal stain, and AFB stain on the primary exudate itself, as well as culture of the specimen for routine, anaerobic, fungal, and acid-fast bacilli. Cytology studies are performed to detect malignancy using immunohistochemical stains, and to identify infectious agents by special stains in addition to use of the Diff-Quik® and Pap smear stains. Other studies may include flow cytometry, tumor marker analysis, immuno-histochemical stains, viral markers, and nucleic acid-based diagnostic techniques. Figures 19.10 through 19.16 depict both normal and abnormal cells that may be found in specific pleural fluids and effusions.

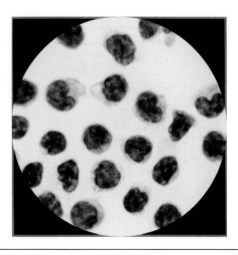

FIGURE 19.12 Pleural effusion in patient with non-Hodgkin's lymphoma, small lymphocytic type. *From DeMay RM.* The Art & Science of Cytopathology. *ASCP Press, American Society of Clinical Pathologists, Chicago 1996, p. 307.*

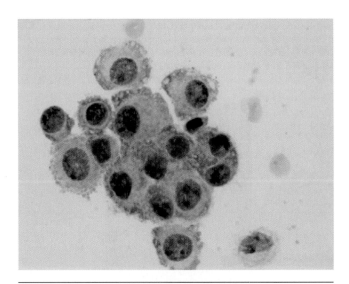

FIGURE 19.10 Benign mesothelial cells. Note the nearly uniform appearances of all cells and their relatively low nuclear:cytoplasmic ratio.

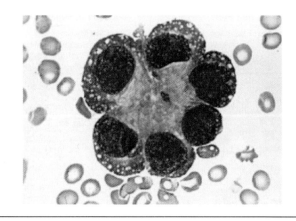

FIGURE 19.13 A cluster of well-differentiated breast carcinoma cells in pleural fluid. *From* Henry's Clinical Diagnosis and Management by Laboratory Methods, *21st ed. Philadelphia, PA: Saunders; 2007.*

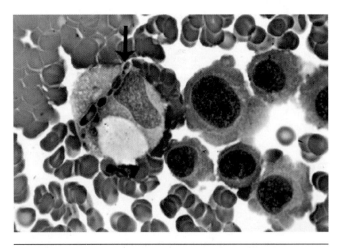

FIGURE 19.11 *Candida albicans* shown replicating into hyphae within a pleural fluid macrophage (arrow). The image also contains numerous red blood cells and benign mesothelial cells as in Fig. 19.10. *From Lichtman MA,* Lichtman's Atlas of Hematology. *New York, NY: McGraw-Hill; 2007.*

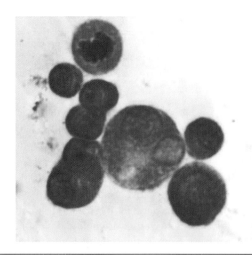

FIGURE 19.14 Plasma cells in the pleural fluid from a patient with multiple myeloma. *From Dhingra KK, Singhai N, Nigam S, Jain S:* Unsuspected multiple myeloma presenting as bilateral pleural effusion - a cytological diagnosis, *Cytojournal Sep 7;4:17, 2007.*

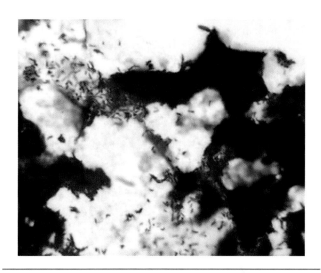

FIGURE 19.15 Smear of broth-cultured pleural fluid, showing growth of acid-fast bacilli using a Kinyoun carbolfuchsin stain. *From Siddiqui TJ and O'keefe P; Brain Abscesses in a Renal Transplant Recipient, 2004. Cliggott Publishing, Division of CMP Healthcare Media.*

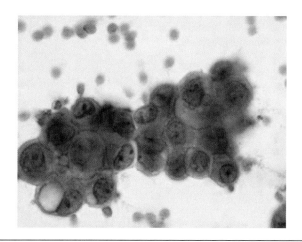

FIGURE 19.16 Pleural fluid containing metastatic adenocarcinoma cells from a previously diagnosed lung carcinoma, visualized using a conventional H&E stain. *Zendehrokh N and Dejmek A:* telomere repeat amplification protocol (TRAP) in situ reveals telomerase activity in three cell Itypes in effusions: malignant cells, proliferative mesothelial cells, and lymphocytes, Modern pathology Feb;18(2):189-196, 2005.

Suggested Readings

1. Galagan KA, Blomberg D, Cornbleet PJ, Glassy EF, eds. *Color Atlas of Body Fluids,* 2006, College of American Pathologists (CAP); 2006. *This concise manual gives an excellent overview on the origins of body fluids, as well as the procedures for collection and testing. It contains numerous color pictures with explanations.*

2. Croft AC, Woods GL. Specimen collection and handling for diagnosis of infectious diseases. In: McPherson RA and Pincus MR, eds. *Henry's Clinical Diagnosis and Management by Laboratory Methods,* 21st ed. Philadelphia, PA: Saunders; 2007. These authors review the collection and analysis of sputum and other clinical specimens.*

3. Knight JA, Kjeldsberg CR. Cerebrospinal, synovial, and serous body fluids. In: McPherson RA and Pincus MR, eds. *Henry's Clinical Diagnosis and Management by Laboratory Methods,* 21st ed. Philadelphia, PA: Saunders; 2007. *This chapter provides a thorough explanation of these laboratory tests, with excellent color images.*

CASE STUDIES AND PRACTICE PROBLEMS

CASE 19.1 A 70-year-old woman is seen in an acute care clinic for fever, chills, shortness of breath, and a cough. She states that her son's family stayed with her over Thanksgiving weekend and they had a respiratory infection from which they recovered. She later contracted the respiratory illness also, but after two weeks her symptoms have worsened. A sputum Gram stain is shown below. Which of the following is the most likely cause of this patient's current symptoms?

a. *Haemophilus influenzae*

b. *Mycoplasma pneumoniae*

c. *Staphylococcus aureus*

d. Respiratory syncytial virus

e. *Streptococcus pneumoniae*

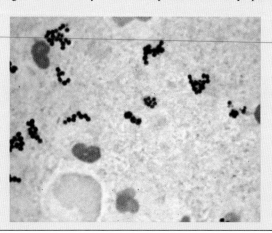

CASE 19.2 A 55-year-old woman presents to the ER with new onset shortness of breath. Her chest x-ray shows a large right pleural effusion. A therapeutic thoracentesis is performed, and the fluid is sent to the laboratory. The pleural fluid/serum total protein ratio is 0.6 and the pleural fluid/serum LDH ratio is 0.7. Amylase and glucose levels are unremarkable on the pleural fluid. The culture and Gram stain are negative and the cytology results are negative for malignancy. Which of the following is most likely correct regarding the type and origin of her pleural fluid?

a. The fluid is a transudate, and congestive heart failure should be excluded.

b. The fluid is an exudate that is probably infected.

c. The fluid is an exudate, and pulmonary embolism should be excluded.

d. The fluid is a transudate, and nephrotic syndrome should be considered.

e. The fluid is an exudate that could be of pancreatic origin.

CASE 19.3 A 53-year-old man with chronic alcoholism and a history of squamous cell carcinoma of the esophagus has a pleural effusion. He has difficulty swallowing and left-sided chest pain on deep inspiration. A small amount of pleural fluid is obtained and the pleural fluid/serum protein ratio is 0.8. A specimen is sent to cytology, but it is Friday night and cytology results will not be ready until Monday. There is sufficient pleural fluid left to perform one more test. Which of the following would be most likely to establish the etiology of the pleural effusion in this patient?

a. [Glucose]

b. Amylase activity

c. Pleural fluid/serum [LDH] ratio

d. Gram stain

e. AFB (acid-fast bacillus) stain

Solutions to Case Studies and Practice Problems

CASE 19.1 The most correct answer is c, *Staphylococcus aureus*.

The Gram stain shows large gram-positive cocci, predominantly in clumps, some with a grape-like appearance that is typical of *Staphylococcus*. *Haemophilus* is a gram-negative coccobacillus; *Mycoplasma pneumoniae* cannot be cultured on routine media; RSV does not take up Gram stain; and *Streptococcus pneumoniae* are typically gram-positive, lancet-shaped diplococci.

CASE 19.2 The most correct answer is c, an exudate and pulmonary embolism should be excluded.

The pleural fluid/serum total [protein] ratio and the fluid/serum [LDH] ratio both indicate the fluid is an exudate. The culture and Gram stain are both negative, so infection is less likely. Amylase levels are unremarkable, as is cytology, so malignancy or pancreatic origin is unlikely. Excluding a pulmonary embolism is the best next diagnostic step among the choices offered.

CASE 19.3 The most correct answer is b, requesting an amylase assay on the pleural effusion.

The patient's history of squamous cell carcinoma of the esophagus, and the pleural fluid/serum [protein] ratio indicate an exudate, with malignancy high on the differential. While awaiting the cytology results, the test that would be most helpful in providing evidence for or against malignancy is for amylase activity, which would be elevated in malignant pleural effusions.

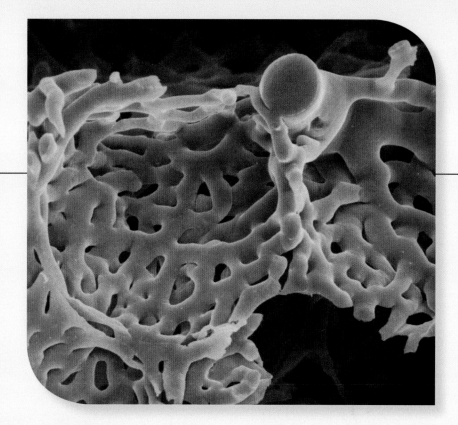

SECTION

III

OBSTRUCTIVE AND RESTRICTIVE LUNG DISEASES

Chapter 20

Pathology of Obstructive Pulmonary Diseases

DAVID S. BRINK, MD AND ANDREW J. LECHNER, PhD

Learning Objectives

- The student will be able to define emphysema and chronic bronchitis and differentiate their various forms, including etiology, pathogenesis, gross and microscopic morphology, and clinical presentation.

- The student will be able to describe the histological presentation of asthma, particularly as it may involve both airways and lung parenchyma.

- The student will be able to describe the development and appearance of bronchiectasis as it evolves from an initial obstructive process.

Introduction

Obstructive lung diseases are characterized by reductions in airflow due to increased resistance from partial or complete airway obstructions at any level. Such obstructions can arise from direct narrowing of the airway lumen or by decreased elastic recoil of the pulmonary parenchyma surrounding the airways, which has the effect of reducing lumen caliber. The many causes of obstructive disease include tumors, aspirated foreign bodies, asthma, emphysema, chronic bronchitis, cystic fibrosis, and bronchiolitis. This chapter will focus on the pathology of **emphysema**, **chronic bronchitis**, **asthma**, and **bronchiectasis**. Bronchiectasis is included here although it occurs as a result of airway obstruction, rather than being a cause in itself. The **chronic obstructive pulmonary diseases (COPDs)** comprise emphysema and chronic bronchitis. Though it is possible to have emphysema without chronic bronchitis or the converse, most patients have some degree of both, though one may dominate the clinical scenario. They share common etiologies, the most significant of which is tobacco smoking. Despite this significant association, most smokers do not develop COPD.

Pathology of Emphysema

Emphysema is defined morphologically as the irreversible enlargement of airspaces distal to the terminal bronchioles, due to destruction of airspace walls and without obvious fibrosis. Emphysema is present in approximately one-half of adults at autopsy, most of whom were asymptomatic. Emphysema is further subdivided into four subtypes based on the anatomic distribution of the airspace enlargement: **centriacinar** (centrilobular), **panacinar** (panlobular), **distal acinar** (paraseptal), and **irregular**.

Centriacinar emphysema (Figs. 20.1 and 20.2) is characterized by airspace enlargement at the level of the respiratory bronchioles, sparing the distal alveoli. Anatomically, the several acini that comprise a lobule (Chap. 2) are arranged such that their respiratory bronchioles are grouped in the center of the lobule. This anatomic arrangement underlies the alternate name, centrilobular emphysema. Centriacinar emphysema accounts for more than 95% of those cases of emphysema with clinically significant airway obstruction. It is more pronounced in the upper lobes and is the type of emphysema most strongly associated with smoking. *(# 60)*

Panacinar emphysema (Figs. 20.1 and 20.3) is characterized by airspace enlargement at the level of the alveolar ducts and more distally. At the gross level, airspace enlargement appears to affect the entire lobule, giving rise to the alternate name, panlobular emphysema. Panacinar emphysema accounts for less than 5% of cases of emphysema with clinically significant airway obstruction and is more pronounced in the lower lung zones. It is the type of emphysema most strongly associated with α_1-antiprotease (α_1-PI) deficiency (Chap. 22).

Distal acinar emphysema (Fig. 20.4) involves distal airspaces and is most prominent adjacent to the visceral pleura and to the connective tissue septa that define the lobules. Distal acinar emphysema typically does not result in clinically significant airway obstruction. It is more severe in the upper half of the lungs and likely represents the underlying lesion resulting in spontaneous pneumothorax in young adults.

Emphysema that does not show centriacinar, panacinar, or distal acinar distribution is called **irregular emphysema**. Irregular emphysema is very common adjacent to foci of scarring and does not typically cause significant airway obstruction. In any form of emphysema, large, distended sacs of air or **bullae** can form. Any subtype of emphysema with bullae is likely to be referred to as **bullous emphysema** (Fig. 20.5). In its most severe forms, emphysema is difficult to subclassify (Fig. 20.6).

The pathogenesis of emphysema is generally considered to involve excess protease and/or elastase activity that is insufficiently opposed by antiprotease regulation (Fig. 20.7). The probable sequence begins with neutrophil sequestration in capillaries, migration into airways and alveoli, and

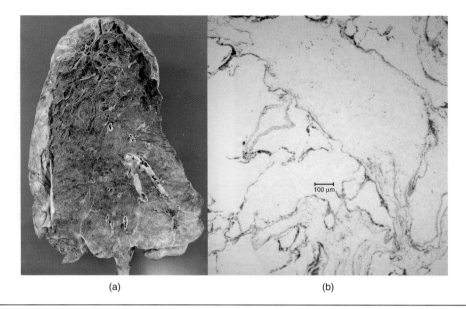

(a)   (b)

FIGURE 20.6 (a): Severe emphysema. Particularly evident in the upper portion of the cut surface of the lung, the pulmonary parenchyma droops below the plane of section, imparting a web like appearance. *From Kemp WL,* Pathology: The Big Picture, *McGraw-Hill, 2008.* (b): Low power photomicrograph of severe emphysema. The main finding is the absence of tissue. Note how large airspaces are and how few alveolar septa are present. When severe as here, one cannot determine whether the morphology reflects the centriacinar, panacinar, distal acinar, or irregular form.

Chronic bronchitis, despite its suffix, does not always show severe inflammation. In the absence of superimposed infection, the inflammatory infiltrate is predominantly mononuclear (Fig. 20.9) as would be expected based on normal lung host defense mechanisms (Chap. 10). When superimposed infection is present, variable numbers of neutrophils are likely. In the setting of chronic bronchitis, there is typically small airway disease (**chronic bronchiolitis**) featuring goblet cell metaplasia, inflammation, smooth muscle hyperplasia, thickened basement membranes, and fibrosis. In the most severe

forms, the fibrosis occludes the bronchiolar lumen to cause **bronchiolitis obliterans**.

Pathology of Asthma   ＊68

Asthma is a chronic inflammatory airway disease characterized by episodic bronchospasm which is clinically manifest as an asthma attack comprising dyspnea, chest tightness, cough, and wheezing (Chap. 21). The airway luminal narrowing is partially reversible, and inflammation likely plays a role in

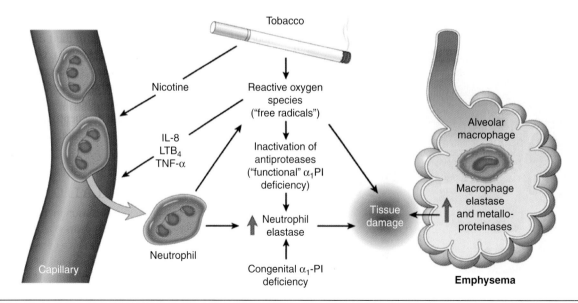

FIGURE 20.7 Model of the pathogenesis of emphysema, in which protease activity exceeds antiprotease regulation. Tissue damage worsens with congenital α_1-PI deficiency or its functional impairment. Tobacco smoke inactivates antiproteases and recruits neutrophils, enhancing release of elastase. *From* Robbins and Cotran Pathologic Basis of Disease, *8th ed. 2009.*

Main factors underlying the pathogenesis of asthma are a genetic predisposition to type I hypersensitivity reactions, airway inflammation, and bronchial hyperresponsiveness. Many inflammatory cells play roles in the pathogenesis of asthma: eosinophils, mast cells, macrophages, neutrophils, and lymphocytes. Among these lymphocytes, the CD4+ T-cells include T_H1 and T_H2 phenotypes. A number of T_H1-derived cytokines (eg, IFN-γ, IL-2) activate macrophages and CD8+ cytotoxic T-cells to kill viruses and other intracellular pathogens. T_H1 cells also inhibit the action of T_H2 cells. In contrast, the T_H2-derived mediators promote allergic inflammation and stimulate production of IgE by B-cells. Additionally, T_H2 cells inhibit T_H1 cells. In asthma, it appears that this mutual inhibition of T_H1 cells and T_H2 cells is altered to favor T_H2 cell-mediated effects. The transcription factor **T-bet** that is required for T_H1 cell differentiation has been found to be diminished or lacking in pulmonary lymphocytes in the setting of asthma. Thus, a future approach to asthma may be to up-regulate *T-bet* expression (Chap. 21). Despite the role of lymphocytes in the pathogenesis of asthma, the inflammatory infiltrate in asthma is typically rich in eosinophils.

Morphologically, asthma is characterized by **airway remodeling**, including bronchial smooth muscle hypertrophy and subepithelial collagen deposition. Recently, the gene **ADAM-33** that encodes a metalloproteinase has been linked to asthma. Polymorphisms in *ADAM-33* accelerate bronchial smooth muscle cell proliferation, resulting in bronchial hyperreactivity, and accelerate fibroblast proliferation, leading to subepithelial fibrosis.

Pathogenetically, asthma can be subdivided into extrinsic and intrinsic categories. All forms of **extrinsic asthma** involve initiation of an asthmatic crisis by a **type I hypersensitivity reaction** to an extrinsic antigen, which in this setting can be called an **allergen**. The most common form of extrinsic asthma is **atopic asthma**; other forms of extrinsic asthma include some types of **occupational asthma** as well

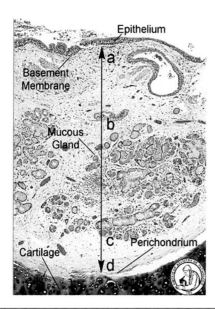

FIGURE 20.8 Chronic bronchitis. Though defined clinically, chronic bronchitis does have a characteristic morphology, which includes such features as mucous gland hyperplasia, goblet cell hyperplasia, and thickened basement membrane. Morphologically, severity of chronic bronchitis can be expressed through the Reid index, a ratio of the mucous gland thickness (b to c) to the distance between epithelium and cartilage (a to d). *From Travis et al. Non-Neoplastic Disorders of the Lower Respiratory Tract. American Registry of Pathology: 2002.*

causing exaggerated bronchoconstriction. Asthma affects approximately 5% of adults and 7%-10% of children in the United States. There are several approaches to classifying asthma (Table 20.1); regardless of the system used, many patients will have features overlapping two or more categories (Chap. 21). Asthma can be complicated by *Aspergillus* ssp. colonization of the bronchial mucosa which, in a patient with allergy to the fungus, is called **allergic bronchopulmonary aspergillosis**.

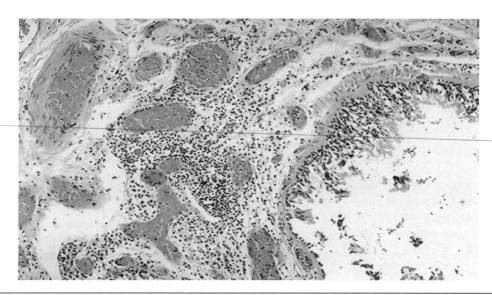

FIGURE 20.9 Chronic bronchitis. Medium power photomicrograph showing thickening of the basement membrane beneath the airway lumen and adjacent mononuclear inflammation. *From Robbins and Cotran Atlas of Pathology, 2nd ed. 2010.*

Table **20.1** Various approaches to the classification of asthma[a]

By Frequency of Signs and Symptoms	By Response to Therapy	By Triggers of Attack	By Pathophysiology
Mild intermittent	Steroid-dependent	Seasonal	Extrinsic
Mild persistent	Steroid-resistant	Exercise-induced	Intrinsic
Moderate persistent	Difficult	Occupational	
Severe persistent	Brittle	Asthmatic bronchitis (in smokers)	

[a]There is considerable overlap regardless of the classification system used.

as allergic bronchopulmonary aspergillosis. Sensitization occurs when inhaled allergens stimulate an inflammatory response dominated by T_H2 cells, favoring the production of IgE and recruiting eosinophils. The IgE released by B-cells attaches to the surface of resident mast cells. Once sensitized, reexposure to the allergen can trigger the asthma attack, classically described as having an early phase and late phase. The **early phase** occurs 30-60 minutes after exposure as the inhaled antigen binds to IgE on mast cells, stimulating release of their mediators that cause bronchoconstriction, edema, mucus secretion, and recruitment of granulocytes, especially eosinophils. The **late phase** begins 4-8 hours after the early phase and is dominated by eosinophil release of mediators that activate mast cells. During the late phase, these eosinophil-derived mediators increase and sustain the inflammatory response that damages airway epithelia, even in the absence of additional allergen exposure. If exposure persists, the epithelial injury facilitates translocation of inhaled allergen from the airway lumen into the subepithelial connective tissue, where more inflammatory cells reside.

Intrinsic asthma involves nonimmune triggers of an asthma attack. Its subtypes include **non-atopic asthma** that is usually initiated by viral respiratory infections. The ensuing infectious inflammation stimulates subepithelial vagus receptors, causing bronchospasm. A classic example of **drug-induced asthma** is initiated by aspirin, in which cyclooxygenase inhibition leads to leukotriene synthesis that stimulates bronchoconstriction.

▶▶ C L I N I C A L   C O R R E L A T I O N   2 0 . 3

Intrinsic asthma can be triggered by aspirin, viral infection, inhalation of cold air or chemical irritants, psychological stimuli including stress, and exercise. Notably, triggers of intrinsic asthma also cause bronchospasm in non-asthmatics, and bronchospasms in intrinsic asthma are more pronounced and persistent than those associated with extrinsic asthma.

Morphologically, asthma is characterized by bronchial wall edema, erythema due to hyperemia, and inflammation, with 5%-50% eosinophils. These are accompanied by patchy

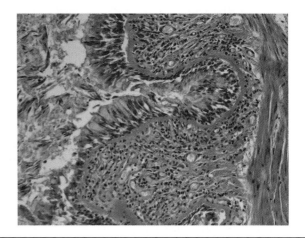

FIGURE 20.10 Atopic asthma, showing a mucous plug obscuring the airway lumen (left). Also seen are numerous epithelial goblet cells, thickened basement membrane, an eosinophilic inflammatory infiltrate, and smooth muscle hyperplasia (right). *From Kemp WL,* Pathology: the Big Picture, *McGraw-Hill, 2008.*

epithelial necrosis and cell shedding, with basement membrane thickening due to subepithelial deposition of collagen. Hyperplasia of submucosal mucous glands and goblet cells is evident, as well as hypertrophy and hyperplasia of bronchial smooth muscle (Fig. 20.10).

Microscopic features of asthma overlap with those of chronic bronchitis. Clues that help distinguish asthma from chronic bronchitis morphologically include whorls of shed epithelium termed **Curschmann spirals**, and eosinophil-dominant inflammation that produces **Charcot-Leyden crystals** composed of eosinophil proteins (Fig. 20.11).

Clinically, the asthma attack includes wheezing and dyspnea, with more difficult expiration. Symptoms can last several hours and are followed by prolonged coughing. Though the asthma attack can spontaneously resolve, medical therapy with bronchodilators and/or corticosteroids can expedite resolution (Chap. 21). In some patients, a severe and treatment-resistant asthma attack can persist for days to weeks, resulting in **status asthmaticus** and leading to hypoxemia, acidosis, and death. In the event of such a death, autopsy would show plugging of airways by viscous mucus.

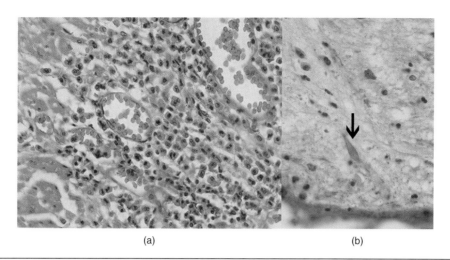

(a)   (b)

FIGURE 20.11 (a) The eosinophil-rich inflammatory infiltrate that typifies atopic asthma. Although thickening of the basement membrane, hyperplasia of submucosal glands, increase in goblet cells and smooth muscle hyperplasia all mimic findings in chronic bronchitis, the inflammatory infiltrate in chronic bronchitis is not eosinophil-rich. (b) While Charcot-Leyden crystals (arrow) are frequently seen in asthma, they are not specific for asthma but rather are common in many inflammatory disorders with prominent **eosinophilia**. The crystals are composed of **major basic protein** from degranulated eosinophils. (a): *From* Robbins and Cotran Atlas of Pathology, *2nd ed. 2010.* (b): *From Kemp WL,* Pathology: the Big Picture, *McGraw-Hill, 2008.*

Pathology of Bronchiectasis

Bronchiectasis is defined as the permanent dilatation of airways due to the destruction of tissue caused by chronic necrotizing inflammation and obstruction (Fig. 20.12). Bronchiectasis is not a primary disease but rather occurs secondarily to chronic infection and/or chronic obstruction. There are many predispositions to the development of bronchiectasis: bronchial obstruction; congenital and hereditary conditions such as cystic fibrosis, immunodeficiency, ciliary dyskinesia, and intralobar sequestration; necrotizing or suppurative pneumonia; and allergic bronchopulmonary aspergillosis. The pathogenesis of bronchiectasis involves obstruction and persistent infection, occurring in either order and frequently overlapping. The infection usually involves mixed flora.

Morphologically, there is by definition bronchial dilatation up to fourfold normal airway diameters. Such bronchial dilatation is usually more prominent in lower lung lobes and can be cylindroid, fusiform, or saccular. In the setting of active infection, there is typically a dense mixed inflammatory exudate with epithelial ulceration. The chronic nature of the inflammation is reflected in bronchial, bronchiolar, and peribronchial fibrosis. Bronchiectasis can be complicated by abscess formation. Clinically, the patient with bronchiectasis presents with severe, persistent cough and mucopurulent sputum that is occasionally bloody. Additional clinical findings may include frank hemoptysis, digital clubbing, and the blood gas sequelae expected with pulmonary obstruction as well as disseminated infection and reactive amyloidosis.

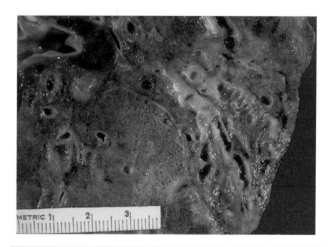

FIGURE 20.12 In bronchiectasis, the cut surface of the lung shows dilated airways (right) that are too large to be normal when this close to the pleural surface. Indeed, airways of this size would normally be proximal segments near the hilum. *From* Robbins and Cotran Atlas of Pathology, *2nd ed. 2010.*

Suggested Readings

1. Kumar V, Abbas AK, Fausto N. *Robbins and Cotran Pathologic Basis of Disease,* 8th ed. Philadelphia, PA: Elsevier; 2009. *Throughout its many editions, this reference work is the most definitive and approachable compendium of pathology images available to students.*

2. Kemp WL. *Pathology – the Big Picture,* 1st ed. New York, NY: Lange/McGraw-Hill; 2008. *As several images in this chapter illustrate, this text is an excellent addition to the study materials available, and it includes a wealth of practice problems and review slides.*

CASE STUDIES AND PRACTICE PROBLEMS

CASE 20.1 A 62-year-old man worked most of his adult life in a metals foundry before becoming eligible for permanent disability three years ago due to extreme exertional dyspnea and PFT results that included an $FEV_1/FVC = 34\%$ of predicted. He began smoking as a teenager and continued until his death last week from a heart attack. A 2-cm thick slice of his right middle lobe is shown on the right. What is the most likely diagnosis of his underlying pulmonary disease?

a. Bronchiectasis

b. Occupational asthma

c. Centriacinar emphysema

d. Chronic bronchitis

e. Bullous emphysema

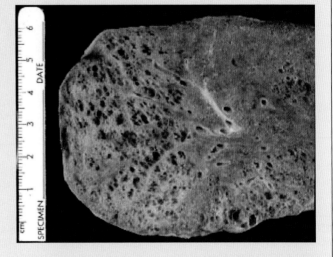

CASE 20.2 This image of lung tissue was labeled, but its patient source has been misplaced. To which of the following cases does it most likely belong?

a. Postmortem tissue of a 10-year-old boy dying of status asthmaticus

b. Biopsy of a 45-year-old nonsmoking man with simple chronic bronchitis

c. Autopsy specimen of a 72-year-old woman dying with bronchiectasis

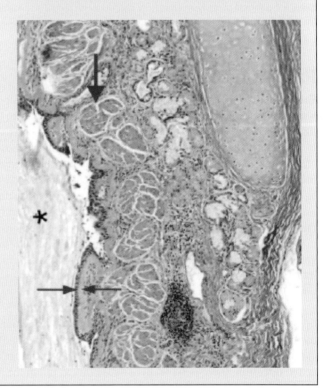

Solutions to Case Studies and Practice Problems

CASE 20.1 The most correct answer is c, centriacinar emphysema.

The distribution of the dilated airspaces is a centrilobular distribution, which corresponds microscopically to a centriacinar distribution. Furthermore, this patient's history and PFT data are most consistent with a smoking-induced disability, which in his case may have had cardiovascular as well as pulmonary consequences.

The absence of any remarkable cough or sputum production makes chronic bronchitis less a feature of his obstructive pattern (*answer d*), and thus bronchiectasis is also less likely to have developed (*answer a*). Foundry work is more often associated with metal toxicity than asthma (*answer b*). The gross appearance of his lung is not a convincing demonstration of the numerous bullae that are common in bullous emphysema (*answer e*).

CASE 20.2 The most correct answer is a.

A 10-year-old child dying of status asthmaticus. The high-resolution CT and histopathology of this patient were evaluated by Dr. Silva and her colleagues in the Department of Radiology at Vancouver General Hospital (*Am J Radiology*. 2004;183:817-824. ©American Roentgen Ray Society). Using the thick segment of cartilage at right as a point of reference to identify a large bronchus (Chap. 2), the labeled image is noteworthy in showing impressive thickening of the basement membranes (opposing thin arrows), muscle layer hypertrophy (thick arrow), and a thick bronchial plug of mucus (asterisk). A patient with simple chronic bronchitis (*answer b*) would not likely have such an obstructive accumulation of airway mucus. Neither mucus plugging nor smooth muscle hyperplasia are consistent findings in patients dying with bronchiectasis (*answer c*).

Chapter 21

Diagnosis and Management of Asthma

JOSEPH R. D. ESPIRITU, MD AND
GEORGE M. MATUSCHAK, MD

Learning Objectives

- The student will be able to describe the epidemiology of asthma in the United States, and list the known or suspected risk factors and triggers for asthma.

- The student will be able to explain the immunopathogenesis of asthma.

- The student will be able to distinguish the clinical features of asthma from other cardiopulmonary disorders.

- The student will be able to develop an evidence-based evaluation and management plan for patients with asthma.

Introduction to Asthma and Its Epidemiology

Asthma is a complex disorder characterized by variable and recurring symptoms, airflow obstruction, bronchial hyperresponsiveness, and underlying airway inflammation. Asthma is one of the most common chronic diseases globally and domestically, affecting 23 million individuals and including 7 million in the United States alone. The prevalence of asthma has been increasing since the early 1980s across all age, gender, and racial groups. Asthma is the most common chronic disease in children and affects more children (7%-10%) than adults (3%-5%). Prevalence by gender varies by age, being more common in boys than girls in childhood but more common in women than men in adulthood. The slightly higher prevalence of asthma among African Americans and Puerto Ricans than Caucasians is highly correlated with socioeconomic status (ie, poverty, urban air quality, indoor allergens, lack of patient education, and inadequate medical care).

Asthma is associated with increased morbidity. Approximately 10 million ambulatory care visits, 2 million emergency department visits, and half a million hospitalizations annually are attributed to asthma. In fact, asthma is the third-ranking cause of hospitalization in children. It is also the leading cause of school absenteeism among children, accounting for >14 million total missed days of school. Meanwhile, in terms of risk by ethnicity, African Americans are also three times more likely to be hospitalized from asthma.

Asthma is also a major cause of mortality. It is the primary cause of more than 4,000 United States annual deaths due to asthma and is a contributing factor for nearly 7,000 other deaths annually. Despite improvements in the understanding of the pathophysiology and the expansion of available effective therapies, overall asthma death rates continue to increase by 50% among all genders, age groups, and ethnic groups since the 1980s. In addition, mortality rates for children younger than 19 years old have increased by nearly 80% percent since then. Mortality rates are higher in women, accounting for nearly 65% of all asthma deaths. African Americans are also three times more likely to die from asthma. In fact, mortality rates are highest in African-American women, whose rate is 2.5 times higher than that of Caucasian women. Aside from gender and ethnicity, risk factors for increased asthma mortality include severe airflow obstruction, multiple recent emergency department visits or hospitalizations in the past year, history of intubation or ICU admission in the past five years, nonuse of inhaled corticosteroids, current smoking, psychosocial stress and depression, socioeconomic factors, and attitudes and beliefs regarding medications.

The adverse health outcomes from asthma also impose a major socioeconomic burden. It is estimated that asthma costs the United States $18 billion dollars, $10 billion from direct health care costs and $8 billion from lost productivity due to illness and death. Thus, public health efforts to improve socioeconomic conditions and access to medical care are needed to address this disparity in asthma health outcomes.

Etiology of Asthma

There are myriad factors that precipitate and aggravate asthma (Table 21.1). Indoor airborne allergens such as house dust mites, molds, cockroaches, animal/pet dander are well known triggers that may be amenable to environmental modification. Acute viral bronchiolitis due to rhinoviruses not only increase the number of wheezing episodes early in life but also increase the risk of asthma at the age of 6 years. Viral respiratory infections also commonly precipitate exacerbations in asthmatic patients, who may be vulnerable based on epithelial deficiencies in antiviral activity and the integrity of the airway epithelial barrier. Fetal exposure to **environmental tobacco smoke (ETS)** is an independent risk factor for poor lung function, wheezing,

Table **21.1** Factors that trigger asthma[a]

Airborne Allergens	Occupational Exposures	Diet, Lifestyle
House dust mite (*Dermatophagoides*)	Dusts (mineral, plant, etc)	Specific foods
Mold (*Alternaria, Aspergillus, etc*)	Vapors and fumes	Additives, preservatives
Cockroach (including feces)	Other irritants	Tobacco smoke
Animal dander	Air pollution	Exercise
Pollen (seasonal)		
Drugs	**Endocrine Factors**	**Co-morbidities**
Aspirin, NSAIDs	Menstruation	Rhinosinusitis
β-blockers	Pregnancy	Gastroesophageal reflux
Psychological Factors	**Respiratory Viruses**	

[a]*Data from the National Asthma Education and Prevention Program Expert Panel Report 3.* "Guidelines for the Diagnosis and Management of Asthma." *US Dept. H&HS; 2007.*

and the development of asthma. Both ETS and personal smoking were significantly related to asthma and wheeze in teenagers. In addition, smoking is associated with decreased asthma control and increased risk of mortality and asthma attacks and exacerbations in adults. Asthmatics should be encouraged to abstain from smoking since cessation is associated with improvements in both asthma and lung function. Heavy exertion (eg, sports activity), particularly in cold, dry weather conditions, can trigger bronchospasm in patients with exercise-induced asthma.

Occupational asthma (OA) is defined as new asthma, or the recurrence of previously quiescent asthma induced by either sensitization to a specific substance (eg, an inhaled protein) or a chemical at work (**sensitizer-induced OA**) or by exposure to an inhaled irritant at work (**irritant-induced OA**). Epidemiological studies reveal an association between the increase in the incidence of allergic respiratory diseases and bronchial asthma in urban populations and the increased presence of outdoor air pollutants resulting from more intense energy consumption and exhaust emissions from cars and other vehicles. Psychogenic stress not only influences the symptoms but also complicates the management of asthma. For example, depressed patients may lack the motivation to adhere to an asthma action plan, while anxious asthmatics who hyperventilate can develop bronchospasm. Five percent of asthmatics are allergic to aspirin or **nonsteroidal anti-inflammatory drugs (NSAIDs)** and when combined with nasal polyposis is a condition known as the **Samter triad**. Meanwhile, asthma symptoms appear to worsen in 30%-40% of asthmatic women during the perimenstrual period. During pregnancy, a third of asthmatic women develop worse symptoms while another third report an improvement in symptoms. Pregnant women with uncontrolled asthma have been reported to have higher risks of several complications of pregnancy, including preeclampsia, preterm birth, infants with low birth weight or intrauterine growth restriction, infants with congenital malformations, and

perinatal death. Dietary intake of certain foods (eg, shellfish), food additives, and preservatives (eg, sulfites) trigger asthma in hypersensitive individuals. Comorbid conditions such as allergic rhinitis and gastroesophageal acid reflux commonly play an aggravating role in asthma symptoms.

Immunology of Asthma

The immunopathogenesis of asthma is thought to be due to the promotion of the allergic asthmatic phenotype resulting from the predominance of Th2 over Th1 cytokine response during early life, also referred to as the **Hygiene Hypothesis** (Fig. 21.1). This theory stemmed from the observation of increasing prevalence of asthma in industrialized Western societies. Early childhood exposures in these industrialized countries favoring the Th2 response include widespread use of antibiotics, an urban rather than rural environment, and sensitization to cockroaches, which are believed to lead to the development of the allergic asthmatic phenotype. On the other hand, the higher propensity for microbial exposure in developing countries with increased prevalence of infections from *Mycobacterium tuberculosis*, measles virus, and hepatitis A virus all enhance Th-1 mediated responses which reduce the development of an atopic/allergic immunologic phenotype. Other factors believed to be protective against the asthma phenotype include contact with other siblings and attendance at a day-care facility during the first 6 months of life.

Diagnosing Asthma

The diagnosis of asthma is based on the presence of episodic symptoms of completely or partially reversible airflow obstruction and/or airway hyperresponsiveness, and only with exclusion of alternative diagnoses. The evaluation includes at least a detailed medical history, physical exam, and spirometry. Additional studies may also be indicated, such as a full pulmonary function test (PFT) combined with a **methacholine**

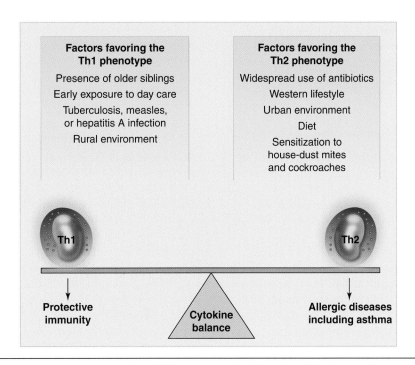

Factors favoring the Th1 phenotype	Factors favoring the Th2 phenotype
Presence of older siblings	Widespread use of antibiotics
Early exposure to day care	Western lifestyle
Tuberculosis, measles, or hepatitis A infection	Urban environment
Rural environment	Diet
	Sensitization to house-dust mites and cockroaches

Th1 → Protective immunity

Cytokine balance

Th2 → Allergic diseases including asthma

FIGURE 21.1 The **Hygiene Hypothesis** in which it is argued that factors that promote predominance of a Th2 versus Th1 cytokine response leads to the allergic asthma phenotype. *From Busse WW, Lemanske RF Jr.: Asthma, NEJM Feb 1;344(5):350-362, 2001.*

bronchoprovocation challenge (see below) and chest imaging studies (Chaps. 15 and 16). Symptoms consistent with asthma include: chronic episodic cough that is worse particularly at night; recurrent difficulty in breathing or chest tightness; and recurrent wheezing upon expiration (Chap. 14). However, symptoms may vary depending on the severity of asthma. Severe asthmatics may present having all of the symptoms listed, while patients with mild asthma may complain of just one symptom such as intermittent cough (the so-called **cough-variant asthma**).

Physical examination findings in patients with uncontrolled asthma or an acute asthma exacerbation include tachypnea, use of the accessory muscles of respiration, audible wheezing, and a prolonged forced expiratory phase. However, given the episodic nature of the airflow limitation in asthma, many patients with intermittent, mild, or even moderate asthma may have a completely normal physical exam. It is also important to emphasize that even in patients with severe disease, lack of wheezing does not exclude asthma, since reduced airflow may attenuate chest physical findings. Physical signs of **atopy** such as nasal congestion and drainage and/or nasal polyps and eczema may help support a diagnosis of allergic asthma.

Spirometry is the clinical mainstay to objectively confirm the reversibility of airflow obstruction in patients with asthma (Chap. 16). Given the normal decline in spirometric airflow measures with aging, the **National Asthma Education and Prevention Program (NAEPP)** guidelines recommend using age-adjusted FEV_1/FVC thresholds for determining the presence of airflow obstruction (Table 21.2). The FEV_1/FVC is calculated by dividing the actual FEV_1 in liters (not the percent

of predicted) by the actual FVC in liters and multiplying the resulting ratio by 100%. An FEV_1/FVC below the **lower limits of normal (LLN)** for a patient's age confirms the presence of airflow obstruction, and also indicates asthma that is not well-controlled. To confirm the reversibility of airflow obstruction after baseline spirometry shows airflow obstruction, a short-acting bronchodilator such as albuterol is administered at a dose of up to 500 μg either by metered-dose inhaler or by nebulization. A postbronchodilator increase in the actual FEV_1 of ≥12% and ≥200 mL above the pre-bronchodilator baseline indicates at least partial reversibility of airflow obstruction.

Measurement of **peak expiratory flow rate (PEFR)** using an inexpensive portable device has been employed in the diagnosis and monitoring of asthma. An improvement in PEFR before and after bronchodilator administration of 60 L/min or 20%, a 20% day-to-day PEFR variability, or a >10% intraday PEFR variability when measured twice daily are suggestive evidence of asthma. However, peak flows are highly effort-dependent and variable, making them less reliable than spirometrically derived airflow measurements. Despite its limitations, PEFR measurement may be useful for monitoring airflow limitation in patients with poor perception of their asthma symptoms. The PEFR is also useful in identifying environmental triggers, and in documenting work-related asthma. Additional pulmonary function tests are not routinely necessary unless other pulmonary conditions are suspected, for example, a reduced DL_{CO} in COPD or a limitation of the inspiratory flow-volume loop in vocal chord dysfunction (Chaps. 16 and 33).

In patients with normal baseline spirometry, a broncho-provocation challenge test can be employed to demonstrate the

Table **21.2** Age-adjusted FEV₁/FVC threshold for airflow obstruction in asthmaᵃ

Age (years)	Lower Limit of Normal (LLN, in %) for FEV_1/FVC
8-19	85%
20-39	80%
40-59	75%
60-80	70%

ᵃData from the National Asthma Education and Prevention Program Expert Panel Report 3. "Guidelines for the Diagnosis and Management of Asthma." US Dept. H&HS; 2007.

bronchial hyperresponsiveness or airway hyperreactivity typical of asthma. The degree of bronchial hyperresponsiveness is classified based on the **[methacholine] provoking a ≥20% reduction in FEV₁ or FVC (PC₂₀)**. A PC_{20} <4.0 mg/mL indicates positive bronchial hyperresponsiveness, although some asthmatics may have values in the borderline range <16.0 mg/mL (Table 21.3). Although methacholine broncho-provocation challenge is a highly sensitive test in diagnosing asthma, it has a low specificity; a positive test can also be present in allergic rhinitis, COPD, bronchiectasis, and cystic fibrosis. Aside from methacholine, other bronchoprovocating agents such as histamine, mannitol, patient-specific aeroallergens, exercise, and dry air also are used to detect bronchial hyperresponsive/airway reactivity.

Allergy testing may be indicated in some asthmatics with persistent asthma and can help identify asthma environmental triggers that may be amenable to environmental control or desensitization therapy. Skin allergy (pin-prick) testing is considered the first-line method for determining allergic status because of its simplicity, efficiency, relatively lower cost, and high sensitivity. Despite its cost, serum [IgE] testing for regional and indoor allergens is more commonly being employed as the initial test to determine allergy status.

Table **21.3** Bronchial hyperresponsiveness based on a methacholine challenge testᵃ

PC₂₀ (mg/mL)	Interpretation	Result
>16.0	Normal bronchial hyperresponsiveness	Negative
4.0-16.0	Borderline bronchial hyperresponsiveness	Borderline
1.0-4.0	Mild bronchial hyperresponsiveness	Positive
<1.0	Moderate-to-severe hyperresponsiveness	Positive

ᵃAdapted from From Crapo RO et al: Guidelines for methacholine and exercise challenge testing-1999. This official statement of the American Thoracic Society was adopted by the ATS Board of Directors, July 1999, Am J Respir Crit Care Med 2000 Jan;161(1):309-329.

This approach is taken particularly by physicians not trained in skin testing, or for certain patients with severe persistent asthma requiring moderate-to-high doses of corticosteroids or even systemic corticosteroids. In this subset of patients, measurement of total serum [IgE] and documentation of hypersensitivity to an aeroallergen is a prerequisite to prescribing therapy with a monoclonal anti-IgE antibody.

Measurement of the **fractional excretion of nitric oxide (F$_e$NO)** is a well-studied non-invasive method of gauging the presence of active airway inflammation. An F$_e$NO >45 parts per billion (ppb) is considered a marker for active eosinophilic airway inflammation, while an F$_e$NO <25 ppb is highly predictive of its absence. These F$_e$NO levels increase during exacerbations of asthma and vary with titration of inhaled corticosteroid therapy. However, recent randomized control trials reached inconclusive results when evaluating whether the use of F$_e$NO to guide anti-inflammatory therapy in predominantly mild-to-moderate asthma improves clinical outcomes.

Chest imaging studies are not routinely recommended for the diagnosis of asthma. However, in patients with recent onset of asthma symptoms or in those with moderate-to-severe symptoms who are not responding to recommended therapy, obtaining a chest radiograph is prudent practice to exclude other diagnoses such as pneumonitis, pulmonary vascular congestion, and pneumothorax (Chaps. 15 and 37). In patients with poorly controlled, severe persistent asthma, and with fixed airway obstruction despite maximal therapy, a chest HRCT may reveal the presence of bronchiectasis, obliterative bronchiolitis due to environmental chemical exposure, or other serious pulmonary conditions.

Various cardiopulmonary diseases can mimic asthma. **Chronic obstructive pulmonary disease** is at times difficult to distinguish from asthma, but COPD usually affects smokers older than 40 years and presents with progressive rather than episodic symptoms. COPD patients, particularly those with emphysema, show by PFT an incompletely reversible airflow obstruction and low DL$_{CO}$, as opposed to asthmatics whose airflow limitation can normalize with optimal therapy and whose DL$_{CO}$ is typically normal or even elevated. **Congestive heart failure (CHF)** can manifest as **cardiac asthma** with dyspnea, cough, and wheezing from pulmonary vascular congestion and associated interstitial pulmonary edema. In this setting, chest radiography distinguishes the pulmonary vascular congestion and edema of CHF from the normal or hyperinflated lungs of asthmatics. Focal wheezing may be a clue to mechanical obstruction of the airways, as from a tumor or foreign body, which may be detected by chest imaging or bronchoscopy. During an acute episode of **vocal chord dysfunction syndrome**, routine spirometry can detect the variable airflow limitation of the inspiratory limb of the flow-volume loop, while **laryngoscopy** can show the paradoxical closure of the vocal chords during inspiration. Complete resolution of unexplained cough after discontinuation of **angiotensin converting enzyme** (ACE) inhibitor medication effectively rules out asthma etiologically. Pulmonary infiltrates on chest imaging studies suggest an infectious pneumonitis or some other interstitial lung disease rather than asthma. If radiographic infiltrates are coupled with an elevated eosinophil count in the peripheral blood or bronchoalveolar lavage fluid (BALF), an eosinophilic pneumonia should be suspected, either idiopathic or secondary to drugs or parasitic infection. Finally, in individuals with unexplained dyspnea who have a normal chest-ray but risk factors for thromboembolic disorders (eg, postsurgery, medical debility, malignancy, hereditary thrombophilia), pulmonary embolism should be ruled out with chest computed tomographic angiography or a ventilation-perfusion scan (Chap. 27).

Management Strategies for Asthma
First-Line Pharmacotherapies

The pharmacological treatment of asthma invariably involves selection of a **rescue bronchodilator**, usually a **short-acting β_2 adrenergic receptor agonist**. In patients with persistent asthma, one or more **controller medications** are usually required, such as **inhaled corticosteroids**, **long-acting β_2 agonists**, **leukotriene modifiers**, and other immunomodulators.

Bronchodilators reverse the airflow limitation from contraction of airway smooth muscles. Bronchodilation is mediated via two receptor types: β_2 adrenergic receptor agonists and the anticholinergic pathway via muscarinic receptor antagonists. Stimulation of β_2 receptors enhances adenylate cyclase activity via a stimulatory G_s protein, increasing **[cyclic AMP]** in airway smooth muscle cells. This increase in cyclic AMP activates **protein kinase A** that phosphorylates several target proteins, leading to Ca^{2+} efflux from the cell and its intracellular sequestration, and K^+ influx through Ca^{2+}-activated K^+ channels. These changes in intracellular Ca^{2+} lead to smooth muscle relaxation, while the K^+ influx hyperpolarizes cell membranes; both effects lead to bronchodilation.

Pharmacokinetically, the β_2 adrenergic agonists are classified based on their selectivity, onset of action, and duration of action (Table 21.4). For example, **albuterol** is the most widely used rescue bronchodilator for asthma because its β_2 selectivity causes fewer cardiovascular β_1 side effects like tachycardia than do the nonselective β-agents terbutaline and epinephrine. Albuterol has a rapid onset of action (10-15 min) but a short duration, lasting only 4-6 hours. **Long-acting β_2-adrenergic receptor agonists (LABAs)** have durations of ~12 hours and thereby allow twice-daily dosing. Of the two clinically available LABA formulations, **formoterol** has a more rapid onset of action (as early as 5 min) than does **salmeterol** (30 min).

Anticholinergics play a secondary role as bronchodilator therapy for asthma by blocking the **acetylcholine** released from vagal parasympathetic nerves from activating **muscarinic type 3 (M_3)**-receptors on airway smooth muscle cells, thereby reversing bronchoconstriction. **Ipratropium** is an inhaled short-acting anticholinergic that may be combined with a short-acting β_2-agonist during the first 24 hours of treatment for a severe asthma exacerbation. Meanwhile, there is preliminary evidence that the inhaled long-acting M_3 anticholinergic **tiotropium** may have a role as an adjunctive bronchodilator in patients with persistent asthma.

Inhaled corticosteroids are the first-line treatment for persistent asthma and are primarily responsible for controlling airway inflammation (Table 21.5). Corticosteroids enter the cell nucleus to inhibit gene transcription and synthesis of inflammatory cytokines, enzymes, and other mediators of asthma. By such actions, corticosteroids reduce the number of inflammatory cells (eosinophils, mast cells, T-lymphocytes, macrophages, and dendritic cells) in the airway. These anti-inflammatory agents also increase β-adrenergic responsiveness and reduce mucus hypersecretion and endothelial leakage. Inhaled corticosteroids are effective in controlling asthma symptoms, reducing frequency of exacerbations, and improving health-related quality of life measures in asthmatics. Side effects of inhaled corticosteroids include **oral thrush (candidiasis)**, respiratory infections, and mild **adrenal suppression**. On the other hand, systemic (oral or parenteral) corticosteroids normally are reserved for patients suffering

Table **21.4** Bronchodilators for (✱기1)
treatment of asthma

β-agonists		Anticholinergics	
Short-acting	**Long-acting**	**Short-acting**	**Long-acting**
Albuterol	Formoterol	Ipratropium	Tiotropium
Fenoterol	Salmeterol	Oxitropium	
Levalbuterol			
Terbutaline			

Table **21.5** Corticosteroids for
treatment of asthma

Inhaled Corticosteroids	Systemic Corticosteroids
Beclomethasone	Methylprednisolone
Budesonide	Prednisone
Ciclesonide	
Fluticasone	
Mometasone	

from an acute asthma exacerbation. They are also useful to treat patients with severe persistent asthma that is uncontrolled despite maximal therapy with high dose inhaled corticosteroid, bronchodilators, and other immunomodulators.

Leukotriene modifiers are secondary or add-on anti-inflammatory controller medications for persistent asthma. Elevated **cysteinyl-leukotriene** levels in asthmatic airways cause bronchoconstriction, airway hyperresponsiveness, mucus hypersecretion, and plasma transudation. In this context, the leukotriene modifiers improve asthma airway inflammation by inhibiting **5-lipoxygenase** as with **zileuton**, or by binding to cysteinyl-leukotriene receptors, as do **montelukast** and **zafirlukast**. Leukotriene modifiers have been shown to significantly improve the FEV_1, although they do so with less potency than either inhaled corticosteroids or bronchodilators.

Combining First-Line Pharmacotherapies

Several studies have demonstrated that combining two or more types of anti-inflammatory agents and bronchodilators may provide additive benefits in terms of improvements in lung function and symptom control. Combinations of inhaled corticosteroids and LABAs are delivered via special inhalational devices, with several of the more common pairings being salmeterol/fluticasone, budesonide/formoterol, and mometasone/formoterol. These combinations also may help improve a patient's adherence to a simplified asthma regimen.

Other Pharmacotherapeutics

Allergic asthma is characterized by elevation of specific IgE levels against one or more aeroallergens, contributing to airway inflammation and bronchial hyperresponsiveness. **Omalizumab** is a humanized monoclonal antibody that blocks the binding of IgE to the **high-affinity IgE receptors** found on mast cells, thus preventing their activation and release of histamine and other inflammatory mediators. Omalizumab has been shown to significantly reduce the number of asthma exacerbations, as well as the dose of inhaled or oral corticosteroids in patients with steroid-dependent persistent allergic asthma.

Methylxanthines and **cromones** are rapidly becoming less utilized for asthma therapy, as the more effective therapies described above have become clinically available. The methylxanthines **theophylline** and aminophylline are non-selective phosphodiesterase inhibitors that have been administered as bronchodilators since the 1930s. There is evidence that theophylline has additional anti-inflammatory and immunomodulatory effects in asthma. As such, some clinicians still prescribe methylxanthines in difficult clinical situations, for example, the use of IV aminophylline in patients with **status asthmaticus** and oral theophylline in patients with refractory severe persistent asthma. In the United States however, use of methylxanthines has declined due to their side effects at higher plasma concentrations such as nausea, vomiting, headaches, cardiac arrhythmias, seizures, and their propensity for serious drug interactions.

Cromones such as **cromolyn sodium** and **nedocromil**, are mast-cell membrane stabilizers that inhibit the release of histamine and other inflammatory mediators in asthma. Cromones were previously prescribed as prophylactic treatments in children with mild asthma to prevent bronchoconstriction from various stimuli, including exercise and cold air. However, because of their low potency as controller medications, cromones are quickly becoming drugs of only historical interest.

The Stepwise Approach to Asthma Therapy

The choice of asthma regimen depends upon its severity as defined by the National Asthma Education and Prevention Program (NAEPP), which classified asthma into **intermittent, mild persistent, moderate persistent**, and **severe persistent** forms. These levels are in turn based on the frequency and intensity of symptoms and resulting functional limitations, the degree of lung function impairment, and the frequency of exacerbations (Table 21.6).

The degree of airflow limitation, based on the FEV_1 expressed as the percentage predicted and the FEV_1/FVC ratio, parallels these asthma severity levels and provides a more objective measure of impairment. The NAEPP updated its treatment guidelines in 2007 and recommends a stepwise approach based on initial disease severity and subsequent degree of control of asthma (Table 21.7).

Intermittent asthma only requires the as-needed use of a short-acting β-agonist bronchodilator such as albuterol. **Persistent asthma** describes patients with daytime symptoms more than twice per week, as well as those who experience nocturnal awakenings 3-4 times per week or use their rescue bronchodilator (eg, albuterol) more than twice per week. Persistent asthma also includes those patients with functional limitations at home, school, or work, or who require oral/systemic corticosteroids for exacerbations at least twice a year. Such persistent asthma patients require controller anti-inflammatory medications, particularly inhaled corticosteroids. For patients with moderate-to-severe degrees of persistent asthma, adding other initial therapies may be necessary, such as long-acting bronchodilators, leukotriene modifiers, monoclonal anti-IgE antibodies, and even oral corticosteroids. All patients should be assessed periodically for their asthma control based on symptom frequency, use of rescue bronchodilators, and periodic spirometry or daily self-reported peak airflow measurements. Therapy should be "stepped up" using the NAEPP guidelines if asthma is not well controlled by adding one or more controller medications. If a patient's asthma has been well-controlled for at least three months, then a "step-down" along the same guidelines should be considered, such as reducing their inhaled corticosteroid dosing.

Immunotherapy for Asthma

Asthma immunotherapy, or the injection of increasing concentrations of a specific allergen over time, has long been employed by allergists, otorhinolaryngologists, and some pulmonologists in the treatment of allergic asthma. Such immunotherapy stimulates the patient's synthesis of **IgE-blocking antibodies** as well as **allergen-specific IgG**, thereby reducing IgE-mediated allergic asthma responses. Such **injection allergen**

Table **21.6**   Classification of asthma severity[a]

Components of Severity		Classification of Asthma Severity ≥12 years of age				
				Persistent		
		Intermittent	Mild	Moderate	Severe
Impairment Normal FEV_1/FVC: 8-19 yr 85% 20-39 yr 80% 40-59 yr 75% 60-80 yr 70%	Symptoms	≤2 days/week	>2 days/week but not daily	Daily	Throughout the day
	Nighttime awakenings	≤2×/month	3-4×/month	>1×/week but not nightly	Often 7×/week
	Short-acting beta$_2$-agonist use for symptom control [not prevention of exercise-induced bronchospasm (EIB)]	≤2 days/week	>2 days/week but not daily, and not more than 1× on any day	Daily	Several times per day
	Interference with normal activity	None	Minor limitation	Some limitation	Extremely limited
	Lung function	Normal FEV_1 between exacerbations FEV_1 >80% predicted FEV_1/FVC normal	FEV_1 >80% predicted FEV_1/FVC normal	FEV_1 >60% but <80% predicted FEV_1/FVC reduced 5%	FEV_1 <60% predicted FEV_1/FVC reduced >5%

[a]Data from the National Asthma Education and Prevention Program Expert Panel Report 3. "Guidelines for the Diagnosis and Management of Asthma." US Dept. H&HS; 2007.

immunotherapy reduces asthma symptoms and bronchial hyperresponsiveness, as well as the need for asthma medications. **Sublingual allergen immunotherapy** is also available for patients who are averse to injection immunotherapy. Patients undergoing immunotherapy should be monitored for side effects that can include local and systemic hypersensitivity reactions. An **epinephrine injection kit** and resuscitation equipment should be available for use by a trained personnel in case of an **anaphylactic reaction**.

Bronchial Thermoplasty

In patients with persistent asthma that is refractory despite maximal medical therapy, bronchial thermoplasty is emerging as a minimally invasive bronchoscopic procedure and promising therapeutic option. Bronchial thermoplasty involves the delivery of controlled thermal energy to the bronchial wall via serial bronchoscopies in order to achieve a reduction in airway smooth muscle mass. Bronchial thermoplasty has been

Table **21.7**   The NAEPP stepwise approach to asthma therapy[a]

Intermittent Asthma	Persistent Asthma: Daily Medication. Consult with asthma specialist if step 4 care or higher is required. Consider consultation at step 3.

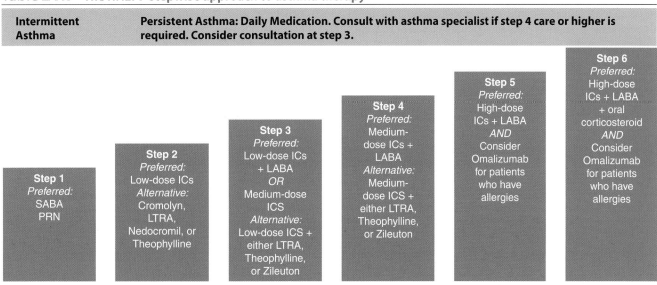

Step 1
Preferred:
SABA PRN

Step 2
Preferred:
Low-dose ICs
Alternative:
Cromolyn, LTRA, Nedocromil, or Theophylline

Step 3
Preferred:
Low-dose ICs + LABA
OR
Medium-dose ICS
Alternative:
Low-dose ICS + either LTRA, Theophylline, or Zileuton

Step 4
Preferred:
Medium-dose ICs + LABA
Alternative:
Medium-dose ICS + either LTRA, Theophylline, or Zileuton

Step 5
Preferred:
High-dose ICs + LABA
AND
Consider Omalizumab for patients who have allergies

Step 6
Preferred:
High-dose ICs + LABA + oral corticosteroid
AND
Consider Omalizumab for patients who have allergies

[a]Data from the National Asthma Education and Prevention Program; 2007.

associated with an improvement in overall asthma control and health-related quality of life, as well as a reduction in symptoms and exacerbations, health care utilization, and absences from occupational or academic settings.

Management of Asthma Exacerbations

An **asthma exacerbation** is defined as an episode of progressively increasing dyspnea, cough, wheezing, and/or chest tightness associated with a significant reduction in airflow parameters by spirometry or peak flow measurement. Asthma exacerbations are treated with an increase in the dose and/or frequency of short-acting bronchodilator therapy, combined with oral or IV corticosteroids at a dose equivalent to 0.5-1 mg of prednisone/kg/day (usually not exceeding 60-80 mg/day). Severe exacerbations not responding to initial therapy, or **status asthmaticus**, require in-hospital therapy. Although robust supportive evidence is lacking, IV aminophylline and/or magnesium sulfate have been employed as adjunctive bronchodilators in severe exacerbations. **Heliox** (helium-enriched air; see Chap. 13) increases laminar airflow and reduces airway turbulence by its reduced density and viscosity, and thus may help ameliorate dyspnea and decrease the work of breathing in patients with status asthmaticus. Non-invasive ventilation can be attempted in patients experiencing respiratory distress and impending respiratory failure; it may obviate the need for intubation and mechanical ventilation in status asthmaticus (Chaps. 25 and 30). For patients requiring invasive mechanical ventilation, **permissive hypercapnia** can be used to maintain adequate S_aO_2 and low peak P_{AW} at the expense of a mild respiratory acidosis with elevated P_aCO_2 values (Chaps. 28 and 30). This particular approach has been associated with a decrease in asthma mortality compared to historical controls.

Environmental Measures

Although there are no proven methods to prevent the development of asthma in persons with genetic or familial predispositions, identifying and avoiding asthma triggers using environmental control measures may improve symptoms and prevent asthma attacks. Measures that reduce indoor dust mite burden include encasing the mattress and pillows in mite-impermeable materials, removing bedroom carpets and upholstered furniture as well as furry toys, washing the beddings weekly in hot water, and using dehumidifiers. Dehumidifiers and proper ventilation systems also prevent the growth of mold in damp areas such as basements and bathrooms. Mold damage in homes and work areas should be rectified. Removal or distancing of pets from the living areas or at least the bedroom can improve asthma symptoms in a pet-sensitized asthmatic. Keeping doors and windows closed year-round can prevent outdoor aeroallergens from entering the home. Public health policies should be promoted that prohibit smoking in public areas and improve indoor and outdoor air quality.

Immunization

Yearly **influenza vaccination** is recommended by the **Centers for Disease Control and Prevention (CDC)** for asthma patients to reduce their frequency of exacerbations associated with the flu, although strong proof of this efficacy in asthmatics is lacking. Immunization of all asthmatics with the **23-valent pneumococcal vaccine** has also been recommended by the CDC, again despite the lack of robust evidence of its clinical efficacy in preventing pneumococcal pneumonia in this cohort (Chaps. 35 and 40).

Conclusions

Asthma is a complex disorder characterized by variable and recurring symptoms, airflow obstruction, bronchial hyperresponsiveness, and underlying inflammation. Airway inflammation as a response to allergens and irritants plays a predominant role in the pathogenesis and pathophysiology of asthma. The diagnosis of asthma is based upon the presence of recurrent symptoms combined with spirometric measures that are consistent with at least a partially reversible airflow obstruction and bronchial hyperresponsiveness. Current management of asthma utilizes the stepwise approach based on the assessment of initial severity and frequency of symptoms and on their subsequent control. Preventive measures that involve environmental modifications to reduce exposure to indoor and outdoor aeroallergens may help improve asthma symptoms and reduce its potentially serious exacerbations.

Suggested Readings

1. National Asthma Education and Prevention Program Expert Panel Report 3. *Guidelines for the Diagnosis and Management of Asthma.* US Department of Health and Human Services, 2007. http://www.nhlbi.nih.gov/guidelines/asthma/asthgdln.htm. *This NAEPP Report is a comprehensive guide for systematic evaluation and management of asthma based on risk, impairment, and control. Its recommendations are tailored to address the burden of asthma and utilize the health resources available in the United States.*

2. The Global Initiative for Asthma Report, *Global Strategy for Asthma Management and Prevention.* http://www.ginasthma. com/. *The GINA guidelines are updated annually by a panel of international experts in asthma. More global than the NAEPP guidelines, the GINA recommendations take into account the variable availability of diagnostic and therapeutic resources worldwide.*

3. Fanta CH. Drug therapy: Asthma. *N Engl J Med.* 2009; 360:1002-1014. *Succinct and well-referenced clinical review of the current recommended pharmacotherapy of asthma.*

CASE STUDIES AND PRACTICE PROBLEMS

CASE 21.1 A 17-year-old woman presents to clinic for cough and wheeze. Her symptoms have been present for the past 12 weeks, and she has not received any medications for these symptoms in the past. She states her symptoms are present daily, but not throughout the day, and denies nocturnal symptoms; she has only minor limitation with physical activity. Her baseline FEV_1 = 62% of predicted, which increases 10 minutes later by 14% and 240 mL after a one-time bronchodilator use. What is the appropriate classification of her asthma severity?

   a. Intermittent

   b. Mild persistent

   c. Moderate persistent

   d. Severe persistent

   e. Very severe persistent

CASE 21.2 A 27-year-old woman presents to clinic for follow-up of her asthma. Over the past 6 months, she has been on fluticasone 100 µg/salmeterol 50 µg, one puff b.i.d. She reports no daytime symptoms, no nocturnal symptoms, and has not used albuterol for rescue in the past 3 months. She reports no interference with daily activities from her asthma and has not required any systemic steroids for asthma over the past year. Spirometry reveals an FEV_1 = 97% predicted, FVC = 100% predicted, and an FEV_1/FVC = 0.84. What is the most appropriate next step in this patient's care?

   a. Discontinue salmeterol and continue fluticasone

   b. Discontinue fluticasone and continue salmeterol

   c. Continue current medications and reassess her symptoms in 3 months

   d. Continue current medications and reassess her symptoms in 6 months

   e. Discontinue current medications and conduct methacholine challenge to verify that patient has asthma

CASE 21.3 A 42-year-old woman presents to a new clinic and reports a 30-year history of asthma that has only ever been treated with inhaled albuterol, and which she uses at least 2-3 times per day. Pulmonary function testing (PFT) pre- and post-bronchodilator treatment is performed. Which of the following patterns would be most likely in her case if the physician suspects airway remodeling from asthma?

Pre-albuterol FEV$_1$ (% predicted)	Post-albuterol FEV$_1$ (% predicted)
a. 60%	95%
b. 80%	100%
c. 60%	65%
d. 95%	95%

Solutions to Case Studies and Practice Problems

CASE 21.1 The most correct answer is c, moderate persistent.

The NAEPP recommends classifying the initial severity of asthma based on the frequency of symptoms, nocturnal awakenings, use of rescue bronchodilator and functional impairment (Table 21.6). The patient has moderate persistent asthma since the patient has daily symptoms and an FEV_1 = 62% of predicted.

CASE 21.2 The most correct answer is a, discontinue salmeterol and continue fluticasone.

Based on the "Stepwise Approach to Asthma Therapy," this patient has had good asthma control for at least 3 months on the lowest dose of fluticasone plus salmeterol and should have her therapy de-escalated. Since the patient has persistent asthma, she still requires a controller anti-inflammatory medication, here fluticasone. Thus, salmeterol should be discontinued since it has no anti-inflammatory

action and has been associated with increased mortality when used as monotherapy for asthma.

CASE 21.3 The most correct answer is c, from 60% to 65%.

Persistent asthma treated only with a short acting bronchodilator without a controller anti-inflammatory medication such as an inhaled corticosteroid puts the patient at risk for developing chronic airflow limitation due to airway remodeling. *Answer c* is consistent with a lack of bronchial reversibility with bronchodilator therapy alone and thus consistent with chronic airflow limitation that makes it the correct choice. *Answer a* demonstrates normalization of airflow obstruction with bronchodilator therapy. *Answer b* also indicates normal or close to normal airflow with likely a positive bronchodilator response. *Answer d* is not consistent with airway obstruction both pre- and post-bronchodilator therapy.

Chapter 22

Management of Chronic Obstructive Pulmonary Diseases

JOSEPH R. D. ESPIRITU, MD AND
GEORGE M. MATUSCHAK, MD

Learning Objectives

- The student will be able to summarize the definition, prevalence, and impact of chronic obstructive pulmonary disease (COPD) in the United States and worldwide.

- The student will be able to list the primary host and environmental risk factors for development of COPD.

- The student will be able to describe the pathophysiology of COPD, distinguish its clinical features, and the guidelines for its treatment and prevention.

Introduction

The **World Health Organization (WHO)** estimates that 210 million people have **chronic obstructive pulmonary disease (COPD)** worldwide, with more than 3 million dying from the disease annually. COPD is the fourth leading cause of mortality in the United States among patients older than 45 years of age, and causes 5% of deaths worldwide. Moreover, COPD mortality is expected to increase by more than 30% over the next decade if current trends in tobacco smoking persist. Despite its increasing prevalence, COPD remains undiagnosed in many patients, thereby delaying important interventions that can prevent death and ameliorate symptoms and disability in those affected.

Working Definition of COPD

The **Global Initiative for Obstructive Lung Disease (GOLD) Guidelines** define COPD as a *"preventable and treatable disease with some cardiopulmonary effects that may contribute to the severity in individual patients. Its pulmonary component is characterized by airflow limitation that is not fully reversible. The airflow limitation is usually progressive and associated with an abnormal inflammatory response of the lung to noxious particles and gases."* Clinically, COPD encompasses the disorders of **chronic bronchitis** and **emphysema**, features of which may overlap with one another in individual patients. Chronic bronchitis is clinically defined as a cough productive of sputum most days of the month, at least 3 months of the year for two successive years without other explanations. In contrast, emphysema is anatomically defined by inflammation and abnormal enlargement of alveolar sacs, ducts, and walls distal to the terminal bronchioles of the small airways. Application of these histopathologic guidelines is summarized in Chap. 20.

Epidemiology of COPD

A meta-analysis of multiple trials and studies that was conducted in 2004 estimated the worldwide prevalence of COPD to be approximately 7.6%. In the United States, where there are up to 24 million individuals with active or previous smoking histories, the estimated prevalence in adults aged 25-75 years is 6.9% for mild COPD (defined as FEV_1/FVC <70% and FEV_1 ≥80% predicted), and 6.6% for moderate COPD (FEV_1/FVC <70% and FEV_1 <80% predicted). These prevalences were established by the **National Health and Nutrition Examination Survey III (NHANES-III)**. Furthermore, the Global Burden of Disease Study has projected that COPD will become the fifth leading cause of disability-adjusted life years lost by the year 2020.

Major Risk Factors for Development of COPD (#72)

The risk factors for COPD include both host and environmental factors (Table 22.1). With respect to host factors, **alpha₁ proteinase inhibitor (α_1-PI) deficiency** is the most well studied **genetic predisposition** to COPD. Inherited α_1-PI deficiency has a prevalence of approximately 1% in COPD populations, although this may underestimate its true incidence. Patients with α_1-PI deficiency may develop **panacinar emphysema** at relatively young ages (in the third to fourth decades of life), particularly in conjunction with exposure to tobacco smoke that greatly amplifies the likelihood of lung damage. The α_1-PI is a glycoprotein that inhibits the activities of proteolytic enzymes, especially **neutrophil elastase**. The normal homozygous **PiMM phenotype** is associated with a circulating [α_1-PI] of 20.0-53.0 µM, whereas the abnormal homozygous **PiZZ phenotype** is associated with severely deficient levels that are <15% of normal (ie, 2.5-7.0 µM). Other proteases, like the serine proteinases, matrix metalloproteinases, and cysteine proteinases, may also be involved in the pathophysiology of COPD. Specifically, it appears that an imbalance of proteinases and antiproteinases in the lungs of patients who

199

significantly reduces the associated weight gain from quitting smoking (1.5 kg in the bupropion SR group vs 2.9 kg in the placebo group). Combining bupropion SR with a nicotine patch also appears to significantly increase abstinence rates versus nicotine patch alone, although not versus bupropion alone.

Varenicline is a selective $\alpha_4\beta_2$ **nicotinic acetylcholine receptor partial agonist**. By binding to this class of nicotinic receptor in the ventral tegmental area, varenicline competitively inhibits binding by nicotine derived from tobacco smoke, and so prevents the release of greater quantities of dopamine associated with the reinforcing effects of smoking. Furthermore, by inducing a regulated release of dopamine (~60% of the maximal response to nicotine), varenicline also ameliorates the withdrawal symptoms from smoking cessation. Varenicline has been shown to have superior efficacy in promoting continuous abstinence rates versus bupropion SR plus placebo at 6 months, and versus placebo at 1 year. Although **nortriptyline** and **clonidine** have been found to be superior in efficacy as compared to placebo in a number of trials, the often serious side-effect profiles of both drugs preclude their widespread use for smoking cessation.

Evidence-based Treatment of COPD

The GOLD Guidelines recommend a treatment approach that is based upon the severity of a patient's airflow obstruction (Table 22.4).

Inhaled bronchodilators include β_2-adrenergic agonists and anticholinergics that provide symptomatic relief. However, as a class of therapeutics these have not been shown to alter the long-term declines in pulmonary function described above (Table 22.5). Use of **theophylline** as a bronchodilator has waned due to its serious side effects including nausea, vomiting, arrhythmia, seizures, and generally a narrow thera-

peutic window. Although **inhaled glucocorticoids** (ICs) (eg, beclomethasone, budesonide, fluticasone, and triamcinolone) also do not ameliorate declines in lung function, they improve airway reactivity and respiratory symptoms that decrease the need for health care utilization. Combining an inhaled glucocorticoid with a long-acting β_2-adrenergic agonist (LABA), such as the budesonide/formoterol or salmeterol/fluticasone formulations available, provides greater improvements in dyspnea and lung function than does each component alone. Systemic steroids are not recommended for maintenance therapy of COPD because of their long-term side effects of osteoporosis, steroid myopathy, adrenal insufficiency, and immunosuppression. Rather, systemic steroids are reserved for significant acute exacerbations of COPD.

Aside from smoking cessation, long-term O_2 therapy (>15 h/day) is the only treatment that has been demonstrated to increase survival in COPD patients with **chronic respiratory failure** or *cor pulmonale*. Chronic respiratory failure is defined as a $P_aO_2 \leq 55$ mm Hg or a $S_aO_2 \leq 88\%$. Cor pulmonale is defined as a P_aO_2 of 55-60 mm Hg or $S_aO_2 \leq 89\%$ with pulmonary hypertension, peripheral edema, or polycythemia. Oxygen therapy has other health benefits, including improved pulmonary hemodynamics, reduced polycythemia, increased exercise capacity, enhanced lung mechanics, and improved neurocognitive function.

Immunization against respiratory infections is recommended in patients with COPD (Table 22.4). Influenza vaccines should be given to all COPD patients, since these can significantly reduce serious illness and death by about 50%. The multivalent **pneumococcal polysaccharide vaccine** that is generally recommended for all persons ≥ 65 years old is indicated for COPD patients <65 years old who have an FEV_1 <40% predicted, since the vaccine can reduce the incidence of **community-acquired pneumonia** (**CAP**) in this cohort.

Table **22.4** **GOLD guidelines: recommended therapies at each stage of COPD[a]**

Stage I: Mild	Stage II: Moderate	Stage III: Severe	Stage IV: Very Severe
FEV_1/FVC <70% + $FEV_1 \geq 80\%$	FEV_1/FVC <70% + 50% $\leq FEV_1$ <80%	FEV_1/FVC <70% + 30% $\leq FEV_1$ <50%	FEV_1/FVC <70% + FEV_1 <30%, or FEV_1 <50% + chronic respiratory failure

Active reduction of risk factor(s); influenza vaccination --→

Add short-acting bronchodilator as needed ---→

Add regular treatment with one or more long-acting bronchodilators ------------------------------→

Add pulmonary rehabilitation --→

Add inhaled glucocorticoid if repeated exacerbations ------------------------------→

Add long-term O_2 if chronic respiratory failure.

Consider surgical treatments

[a]*From the Global Strategy for Diagnosis, Management and Prevention of COPD, updated 2010.* Used with permission from the Global Initiative for Chronic Obstructive Lung Disease (GOLD), www.goldcopd.org.

Table **22.5** Mechanisms and durations of action of bronchodilators for COPD

	β-Agonists	Anticholinergics
Short-acting agents	Albuterol	Ipratropium
	Fenoterol	Oxitropium
	Levalbuterol	
	Terbutaline	
Long-acting agents	Formoterol	Tiotropium
	Salmeterol	

Pulmonary rehabilitation is recommended for patients with moderate COPD and breathlessness (Table 22.4). In this context, such rehabilitation is defined as a combination of patient education plus participation in physical therapy that involves muscle strengthening exercises, including the primary and accessory muscles associated with breathing. Benefits of pulmonary rehabilitation include improvements in a patient's exercise capacity and quality of life, as well as reductions in their dyspnea, anxiety, depression, and health care utilization. The **American Lung Association (ALA)** is one of several nonprofit groups that organizes and/or supervises local pulmonary rehabilitation clinics for COPD patients.

Bullectomy, **lung volume reduction surgery**, and **lung transplantation** are surgical treatment options for selected patients with advanced COPD. Bullectomy may reduce dyspnea and improve lung function in patients with bullous disease (Chap. 37). When lung volume reduction surgery was performed in a subset of patients with very severe COPD (FEV_1 <45%) and predominantly upper lobe emphysema and low exercise capacity, it provided a survival advantage over medical therapy. However, high risk patients with an FEV_1 ≤20% of predicted and/or a DL_{CO} ≤20% of predicted were excluded from the trial. Lung transplantation does not confer a survival benefit in COPD patients, but it has been shown to improve their functional capacity and self-assessed quality of life. The major criteria for referral of a COPD patient for lung transplantation include FEV_1 <35%, P_aO_2 = 55-60 mm Hg, P_aCO_2 >50 mm Hg, and secondary pulmonary hypertension.

Managing Acute Exacerbations in COPD

The GOLD Guidelines define a **COPD exacerbation** as *"an event in the natural course of disease characterized by a change in the patient's baseline dyspnea, cough, and/or sputum that is beyond normal day-to-day variations, is acute in onset, and may warrant a change in regular medications."* Although most COPD exacerbations are triggered by respiratory infectious agents and air pollution, the exact cause is not known in about one-third of these episodes.

Common infectious agents associated with COPD exacerbations include respiratory viruses and bacterial pathogens such as *Haemophilus influenzae, Streptococcus pneumoniae,* and *Moraxella catarrhalis.* Managing acute exacerbations of COPD requires increasing the dosage and frequency of inhaled short-acting β-agonist bronchodilators (eg, albuterol). Adding a short-acting anticholinergic bronchodilator (eg, ipratropium) then is considered if a response to the short-acting β-agonist medication does not occur. Systemic steroid therapy (eg, prednisone, 30-40 mg orally for 7-10 days) has been shown to improve lung function, oxygenation, and time to recovery in COPD patients experiencing acute exacerbations. Systemic steroids should be started in hospitalized patients with COPD, and should be considered in ambulatory patients whose FEV_1 <50% of predicted at the time of presentation.

▶▶ C L I N I C A L   C O R R E L A T I O N   2 2 . 2

COPD patients who are most likely to benefit from antibiotics usually present with at least two of three cardinal symptoms of an acute exacerbation: worsening dyspnea; increased sputum production; and increased sputum purulence. COPD patients in respiratory distress are those with some or all of the following findings: moderate-to-severe dyspnea; tachypnea (*f* >25 breaths/min); accessory respiratory muscle use; paradoxical breathing; severe acidosis (pHa ≤7.35) or hypercapnia (P_aCO_2 >45 mm Hg). Non-invasive ventilation, such as by facial mask with **bilevel positive airway pressure (BiPAP)** as used in patients with **sleep-related hypoventilation/ hypoxemic syndrome** (Chap. 25), has been demonstrated to ameliorate such respiratory failure, decrease hospital length of stay, and reduce mortality. However, for severe life-threatening and/or complicated exacerbation episodes (eg, cardiopulmonary arrest), invasive mechanical ventilation is recommended (Chap. 30).

Summary of Findings and Recommendations in COPD

COPD is a spectrum of preventable and treatable disease states that are characterized by an airflow limitation that is not fully reversible and that result from exposure to noxious gases and particles, primarily tobacco smoke. In COPD, the processes of lung inflammation, dysequilibrium between antiproteases and proteases, and oxidative stress collectively result in airway remodeling and emphysematous parenchymal changes (Chap. 20). Evaluation by spirometry that includes bronchodilator reversibility testing confirms the diagnosis of COPD in patients with respiratory symptoms and known risk factors. Current GOLD and ATS/ERS Guidelines recommend avoidance of exposure, as well as a combination of graded pharmacologic and non-pharmacologic therapies based on the severity of obstructive abnormality. To date, only smoking cessation and long-term oxygen therapy have been shown to ameliorate the decline in lung function and improve survival in patients with COPD.

Suggested Readings

1. NHLBI/WHO Workshop. Global strategy for the diagnosis and management and prevention of chronic obstructive pulmonary disease, (Updated in 2009). http://www.gold.copd.org. *Also known as the GOLD Guidelines, the executive summary is written by COPD experts worldwide and delivers a comprehensive discussion of the epidemiology, pathophysiology, evidence-based evaluation, prevention, and management of COPD.*

2. Celli BR, MacNee W. Standards for the diagnosis and treatment of patients with COPD: a summary of the ATS/ERS position paper. *Eur Respir J.* 2004;23:932-946. *As for the GOLD Guidelines, this excellent article summarizes similar evidence-based recommendations on COPD as formulated by working groups of the American Thoracic Society and the European Respiratory Society.*

CASE STUDIES AND PRACTICE PROBLEMS

CASE 22.1 A 50-year-old female has worsening exertional dyspnea. For 10 years she has coughed up whitish to occasionally yellow-green phlegm most days. Two years ago, she had dyspnea while climbing stairs. Six months ago, she became dyspneic after walking 20 meters on a flat surface. Her past medical history includes childhood asthma, anxiety, and hypertension. She previously smoked two packs of cigarettes/day starting at age 18 years, but reduced that to one pack/day two years ago. Physical exam reveals an alert, thin woman. Vital signs are: BP = 150/90 mm Hg, pulse = 108/min, f = 28/min, T_B = 98.2°F (36.8°C). She has a prolonged expiratory phase, bronchovesicular breath sounds, and low-pitched wheezes bilaterally. Which of the following post-bronchodilator measurements is most consistent with a presumptive diagnosis of COPD in this patient?

a. FEV_1/FVC < lower limit of normal for age, gender, and height
b. FEV_1/FVC <80% of predicted for age, gender, and height
c. TLC <80% of predicted for age, gender, and height
d. DL_{CO} >120%
e. Steep downward slope of the expiratory limb of her flow-volume loop

CASE 22.2 A 55-year-old male is referred by the emergency department (ED) physician to pulmonary clinic for evaluation of dyspnea. He has long-standing progressive dyspnea and minimal cough without sputum production for the past 10 years. He has smoked two packs per day since age 15 years. Physical exam reveals a barrel chest and decreased breath sounds on both lung fields. Spirometry shows his FEV_1 = 40% of predicted with an FEV_1/FVC ratio = 58% of predicted. His S_aO_2 by pulse oximetry is 88%. A high-resolution chest CT reveals diffuse emphysematous changes bilaterally. Which of the following is most associated with improved survival in such a patient?

a. Long-acting β-agonist bronchodilator
b. Long-acting anticholinergic bronchodilator
c. Inhaled corticosteroid
d. Supplemental oxygen
e. Lung volume reduction surgery

CASE 22.3 A 58-year-old woman presents with shortness of breath, and a five-year history of progressive dyspnea on exertion while carrying groceries and going up and down her basement steps. She smoked 1.5 packs of cigarette/day from age 16 until 52 years. She has no other medical problems and has not seen a doctor since giving birth in her mid-twenties. Physical exam reveals a thin woman, not in distress. She has prolonged expiratory phase but no crackles or wheezes; other physical findings are unremarkable. Office spirometry shows FVC = 65%, FEV_1 = 56%, and an FEV_1/FVC = 60%; S_aO_2 on room air = 92%. Her chest x-ray shows severe hyperinflation with flattening of the hemidiaphragms, but no infiltrates. Genetic testing reveals a homozygous PiMM phenotype. Which of the following treatments is most appropriate for her?

a. Pulmonary rehabilitation
b. Inhaled corticosteroid
c. Nocturnal oxygen therapy
d. Lung volume reduction surgery
e. α_1-PI replacement therapy

Solutions to Case Studies and Practice Problems

CASE 22.1 The most correct answer is a.

FEV_1/FVC < lower limit of normal for age, gender, and height. ATS/ERS Guidelines define obstruction as an FEV_1/FVC < lower limit of normal for age, gender, and height. An alternative definition of obstruction used by the GOLD guidelines is an FEV_1/FVC <70% (*answer b incorrect*). A TLC <80% is indicative of restriction and not obstruction (*answer c*) that leads to the hyperinflation (TLC >120%) that is typically found in COPD. DL_{CO} in COPD is typically decreased due to loss of capillary-alveolar membrane surface area (*answer d*), particularly in emphysema. A steep downward slope of the expiratory limb of the flow-volume loop is characteristic of restriction (*answer e*), while the forced expiratory flow-volume curve in obstruction is upwardly concave (Chap. 6).

CASE 22.2 The most correct answer is d, supplemental oxygen.

The Report of the British Medical Research Council Working Party and the Nocturnal O_2 Treatment Trial found that supplemental oxygen improved survival in patients with severe COPD and hypoxemia. Long-acting bronchodilators (*answers a, b*) can significantly relieve symptoms, improve pulmonary function, and reduce exacerbations but they have not been demonstrated to reduce mortality. Likewise, inhaled corticosteroids (*answer c*) improve airway reactivity and reduce exacerbations, but they have not been shown to influence survival in COPD patients. The National Emphysema Treatment Trial found that lung volume reduction surgery reduced mortality only in a subgroup of patients with predominantly upper lobe emphysema and low baseline exercise capacity, but such surgery increased mortality in patients with homogeneous (diffuse) non-upper lobe emphysema of the type this patient's exam findings indicate (*answer e*).

CASE 22.3 The most correct answer is a, pulmonary rehabilitation.

By the GOLD Guidelines criteria in Table 22.4, this woman has Stage II or moderate COPD. Results of genetic testing indicated that she does not have an inherited form of α_1-PI deficiency (*answer e*). Thus, conservative medical management excludes interventions that are normally indicated for more severe COPD disease, such as inhaled corticosteroids, nocturnal O_2 therapy, or surgery (*answers b, c,* and *d*). **Bonus comment:** No mention is made of the patient's immunization status, which should be checked to ensure it includes both influenza and polyvalent pneumococcal vaccines given her age.

Chapter 23

Pathology of Restrictive Lung Diseases

DAVID S. BRINK, MD

Introduction #75

Restrictive lung diseases are characterized by reduced lung compliance that requires greater pressure to inflate the lungs and, clinically, typically are manifest as dyspnea. Restrictive lung disease can result from external compression of the lung parenchyma; examples include severe scoliosis, chest wall tumors, and expansion of the pleural space by fluid or air (Chaps. 26 and 29). This chapter will focus on restrictive lung diseases in which the restriction is intrinsic to the lung rather than due to external compression. Although many different restrictive lung diseases will be discussed, there are some common themes to restrictive lung disease. Many such diseases show thickening of alveolar septa and alveolar epithelial and endothelial injury that lead to $\dot{V}_A/\dot{Q}$ mismatch. With progression of many such diseases, patients develop severe hypoxemia and respiratory failure. These are often complicated with **pulmonary hypertension** and **cor pulmonale** (right ventricular dilatation due to lung disease).

Acute Restrictive Lung Diseases

The **acute respiratory distress syndrome** (ARDS) is a clinical syndrome characterized by the acute onset of respiratory distress with hypoxemia, reduced lung compliance, and diffuse pulmonary infiltrates in the absence of primary left heart failure; a less severe form of the syndrome is **acute lung injury (ALI)** (Chap. 28). **Diffuse alveolar damage** (DAD) is the morphologic counterpart of ALI/ARDS. Though DAD can complicate many conditions (Table 23.1), more than one-half of cases occur in the settings of sepsis, diffuse pulmonary infections, gastric aspiration, and trauma.

The pathogenesis of DAD begins with endothelial damage or, less frequently, epithelial damage. Within 30 minutes, macrophages secrete canonical proinflammatory cytokines including **TNF-α**, **IL-1**, and **IL-8**, leading to neutrophil chemotaxis and activation (Chap. 10). Activated neutrophils secrete oxidants, proteases, **platelet activating factor (PAF)**, and leukotrienes, the results of which are tissue damage, edema, inactivation of pulmonary surfactant, and the formation of hyaline membranes,

the morphologic hallmark of DAD (see below). Later, macrophage secretion of **transforming growth factor-beta (TGF-β)** and **platelet-derived growth factor (PDGF)** causes proliferation of fibroblasts with subsequent synthesis of collagen. The pathogenesis of DAD is further discussed in Chap. 28.

Morphologically, lungs with DAD show reduced **crepitus** and resemble liver in consistency. Early in the course, the lungs are dense and dark red; as collagen deposition occurs, their color changes to gray (Fig. 23.1). Microscopically, DAD shows a spectrum of changes that can be organized into three phases (Fig. 23.2). The earliest of these is the **exudative phase**, with vascular congestion, interstitial and intra-alveolar edema, alveolar epithelial necrosis, neutrophil margination, dilatation and/or collapse of alveolar ducts, fibrin thrombi, and hyaline membranes. **Hyaline membranes**, the hallmark of DAD, are composed of edema fluid and necrotic epithelial cells. Subsequent to this exudative period is the **proliferative phase**, in which there is type 2 pneumocyte hyperplasia as well as fibroblast infiltration of the interstitium and the intra-alveolar exudate (ie, the hyaline membranes). Finally, as fibroblasts synthesize collagen, DAD enters the **fibrotic phase**, with fibrosis of the exudate (also described as **organization**) and expansion of the interstitium by fibrosis.

Clinically, ARDS begins with dyspnea and tachypnea; early in its course, a chest radiograph may be normal. Subsequently, the patient develops cyanosis, hypoxemia, and respiratory failure, at which point a chest radiograph typically shows diffuse bilateral infiltrates. As hypoxemia becomes unresponsive to oxygen therapy, respiratory acidosis often develops. Of note, oxygen therapy can worsen the alveolar epithelial damage. ARDS can be complicated by secondary infection of the hyaline membranes and/or by death, the latter occurring in approximately 40% of cases in the United States.

Acute interstitial pneumonia is a rapidly progressive acute restrictive lung disease with a presentation similar to ARDS but without a known underlying etiology; an alternate name is **idiopathic ALI-DAD**. Morphologically, it closely resembles DAD and may be indistinguishable from DAD. Mortality rates in

Table **23.1** **Conditions associated with development of ALI and ARDS**

Infection	Inhaled Irritants	Physical Injury
Sepsis	Oxygen toxicity	Mechanical trauma, head injury
Diffuse pulmonary infections 　Viral pneumonia 　*Mycoplasma* pneumonia 　*Pneumocystis* pneumonia 　Miliary tuberculosis	Smoke Irritant gases Misc. chemicals	Pulmonary contusion Near-drowning Fractures with fat embolism Burns Ionizing radiation
Gastric aspiration		
Chemical Injury	**Hematologic Conditions**	**Hypersensitivity Reactions**
Heroin or methadone overdose	Multiple transfusions	Organic solvents
Acetylsalicylic acid	Disseminated intravascular coagulation	Misc. drugs
Barbiturate overdose		
Paraquat poisoning		
Pancreatitis	**Uremia**	**Cardiopulmonary Bypass**

Adapted from Kumar et al. Robbins and Cotran Pathologic Basis of Disease, 8th ed. Philadelphia, PA: Elsevier; 2007.

various studies have ranged from 33% to 74%. Survivors often experience complete or near complete recovery.

Chronic Restrictive Lung Diseases

The chronic restrictive lung diseases are also called **diffuse interstitial lung diseases**, because changes in the interstitium dominate the morphologic appearance, and **diffuse infiltrative diseases**, because chest radiographs show diffuse infiltrates.

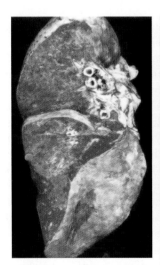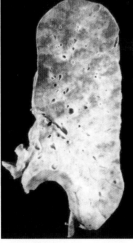

FIGURE 23.1 In diffuse alveolar damage (DAD), lungs are initially dense and dark red (a). As collagen deposition occurs, their color becomes gray (b). *From Travis et al.* Atlas of Nontumor Pathology: Volume 2: Non-Neoplastic Disorders of the Lower Respiratory Tract, *American Registry of Pathology; 2002.*

Chronic restrictive lung diseases are a heterogeneous group of disorders without uniform classification, without uniform terminology, and often without known etiology or pathogenesis. Nevertheless, they share many clinical and morphological features and, at end-stage, they may be indistinguishable from each other. Clinically, patients with chronic restrictive lung diseases have dyspnea, tachypnea, end-inspiratory crackles, and eventual cyanosis (Chap. 24). Later, these patients often develop secondary pulmonary hypertension (Chap. 26) and right heart failure with cor pulmonale. Pathogenetically, many of the chronic restrictive lung diseases begin with **alveolitis**, leading to distortion of alveolar structure and release of mediators that incite cell injury and induce fibrosis. Morphologically, many of the chronic restrictive lung diseases, particularly in later stages, are characterized by **interstitial fibrosis**. The end-stage of many of the chronic restrictive lung diseases is the classic **honeycomb lung**.

　　Idiopathic pulmonary fibrosis (IPF) is a poorly understood, idiopathic, nongranulomatous chronic restrictive lung disease that morphologically is characterized by diffuse interstitial fibrosis. Although many alternate names for the disease exist, **cryptogenic fibrosing alveolitis** is the one most frequently encountered. The pathogenesis of IPF is poorly understood but appears to involve repeated cycles of alveolitis (due to an unidentified agent) that are followed by wound healing with fibroblast proliferation. Grossly, lungs with well-developed IPF have a pleural surface with a **cobblestone** appearance due to wound contraction in interlobular septa. The cut surface of IPF lungs shows rubbery-to-firm, white patches in subpleural regions and in the interlobular septa (Fig. 23.3).

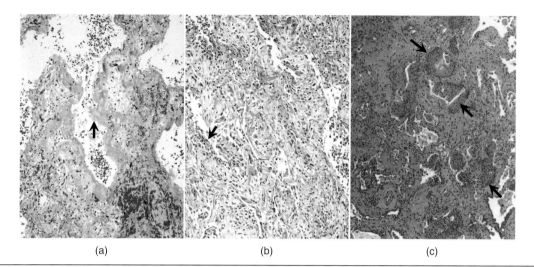

(a)   (b)   (c)

FIGURE 23.2 (a) Hyaline membranes (arrow) dominate the exudative phase of DAD, lining most airspaces in this image. (b) In the proliferative phase, fibroblasts infiltrate the hyaline membranes and expand the interstitium, thickening alveolar septa; type 2 pneumocyte hyperplasia (arrow) is common in the proliferative phase of DAD. (c) As fibroblasts synthesize collagen, DAD enters the fibrotic phase, with marked expansion of the interstitium by collagen; in this example, there is widespread squamous metaplasia (arrows). (c): *From Travis et al.* Atlas of Nontumor Pathology: Volume 2: Non-Neoplastic Disorders of the Lower Respiratory Tract, American Registry of Pathology; *2002.*

Histologically, the morphology of IPF is described as **usual interstitial pneumonia (UIP)** (Fig. 23.4). Although required for a diagnosis of IPF, UIP is not specific and can be seen in other diseases (eg, collagen vascular diseases, asbestosis; see below). UIP is characterized by regional and temporal heterogeneity where different lung foci show different stages of disease. In addition to interstitial fibrosis, magnified in subpleural zones and interlobular septa, UIP includes

characteristic **fibroblastic foci** and typically shows prominent type 2 pneumocyte hyperplasia. End-stage UIP shows dilatated airspaces lined by cuboidal or low columnar epithelium separated by inflamed fibrous tissue. Patients with IPF typically present in the fifth to eighth decade with increasing dyspnea on exertion and dry cough, followed by hypoxemia, cyanosis, and digital clubbing. Progression of IPF is unpredictable, but the mean survival time is approximately three years. The only definitive therapy for IPF is lung transplantation.

▶▶ **CLINICAL CORRELATION 23.1**

By turning up the brightness on a computed tomogram, the resulting CT images of the lungs can demonstrate severity of interstitial disease. The settings used to image lung parenchyma are the **lung windows** and blur detail in surrounding soft tissue. Fig. 23.5(a) is high-resolution CT of UIP, with subpleural distribution of abnormalities. Fig. 23.5(b) is an HRCT of end-stage UIP with honeycombing that is more pronounced on the patient's left side (right side of image).

#76   **Nonspecific interstitial pneumonia (NSIP)** is an idiopathic, nongranulomatous lung disease without the defining diagnostic features of better-characterized diseases. Histologically, NSIP can show a cellular pattern with mild to moderate expansion of the interstitium by lymphocytes and plasma cells with either a uniform or patchy distribution [Fig. 23.6(a)]. Alternatively, a fibrosing pattern with diffuse or patchy interstitial fibrosis is noted [Fig. 23.6(b)]. In contrast to UIP, the fibrosing pattern of NSIP does typically not show fibroblastic foci or the regional/temporal heterogeneity of disease.

Sarcoidosis is an idiopathic multisystem disease characterized by granulomatous inflammation (typically noncaseating) in many tissues and organs. Since there are many causes of granulomatous inflammation—including foreign body,

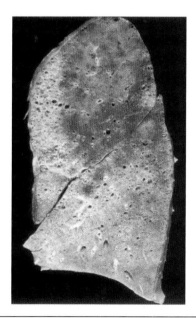

FIGURE 23.3 Usual interstitial pneumonia in idiopathic pulmonary fibrosis. Pale regions represent fibrosis with cystic change (honeycomb pattern) and are concentrated in the lower lobe and in the subpleural zone of the upper lobe (left of image). The darker parenchyma represents portions of lung with little or no fibrosis. *From Travis et al.* Atlas of Nontumor Pathology: Volume 2: Non-Neoplastic Disorders of the Lower Respiratory Tract, American Registry of Pathology; *2002.*

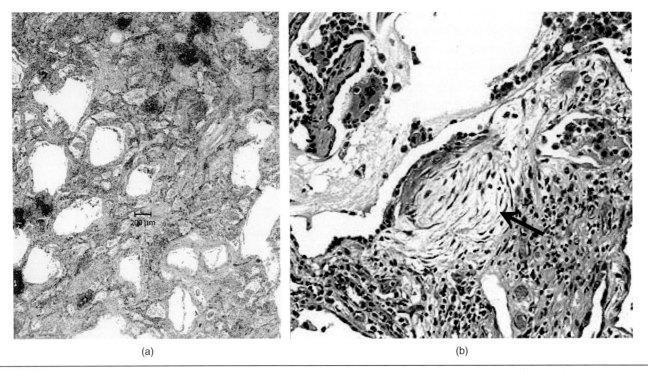

(a)   (b)

FIGURE 23.4 Usual interstitial pneumonia in idiopathic pulmonary fibrosis. (a) Cystically dilatated airspaces are separated by fibrotic and thickened septa. (b) A characteristic finding in UIP is the fibroblastic focus (arrow). (b): *From Travis et al.* Atlas of Nontumor Pathology: Volume 2: Non-Neoplastic Disorders of the Lower Respiratory Tract, American Registry of Pathology; *2002.*

mycobacterial infection, and fungal infection—sarcoidosis is a diagnosis of exclusion. Though its presentation can include involvement of virtually any organ, patients typically have bilateral hilar lymphadenopathy and/or lung involvement. Sarcoidosis shows a racial bias (black:white of about 10:1) and a female gender bias. Though the etiology of sarcoidosis is unknown, its pathogenesis likely involves a **type IV hypersensitivity reaction** (cell-mediated, delayed) to a currently unknown antigen. Familial and racial clustering and association with certain HLA subtypes imply that development of

sarcoidosis may require a genetic predisposition. Many features of sarcoidosis suggest that it is an infectious disease, but there is no unequivocal evidence that sarcoidosis has an infectious etiology. The morphology of sarcoidosis is nonspecific: noncaseating granulomatous inflammation (Fig. 23.7). A **granuloma** is a circumscribed collection of **epithelioid histiocytes** [Fig. 23.7(c)]; the term "epithelioid" is used to describe cells that have more cytoplasm than typical histiocytes, imparting a resemblance to squamous epithelial cells. Epithelioid histiocytes can merge with each other, producing

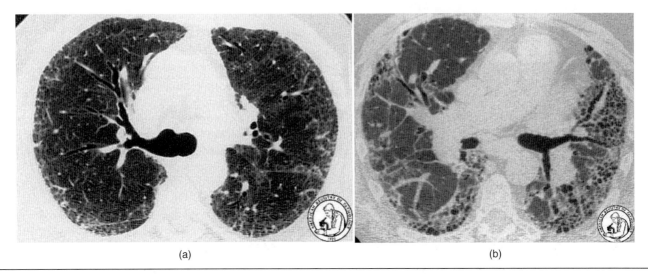

(a)   (b)

FIGURE 23.5 See Clinical Correlation 23.1 for details. *From Travis et al.* Atlas of Nontumor Pathology: Volume 2: Non-Neoplastic Disorders of the Lower Respiratory Tract, American Registry of Pathology; *2002.*

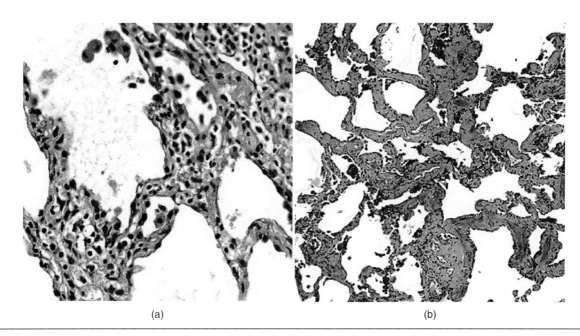

(a)   (b)

FIGURE 23.6 Nonspecific interstitial pneumonia. (a) The cellular pattern of NSIP in which moderate mononuclear inflammatory infiltrate expands the interstitium. (b) The fibrosing pattern of NSIP, in which interstitial fibrosis expands alveolar septa. *From Travis et al.* Atlas of Nontumor Pathology: Volume 2: Non-Neoplastic Disorders of the Lower Respiratory Tract, American Registry of Pathology; *2002.*

a multinucleated giant cell. While multinucleated giant cells are common in granulomata, not all granulomata contain them. In sarcoidosis, the granulomata often contain **Schaumann bodies** [laminated concretions of calcium and protein, Fig. 23.7(d)] and **asteroid bodies** [stellate inclusions within giant cells, Fig. 23.7(e)]. However, neither Schaumann bodies nor asteroid bodies are specific for sarcoidosis.

As mentioned above, the granulomata in sarcoidosis can involve virtually any organ but typically involve the pulmonary interstitium and hilar lymph nodes. Pulmonary involvement is often complicated by interstitial fibrosis. Other organs that are commonly involved include skin, eyes, lacrimal glands, salivary glands, spleen, liver, and skeletal muscle. Clinically, sarcoidosis is often asymptomatic. If symptomatic, sarcoidosis ranges from progressive chronicity to periods of activity separated by periods of remission. Presentation is typically due to

respiratory involvement, with dyspnea, cough, chest pain, and hemoptysis; alternatively, constitutional signs and symptoms (fever, fatigue, weight loss, anorexia, night sweats) may dominate the clinical scenario. Specific symptoms at presentation are markedly variable due to the complex of sites showing involvement. Approximately 65%-70% of patients recover spontaneously or with steroid therapy and have minimal or no residual disease, ~20% of patients develop permanent lung dysfunction or visual impairment, and 10%-15% develop progressive pulmonary fibrosis with subsequent cor pulmonale or central nervous system damage.   #77

Hypersensitivity pneumonitis is typically an occupational disease that begins with alveolar damage from exposure to an organic antigen. The acute phase of the disease occurs 4-6 hours after antigen exposure in a previously sensitized host, likely represents a **type III hypersensitivity reaction** (immune

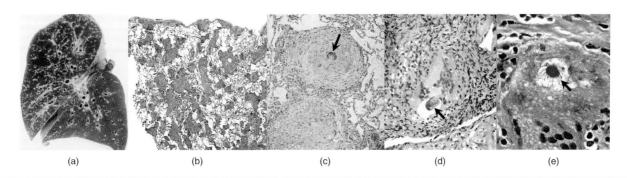

(a)   (b)   (c)   (d)   (e)

FIGURE 23.7 Sarcoidosis. (a) Grossly, numerous white nodules are associated with bronchovascular bundles. (b) At low magnification, the numerous granulomata appear as eosinophilic nodules. (c) At higher magnification, these nodules are seen to be composed of epithelioid histiocytes and multinucleated giant cells (arrow). Though nonspecific, Schaumann bodies [(d), arrow] and asteroid bodies [(e), arrow] also can be present. (a), (b), (d), and (e): *From Travis et al.* Atlas of Nontumor Pathology: Volume 2: Non-Neoplastic Disorders of the Lower Respiratory Tract, American Registry of Pathology; *2002.* (c): *From Klatt.* Robbins and Cotran Atlas of Pathology, *2nd ed. 2010.*

complex), and is typified by diffuse and nodular infiltrates on chest radiograph, restrictive pattern of pulmonary function tests, and neutrophilic inflammation. With continuous antigen exposure, the disease enters its chronic phase with respiratory failure, dyspnea, cyanosis, decreased lung compliance, and decreased total lung capacity. The chronic phase is a type IV hypersensitivity reaction (delayed, cell-mediated) characterized histologically by lymphocytes, plasma cells, and foamy histiocytes in alveoli, alveolar walls, and around terminal bronchioles; interstitial fibrosis; obliterative bronchiolitis; and, in about two-thirds of cases, granulomata. Of note, the eosinophilia that is typical of type I hypersensitivity reactions is not a significant feature of hypersensitivity pneumonitis. If the offending antigen is removed during the acute phase, the disease resolves in weeks. Once the disease has progressed to its chronic phase, resolution can be slow, and approximately 5% of patients develop respiratory failure and die. Table 23.2 summarizes the myriad diseases that represent forms of hypersensitivity pneumonitis.

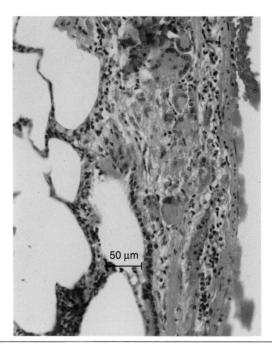

FIGURE 23.8 See Clinical Correlation 23.2 for details.

▶▶CLINICAL CORRELATION 23.2

A 13-year-old boy with a history of congenital heart disease presents with interstitial lung disease of unknown etiology. A wedge biopsy of lung is procured and shows interstitial non-necrotizing granulomatous inflammation with multinucleated giant cells (Fig. 23.8). Special stains for acid-fast microorganisms and fungi are negative. Histologic findings are nonspecific but suggestive of hypersensitivity pneumonitis. Subsequently, additional history is obtained: the patient lives in a home with 17 birds. Combining the clinical scenario with histologic findings, a diagnosis of hypersensitivity pneumonitis (bird fancier's disease) is made, establishing the etiology for the patient's interstitial lung disease.

Table **23.2** Typical presentations of hypersensitivity pneumonitis

Syndrome	Exposure	Antigens
Fungal/Bacterial Antigens		
Farmer's lung	Moldy hay	*Micropolyspora faeni*
Bagassosis	Moldy sugar cane	*Thermoactinomyces sacchari*
Maple bark disease	Moldy maple tree bark	*Cryptostroma corticale*
Humidifier lung	Cool-mist humidifier	Thermophilic *Actinomycetes, Aureobasidium pullulans*
Malt worker's lung	Moldy barley grain	*Aspergillus clavatus*
Cheese washer's lung	Moldy cheeses	*Penicillium casei*
Insect Products		
Miller's lung	Dust-contaminated grain	*Sitophilus granarius* (wheat weevil)
Animal Products		
Bird fancier's lung	Pigeon, parakeet, chicken	Serum proteins in droppings
Chemicals		
Chemical worker's lung	Chemical industries	Trimellitic anhydride, isocyanates

Modified from Kumar et al. Robbins and Cotran Pathologic Basis of Disease, 8th ed. *Philadelphia, PA: Elsevier; 2007.*

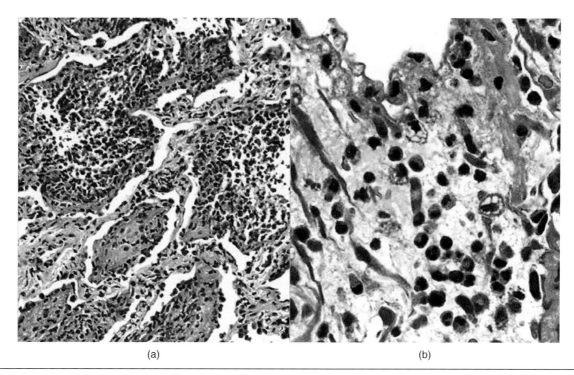

(a)   (b)

FIGURE 23.9   Pulmonary eosinophilia. (a) Intra-alveolar eosinophil-rich exudates dominate this example of idiopathic chronic eosinophilic pneumonia. (b) In this example of acute eosinophilic pneumonia, eosinophils are in the interstitium. *From Travis et al.* Atlas of Nontumor Pathology: Volume 2: Non-Neoplastic Disorders of the Lower Respiratory Tract, American Registry of Pathology; *2002.*

Pulmonary eosinophilia is a collection of diseases with similar morphologies of eosinophilic infiltration of the pulmonary interstitium and/or alveolar spaces (Fig. 23.9) and similar clinical scenarios of corticosteroid-responsive fever, night sweats, and dyspnea. **Acute eosinophilic pneumonia** with respiratory failure is an idiopathic illness with rapid onset of fever, dyspnea, and potentially fatal hypoxemic respiratory failure. **Simple pulmonary eosinophilia (Löffler syndrome)** is characterized by transient pulmonary eosinophilic infiltrates and peripheral blood eosinophilia. **Tropical eosinophilia** represents a microfilarial infection. **Secondary chronic pulmonary eosinophilia** occurs in a number of settings, including certain infections (parasitic, fungal, bacterial), drug allergies, asthma, allergic bronchopulmonary aspergillosis (Chap. 20), and **polyarteritis nodosa**. **Idiopathic chronic eosinophilic pneumonia** is characterized by interstitial and intra-alveolar lymphocytic and eosinophilic infiltrates in peripheral lung fields. From the morphologic perspective, many of these diseases are indistinguishable, thus giving rise to the morphologic term pulmonary eosinophilia.

Though smoking-related lung disease is frequently obstructive (see Chap. 20 for discussions of emphysema and chronic bronchitis), there are several smoking-related restrictive lung diseases. **Desquamative interstitial pneumonitis (DIP)** and **respiratory bronchiolitis-associated interstitial lung disease** are thought of as opposite ends of a spectrum of interstitial lung disease that may develop in smokers; the pathogenesis of both is unknown. In DIP [Fig 23.10(a), (b)], there is mononuclear interstitial inflammation, an abundance of airspace macrophages with dusty brown cytoplasmic pigment, and type 2 pneumocyte hyperplasia. The airspace

macrophages in DIP typically clump together, resulting in an appearance that was historically (and erroneously) interpreted as desquamated alveolar epithelium. In respiratory bronchiolitis-associated interstitial lung disease, there is patchy bronchiolocentric distribution of pigmented macrophages [Fig. 23.10(c)], and there can be histologic overlap with DIP. Both DIP and respiratory bronchiolitis-associated interstitial lung disease present in the fourth to fifth decade, show a male gender bias (male:female ratio of about 2:1), may occur with insidious onset of dyspnea and cough, and improve with cessation of smoking and steroid therapy.

Pulmonary amyloidosis can show diffuse deposition of **amyloid** in alveolar septa, a pattern typically associated with disseminated primary amyloidosis or multiple myeloma, or there may be nodular deposition of amyloid. Pulmonary symptoms are usually not severe. Morphologically, amyloid is hyaline and stains with Congo red stain [Fig. 23.11(a), (b)]. Amyloid shows apple-green birefringence when stained with Congo red and viewed through a polarized light source [Fig. 23.11(c)].

Cryptogenic organizing pneumonia (COP) is a nonspecific pattern of lung injury characterized by polypoid plugs of loose fibrous tissue. In contrast to the majority of diseases discussed in this chapter, in COP the fibrous tissue is not in the interstitium but rather within lumina of alveolar ducts, alveoli, and often bronchioles (Fig. 23.12). The distribution of lesions is typically more peripheral than distal. There are many etiologies of COP including infection (viral, bacterial), collagen vascular diseases, drug toxicity, toxic inhalants, and bronchial obstruction. Most patients show gradual improvement with steroid therapy.

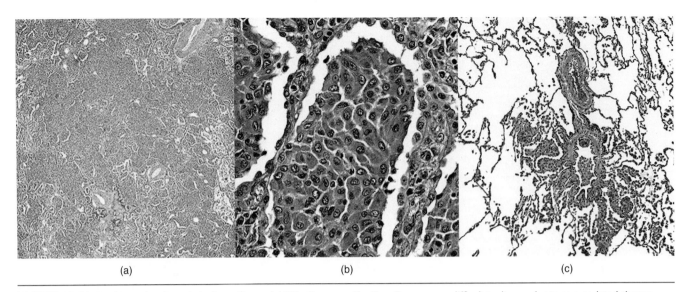

(a)   (b)   (c)

FIGURE 23.10 Smoking-related restrictive lung disease. (a) DIP at low magnification. Airspaces are difficult to discern due to accumulated clumps of intra-alveolar macrophages. (b) DIP at high magnification. Clumping of faintly pigmented intra-alveolar macrophages resembles the cohesion of epithelial cells. (c) In respiratory bronchiolitis, there is patchy distribution of macrophages in the bronchiolar lumen and adjacent airspaces. *From Travis et al. Atlas of Nontumor Pathology: Volume 2: Non-Neoplastic Disorders of the Lower Respiratory Tract, American Registry of Pathology; 2002.*

Pulmonary alveolar proteinosis (PAP) is a rare disease with bilateral, patchy, and asymmetric lung involvement manifesting as opacification on chest radiograph. PAP can be acquired (being most common with ~90% of cases), congenital, or secondary. Acquired PAP appears to result from an autoantibody that inhibits the activity of **GM-CSF**, thereby impairing macrophage clearance of pulmonary surfactant. Congenital PAP is genetically heterogeneous, with the genetic lesion unknown in most cases; alternatively, congenital PAP can arise in the setting of mutations in the genes for **ATP-binding cassette protein member A3 (ABCA3)**, surfactant protein B, GM-CSF, or the GM-CSF receptor β chain. Secondary PAP can arise in the setting of hematopoietic disease, malignancy, immunodeficiency, **lysinuric protein intolerance**, or acute silicosis (and other pneumoconioses, see below). Morphologically, whether acquired, congenital, or secondary, PAP is characterized by enlarged and abnormally heavy lungs which exude turbid fluid on sectioning. Microscopically (Fig. 23.13), there is intra-alveolar accumulation of dense, granular, eosinophilic material containing lipid and PAS-positive material. Clinically, PAP presents with insidious respiratory difficulty and a cough productive of abundant gelatinous chunks. With disease progression, dyspnea, cyanosis, and respiratory insufficiency can develop. Therapy for adult PAP involves lung lavage, and approximately one-half of adults benefit from recombinant GM-CSF therapy. Congenital PAP is fatal in 3-6 months without lung transplantation.

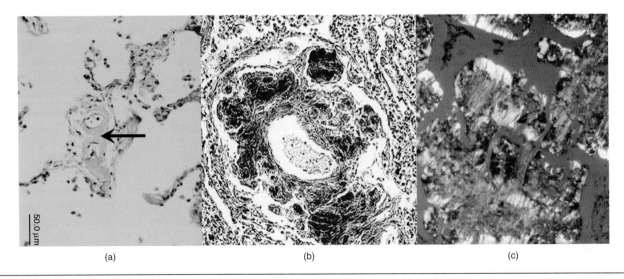

(a)   (b)   (c)

FIGURE 23.11 Pulmonary amyloidosis. (a) By routine H&E staining, amyloid appears as eosinophilic amorphous material, shown here (arrow) surrounding two blood vessels. (b) Amyloid stains deep red with Congo red stain. (c) When stained with Congo red stain and viewed with polarized light, amyloid shows "apple-green" birefringence. (b) and (c): *From Travis et al. Atlas of Nontumor Pathology: Volume 2: Non-Neoplastic Disorders of the Lower Respiratory Tract, American Registry of Pathology; 2002.*

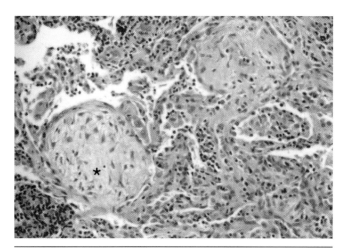

FIGURE 23.12 Cryptogenic organizing pneumonia. Fibrous plugs (*), representing organizing exudate, occlude the lumina of distal airways. *From Klatt.* Robbins & Cotran Atlas of Pathology, *2nd ed. 2010.*

Collagen vascular diseases can be complicated by pulmonary involvement. In **progressive systemic sclerosis (scleroderma)**, pulmonary injury is typified by diffuse interstitial fibrosis. In **systemic lupus erythematosus (SLE)**, pulmonary histopathology typically consists of patchy, transient parenchymal infiltrates. In **rheumatoid arthritis**, pulmonary involvement can manifest as chronic pleuritis (with or without a pleural effusion), diffuse interstitial pneumonitis and

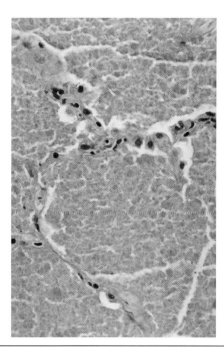

FIGURE 23.13 Pulmonary alveolar proteinosis. Alveolar septa are normal, but airspaces are filled with granular eosinophilic material. Pulmonary edema fluid (Chap. 26) is less granular than PAP material and typically does not contain PAS-positive debris that is present in PAP. *From Klatt.* Robbins & Cotran Atlas of Pathology, *2nd ed. 2010.*

fibrosis, pulmonary hypertension (Chap. 26), or intrapulmonary rheumatoid nodules. The presence of rheumatoid nodules in the setting of pneumoconiosis (see below) is known as **Caplan syndrome**.

Pneumoconioses

The term pneumoconiosis is broad and refers to non-neoplastic lung reactions to the inhalation of irritants to the lung. Nonetheless, many use this term to refer to such lung reactions to the inhalation of nonorganic mineral dusts. The development of pneumoconiosis depends on the amount of dust retained in the lung, particle solubility and physical/chemical reactivity, and the possible additive effects of other irritants such as cigarette smoke. The amount of dust retained in the lung following inhalation has much to do with particle size (Chap. 10). Particles <0.5 μm may remain suspended in inhaled air and are subsequently exhaled. Particles that are 1-5 μm in size are the most dangerous, as these are small enough to pass the vibrissae in the nose and mucociliary clearance action by the conducting portion of the respiratory tract to become deposited in small distal airspaces. Particles exceeding 10 μm are filtered by the vibrissae or are deposited in mucus of the conducting portion of the respiratory tract and cleared through ciliary action. Smaller particles have a greater surface area/volume ratio and so will show more rapid development of toxic levels in fluids. Some dust particles cause direct cell injury, while others can cross the epithelium to directly interact with septal fibroblasts and macrophages.

Coal worker's pneumoconiosis (CWP) can develop with inhalation of carbon dust. Low-level exposure to coal dust leads to **anthracosis**, an asymptomatic accumulation of carbon pigment with no significant cellular response. With moderate coal dust exposure, **simple CWP** can develop that shows little or no pulmonary dysfunction. With heavy exposure, however, simple CWP can progress to complicated CWP with respiratory insufficiency. Morphologically, anthracosis is characterized by accumulation of black pigment in alveolar macrophages, interstitial histiocytes [Fig. 23.14(a)], and lymph nodes, especially hilar. Simple CWP is characterized by 1-2 mm coal macules and larger coal nodules that have a delicate collagen network [Fig. 23.14(b)]. These are found predominantly in the upper lung lobes and the upper portions of lower lobes. The macules and nodules of simple CWP are typically adjacent to respiratory bronchioles. After many years of simple CWP, black scars >2 cm in greatest dimension herald the development of complicated CWP, that can be further complicated by **progressive massive fibrosis (PMF)** [Fig. 23.14(c)]. Microscopically, these black scars represent carbon pigment and dense collagen, often with a region of central necrosis. Most cases of simple CWP and mild complicated CWP show normal pulmonary function tests. In a minority of cases of complicated CWP, PMF leads to pulmonary dysfunction, pulmonary hypertension (Chap. 26), and cor pulmonale. Of note, once PMF has begun, it can progress despite cessation of coal dust exposure.

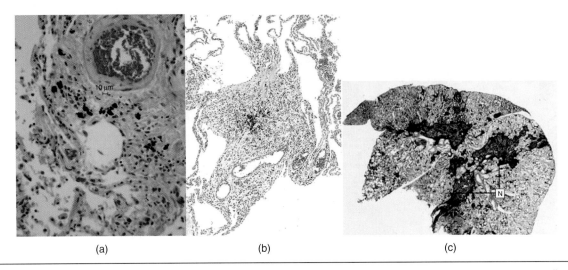

(a)   (b)   (c)

FIGURE 23.14   Carbon-related pulmonary disease. (a) In anthracosis, black pigment (carbon) accumulates in interstitial histiocytes as well as alveolar macrophages (not shown) and regional lymph nodes (not shown). (b) In simple CWP, carbon pigment in macrophages is associated with delicate fibrosis. (c) In complicated CWP, larger black scars, predominantly in the upper lung, are present and can lead to PMF as shown in this thin section of an entire lung (N = large coal nodules with PMF). (b) and (c): *From Stevens et al.* Core Pathology, *3rd ed. 2010.*

Silicosis, the most common chronic occupational disease in the world, is caused by inhalation of silicon dioxide (silica), which can be crystalline or amorphous. Crystalline silica is much more fibrogenic than amorphous silica and exists in the following forms: quartz (the most common), crystobalite, and tridymite. Silicosis manifests as slowly progressive nodular fibrosis developing after decades of exposure. Pathogenetically, the SiOH groups on particle surfaces bind to membrane proteins and phospholipids, leading to protein denaturation and lipid damage. Exposure of macrophages to silica can result in macrophage death or in macrophage activation with release of numerous signaling molecules including IL-1, TNF-α, fibronectin, lipid mediators, oxygen-derived free radicals, and fibrogenic cytokines. Similar to CWP, silicosis lesions localize in the upper lung zones; in contrast,

silicosis lesions are more fibrotic and less cellular than the lesions of CWP. Early in the development of silicosis, small, barely palpable, pale nodules appear in upper lung zones [Fig. 23.15(a)]. With progression, these nodules coalesce into hard, collagenous scars (silicotic nodules) [Fig. 23.15(b)] that can undergo cavitation. Microscopically, the silicotic nodule is composed of concentric layers of hyalinized collagen surrounded by a dense collagen capsule [Fig. 23.15(c)]. The intervening lung parenchyma can be compressed or overexpanded. Silicotic nodules can also develop in regional lymph nodes, where they typically undergo peripheral calcification, imparting an **eggshell appearance** radiographically. In some cases, silicosis evolves into PMF. Clinically, presentation is usually radiographic identification of fine upper lung nodularity in an asymptomatic worker, at which time pulmonary function tests

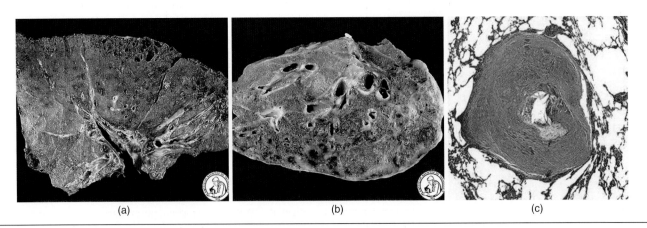

(a)   (b)   (c)

FIGURE 23.15   Silicosis. (a) In early silicosis, small pale nodules appear, predominantly in the upper lung. (b) As silicosis progresses, the nodules coalesce into silicotic nodules. (c) Histologically, silicotic nodules are composed of concentric layers of hyalinized collagen; the fibrotic nodules of silicosis are paucicellular. *From Travis et al.* Atlas of Nontumor Pathology: Volume 2: Non-Neoplastic Disorders of the Lower Respiratory Tract, *American Registry of Pathology; 2002.*

are usually normal or near normal. If complicated by PMF, there can be progression without additional silica exposure. The relationship of silicosis to the development of lung cancer in humans is controversial.

Asbestos represents a family of crystalline hydrated silicates that form fibers of two general forms: serpentine **chrysotile** fibers, which are curly and flexible, and **amphibole** fibers, which are straight, stiff, and brittle. Though less prevalent than chrysotile fibers, amphibole fibers are more pathogenic, likely due to aerodynamic properties that allow straight fibers to align in the airstream and be deposited more deeply in the lung. Amphibole fibers are less soluble than chrysotile fibers, and so chrysotile fibers are leeched from tissue more quickly. Asbestos shows activity as a tumor initiator and tumor promoter, in part due to adsorption of toxic chemicals. Asbestos causes or contributes to the development of many diseases, one of which—**asbestosis**—is characterized by restrictive lung disease with interstitial fibrosis.

Asbestosis begins with inhalation of asbestos fibers, which impact and penetrate tissue at the bifurcation of small airways and ducts. Subsequently, macrophages attempt to ingest and clear the fibers and release chemotactic and fibrogenic mediators. Chronic fiber deposition, causing persistent mediator release, culminates in interstitial fibrosis and interstitial inflammation [Fig. 23.16(a), (b)]. The fibrosis begins around respiratory bronchioles and alveolar ducts. Later fibrosis extends into adjacent alveolar sacs and alveoli, with progressive distortion of the architecture and eventual development of a honeycomb appearance typical of many end-stage chronic restrictive lung diseases. In addition to the interstitial changes, asbestosis is typified by fibrous thickening of the visceral pleura, often leading to adhesions to the parietal pleura with anchoring of the lung to the chest wall. In contrast

to CWP and silicosis, the pathologic findings in asbestosis are more prominent in the lower lung zones but may extend to the middle and upper zones. Microscopically, within the interstitial fibrosis will be **asbestos bodies**, which are golden brown and fusiform or beaded rods with a translucent core [Fig. 23.16(c)]. Asbestos bodies are composed of an asbestos fiber coated with iron-containing, proteinaceous material. Of note, other inorganic material may become coated with similar iron-containing material. When seen outside the setting of asbestos-related disease, such structures are called **ferruginous bodies**, a less specific designation. Clinically, the presentation of asbestosis is usually 10 to more than 20 years after initial exposure and is characterized by dyspnea and productive cough. Though asbestosis can remain static, it may progress and lead to congestive heart failure, cor pulmonale, and death.

In addition to asbestosis, asbestos exposure is implicated in the development of pleural plaques, pleural fibrosis, pleural effusion, bronchogenic carcinoma, malignant mesothelioma, and laryngeal and other extrapulmonary cancer. **Pleural plaques** (Fig. 23.17) are the most common asbestos-related lesion and consist of a well-circumscribed focus of dense collagen, often calcified, on the parietal pleura (usually posterolaterally and over the diaphragm). Such plaques are a morphologic indication of asbestos exposure but otherwise are clinically inconsequential. Asbestos exposure increases the risk of malignant mesothelioma ~1,000-fold and increases the risk of bronchogenic carcinoma fivefold in nonsmokers and 55-fold among smokers; mesothelioma and bronchogenic carcinoma are discussed further in Chap. 31.

Talcosis can result from inhalation of large amounts of talc, a magnesium silicate used widely in industry and cosmetics.

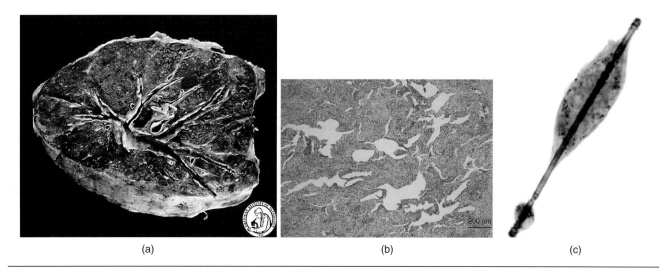

(a)   (b)   (c)

FIGURE 23.16 Asbestosis. (a) Grossly, asbestosis is characterized by interstitial fibrosis that is more pronounced peripherally and especially subpleurally; in contrast to CWP and silicosis, the pathologic findings in asbestosis are more predominant in lower lung zones. (b) Histologically, asbestosis is characterized by expansion of the interstitium by fibrosis. (c) Shown here are macrophages stained green (GMS stain) attempting to phagocytize an asbestos body. (a): *From Travis et al.* Atlas of Nontumor Pathology: Volume 2: Non-Neoplastic Disorders of the Lower Respiratory Tract, American Registry of Pathology; *2002.*

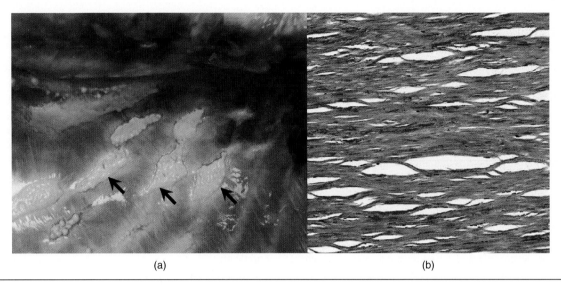

(a)   (b)

FIGURE 23.17 Pleural plaque. (a) Though clinically insignificant, parietal pleural plaques (arrows) indicate prior asbestos exposure. (b) Histologically, pleural plaques are composed of paucicellular fibrous connective tissue, often, as in this image, with a "basket weave" appearance. (a): *From Kemp et al.* Pathology: The Big Picture; 2008. (b): *From Travis et al.* Atlas of Nontumor Pathology: Volume 2: Non-Neoplastic Disorders of the Lower Respiratory Tract, American Registry of Pathology; *2002.*

Morphologically, talcosis is characterized by granulomatous inflammation, hyaline nodules, and interstitial fibrosis (rarely with PMF). Talc is highly birefringent when examined with polarized light.

Berylliosis is caused by exposure to airborne dusts or fumes of metallic beryllium (atomic number 4) or its oxides or salts, many of which are used in the electronics and aviation industries. Acutely, berylliosis is characterized by acute pneumonitis with DAD. Chronically, there is granulomatous inflammation and interstitial fibrosis. Heavy beryllium exposure is associated with bronchogenic carcinoma (Chap. 31).

Additional pneumoconioses include the **hard metal diseases** that are associated with tungsten carbide and cobalt exposure and characterized by giant cell interstitial pneumonitis. **Welder's pneumoconiosis** is most often associated with oxides of aluminum, iron, titanium, or manganese, and patients may show varying degrees of interstitial fibrosis depending on the specific metal oxide involved.

Suggested Readings

1. Travis WD, Colby TV, Koss MN, Rosado-de-Christenson ML, Müller NL, King TE. *Atlas of Nontumor Pathology: Volume 2: Non-Neoplastic Disorders of the Lower Respiratory Tract,* American Registry of Pathology; 2002. *For many years, the Armed Forces Institute of Pathology (AFIP) was responsible for the publication of numerous tumor atlases, frequently referred to as "The Fascicles." Later, the AFIP expanded its atlas publication to include non-neoplastic disease. This text offers well-organized and exceedingly well-illustrated discussions of pulmonary disease with a focus on morphology but with generous clinical and radiographic coverage. In accordance with the 2005 Defense Base Realignment and Closure (BRAC) law, the AFIP is on track to disestablish and permanently close by September 15, 2011.*

2. Katzenstein AL. *Katzenstein and Askin's Surgical Pathology of Non-Neoplastic Lung Disease*, 4th ed. Saunders; 2006. *Prior to the publication of the AFIP nontumor "fascicles," previous editions of this book served surgical pathologists as a sort of "gold standard" for the interpretation of non-neoplastic lung pathology.*

3. Kumar V, Abbas AK, Fausto N. *Robbins and Cotran Pathologic Basis of Disease*, 8th ed. Philadelphia, PA: Elsevier; 2007. *Throughout its many editions, this reference work is the most definitive and approachable compendium of pathology images available to students.*

CASE STUDIES AND PRACTICE PROBLEMS

CASE 23.1 The photograph of lung below (H&E) was obtained from a 60-year-old man with a 7-day history of fever, leukocytosis, systemic hypotension, and evolving multisystem organ failure. With the structure indicated by the arrow, which is the best diagnosis?

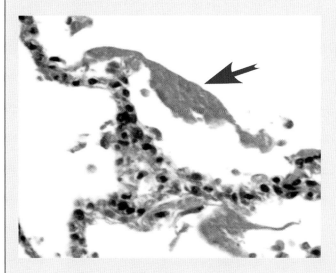

a. Diffuse alveolar damage
b. Hyaline membrane disease
c. Desquamative interstitial pneumonitis
d. Pulmonary alveolar proteinosis
e. *Pneumocystis jiroveci* infection

CASE 23.2 A 33-year-old woman has increasing dyspnea with cough for 10 days. Over the past 48 hours, her cough produced chunks of gelatinous sputum. Physical exam reveals no fever but extensive dullness to percussion over all lung fields. Chest x-ray shows diffuse opacification bilaterally. Biopsy yields the microscopic features shown at upper right (H&E stain); with electron microscopy there are many lamellar bodies. Antibodies directed against which of the following is most likely the cause of her illness?

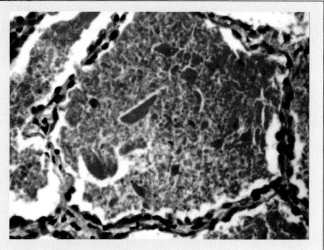

a. Surfactant protein B
b. GM-CSF
c. Pneumocyte epithelial factor 2
d. Surfactant protein C
e. α_3 chain of collagen IV

CASE 23.3 A 60-year-old man shows fine nodularity in the upper lung fields of a chest x-ray. From ages 20-50, he was a miner. Since then he has assisted his son-in-law in contracting work and now averages several hours per day installing insulation in houses. Repeated or chronic inhalation of which of the following substances is most likely to have caused the development of the lesion evident on lung biopsy and shown below (H&E stain)?

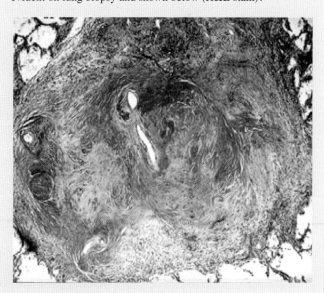

a. Tremolite
b. Crocidolite
c. Chrysotile fibers
d. Coal dust
e. Quartz

Solutions to Case Studies and Practice Problems

CASE 23.1   The most correct answer is a, diffuse alveolar damage.

The arrow is pointing to a hyaline membrane, which could be seen in diffuse alveolar damage (*answer a*) or hyaline membrane disease (*answer b*). Since hyaline membrane disease is a disease of neonates, the patient's age eliminates *answer b*; furthermore, the lung tissue in the image appears more mature than would be expected in a neonate. Desquamative interstitial pneumonitis (*answer c*) is characterized by aggregates of pigmented macrophages rather than the hyaline material shown. In pulmonary alveolar proteinosis (*answer d*), the intra-alveolar material is more granular than a hyaline membrane and typically fills the alveoli. *Pneumocystis jiroveci* infection is characterized by a foamy intra-alveolar exudate rather than the hyaline membrane shown here.

CASE 23.2   The most correct answer is b, GM-CSF.

The patient has pulmonary alveolar proteinosis (PAP), which, in the adult, is frequently caused by autoantibodies directed at GM-CSF. Mutations in surfactant protein B can underlie PAP in the neonate. Autoantibodies directed at the α3 chain of collagen IV are the cause of Goodpasture's syndrome. The name pneumocyte epithelial factor 2 has not been assigned to any known molecule.

CASE 23.3   The most correct answer is e, quartz.

The patient's history of mining puts him at risk for silicosis and, possibly, coal worker's pneumoconiosis, while his exposure to insulation represents a risk factor for asbestosis. Shown is a typical silicosis nodule. Quartz (*answer e*) is a form of silica. *Answers a*, *b*, and *c* are examples of asbestos, which do not typically show nodules of fibrosis but, rather, interstitial fibrosis that is most pronounced subpleurally. Coal dust exposure (*answer d*) could produce nodules of fibrosis, but the nodules would contain abundant black pigment.

Chapter 24

Management of Restrictive Lung Diseases

RAVI P. NAYAK, MD AND
GEORGE M. MATUSCHAK, MD

Learning Objectives

- The student will be able to describe the symptoms and signs of patients presenting with restrictive lung diseases.
- The student will be able to define the pathophysiological mechanisms of specific restrictive lung diseases.
- The student will be able to use clinical, physiological, and chest imaging data to differentiate patients with various forms of restrictive lung diseases.
- The student will be able to provide a stepwise approach to the diagnosis and treatment of patients with selective restrictive lung diseases.

Introduction ✓

Restrictive lung diseases comprise a heterogeneous group of >100 different respiratory disorders whose common denominator is a pathological reduction in lung volume. The reduced volume may result from diffuse inflammatory injury, as well as abnormal fibrotic proliferation and repair within alveolar walls and the lung's interstitial structures. Such disorders are collectively designated **interstitial lung diseases (ILDs)**. Many ILDs not only lead to thickening of alveolar walls and septal interstitium, but also of the lumina and walls of small airways (alveolar ducts, respiratory bronchioles, and terminal bronchioles) and the pulmonary capillary network. **Chest wall disorders** and certain **neuromuscular diseases** that adversely influence the mechanical efficiency of the muscles of respiration also culminate in pulmonary restriction, albeit without ILD-like pathophysiological features in the lung parenchyma. Regardless of the specific etiology of an ILD and its pathophysiological mechanisms, the presenting clinical manifestations usually include three hallmark features: (1) progressive dyspnea on exertion; (2) restrictive physiology on pulmonary function tests; and (3) **diffuse reticular infiltrates** or **ground-glass opacities** on chest radiographs or thoracic CT imaging studies.

Interstitial Lung Diseases

To facilitate a differential diagnosis of ILD, it is helpful to view the condition as associated with ten broad disease categories affecting the respiratory system (Table 24.1). These general categories will be considered in turn.

Idiopathic Interstitial Pneumonias

Idiopathic interstitial pneumonias are a group of lung disorders comprised of: **idiopathic pulmonary fibrosis (IPF)**; **nonspecific interstitial pneumonia (NSIP)**; **cryptogenic organizing pneumonia (COP)**; **acute interstitial pneumonia (AIP)** or **Hamman-Rich syndrome**; **respiratory bronchiolitis-interstitial lung disease (RB-ILD)**; **desquamative interstitial pneumonitis (DIP)**; and **lymphoid interstitial pneumonia (LIP)**. Each of these disorders has characteristic histopathological features which permit their presumptive distinction (Table 24.2; see Chap. 23).

Idiopathic pulmonary fibrosis (IPF) is the most important and common idiopathic interstitial pneumonia and, in many ways is a prototypic ILD and restrictive lung disease with respect to symptoms, physical findings, and laboratory features. IPF affects at least 200,000 persons in the United States, whose median survival is 3-5 years from diagnosis. The exact cause of IPF is not known. Interestingly, 0.5%-3.7% of cases of IPF are familial, and 60% of patients diagnosed with this disorder have a positive history of smoking. The incidence of IPF increases significantly in older adults, being most common between the ages of 50 and 70 years. High-resolution chest CT (HRCT) findings in IPF may be pathognomonic when demonstrating patchy, heterogeneous and subpleural, peripheral reticular opacities and septal thickening usually found in conjunction with honeycombing and traction bronchiectasis (Fig. 24.1). Histopathologically, IPF is a common although not exclusive idiopathic etiology for **usual interstitial pneumonia (UIP)**. Presenting symptoms in IPF include dyspnea on exertion in 90% of patients and nonproductive cough in >70% of subjects. Bibasilar inspiratory **Velcro-like crackles** predominate in 85% of IPF patients on physical examination whereas digital clubbing occurs in at least 25% (Chap. 14). Pulmonary function test abnormalities include restrictive ventilatory limitations characterized

Table **24.1** **General categories of interstitial lung diseases**

Idiopathic interstitial pneumonias	Sarcoidosis
Connective tissue diseases	Eosinophilic lung disorders
Hypersensitivity pneumonitis	Pulmonary vasculitides
Pneumoconioses	Alveolar hemorrhage syndromes
Drug-induced pulmonary disease	Miscellaneous disorders

by a normal or increased FEV_1/FVC ratio together with a TLC that is <80% of predicted or the lower limit of normal (LLN). Characteristically, the single breath DL_{CO} is reduced, and patients manifest mild to moderate arterial hypoxemia or decreasing S_aO_2 during exertion (Chaps. 16 and 17).

Predictors of reduced survival in IPF include coexisting emphysema and the presence of **pulmonary hypertension** as reflected by elevated P_{PA} estimated using transthoracic echocardiography or documented during right heart catheterization. Physiological predictors are reduced FVC, TLC, and DL_{CO} at the time of diagnosis and then further declines in FVC and DL_{CO} over the succeeding 6-12 months. Additionally, a significantly reduced distance during the **six-minute walk test** (**6-MWT**) and exertional decline in S_aO_2 correlate with increased mortality. Causes of death in IPF include coronary artery disease, lung cancer, infection, and pulmonary embolism.

Table **24.2** **Classification of idiopathic interstitial pneumonias**

Histological pattern	Clinical/Radiologic/ Pathologic Diagnosis
Usual interstitial pneumonia	Idiopathic pulmonary fibrosis
Nonspecific interstitial pneumonia	Nonspecific interstitial pneumonia
Organizing pneumonia	Cryptogenic organizing pneumonia
Diffuse alveolar damage	Acute interstitial pneumonia
Respiratory bronchiolitis	Respiratory bronchiolitis interstitial lung disease
Desquamative interstitial pneumonia	Desquamative interstitial pneumonia
Lymphoid interstitial pneumonia	Lymphoid interstitial pneumonia

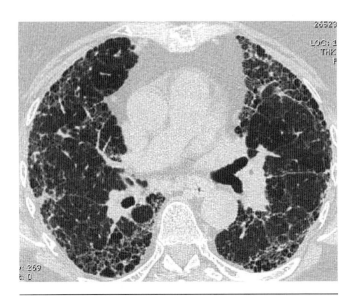

FIGURE 24.1 Representative chest CT scan in a patient with IPF showing increased coarse reticular markings, widespread septal thickening, and honeycombing especially notable in subpleural locations.

IPF is generally a chronic and relentlessly progressive disorder. However, **acute and frequently fatal exacerbations** can occur at any time and are increasingly recognized as a major cause of death during which rapid progression of disease occurs within 4 weeks. Such acute exacerbations of IPF are not related to the severity of underlying PFT abnormalities, and are often heralded by low-grade fever, flu-like symptoms, and worsening cough with dyspnea. Such findings occur in association with severe arterial hypoxemia and newly developing diffuse radiographic opacities that are superimposed on the baseline reticular pattern, often in the absence of infectious pneumonia, heart failure, pulmonary thromboembolism, or sepsis. Histopathologically, **diffuse alveolar damage (DAD)** is generally found in patients with a background of UIP. The rate of acute exacerbations ranges from 10% to 15% per year and the risk factors are unknown. These exacerbations carry a hospital mortality rate of 78%, and recurrence among survivors of another acute exacerbation is common and usually results in death.

Sarcoidosis

Sarcoidosis is a systemic disorder that is characterized by the formation of non-necrotizing, well-formed granulomas in multiple organ systems. With respect to the lungs, **T-helper cell (CD4⁺) lymphocyte-mediated inflammation** plays a key pathogenetic role. Sarcoidosis is a relatively common cause of ILD in young and middle-aged adults, but not all patients with sarcoidosis have pulmonary symptoms. Regardless, there is usually incidental radiographical evidence of lung and intrathoracic lymph node involvement, which is classically distinguished by four stages using standard chest x-rays (Table 24.3; Figs. 24.2 through 24.5).

Table **24.3** Chest radiographic stages of sarcoidosis

Stage	Intrathoracic Manifestations
I	Bilateral hilar adenopathy
II	Bilateral lymphadenopathy and reticulonodular infiltrates/opacities
III	Bilateral reticulonodular infiltrates/opacities
IV	Fibrocystic changes with bullae, upper lobe fibrotic scarring, and upward hilar retraction

▶▶CLINICAL CORRELATION 24.1

The clinical, laboratory, radiographic, and histopathological characteristics of sarcoidosis are closely simulated by **berylliosis (chronic beryllium disease)**, a chronic hypersensitivity response of the lungs to beryllium fumes or dust that results in granulomatous inflammation (Chap. 23). Lung specimens in berylliosis showing non-necrotizing (noncaseating) granulomas are indistinguishable from lungs of patients with sarcoidosis and occasionally, tuberculosis. The diagnosis requires lung biopsy and evidence of sensitivity to beryllium by **lymphocyte proliferation testing** of the patient's blood or bronchoalveolar lavage fluid. Occupations associated with beryllium exposures include scrap metal working, automotive or aircraft electronics, and some oil and gas industries.

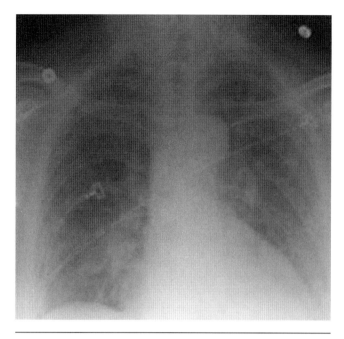

FIGURE 24.3 Stage II pulmonary sarcoidosis with chest x-ray showing bilateral hilar adenopathy in conjunction with bilateral lung interstitial infiltrates.

Connective Tissue Disorders

The radiographical and histopathological spectra of ILD associated with the connective tissue diseases **systemic lupus erythematosis (SLE)**, **polymyositis-dermatomyositis (PM-DM)**, **mixed connective tissue disease, rheumatoid arthritis (RA)**, **progressive systemic sclerosis (PSS**; either the diffuse form or CREST variant), **Sjögren's syndrome**, and **ankylosing**

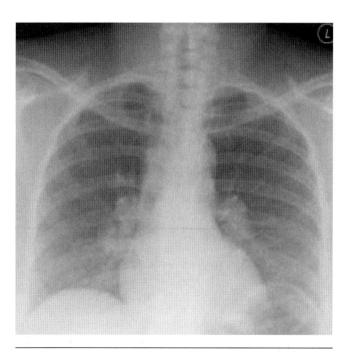

FIGURE 24.2 Stage I pulmonary sarcoidosis with chest x-ray demonstrating bilateral hilar adenopathy in the absence of lung parenchymal abnormalities.

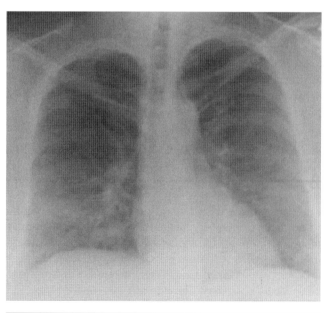

FIGURE 24.4 Stage III pulmonary sarcoidosis with chest x-ray exhibiting right basal interstitial infiltrates.

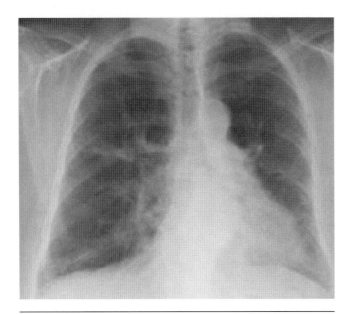

FIGURE 24.5 Stage IV pulmonary sarcoidosis with chest x-ray demonstrating chronic bilateral fibrotic changes.

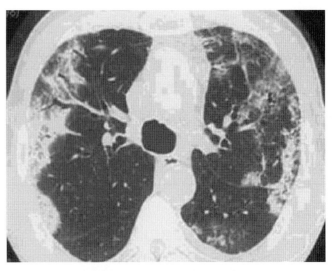

FIGURE 24.6 Chest CT scan image of the upper lung fields in a patient with chronic eosinophilic pneumonia demonstrating peripheral, bilateral subpleural interstitial infiltrates that are the reverse of the central perihilar shadows of pulmonary edema.

spondylitis encompass all of the patterns observed in the idiopathic interstitial pneumonias. Consequently, the clinical history, physical examination and results of specific laboratory serologic tests are especially important.

Generally speaking, development of ILD in patients with connective tissue diseases may precede rheumatological symptoms and signs; alternatively, pulmonary involvement may occur concomitantly with, or follow, the onset of rheumatic disease. **Nonspecific interstitial pneumonia** is the most common form of ILD found in the setting of connective tissue diseases, occurring in up to 80% of patients with PSS, Sjögren's syndrome, and PM-DM. However, a UIP-like pattern as also seen in IPF frequently predominates in RA. Although ILD secondary to connective tissue diseases is generally a chronic process, acute, rapidly progressive presentations of ILD may complicate the clinical picture, especially SLE and PM-DM. Such rapid-onset ILD, typified by acute SLE pneumonitis, may simulate infectious pneumonia and/or acute lung injury/acute respiratory distress syndrome.

Eosinophilic Lung Disorders

These chronic ILD disorders are characterized by a pathological influx of eosinophils into the pulmonary interstitium and distal airspaces and are exemplified by **acute eosinophilic pneumonia, Löffler's syndrome** and by **chronic eosinophilic pneumonia.** Löffler's syndrome, also termed **simple pulmonary eosinophilia**, is the commonest eosinophilic lung disorder. It frequently complicates **helminthic infection** or drug reactions and manifests clinically by cough, wheeze, and dyspnea with peripheral blood eosinophilia and transitory pulmonary infiltrates that resolve spontaneously and do not recur. In contrast, chronic eosinophilic pneumonia classically occurs in middle-aged female asthmatic patients, usually in conjunction

with fever, blood eosinophilia, and interstitial pulmonary infiltrates. In at least 25% of patients with chronic eosinophilic pneumonia, pulmonary infiltrates occur in a pattern that is the reversal of shadows typically seen in pulmonary edema. Here the infiltrates occur in the peripheral and subpleural locations of the lungs, with relative sparing of the central and perihilar areas, where pulmonary edema from other causes is usually first manifest (Fig. 24.6).

Hypersensitivity Pneumonitis

ILD from chronic hypersensitivity pneumonitis, also known as **extrinsic allergic alveolitis**, is a granulomatous process that results from repeated inhalation and sensitization to a large number of diverse organic antigens including, for example, those related to specific bacteria as typified by farmer's lung, mushroom worker's lung, and bagassosis involving moldy sugar cane in which thermophilic bacteria play a role, or animal proteins from feathers or avian droppings as in bird breeder's disease. This ILD can also result from inhalation and sensitization to low molecular weight chemical antigens such as isothiocyanates in industrial workers. The development of chronic hypersensitivity pneumonitis may be occult and slowly progresses over time with continuing inhalational exposures until symptoms occur, or may follow episodes of acute hypersensitivity pneumonitis which typically occur 4-12 hours after exposures.

Pulmonary Vasculitides

Systemic disorders of immune regulation characterized by necrotizing vasculitis may involve the lungs to result in ILD and restrictive pulmonary dysfunction. Examples of such disorders include necrotizing granulomatous vasculitis (**Wegener's granulomatosis**) and microscopic polyangiitis. Notably, patients with these disorders may have more than one cause of ILD,

Table **24.4** Clinical features of (#79)
selected pneumoconioses

Inorganic Dust	Clinical Features
Asbestos	Lower lobe interstitial infiltrates
	Pleural, pericardial calcification
Silica	Nodular coalescing infiltrates mid-upper lungs
	Increased susceptibility to tuberculosis
Coal dust	Small rounded opacities
	May develop into progressive massive fibrosis
Beryllium	Interstitial infiltrates & intrathoracic adenopathy
	Similarity to sarcoidosis
Hard metal dusts (eg, cobalt, tungsten)	Lower lobe interstitial infiltrates
	Multinucleated giant cells on histopathology

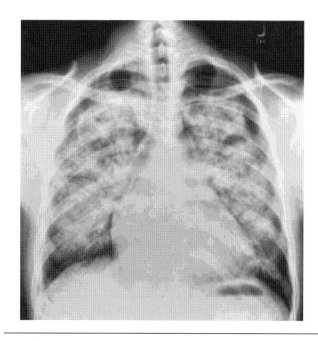

FIGURE 24.7 Diffuse alveolar hemorrhage with bilateral pulmonary infiltrates in a patient with rheumatic heart disease. *From Woolley K, Stark P:* Pulmonary parenchymal manifestations of mitral valve disease, Radiographics Jul-Aug;*19(4)965-972, 1999.*

since the clinical course may include episodes of diffuse alveolar hemorrhage and pulmonary drug toxicity.

Pneumoconioses

Occupational and environmental inhalational exposures to inorganic dusts are the primary causes of pneumoconiosis manifesting as ILD (Table 24.4), the majority of which occur in men. An important concept is that ILD from pneumoconiosis may have a **prolonged latency interval**, which in the case of asbestosis may be 15-20 years following initial exposure.

Alveolar Hemorrhage Syndromes

Diffuse alveolar hemorrhage (DAH) associated with either alveolar inflammatory **capillaritis** or bland DAH simulates ILD by causing dyspnea and radiographically by producing interstitial infiltrates and/or increased ground glass opacities on chest CT scans. DAH is a common interstitial process in SLE as well as in other "pulmonary-renal syndromes" such as mixed connective tissue disease, **Goodpasture's syndrome**, and pulmonary vasculitides including microscopic angiitis (Fig. 24.7). DAH may occur with minimal or absent hemoptysis in as many as one-third of patients, since the bleeding may remain localized to the respiratory (alveolar) zone of the lungs. The diagnosis of DAH is supported by **progressively greater bloody recovery** of sequentially instilled bronchoalveolar lavage fluid during fiberoptic bronchoscopy (Chap. 18).

Drug-Induced Pulmonary Disease

Drug-induced pulmonary disease covers a broad spectrum of reactions of the lungs that includes parenchymal scarring culminating in ILD. Adverse pulmonary reactions may occur: to **chemotherapeutic agents** (bleomycin, busulfan, cyclophosphamide, etc);

to **antibiotics** such as nitrofurantoin; to **anti-inflammatory agents** including gold, penicillamine, and methotrexate; and to other agents. Apart from a history of receiving one of these or other agents, there are no unique clinical findings, radiographic features, or physiological abnormalities to distinguish drug-induced ILD from other categories of ILD. Consequently, careful attention must be given to all current and previous drugs the patient with ILD has received in order to make a timely diagnosis.

▶▶ CLINICAL CORRELATION 24.2

Among drugs associated with diffuse ILD, the anti-arrhythmic **amiodarone** is important given its frequency of clinical use, very long mean elimination half-life (58 days), and lack of significant metabolism by liver or kidneys. Based on the daily dose, up to 4%-6% of patients receiving amiodarone may develop pulmonary toxicity in the form of interstitial pneumonitis that progresses to pulmonary fibrosis. Chief symptoms are insidious onset of nonproductive cough, progressive dyspnea on exertion, and low-grade fever; physical exam reveals inspiratory crackles. Radiological findings include initial asymmetric or unilateral interstitial or alveolar infiltrates; these progress to diffusely involve the lungs. Characteristically, a bronchoalveolar lavage or lung biopsy reveals **foamy, phospholipid-laden macrophages**, but such findings indicate only exposure to the drug and not toxicity. Treatment consists of drug withdrawal and in selected instances, administration of corticosteroids. Despite these therapeutic maneuvers, fatal outcomes remain common.

Miscellaneous

Lymphangioleiomyomatosis (LAM) is a rare form of ILD caused by abnormal smooth muscle proliferation involving the alveolar septae, bronchioles, and lymphatic vessels that occurs sporadically in females of child-bearing age. Of note, despite the apparent ILD, LAM results in small airways obstruction and thus, an obstructive pattern on pulmonary function tests rather than the anticipated restrictive pattern. A characteristic radiographic feature is the combination of bilateral interstitial opacities and generalized pulmonary cyst formation.

Pulmonary Langerhans' cell histiocytosis (granulomatosis) is a rare disorder accounting for <5% of ILD cases and characterized by interstitial pulmonary fibrosis or extensive cyst formation that is usually seen in smokers. Chest x-rays typically show diffuse reticular markings, reticulonodular infiltrates, and/or cysts representing dilated bronchi or bronchioles; there is a predilection for middle and upper lung zones. **Pneumothoraces** develop frequently. In later stages of the disease, the fibrosis can be extensive.

Pulmonary alveolar proteinosis (PAP) is an unusual ILD in which there is increased secretion and/or abnormal processing by alveolar macrophages of surfactant-derived phospholipids which accumulate in alveolar spaces and stain positive by the **periodic acid-Schiff (PAS)** reagent. Deficiency or inactivation of **GM-CSF** plays a causal role in autoimmune forms of the disease. PAP is not a specific disease but rather a syndrome depending on whether an underlying disease associated with **surfactant dysfunction** is present. Radiographically, PAP shows **geographic regional variation** in its interstitial involvement, with map-like alternations of increased and decreased tissue density (Fig. 24.8).

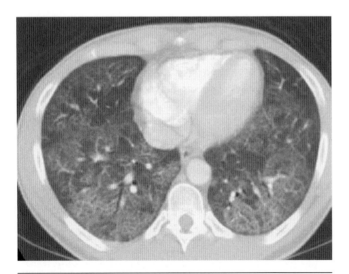

FIGURE 24.8 Chest CT scan of a patient with pulmonary alveolar proteinosis demonstrating areas of increased ground glass attenuation alternating in a geographically regional manner with areas of normal (darker) lung density.

Clinical Features

Regardless of etiology, patients with restrictive lung disease present with progressive dyspnea on exertion and nonproductive cough. Dyspnea in ILD results from restrictive lung impairment with **decreased lung compliance** secondary to interstitial fibrosis, along with increased inspiratory muscle work and O_2 consumption during breathing, particularly during exertion. Constitutional symptoms such as low-grade fever and malaise may also be present at the onset of disease.

The classic finding on physical exam in most forms of ILD is **bibasilar inspiratory crackles** and may be present in a symptomatic patient with even an apparently normal chest radiograph. Clubbing of the digits usually indicates advanced fibrotic lung disease and is present in 25%-50% of patients with ILD at initial presentation. An important exception however is drug-induced ILD, in which clubbing is generally not observed. In known cases of ILD, the new onset of clubbing may indicate the concomitant development of lung cancer. Cyanosis accompanying severe hypoxemia may occur in advanced restrictive lung disease. Because of chronic arterial hypoxemia, patients with restrictive lung disorders are at risk for development of **pulmonary hypertension** and resultant right ventricular hypertrophy.

Diagnostic Approach

Medical History

Considering the impact of environmental inhalational exposures, pneumoconioses, and drug-induced pulmonary reactions in the pathogenesis of restrictive lung diseases, a comprehensive medical history with a special focus on the patient's environmental and occupational history is important. So too is an evaluation of all the patient's current medications and their duration of use. Likewise, determining the tempo of progression of respiratory symptoms is helpful with respect to differential diagnostic considerations. For example, alveolar hemorrhage syndromes are likely to present in an acute manner, whereas IPF or sarcoidosis typically evolve more chronically.

Laboratory Tests

By themselves, laboratory tests are of limited utility in establishing a diagnosis of ILD. Results must be integrated with clinical findings, thoracic imaging studies, and histopathological results when available. Nonetheless, focused testing can be useful in narrowing the differential diagnosis in the appropriate setting. For example, **peripheral blood eosinophilia** may be an important clue to the presence of an underlying eosinophilic lung disorder or drug-induced pulmonary reaction. Serological blood testing for specific connective tissue disorders such as **rheumatoid arthritis** and **SLE** is similarly helpful, whereas **anti-neutrophil cystoplasmic antibody (ANCA)** studies to diagnose **Wegener's granulomatosis** and **microscopic polyangiitis**, respectively, and **anti-glomerular basement membrane antibody** determination to diagnose

Goodpasture's syndrome assist in pinpointing the cause of alveolar hemorrhage syndromes.

Pulmonary Function Tests

The classic findings of ILD are a restrictive ventilatory pattern and a decrease in the DL_{CO} (Chap. 16). This restrictive ventilatory limitation is characterized by a dual reduction in the FEV_1 and FVC with a correspondingly normal or elevated FEV_1/FVC ratio. In this setting, a total lung capacity (TLC) finding ≤80% of predicted values confirms the diagnosis of restrictive lung disease. Whereas the presence of ILD is consistent with a reduction in both the TLC and the DL_{CO}, chest wall and neuromuscular disorders are generally associated with a reduced TLC but a normal DL_{CO}.

Arterial blood gases and specifically the P_aO_2 or S_aO_2 may be normal at rest in patients with ILD. However, respiratory alkalosis with hypocapnia and mild-to-moderate arterial hypoxemia and widening of the (A − a) Po_2 gradient develop with progressive disease. In patients who have normal gas exchange at rest, cardiopulmonary exercise tests are especially useful in unmasking gas exchange abnormalities, principally exertional O_2 deoxygenation by oximetry. Exercise physiology studies may further reveal an elevation in the V_D/V_T, a widened (A − a) Po_2 gradient, and arterial hypoxemia in conjunction with progressive tachypnea.

Radiological Studies

One of the main features of ILD is an abnormal chest radiograph showing reticular, nodular, or reticulonodular opacities. Notably, the differential diagnosis should include ILD when individuals with dyspnea, cough, and an abnormal chest radiograph who are suspected of having infectious pneumonia do not respond to empiric antimicrobial therapy. However, the standard chest radiograph may appear normal in up to 10% of patients with symptomatic ILD. Thus HRCT is the imaging modality of choice in patients with suspected ILD, since it will reveal abnormalities in all patients with symptomatic ILD. These would include reticular opacities as well as honeycombing consistent with pulmonary fibrosis, and architectural distortion with **traction bronchiectasis**.

▶▶**CLINICAL CORRELATION 24.3**

The geographic regional distribution and type of radiographic abnormalities on chest imaging studies yield useful clues for diagnosis of specific forms of ILD. Thus, predominant abnormal radiographical involvement of the mid-upper lung zones should raise the possibility of sarcoidosis, pulmonary Langerhans' cell histiocytosis, silicosis, and hypersensitivity pneumonitis. In contrast, IPF usually presents with pleural-based reticular infiltrates in the lung bases. **Intrathoracic lymphadenopathy** is frequently encountered in patients with sarcoidosis,

lymphangitic spread of lung cancer, lymphocytic interstitial pneumonia, berylliosis, and amyloidosis. **Spontaneous pneumothorax** associated with a cystic ILD suggests underlying LAM (Fig. 24.9) and pulmonary Langerhans' cell histiocytosis (Fig. 24.10).

Fiberoptic Bronchoscopy

Fiberoptic bronchoscopy with BAL is useful in the diagnostic evaluation of several forms of restrictive lung diseases, most notably to confirm diffuse alveolar hemorrhage syndromes and eosinophilic pneumonia. It also is valuable in excluding pulmonary infections associated with diffuse infiltrates such as *Pneumocystis jiroveci* **pneumonia**. Bronchoscopy with transbronchial lung biopsy is also simpler and safer than surgical lung biopsy in selected patients suspected of having infections, and for granulomatous disorders such as sarcoidosis and berylliosis, and lymphangitic spread of lung cancer (Chap. 18). In contrast, **transbronchial lung biopsy** is not useful in establishing a diagnosis or discriminating among different types of idiopathic interstitial pneumonia, including IPF, because of the technique's limitations of lung sample size.

Surgical Lung Biopsy

Surgical lung biopsy is a key diagnostic modality in patients with ILD and is the procedure of choice in establishing a diagnosis in patients with ILD secondary to suspected idiopathic interstitial pneumonia. The location of the surgical lung biopsy is guided by the distribution of disease on HRCT images. The larger lung specimens afforded by this technique are ideally obtained for pathological analysis from a region that is radiographically normal, as well as from an area with

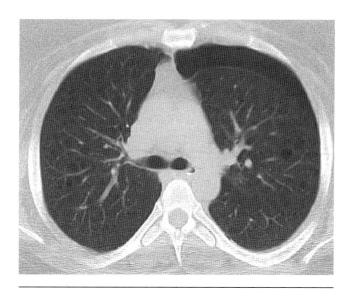

FIGURE 24.9 Chest CT scan in a patient with lymphangioleiomyomatosis demonstrating multiple parenchymal lung cysts and a left pneumothorax.

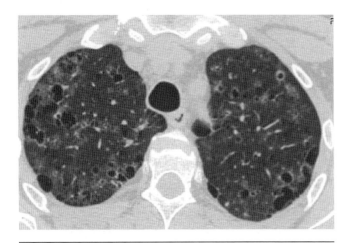

FIGURE 24.10 Chest CT scan of a patient with pulmonary Langerhans' cell histiocytosis demonstrating the combination of upper lung zone parenchymal lung cysts and nodular interstitial opacities.

mild-to-moderate disease. **Video-assisted thoracoscopic surgery** (**VATS**) biopsy causes less morbidity than open thoracotomy and is better tolerated (Chap. 18). In certain instances of idiopathic interstitial pneumonia suspected of being IPF, a confident clinical diagnosis may be made without subjecting the patient to surgical lung biopsy, when both clinical findings and the HRCT features are supportive (Table 24.5). All major criteria and at least three minor criteria must be present to increase the likelihood of a correct IPF diagnosis.

Treatment

Considering the diversity of restrictive lung diseases, treatment depends on the cause. For most restrictive disorders, mechanism-specific therapy is not available. With respect to the idiopathic interstitial pneumonias and IPF in particular,

Table **24.5** **Diagnostic criteria for IPF in the absence of a surgical lung biopsy**

Major Criteria	Minor Criteria
Exclusion of other known causes of ILD	Age >50 years
PFT results showing restriction and impaired gas exchange	Onset of otherwise unexplained dyspnea on exertion
Bibasilar reticular abnormalities with minimal ground glass opacities on HRCT scan	Duration of illness >3 months
Transbronchial lung biopsy or BAL do not support alternative diagnosis	Bibasilar inspiratory Velcro-like crackles

there is insufficient evidence-based support for any specific treatment to improve survival or the quality of life. Selected patients with IPF of mild-to-moderate severity receive combination therapy with corticosteroids, immunosuppressive drugs typified by **azathioprine**, and **N-acetylcysteine**. However, this approach is based on expert opinion rather than clinical trials. Since pharmacological therapy may be toxic, potential benefits may be outweighed by increased risk of treatment-related complications. This is especially likely to occur in patients >70 years of age, subjects with morbid obesity, or those having comorbidities such as cardiac disease, diabetes mellitus, osteoporosis, and end-stage honeycomb fibrotic changes that are unlikely to be reversed by any drug treatment.

It is best to enroll patients with IPF in ongoing clinical studies so that beneficial pharmacological therapy will be developed. Patients with IPF should be encouraged to enroll in a **pulmonary rehabilitation** program to avoid deconditioning. Severe hypoxemia ($P_{a}O_{2}$ <55 mm Hg at rest or during exercise) is managed by providing supplemental O_2 therapy. **Antitussive agents** assist in controlling cough and avoiding complications such as rib fractures in the elderly.

Concerning other idiopathic interstitial pneumonias, the cellular form of NSIP has an excellent prognosis compared to the fibrotic subtype NSIP. In contrast to IPF, the response to steroids in cellular NSIP is good with an overall 5-year survival >80%. In the smoking-related idiopathic interstitial pneumonias (RB-ILD and DIP), the prognosis is generally good although complete recovery requires smoking cessation. Acute interstitial pneumonia has a high mortality rate, but remission is possible with high-dose corticosteroids; however, supportive data are limited. Cryptogenic organizing pneumonia (COP) shows excellent response to corticosteroid therapy.

Anti-inflammatory corticosteroid therapy occasionally combined with immunosuppressive therapy is similarly utilized in other forms of ILD with varying results, including sarcoidosis, connective tissue diseases, eosinophilic lung disorders, hypersensitivity pneumonitis, pulmonary vasculitides, alveolar hemorrhage syndromes, and drug-induced pulmonary disease. In sarcoidosis, therapy with the corticosteroid **prednisone** depends on a firm diagnosis of the disease with supportive clinical features, chest radiographic evidence, and noncaseating granulomas on lung biopsy with all other causes of granulomas ruled out. Initial treatment for pulmonary sarcoidosis with 20-40 mg of prednisone per day is generally begun for dyspnea, cough, and wheezing in conjunction with reductions in the FEV_1 and FVC <70% of predicted values. Steroid-sparing agents including **hydroxychloroquine**, **methotrexate**, and **tumor necrosis factor-α antagonists** such as infliximab are also utilized in selected instances depending on disease severity and pattern of organ involvement. Pharmacological therapy is not employed in patients with pneumoconiosis.

Lung Transplantation

Transplantation is considered for patients with ILD exhibiting progressive physiological deterioration who meet established criteria. Current criteria for referral of patients for single lung transplantation are age <70 years, histological or radiographic evidence of UIP, and any of the following: DL_{CO} <39% pre-

dicted, 10% or greater decrement in the FVC during 6 months of follow-up, a decrease in pulse oximetry to <88% during a 6-MWT, and honeycombing on HRCT scan.

Suggested Readings

1. American Thoracic Society/European Respiratory Society. International multidisciplinary consensus classification of the idiopathic interstitial pneumonias. *Am J Respir Crit Care Med.* 2002;165:277. *This consensus statement provides an integrated clinical, radiologic, and pathologic approach to classification of the clinicopathological entities within the Idiopathic Interstitial Pneumonia group that has a bearing on clinical course and prognosis.*

2. American Thoracic Society. Idiopathic pulmonary fibrosis: diagnosis and treatment; International consensus statement. *Am J Respir Crit Care Med.* 2000;161:646. *This consensus statement provides guidance to clinicians in the diagnosis and management of IPF.*

3. Ley B, Collard HR, King Jr TE. Clinical course and prediction of survival in idiopathic pulmonary fibrosis. *Am J Respir Crit Care Med.* Oct 8; 2010 (published ahead of print). *This concise clinical review deals with current data on the clinical course, individual predictors of survival, and proposed clinical prediction models in IPF. It also discusses the challenges and future directions related to predicting survival in IPF.*

4. Iannuzzi MC, Rybicki BA, Teirstein AS. Sarcoidosis. *New Engl J Med.* 2007;357:2153-2165. *This outstanding review article summarizes recent advances and addresses pitfalls in the diagnosis and treatment of sarcoidosis.*

CASE STUDIES AND PRACTICE PROBLEMS

CASE 24.1 A 55-year-old black woman presents with fatigue, nonproductive cough, and dyspnea when walking two blocks on level ground or climbing twelve steps for the past three months. She has mild pain but no swelling in the small joints of her hands. She has no history of fever, night sweats, or chest pain, has never smoked, and has worked many years as a front desk secretary in a physician's office. She has no pets at home and is not taking any medications. A new chest x-ray and CT scan show upper lobe predominant ground-glass opacities, and bilateral hilar and subcarinal lymphadenopathy. PFTs today show TLC = 70% predicted, and DL_{CO} = 65% predicted. What is the best test to confirm the diagnosis?

a. Bronchoscopy with transbronchial lung biopsy
b. Lymphocyte proliferation testing of her blood or bronchoalveolar lavage fluid
c. Peripheral blood or bronchoalveolar lavage eosinophilic count
d. Serological studies for connective tissue disease
e. Video-assisted thoracoscopic surgery (VATS) biopsy

CASE 24.2 A 48-year-old white man with a history of severe depression presents with shortness of breath and nonproductive cough of 1-year duration. He has smoked two packs of cigarettes daily since 16 years old, but has no significant occupational exposures. He denies joint pains, skin rashes, fever, loss of weight or appetite, or chest pain. Physical exam reveals bilateral basilar crackles. A chest CT scan shows diffuse ground-glass appearance in middle and lower lung zones with reticular infiltrates in the bases. A previous chest x-ray from 2 years ago revealed mild reticular markings at the bases of the lungs. Pulmonary function tests indicate FVC = 69%, FEV_1 = 68%, FEV_1/FVC = 84%, TLC = 65%, and DL_{CO} = 64%, all of predicted. Bronchoscopy with bronchoalveolar lavage is unremarkable. Which of the following is most likely to improve this patient's disease?

a. Corticosteroids
b. Cytotoxic therapy with cyclophosphamide
c. Lung transplantation
d. Pulmonary rehabilitation
e. Smoking cessation

Solutions to Case Studies and Practice Problems

CASE 24.1 The most correct answer is a, bronchoscopy with transbronchial lung biopsy.

The patient presents with classic clinical features of sarcoidosis, including fatigue and joint pains. The adjusted annual incidence among black Americans is roughly three times that among white Americans. The patient has radiological Stage III pulmonary sarcoidosis, and restrictive ventilatory limitation with impairment of the DL_{CO}. Unlike idiopathic interstitial pneumonias, bronchoscopy

with transbronchial biopsy confirms the presence of non-necrotizing granulomatous inflammation. In most cases, VATS is not warranted. Her overall clinical presentation and radiological features are not suggestive of eosinophilic lung diseases; hence, the eosinophilic count is not helpful in arriving at a diagnosis. Although the patient has mild joint pain or arthralgia, she does not have any joint swelling or other evidence of a connective tissue disease.

CASE 24.2 The most correct answer is e, smoking cessation.

The patient has smoking-related interstitial lung disease. There is nothing in the history to suggest that he is immunocompromised, and there is no other organ involvement to suggest the presence of connective tissue disuse. His normal bronchoalveolar lavage reduces the likelihood of an infectious etiology, and it also excludes diffuse alveolar hemorrhage and eosinophilic lung diseases. The patient appears to have chronic ILD based on the radiological features, while his younger age and the ground-glass appearance on CT scan are not consistent with IPF but are rather suggestive of either desquamative interstitial pneumonia or respiratory bronchiolitis interstitial lung disease. These two diseases are similar clinically, and both have a good prognosis with smoking cessation.

Chapter 25

Management of Sleep-Related Breathing Disorders

JOSEPH R. D. ESPIRITU, MD AND
GEORGE M. MATUSCHAK, MD

Learning Objectives

- The student will be able to use clinical and polysomnographic data to differentiate patients showing obstructive sleep apnea, central sleep apnea, complex sleep apnea, and sleep-related hypoventilation/hypoxemic syndromes.

- The student will be able to describe the pathophysiological mechanisms underlying each of these classes of sleep-related breathing disorders.

- The student will be able to summarize the most effective therapies for each type of sleep-related breathing disorder.

Obstructive Sleep Apnea Syndromes

#81

Introduction

The three major types of sleep-related breathing disorders are **obstructive sleep apnea syndrome** (OSAS), **central sleep apnea syndrome**, and **sleep-related hypoventilation hypoxemic syndromes**. Of these, OSAS is the most common type of sleep-related breathing disorder and is characterized by repetitive episodes of complete **apnea** or partial **hypopnea** caused by upper airway obstruction. Episodes last at least 10 seconds, occur during sleep, are usually associated with decreased $S_{a_{O_2}}\%$, and are terminated by brief arousals. OSAS is associated not only with neurocognitive dysfunction but also with increased cardiovascular morbidity and mortality.

Epidemiology of OSAS

OSAS is relatively common, with a prevalence of 4% in men and 2% in women when defined by an **apnea-hypopnea index (AHI)** ≥5 events/h plus a complaint of excessive daytime sleepiness. Features predisposing to OSAS include male sex, age, obesity, menopausal state, race, craniofacial abnormalities with decreased orohypopharyngeal space, endocrine disorders, and certain congenital disorders (Table 25.1).

The high male-to-female prevalence ratio for OSAS of 2:1 is attributed to the protective effect of female sex hormones predominant in premenopausal women; the prevalence of OSAS in women triples after menopause and is reduced to premenopausal levels with hormone replacement therapy. Meanwhile, increased **body mass index (BMI)** is the major risk factor for OSAS in adults (Chap. 12). There appears to be a linear relationship between BMI and OSAS severity: Each 10% increase in body weight results in a 30% increase in AHI. On the other hand, adenotonsillar hypertrophy is the major cause of OSAS in children. For patients who are not overweight or obese, certain craniofacial features (eg,

retrognathia, long uvula) can predispose to OSAS. Increased nasal resistance from rhinitis or a deviated nasal septum can worsen airway collapse due to the greater inspiratory effort required to breathe through such nasal passages. Asians may be at a higher risk for OSAS due to crowding of the posterior oropharynx and a steep thyromental plane. Smoking causes nasal and oropharyngeal mucosal edema that can aggravate upper airway obstruction. Hormonal abnormalities may alter craniofacial skeletal and soft tissue structure, thereby promoting oropharyngeal crowding, as seen in the macroglossia of **hypothyroidism** and **acromegaly**. Up to 50% of patients with **Down syndrome** suffer from OSAS due to multiple risk factors. These can include midfacial and mandibular hypoplasia, small upper airways with superficially positioned tonsils and relative tonsillar and adenoidal encroachment, generalized hypotonia, and an increased prevalence of obesity and hypothyroidism.

Pathophysiology of OSAS ✓ #82

OSAS occurs due to dynamic upper airway closure or narrowing. These may be secondary to excessive pharyngeal tissue volume from obesity, adenotonsillar hypertrophy, craniofacial anatomy, and can accompany attenuated tone of the pharyngeal dilating muscles during sleep (Fig. 25.1).

Adverse Health Effects of OSAS

Left untreated, OSAS is associated with neurocognitive impairment, cardiovascular dysfunction, endocrine abnormalities, and mortality (Table 25.2). In prospective cohort studies, moderate-to-severe OSAS has been associated with an increased incidence in systemic hypertension and diabetes mellitus, as

Table **25.3** **Diagnostic criteria for obstructive sleep apnea in adults**[a]

The combination of either (A + B + D) or of (C + D) satisfies the criteria for OSA
A. *At least one of the following applies:*   1. Patient complains of unintentional sleep episodes, daytime sleepiness, unrefreshing sleep, fatigue, or insomnia.   2. Patient awakens with breath-holding, gasping, or choking.   3. Bed partner reports loud snoring, interrupted breathing, or both as patient sleeps.
B. *Polysomnography recording shows the following:*   1. ≥5 scoreable respiratory events (apneas, hypopneas, or RERAs) per hour of sleep.   2. Evidence of respiratory effort during all, or a portion of each, respiratory event. In the case of RERAs, this is best revealed with the use of esophageal manometry.
C. *Polysomnography recording shows the following:*   1. ≥15 scoreable respiratory events (apneas, hypopneas, RERAs) per hour of sleep.   2. Evidence of respiratory effort during all, or a portion of each, respiratory event. In the case of RERAs, this is best revealed with the use of esophageal manometry.
D. *The disorder is not better explained by another current sleep disorder, medical or neurological disorder, medication use, or substance abuse disorder.*

[a]*Data From* The International Classification of Sleep Disorders, *2nd ed.*

Oral appliances have been demonstrated to moderately decrease the AHI in patients with mild-to-moderate OSA and, to a lesser extent, their systemic blood pressure if they are hypertensive.

Tonsillectomy and **adenoidectomy** is the treatment of choice for children with OSAS and adenotonsillar hypertrophy (Clinical Correlation 25.1). **Uvulopalatopharyngoplasty** (UPPP) is the most commonly performed surgical procedure for adult patients with OSAS, and involves the surgical removal of the tonsils and redundant soft palate and tonsillar pillars. UPPP has been found to have an overall success rate of 40% when defined as reducing the severity of patients' OSA by at least 50%. Other surgical procedures for OSAS may help correct specific anatomic abnormalities responsible for causing upper airway obstruction (Table 25.6).

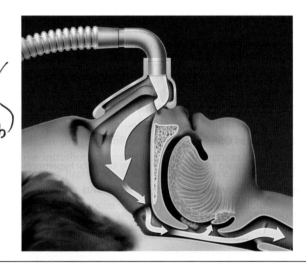

FIGURE 25.3 Continuous positive airway pressure (CPAP) therapy for obstructive sleep apnea.

Table **25.4** **Definitions of scoreable respiratory events in adults**

Respiratory disturbance index (RDI)[1] = mean number of episodes of apnea, hypopnea, and RERAs per hour of sleep.
Apnea-hypopnea index (AHI)[2] = mean number of episodes of apnea and hypopnea per hour of sleep, based on at least 2 hours of sleep recorded by polysomnography.
Apnea[3] = a cessation of airflow lasting at least 10 seconds.
Hypopnea[4,5] = an abnormal respiratory event lasting at least 10 seconds with at least a 30% reduction in thoracoabdominal movement or airflow compared to baseline, and with at least a 4% decline in $S_{a}O_{2}$%. Alternatively, a 50% reduction in airflow lasting for 10 seconds accompanied by either a ≥3% decline in $S_{a}O_{2}$% or an arousal.
Respiratory effort-related arousal (RERA)[5] = an abnormal respiratory event characterized by a clear drop in inspiratory airflow, an increased inspiratory effort (by esophageal manometry), associated with an arousal but not with a discernible drop in $S_{a}O_{2}$%.

[1]*Data from International Classification of Sleep Disorders*, 2nd ed.
[2,3,4]*Centers for Medicare & Medicaid Services' Medicare Coverage Issues Manual*, December; 2001.
[5]Modified from *The AASM Manual for the Scoring of Sleep and Associated Events, Rules, Terminology and Technical Specifications.*

Table 25.5 Multisystem benefits of CPAP therapy for OSAS

Improved sleep quality:
   ↓ Arousal index, ↑ sleep efficiency
   ↓ Stage 1 sleep, ↑ stages 3 & 4 sleep

Decreased daytime somnolence

Improved cardiovascular function:
   ↑ Left ventricular function
   ↓ Systemic & pulmonary hypertension
   ↑ Exercise performance
   ↓ Endothelial dysfunction
   ↑ Transplant-free survival time (?)

Improved neurocognitive function:
   ↑ Driving simulator performance
   ↑ Vigilance

Improved subjective work performance

Improved self-reported health status

Improved glycemic control, insulin sensitivity

Reversed deficiencies in:
   Plasma IGF-1, SHBG
   Serum testosterone

Central Sleep Apnea Syndromes

Definitions

Central sleep apnea (**CSA**) is a condition characterized by recurrent cessation of respiration during sleep, with the observed apnea having no associated ventilatory effort (Fig. 25.4). A CSA may be due to idiopathic/primary disorders, or be caused by medical and neurological conditions, drugs, or ascent to high altitude (Table 25.7).

     Cheyne-Stokes respiration (**CSR**) is a subtype of CSA in which a breathing pattern consists of hypopneas alternating with hyperpneas. During such episodes, the patient's V_T gradually waxes and wanes in a crescendo-decrescendo pattern (Fig. 25.5).

Epidemiology of Central Sleep Apnea Syndromes

Primary CSA is a rare idiopathic subtype of CSA diagnosed after ruling out other secondary causes of CSA or CSR, and it typically affects middle-age to elderly individuals. CSA due to Cheyne-Stokes respiration occurs in subjects 60 years and older with congestive heart failure, cerebrovascular disease, and renal insufficiency, with a male predominance. High-altitude periodic breathing occurs more commonly in men who recently ascended to high altitude (≥4,000 m). The increased prevalence of both CSR and high-altitude periodic breathing in men compared to women is attributed not only to

their higher prevalence of cardiovascular disease and outdoor activity participation but also to greater ventilatory chemoresponsiveness in men. **Long-acting opioids** (eg, methadone, time-released morphine, and hydrocodone) taken for at least 2 months are the most common drugs associated with CSA.

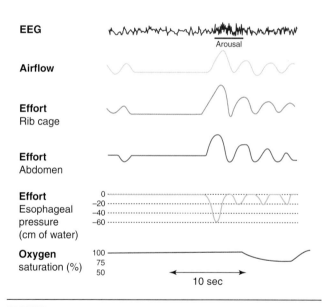

FIGURE 25.4 A polysomnogram (PSG) showing complete absence of airflow in the nasal-oral channel with an accompanying absence of respiratory effort lasting for at least 10 seconds, consistent with a central sleep apnea episode.

Table 25.6 Potential surgical techniques for treating OSAS

Nasal reconstruction	Maxillomandibular advancement
Temperature-controlled radiofrequency tissue ablation	Base of tongue resection
Laser-assisted uvulopalatoplasty (LAUP)	Uvulopalatopharyngoplasty (UPPP)
Genioglossus advancement plus hyoid myotomy and suspension (GAHMS)	Bariatric surgery
Mandibular osteotomy with genioglossus advancement	Tracheotomy

Table **25.7** Classification of central sleep apnea syndromes[a]

Primary/Idiopathic	Secondary Causes

Primary central sleep apnea (adult)
Primary sleep apnea of infancy
	Cheyne-Stokes breathing pattern:
	   Congestive heart failure
	   Cerebrovascular disease
	   Renal failure
	High-altitude periodic breathing
	Drug or substance (eg, long-acting opioids)
	Medical condition not involving Cheyne-Stokes

[a]*From* The International Classification of Sleep Disorders, *2nd ed.*

Pathophysiology of CSAS

A high ventilatory chemoresponsiveness to P_aCO_2 is believed to be the underlying predisposing factor for the development of CSA and CSR. In CSA patients with such increased ventilatory chemoresponsiveness, sleep-related rises in P_aCO_2 stimulate an exaggerated ventilatory response, resulting in subsequent decrements of the P_aCO_2 to below the patient's apneic threshold. This exaggerated hyperpnea for a given disturbance (apnea or hypopnea with resulting $\uparrow P_aCO_2$ and/or $\downarrow P_aO_2$), or **high loop gain**, is considered most likely to produce these sustained oscillations in the system leading to periodic breathing or CSR (Fig. 25.6).

In patients with CSR due to congestive heart failure, the **circulatory delay time**, measured from the termination of the central apnea to the nadir of $S_aO_2\%$, is inversely related to $\dot{Q}$. The prolonged circulatory delays in patients with heart failure reflect the longer time required for oxygenated blood to travel from the pulmonary veins and left ventricle to a pulse oximeter probe attached to the finger or ear because of their cardiac pump failure. Heart transplantation has been demonstrated to reduce circulatory delay time in patients with congestive heart failure and CSA-CSR. However, their high ventilatory chemoresponsiveness and dysregulated control of breathing seem to persist post-transplantation in this cohort.

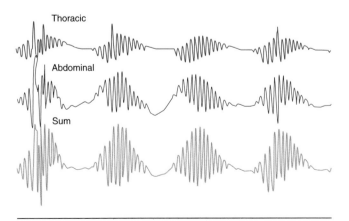

FIGURE 25.5 Cheyne-Stokes breathing is characterized by **crescendo-decrescendo** oscillations in V_T shown by inductive plethysmography of a patient's chest and abdominal motions.

Diagnosis of CSAS

A diagnosis of CSAS requires clinical features (excessive daytime sleepiness, frequent arousals and awakenings, insomnia complaints, or awakenings due to dyspnea), plus a polysomnogram showing a central apnea index of ≥5 scoreable events per hour of sleep. A **central apnea** is a respiratory event characterized by cessation of airflow lasting at least 10 seconds that is unaccompanied by respiratory effort. The diagnosis of CSR is confirmed by a polysomnogram showing at least 10 central apneas and hypopneas per hour of sleep, occurring in a crescendo-decrescendo pattern of V_T accompanied by frequent arousals from sleep and derangement of sleep structure.

Therapeutic Approaches to CSAS

Most published clinical trials for CSAS focus on the treatment of CSA-CSR that is due to congestive heart failure. Optimizing treatment of such patients with congestive heart failure (eg, antihypertensives/vasodilators, diuretics, and inotropes, coronary revascularization, etc) is the first step in treating their CSA-CSR. Supplemental O_2 therapy increases body O_2 reserves and blunts hypoxemic respiratory drive, thereby reducing central apneas and periodic breathing pattern and enhancing quality of life in patients with CSR due to CHF. **Acetazolamide**, a **carbonic anhydrase inhibitor**, induces a mild metabolic acidosis that stimulates respiration by increasing the difference between the subject's prevailing P_aCO_2 and their apneic P_aCO_2 threshold. Acetazolamide improves central sleep apnea, nocturnal oxygenation, and related daytime symptoms. **Theophylline**, a **phosphodiesterase inhibitor**, has excitatory effects on breathing, enhances ventilation, reduces respiratory disturbances, and increases nocturnal oxygenation. However, theophylline also nearly doubles circulating renin levels in CHF patients. As for OSA patients, the use of CPAP has been shown to improve left ventricular ejection fraction, mitral regurgitant fraction, atrial natriuretic peptide level, and ventilation efficiency in patients with CSA-CSR due to CHF. However, a large, randomized controlled trial conducted in Canada found that CPAP did not affect overall survival in all patients with CSA-CSR due to CHF, except in those whose central apneas are suppressed soon after CPAP initiation.

Variable or **bilevel positive airway pressure (BiPAP)** ventilation, in which the positive airway pressure applied is

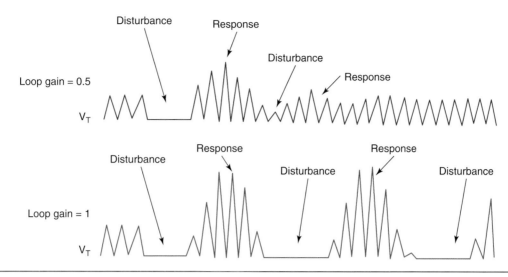

FIGURE 25.6 The ventilatory response to an apnea (disturbance) with a normal loop gain or LG (upper trace), and with the high loop gain (lower trace) characteristic of the increased ventilatory chemoresponsiveness among patients with CSA/Cheyne-Stokes breathing. *From White DP.* Am J Respir Crit Care Med. *Dec 1, 2005;172 (11):1363-1370.*

higher during inspiration than during expiration, appears to be as effective as CPAP in improving respiratory disturbances, nocturnal oxygenation, and sleep architecture in patients with CSR due to CHF (Chap. 30). **Adaptive support servo-ventilation (ASV)** suppresses CSA and/or CSR in CHF patients and improves their sleep quality better than CPAP or O_2 supplementation. Use of ASV automatically adjusts the positive inspiratory P_{AW} according to the patient's fluctuating V_T pattern. In patients with symptomatic **sinus bradycardia**, the use of **atrial overdrive pacing** significantly reduced central apneas in one study, presumably by increasing $\dot{Q}$ via an increase in heart rate. Low-flow supplemental CO_2 raises the patient's P_aCO_2 above their apnea threshold and has been demonstrated to improve CSA and CSR in patients with CHF. However, such CO_2 supplementation is ineffective in reducing arousals and is associated with sympathetic activation that may be detrimental in CHF.

Descending just 500-1,000 m of elevation can ameliorate most high altitude clinical syndromes, including acute mountain sickness, high-altitude periodic breathing, and high-altitude pulmonary edema (Chap. 13). At altitude, nocturnal O_2 enrichment of the ambient air to an effective $F_IO_2 = 0.25$ can ameliorate the central apneas and periodic breathing and improve both sleep quality and daytime function. As mentioned above, theophylline and acetazolamide both normalize sleep disordered breathing at high altitude. **Temazepam**, a **benzodiazepine receptor agonist**, reduces periodic breathing at high altitude by consolidating sleep. However, its use has been associated with a small decrease in nocturnal $S_aO_2\%$. **Zolpidem**, a **non-benzodiazepine receptor agonist**, improves sleep quality without affecting respiration at high altitude.

In patients with known or suspected drug-related CSA, the discontinuation of long-acting opioid medications, their substitution with non-narcotic medications, or reduction of the narcotic dose may each help ameliorate periodic breathing.

Complex Sleep Apnea Syndrome

Definition

Complex sleep apnea syndrome (CompSAS) is a form of sleep apnea specifically identified by the persistence or emergence of central apneas or hypopneas upon exposure of a patient to CPAP when any obstructive events have disappeared.

> ▶▶ **CLINICAL CORRELATION 25.2**
>
> CompSAS should be distinguished from the term **mixed apnea**. While CompSAS is diagnosed by unmasking central apneas when using CPAP in a patient with OSA, a mixed apnea is a specific respiratory pattern that begins as a central apnea but ends as an obstructive event (Fig. 25.7). Mixed apneas are traditionally considered as "obstructive" respiratory events, although mixed apneas can also be present in CompSAS.

Epidemiology of CompSAS

The reported estimate of the prevalence of CompSAS among sleep apnea patients in the United States is 16%, although it is derived from a relatively small clinical cohort study. A larger study of >1,200 Japanese patients with all forms of sleep apnea syndromes revealed a CompSAS prevalence of 5%. There appears to be an overwhelming male predominance in CompSAS, approaching 80%-90% across racial and national borders.

Pathophysiology of CompSAS

The pathophysiology of this disorder involves the combination of an anatomically narrow and excessively collapsible airway with a highly sensitive hypocapnia-induced apneic threshold.

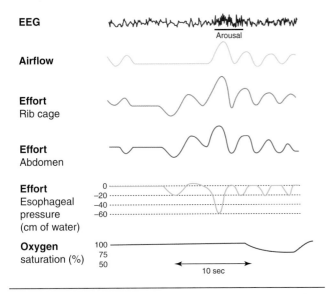

EEG

Airflow

Effort
Rib cage

Effort
Abdomen

Effort
Esophageal
pressure
(cm of water)

Oxygen
saturation (%)

FIGURE 25.7 Demonstration of a mixed apnea by polysomnographic evaluation. See text for additional details.

Baseline polysomnography in CompSAS patients typically demonstrates OSAS, and features predominantly obstructive respiratory events (apnea, hypopneas, and respiratory-effort related arousals). With administration of CPAP to eliminate upper airway obstruction, however, the dysregulated central control of ventilation is unmasked, causing the emergence of central apneas and a Cheyne-Stokes breathing pattern. The lowering by CPAP of P_aCO_2 below the patient's apneic threshold likely precipitates the central apneas in those CompSAS patients with highly sensitive hypocapnia-induced ventilatory control system. Meanwhile, excessive CPAP that increases intrathoracic pressures and hyperinflation may also trigger central apneas via the **Hering-Breuer reflex** (Chap. 11).

Diagnosis of CompSAS

In a patient presenting with clinical features of a sleep apnea syndrome, the diagnosis of CompSAS is based upon an initial baseline polysomnogram that demonstrates predominately obstructive respiratory events occurring at least five times per hour. Then a subsequent therapeutic CPAP trial should demonstrate the resolution of obstructive respiratory events and the

emergence of prominent or disruptive central apneas (again ≥5/h) and/or a Cheyne-Stokes respiratory pattern.

Treatment of CompSAS

As mentioned above, the use of adaptive support servo-ventilation (ASV) appears to be superior to other PAP therapies in controlling the respiratory disturbances in CompSAS. Several promising therapies, including positive airway pressure with gas modulation using a low F_ICO_2 (PAPGAM), artificially enhanced dead space, and prescription of acetazolamide, all aim to stabilize chemoreceptor control of respiration by inducing metabolic acidosis or raising P_aCO_2 above a patient's apneic threshold.

Sleep-Related Hypoventilation/ Hypoxemic Syndrome

Definition

Sleep-related hypoventilation/hypoxemic syndrome (SRH) is a group of breathing disorders characterized by decreased $\dot{V}_A$ from various causes that exclude OSA, all of which decrease $S_aO_2\%$ and increase P_aCO_2 during sleep. Most authors divide SRH into two categories based on their underlying etiologies. These include primary or idiopathic disorders, namely the sleep-related non-obstructive alveolar hypoventilation syndrome, and **congenital central alveolar hypoventilation syndrome (CCAHS)**. CCAHS is also known as **Ondine's curse**, from the German folktale of Ondine, a water nymph who cursed her unfaithful husband to cease breathing should he ever fall asleep again. Other cases of SRH develop secondarily to an underlying pulmonary, neuromuscular, or skeletal abnormality (Table 25.8).

Epidemiology of SRH

The demographics of patients with secondary SRH parallel those of the underlying causative medical conditions. The primary SRH syndromes occur very rarely, with only 160-180 confirmed cases of CCAHS having been reported worldwide. CCAHS affects newborns and infants, and is associated with other congenital abnormalities including **Hirschsprung disease**, autonomic dysfunction, neural tumors, swallowing dysfunctions,

Table **25.8** Classification of sleep-related hypoventilation/hypoxemic syndromes[a]

Primary or idiopathic
Sleep related non-obstructive alveolar hypoventilation
Congenital central alveolar hypoventilation syndrome (Ondine's curse)

Secondary sleep related hypoventilation/hypoxemia due to a medical condition
Pulmonary parenchymal abnormalities, eg, interstitial lung disease
Pulmonary vascular abnormalities, eg, pulmonary embolism, right-to-left shunt
Lower airways obstruction, eg, chronic obstructive pulmonary disease
Neuromuscular disorder, eg, amyotrophic lateral sclerosis
Chest wall disorders, eg, kyphoscoliosis, obesity-related hypoventilation

[a]*From* The International Classification of Sleep Disorders, *2nd ed.*

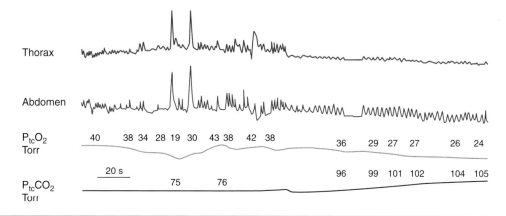

FIGURE 25.8 Respiratory monitoring in a newborn with congenital central alveolar hypoventilation syndrome. Note the erratic thoracoabdominal respiratory pattern that is associated with profound decline in arterial oxygenation and progressive hypercapnia as detected by transcutaneous exhaled gas monitoring ($P_{tc}O_2$ and $P_{tc}CO_2$, respectively).

and ocular abnormalities. CCAHS usually occurs sporadically but some cases are related to *de novo* mutations of the ***PHOX2B* gene**. In contrast, little is known about the epidemiology of adult idiopathic sleep-related non-obstructive alveolar hypoventilation syndrome, whose onset is during adolescence and early adulthood.

Pathophysiology of SRH

Idiopathic and congenital forms of SRH are characterized by decreased ventilatory responsiveness to hypercapnia or hypoxia during both wakefulness and sleep. Such altered responsiveness is due to a postulated lesion in the medullary chemoreceptors (adult idiopathic type) or to an abnormality in brainstem integration of chemoreceptor afferents (congenital type). Mutations of *PHOX2B*, which has an autosomal dominant mode of transmission with incomplete penetrance, appear to impair respiratory control function of the **retrotrapezoid nucleus** in the rostral medulla in infants with CCAHS (Chap. 11). By comparison, SRH due to medical conditions most often is traceable to ventilation-perfusion abnormalities (Chap. 8) including mechanical ventilatory insufficiencies that are associated with these serious conditions.

Differential Diagnosis of SRH

CCAHS is suspected in a newborn who presents with sustained shallow breathing, cyanosis, and apnea during sleep (Fig. 25.8). In older patients, a diagnosis of idiopathic SRH is made in adolescents and adults only after excluding medical conditions that can cause secondary SRH. The syndrome is characterized by blunted chemoresponsiveness that causes daytime hypercapnia and hypoxemia despite normal mechanical properties of the lungs and chest. When left untreated, these primary alveolar hypoventilation syndromes can progress to pulmonary hypertension and death.

In SRH secondary to medical conditions, the diagnosis requires a polysomnogram and/or arterial blood gases that demonstrate persistent nocturnal hypoxemia and/or hypercapnia in the absence of obvious obstructive apneas or periodic breathing in a patient with a predisposing medical, neurologic, or muscular condition (Table 25.9).

▶▶ CLINICAL CORRELATION 25.3

An increasing cause of secondary SRH is the **obesity-hypoventilation syndrome (OHS)**, formerly the **Pickwickian syndrome** for the "fat and red-faced sleepy boy" in Dickens' *The Pickwick Papers*. OHS occurs in the morbidly obese with daytime hypersomnolence, hypercapnia, and hypoxemia that worsen in sleep, polycythemia, and if untreated, pulmonary hypertension. Independent clinical predictors of OHS in a patient with known OSAS include a serum [HCO_3^-] ≥27 mM/L, an elevated AHI (nominally ≥100 events/h), and an abnormally low $S_{a}O_2$%.

Table **25.9** **Polysomnographic and arterial blood gas criteria for SRH**[a]

Polysomnograms or ABGs obtained during sleep showing at least one of the following:
An $S_{a}O_2$ during sleep of <90% lasting >5 minutes with a nadir of ≤85%; *OR*
>30% of total sleep time with $S_{a}O_2$ of <90%; *OR*
Sleeping ABGs with a $P_{a}CO_2$ that is abnormally high or disproportionately increased relative to levels during wakefulness.

[a]*From* The International Classification of Sleep Disorders, *2nd ed.*

Therapeutic Approaches to SRH

Optimal therapy of underlying medical conditions ameliorates many secondary SRH, including nocturnal O_2 and long-acting bronchodilators in COPD patients. Drugs that improve ventilatory drive (theophylline, progesterone, acetazolamide) or enhance muscle strength such as anabolic steroids, growth hormone, and insulin-like growth factor-1 (IGF-1), have not been reliably effective in ameliorating the chronic hypoventilation of SRH. Non-invasive positive pressure ventilation, either via a nasal or orofacial mask using a BiPAP device or by mechanical ventilator, is indicated in patients with fatigue, dyspnea, morning headache, or chronic respiratory failure. In a subgroup of OHS patients, both CPAP and BiPAP are effective in reducing daytime hypercapnia, and BIPAP substantially improves oxygenation, sleep quality, and health-related quality of life. **Average volume-assured pressure support (AVAPS)** ventilation combines the pressure-limited and volume-limited modes of assisted ventilation to ensure a more consistent V_T while delivering the comfort and advantages of pressure support (Chap. 30). While AVAPS and BiPAP provide similar sleep and health quality benefits, AVAPS achieves better ventilatory efficacy as assessed by $P_{tc}CO_2$ in OHS patients.

Suggested Readings

1. Sateia, MJ, ed. *International Classification of Sleep Disorders*, 2nd ed. Westchester, IL: American Academy of Sleep Medicine; 2005;33-77. *The comprehensive ICSD-2 manual provides standardized definitions and diagnostic criteria, and also summarizes information regarding their epidemiology and distinguishing clinical features.*

2. Epstein LJ, Kristo D, Strollo PJ, et al. Clinical guideline for the evaluation, management, and long-term care of obstructive sleep apnea in adults. *J Clin Sleep Med.* 2009;5:263-276; Yumino D, Bradley TD. Central sleep apnea and Cheyne-Stokes respiration. *Proc Am Thorac Soc.* 2008;226-236; Gilmartin GS, Daly RW, Thomas RJ. Recognition and management of complex sleep-disordered breathing. *Curr Opin Pulm Med.* 2005;11:485-493; Casey KR, Cantillo KO, Brown LK. Sleep-related hypoventilation/hypoxemic syndromes. *Chest.* 2007;131:1936-1948. *Collectively, these four articles review the clinical features, diagnosis, and management of the three major types of sleep-related breathing disorders.*

CASE STUDIES AND PRACTICE PROBLEMS

CASE 25.1 A 38-year-old man presents with paroxysmal nocturnal dyspnea. He is experiencing progressive muscle weakness of the arms and legs secondary to amyotrophic lateral sclerosis. He also complains of early morning headaches lasting about 30 minutes. Pulmonary function testing shows an FVC = 48% of predicted and a maximum inspiratory pressure of −15 cm H_2O. His resting awake arterial blood gases show pH_a = 7.35, P_aCO_2 = 55 mm Hg, and P_aO_2 = 78 mm Hg. Use of an overnight earlobe pulse oximeter reveals sustained episodes of S_aO_2 <88% lasting 15 minutes. What is the most likely cause of his sleep-related breathing disorder?

a. Complex sleep apnea

b. Sleep-related hypoventilation/hypoxemic syndrome

c. Central sleep apnea

d. Cheyne-Stokes hypoventilation

e. Mixed sleep apnea

CASE 25.2 A 75-year-old man is brought to the physician by his wife who witnessed frequent episodes of pauses in his breathing. She reports that the patient snores only mildly and intermittently. The patient's **Epworth Sleepiness Scale** score is at 12 [range: 0 (never sleepy) to 24 (very sleepy)] denoting mild hypersomnolence. His polysomnogram reveals frequent episodes of the event (double-headed arrow) seen below:

Which of the following conditions is most often associated with this event?

a. Congestive heart failure

b. Chronic obstructive pulmonary disease

c. Obesity

d. Severe kyphoscoliosis

e. Adenotonsillar hypertrophy

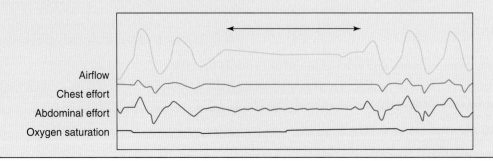

Airflow
Chest effort
Abdominal effort
Oxygen saturation

CASE 25.3 A 32-year-old man with no known medical problems undergoes polysomnography for suspected OSA. He was reported by his wife to have loud persistent snoring as well as nocturnal choking and gagging. His sleep study reveals an apnea-hypopnea index (AHI) of 35 events/h with a minimal $S_aO_2 = 84\%$. The patient is reluctant to try CPAP therapy, but his physician wants to use evidence-based medicine to convince the patient to try it. Which of the following is a known effect of CPAP therapy for OSA?

a. Increased Epworth Sleepiness Score

b. Increased arousal index

c. Increased delta (slow wave) sleep

d. Decreased sleep latency during naps

e. Decreased rapid eye movement (REM) sleep

Solutions to Case Studies and Practice Problems

CASE 25.1 The most correct answer is b, the sleep-related hypoventilation/hypoxemic syndrome (SRH).

This patient has neuromuscular weakness (reduced FVC and MIP) due to amyotrophic lateral sclerosis, as well as hypercapnia (P_aCO_2 >45 mm Hg), and polysomnography that confirms sustained hypoxemia (S_aO_2 <90% for ≥5 minutes). These results are most consistent with secondary SRH due to neuromuscular disease.

CASE 25.2 The most correct answer is a, congestive heart failure (CHF).

The polysomnogram depicts absent airflow accompanied by absent respiratory effort that are consistent with a central sleep apnea syndrome. CHF, chronic kidney disease, and cerebrovascular disease are medical conditions associated with central sleep apnea and/or Cheyne-Stokes breathing. Very severe COPD is associated with

nocturnal hypoventilation and hypoxemia, especially worse during REM sleep. Chest wall abnormalities from morbid obesity and severe kyphoscoliosis can also result in sleep-related hypoventilation/hypoxemia. Adenotonsillar hypertrophy is the major cause of obstructive sleep apnea syndrome in children.

CASE 25.3 The most correct answer is c, increased delta (slow wave) sleep.

Indicators of a successful CPAP trial include improved sleep architecture with fewer arousals and sleep stage shifts, increased proportion of delta sleep, and increased REM sleep. Long-term CPAP use has also been demonstrated to reduce daytime hypersomnolence, both subjectively (a reduced Epworth Sleepiness Scale score) and objectively (increased latency during a multiple sleep latency test).

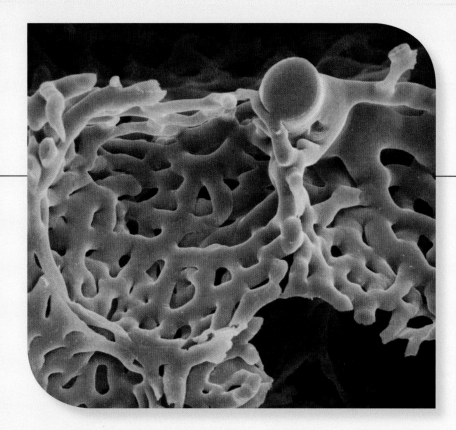

INFLAMMATORY, VASCULAR, AND PLEURAL DISEASES

Pathology of Atelectatic, Vascular, and Iatrogenic Diseases of the Lungs and Pleural Space

DAVID S. BRINK, MD

(#84)

Atelectasis

Atelectasis describes a reduction in lung volume due to incomplete expansion of airspaces or, more commonly, the collapse of previously inflated pulmonary parenchyma. In atelectasis, perfusion of such nonventilated lung creates a physiological shunt that mixes inadequately oxygenated blood from pulmonary arteries with better oxygenated blood in the pulmonary veins (Chap. 9). If the ventilation-perfusion mismatch is sufficiently severe, systemic hypoxemia results. Additionally, atelectatic lung is more likely to become infected. Atelectasis can be subdivided by its pathogenesis.

In **resorption atelectasis** (also known as **obstruction atelectasis**), air is prevented from reaching distal airspaces because of airway obstruction. Then, as more distal air is absorbed, the previously expanded lung collapses. The extent of involvement is determined by the level of obstruction: Obstruction of a major airway can result in collapse of an entire lobe. Most commonly, a mucous or mucopurulent plug is responsible for the obstruction, although any physical obstruction will suffice. In resorption atelectasis, the mediastinum shifts toward the affected side.

In **compression atelectasis** (also known as **passive atelectasis** and as **relaxation atelectasis**), accumulation of space-occupying material within the pleural space mechanically compresses the lung parenchyma (Fig. 26.1). Compression atelectasis complicates pleural effusion and pneumothorax (see below), as well as pleural tumors (Chap. 31). Additionally, compression atelectasis of basal lung zones complicates peritoneal effusion (**ascites**) and frequently occurs in bedridden patients due to diaphragmatic elevation. In compression atelectasis, the mediastinum shifts away from the affected side.

Microatelectasis complicates adult and neonatal respiratory distress syndromes (Chaps. 23 and 39) as well as interstitial inflammatory lung diseases (Chap. 23). Its pathogenesis involves a complex set of events, the most important being deactivation of surfactant in the mature lung or its inadequate synthesis in neonatal lung.

In the setting of localized or generalized **pulmonary fibrosis**, the foci of fibrosis contract largely due to the action of myofibroblasts, collapsing adjacent lung tissue and resulting in **contraction atelectasis** or **cicatrization atelectasis**.

Generally, resorption atelectasis, compression atelectasis, and microatelectasis are reversible, while contraction atelectasis is not.

Pulmonary Edema

When edema develops in the lung, the excess fluid rapidly moves from the interstitium to the airspaces (Chaps. 7 and 28). While there are many specific causes of **pulmonary edema** (see Table 7.2), it is generally due to a change in hemodynamics (perfusion vs interstitial pressures) or to microvascular injury. Congestive heart failure is the most common cause of an increase in pulmonary venous pressure and the resultant pulmonary edema. Less commonly, reduction of plasma oncotic pressure will result in egress of fluid from the vascular space into the interstitium and then the alveoli. Alternatively, an increase in the permeability of capillaries, as occurs in the setting of alveolar and microvascular injury, can result in edema (Chap. 28).

Gross manifestations of pulmonary edema include increase in lung weight and a wet cut surface with frothy fluid visible in larger airways. Microscopically, pulmonary edema is characterized by pale, eosinophilic, glassy or finely granular

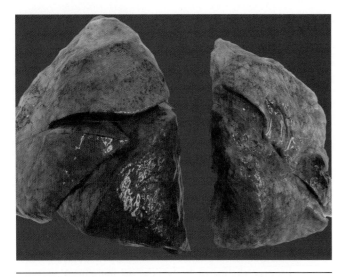

FIGURE 26.1 Compression atelectasis. The left lung (right side of image) is atelectatic due to a left-sided hemothorax caused by a gunshot wound. Note that the left lung is significantly smaller than the right and has a wrinkled pleural surface. *From* Kemp *et al.* Pathology: The Big Picture, *McGraw-Hill; 2008.*

rupture of capillaries, resulting in microhemorrhages that release formed blood elements into alveolar spaces. As erythrocytes are cleared by macrophages, hemoglobin is progressively catabolized to hemosiderin, which persists in macrophage cytoplasm. Thus, the presence of hemosiderin-laden macrophages (or **siderophages**) reflects remote hemorrhage and implies chronic congestion [Fig. 26.2 (b)]. While any form of pulmonary hemorrhage will eventually show siderophages, the most common cause of pulmonary congestion and hemorrhage is congestive heart failure. This has led to widespread usage of the term "**heart failure cells**" to describe such intra-alveolar hemosiderin-laden macrophages.

Pulmonary Embolus

A large majority of pulmonary emboli are thrombotic in origin. Therefore, unless otherwise specified, the term "pulmonary embolus" typically refers to **pulmonary thromboembolus**. Pulmonary thromboembolism is involved in approximately 10% of hospital deaths. In more than 95% of cases, the source of pulmonary thromboemboli is a thrombus in a deep vein of the lower extremity (Chap. 27). Risk factors for venous thrombosis and pulmonary thromboembolus include prolonged bed rest (especially in the setting of lower extremity immobilization), severe trauma, burns, congestive heart failure, and hypercoagulable states (Table 26.1).

When a venous thrombus embolizes, it travels in progressively larger systemic veins toward the right heart. Upon ejection from the right ventricle, fragments of the embolism

intra-alveolar precipitate [Fig. 26.2 (a)]. In the setting of pulmonary edema secondary to elevation of venous pressure, alveolar septal capillaries will show congestion characterized by engorgement with blood. Due to the delicate nature of alveolar septa, congestion is typically accompanied by occasional

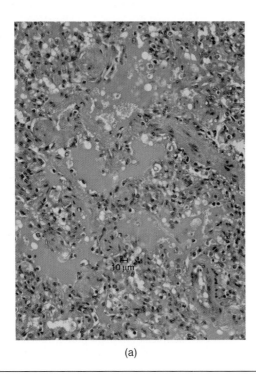

(a)

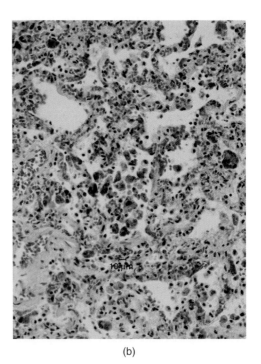

(b)

FIGURE 26.2 (a) Pulmonary edema is recognizable microscopically as a pale, eosinophilic, glassy or finely granular precipitate filling airspaces. (b) In pulmonary congestion, alveolar capillaries are engorged with blood. Additionally, numerous hemosiderin-laden macrophages ("heart failure cells") are present within alveoli, reflective of remote hemorrhage.

Table **26.1** Causes of hypercoagulable states

Primary	Secondary
Antithrombin III deficiency	Obesity
Protein C deficiency	Recent surgery
Defective fibrinolysis	Pregnancy
Factor V Leiden	Oral contraceptive with high estrogen content
Prothrombin 20210A	Cancer
Hyperhomocysteinemia	
Antiphospholipid syndrome	

move into progressively smaller branches of the pulmonary artery until they reach vessels too small to allow passage. At that point the thromboemboli occlude a pulmonary artery or arteriole and increase pulmonary vascular resistance and can induce vasospasm. When a major vessel is occluded, the resulting pulmonary hypertension can reduce cardiac output and induce cor pulmonale and death. If death does not result, pulmonary thromboembolism results in hypoxemia due to ventilation-perfusion mismatch with increased dead space ventilation (Chap. 8). The ischemia may also reduce surfactant release and cause pleuritic pain that add to the work of breathing (Chaps. 5 and 6). Despite the lung's systemic blood supply (Chap. 2), pulmonary thromboembolism can result in lung parenchymal ischemia and **pulmonary infarction**. In patients with **patent foramen ovale** (~30% of all

people), pulmonary arterial thrombotic occlusion can cause right-to-left shunting and subsequent **paradoxic embolism**, in which a venous thrombus enters and embolizes systemic arteries and cause distal ischemia.

Grossly, a pulmonary thromboembolus is a serpentine blood clot impacted in a pulmonary arterial branch [Fig. 26.3 (a)]. A very large thromboembolus occluding the main pulmonary arteries is typically referred to as a "saddle embolus." Microscopically, the thromboembolus is characterized by alternating layers of fibrin (eosinophilic) and erythrocytes. Ischemic lung damage is characterized by intra-alveolar hemorrhage [Fig. 26.3 (b)]. A pulmonary infarct will be conical (or, on cut section, wedge-shaped) and hemorrhagic [Fig. 26.4 (a)]. Initially, the infarct is red-blue. It becomes paler and later red-brown as erythrocytes lyse and hemoglobin is degraded to hemosiderin. Next, as fibroblasts progressively replace necrotic tissue with scar, the infarct shows a gray-white peripheral zone. Microscopically, infarcted lung tissue shows **coagulative necrosis** with loss of nuclear basophilia, although alveolar hemorrhage often dominates the microscopic appearance [Fig. 26.4 (b), (c)]. In cases of sudden death due to saddle embolus, there are typically no gross or microscopic changes to the lung.

Clinically, 60%-80% of pulmonary thromboemboli are asymptomatic; approximately 5% cause acute cor pulmonale, shock, or sudden death; and 10%-15% affect medium-sized arteries and, through an unknown mechanism, cause dyspnea. In the presence of an underlying risk factor, a patient who has had pulmonary thromboembolism has a 30% chance of recurrent pulmonary thromboembolism. A minority (<3% of patients with recurrent pulmonary thromboembolism develop pulmonary hypertension (see below), chronic cor pulmonale, vascular

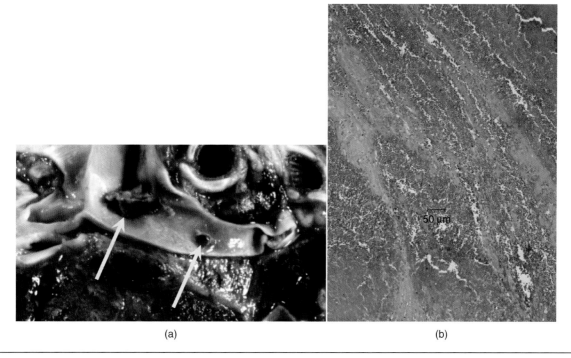

(a) (b)

FIGURE 26.3 Pulmonary thromboembolism. (a) The arrows indicate fragments of a pulmonary thromboembolus within a pulmonary artery, which has been opened longitudinally. (b) Microscopically, a thrombus shows lamellae of platelets with fibrin (pink), and erythrocytes (red).

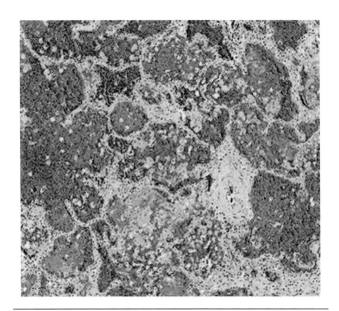

FIGURE 26.6 In this example of Goodpasture syndrome, the lung shows extensive acute hemorrhage with focal interstitial thickening. *From Travis et al. Atlas of Nontumor Pathology: Volume 2: Non-Neoplastic Disorders of the Lower Respiratory Tract, American Registry of Pathology; 2002.*

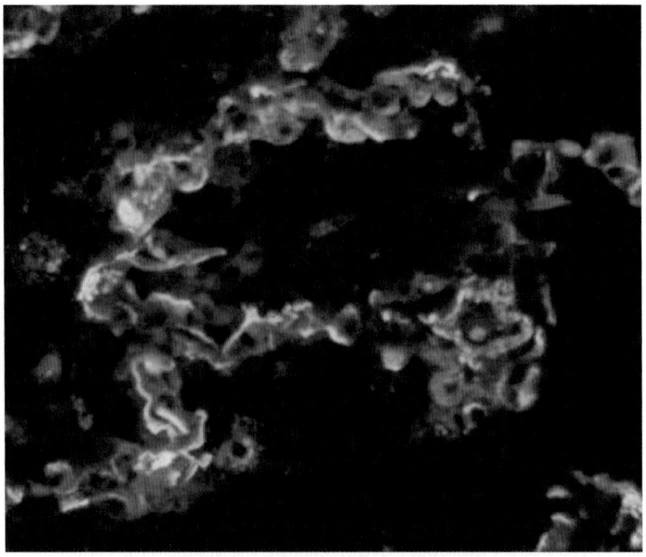

FIGURE 26.7 Immunofluorescent labeling of alveolar parenchyma with IgG. See Clinical Correlation 26.2 for more details. *From Travis et al. Atlas of Nontumor Pathology: Volume 2: Non-Neoplastic Disorders of the Lower Respiratory Tract, American Registry of Pathology; 2002.*

▶▶ CLINICAL CORRELATION 26.2

In the setting of suspected Goodpasture syndrome, immunofluorescence analysis of lung and/or kidney can be informative. In this disease, immunofluorescent labeling with IgG will show a **linear basement membrane label** of alveoli (Fig. 26.7) and glomeruli, rather than a **granular basement membrane label** typical of immune complex deposition. Immunofluorescence analysis requires frozen, nonfixed tissue. Consequently, in any situation in which immunofluorescence analysis would be helpful, it is important to promptly deliver fresh tissue to the pathologist to be frozen and sectioned for immunofluorescence labeling rather than placing the tissue in a fixative (eg, 10% formalin), as is typically done with biopsy specimens.

Clinically, the presentation of Goodpasture syndrome typically involves **hemoptysis** with the subsequent development of rapidly progressive renal insufficiency. Therapy involves removal of the pathologic autoantibodies by **plasmapheresis** and reduction of autoantibody production through immunosuppression.

Wegener's granulomatosis is a systemic vasculitis with a peak incidence in the fifth decade. Pathogenetically, it is likely a form of hypersensitivity, and patients typically have **anti-neutrophil cytoplasmic antibodies** with cytoplasmic localization (**c-ANCA**). Simplistically, the antibodies activate neutrophils, which then attack vascular luminal surfaces, resulting in vasculitis of small and medium-sized vessels. Like Goodpasture syndrome, the clinical scenario in Wegener's granulomatosis is dominated by simultaneous pulmonary and renal disease. Morphologically, respiratory tract involvement in Wegener's granulomatosis includes upper tract vasculitis,

mucosal granulomata, and ulcers rimmed by granulomatous inflammation as well as lower tract **necrotizing granulomatous inflammation** (often with cavitation) and necrotizing or granulomatous vasculitis (Fig. 26.8). Renal involvement is typified by **necrotizing glomerulonephritis**, typically with crescent formation (extracapillary proliferation).

Idiopathic pulmonary hemosiderosis is a disease of children and young adults characterized by the insidious development of hemoptysis, anemia, and weight loss. Morphologically, lungs are heavy, consolidated, and discolored red to red-brown. Microscopically, lungs show alveolar

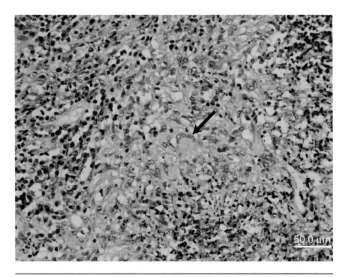

FIGURE 26.8 Wegener's granulomatosis. Granulomatous inflammation with a multinucleated giant cell (arrow) is in the center of the image. To the left is a mononuclear inflammatory infiltrate; to the right is necrosis infiltrated by neutrophils.

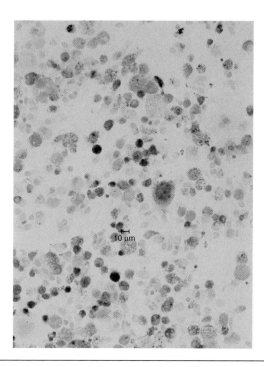

10 µm

FIGURE 26.9 Prussian blue staining of the cytospin of cells recovered by bronchoalveolar lavage. See Clinical Correlation 26.3 for details.

epithelial degeneration, shedding, and hyperplasia; intra-alveolar siderophages; marked congestion of alveolar septal capillaries; and varying degrees of fibrosis.

▶▶ CLINICAL CORRELATION 26.3

Figure 26.9 shows Prussian blue staining (Pearl reaction, iron stain) of the **cytospin** preparation from bronchoalveolar lavage fluid in the setting of idiopathic pulmonary hemosiderosis. Numerous hemosiderin-laden macrophages are seen, from which the disease takes its name. With this stain, hemosiderin is blue.

Iatrogenic Lung Diseases

Many drugs induce lung disease, the morphology of which varies with each compound. The most significant among these are summarized in Table 26.5.

Ionizing radiation injury to the lung can complicate therapeutic irradiation of the lungs, mediastinum, esophagus, and breast. **Acute radiation pneumonitis** occurs 1-6 months after radiation therapy in 10%-20% of patients receiving therapeutic irradiation involving the lung fields. The pneumonitis in these patients is characterized clinically by fever, dyspnea, and infiltrates on chest x-rays corresponding to the site of previous irradiation. Morphologically, lungs show diffuse alveolar damage (Chap. 23), often with severe atypia of hyperplastic type II alveolar epithelial cells. Some patients with acute radiation pneumonitis will, after about 6 months, progress to

Table 26.5 Drug-induced pulmonary disease

Drug	Pathological Type of Pulmonary Disease
Bleomycin	Pneumonitis and fibrosis
Methotrexate	Hypersensitivity pneumonitis
Amiodarone	Pneumonitis and fibrosis
Nitrofurantoin	Hypersensitivity pneumonitis
Aspirin	Bronchospasm
β-Antagonists	Bronchospasm

From Kumar et al. Robbins and Cotran Pathologic Basis of Disease, 8th ed. Philadelphia, PA: Elsevier; 2007.

chronic radiation pneumonitis that is characterized by interstitial fibrosis in the previously irradiated areas (Fig. 26.10).

▶▶ CLINICAL CORRELATION 26.4

Radiation-induced **cytologic atypia** in the lung (and elsewhere in the body) can morphologically mimic cytologic atypia in malignant neoplasia. Consequently, communicating to the pathologist a history of irradiation can help prevent an erroneous diagnosis of cancer in the setting of radiation atypia.

With lung transplantation, maintaining graft survival and function involves balancing the two major complications of transplantation: infection and rejection. Powerful immune suppression reduces the incidence of rejection while raising the incidence of infection. Decreased immunosuppression reduces the incidence of infection while raising the incidence of rejection. Lung transplant patients are at risk for bacterial, viral (especially CMV), and fungal infections (including candidiasis, aspergillosis, and *Pneumocystis jiroveci* pneumonia; Chap. 34). **Acute rejection** typically occurs within 3 months of transplantation and is characterized by fever, dyspnea, cough, and chest radiograph infiltrate. Since the symptoms and signs of acute rejection mimic those of infection, lung biopsy may be required to establish the diagnosis. The histologic hallmark of acute rejection in the pulmonary allograft is a perivascular lymphocytic inflammatory infiltrate [Fig. 26.11 (a)]. **Chronic rejection** can present 6-12 months after transplantation and is present in more than one-half of lung transplant recipients within 5 years of transplantation. The histologic hallmark of chronic rejection is bronchiolitis obliterans, in which bronchiolar lumina are obstructed by an inflammatory fibrous exudate [Fig. 26.11 (b)]. Long-standing chronic rejection can result in bronchiectasis (Chap. 20).

Abnormalities of the Pleural Space

A **pleural effusion** is excess fluid in the pleural space and can be inflammatory or non-inflammatory (Chap. 19). Inflammatory pleural effusions typically occur in the setting of pleuritis,

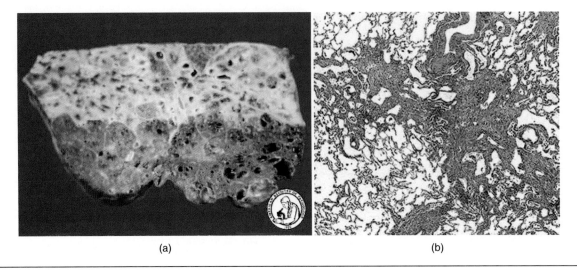

(a)   (b)

FIGURE 26.10   Chronic radiation pneumonitis. (a) The top portion of the lung shows striking fibrosis that is well demarcated from more normal lung tissue. The fibrotic area corresponds to a site of previous irradiation for lung cancer. (b) Microscopically, chronic radiation pneumonitis shows interstitial fibrosis. *From Travis et al.* Atlas of Nontumor Pathology: Volume 2: Non-Neoplastic Disorders of the Lower Respiratory Tract, *American Registry of Pathology; 2002.*

which can be due to infection of the lung (Chap. 34), collagen vascular disorders, uremia, systemic infection, or metastatic cancer. **Empyema** is a purulent pleural effusion and can be due to spread of an intrapulmonary infection to the pleural space or from **lymphohematogenous spread of infection**. Typically, empyema undergoes organization, with the development of fibrous adhesions that obliterate the pleural space. In hemorrhagic pleuritis, pleural effusion is sanguineous; underlying conditions include hemorrhagic diathesis, rickettsial disease, and neoplastic involvement of the pleural space. Other pleural effusions include **hydrothorax** (typically in the setting of congestive heart failure), **hemothorax** (blood in pleural space), and **chylothorax** (lymph fluid in pleural space; typically left-sided and due to thoracic duct trauma or obstruction).

Pneumothorax describes air in the pleural space and can be secondary to trauma, interstitial emphysema (Chap. 20), asthma (Chap. 21), tuberculosis (Chap. 36), or a lung abscess (Chap. 34) communicating with the pleural space. **Tension pneumothorax**, a medical emergency, is a pneumothorax wherein the defect acts as a valve, such that air enters the pleural cavity on inspiration but is prevented from leaving the pleural cavity on expiration.

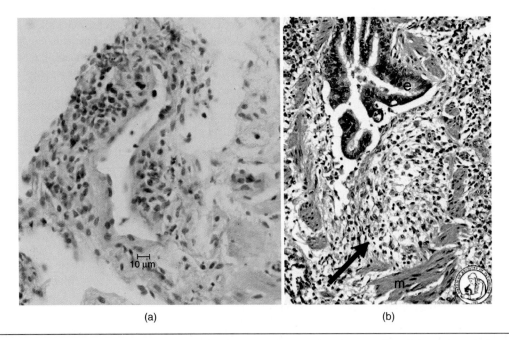

(a)   (b)

FIGURE 26.11   **Pathology of lung transplantation.** (a) The hallmark of acute rejection of a pulmonary allograft is a perivascular lymphocytic inflammatory infiltrate. (b) Chronic rejection is characterized by obliterative bronchiolitis that features an inflammatory fibrous exudate (arrow) between the smooth muscle (m) and bronchiolar epithelium (e). (b): *From Travis et al.* Atlas of Nontumor Pathology: Volume 2: Non-Neoplastic Disorders of the Lower Respiratory Tract, *American Registry of Pathology; 2002.*

Suggested Readings

1. Travis WD, Colby TV, Koss MN, Rosado-de-Christenson ML, Müller NL, King TE. *Atlas of Nontumor Pathology: Volume 2: Non-Neoplastic Disorders of the Lower Respiratory Tract,* American Registry of Pathology; 2002. *For many years, the Armed Forces Institute of Pathology (AFIP) was responsible for the publication of numerous tumor atlases, frequently referred to as "The Fascicles." Later, the AFIP expanded its atlas publication to include non-neoplastic disease. This text offers well-organized and exceedingly well-illustrated discussions of pulmonary disease with a focus on morphology but with generous clinical and radiographic coverage. In accordance with the 2005 Defense Base Realignment and Closure (BRAC) law, the AFIP is on track to disestablish and permanently close by September 15, 2011.*

2. Katzenstein AL. *Katzenstein and Askin's Surgical Pathology of Non-Neoplastic Lung Disease,* 4th ed. Philadelphia, PA: Saunders; 2006. *Prior to the publication of the AFIP nontumor "fascicles," previous editions of this book served surgical pathologists as a sort of "gold standard" for the interpretation of non-neoplastic lung pathology.*

3. Kumar V, Abbas AK, Fausto N. *Robbins and Cotran Pathologic Basis of Disease,* 8th ed. Philadelphia, PA: Elsevier; 2007. *Throughout its many editions, this reference work is the most definitive and approachable compendium of pathology images available to students.*

CASE STUDIES AND PRACTICE PROBLEMS

CASE 26.1 A 40-year-old African-American man is diagnosed with nephrotic syndrome due to collapsing glomerulopathy, a renal disease in which proteinuria is severe. Although he does not have heart failure, he does have pulmonary edema. Which of the following is likely involved in the mechanism of his pulmonary edema?

  a. Lymphatic obstruction
  b. Liquid aspiration
  c. Shock
  d. Decreased oncotic pressure
  e. Pulmonary vein obstruction

CASE 26.2 A forensic pathologist performs an autopsy on an unidentified woman with an unknown medical history. She appears to be approximately 35-40 years old. The cut surface of the lung shows atheromata in pulmonary arteries. Which of the following was most likely present prior to the woman's death?

  a. Pulmonary hypertension
  b. Idiopathic pulmonary hemosiderosis

  c. Wegener's granulomatosis
  d. Goodpasture's syndrome
  e. Deep vein thrombosis in the lower extremity

CASE 26.3 Three months after undergoing irradiation therapy for breast cancer, a 50-year-old woman develops fever and dyspnea. Chest radiograph shows infiltrates corresponding to the irradiation field. The clinician is considering a diagnosis of acute radiation pneumonitis but cannot exclude the possibility of infection. Consequently, a lung biopsy is performed, and a diagnosis of acute radiation pneumonitis is made by the pathologist. Which of the following was most likely present in the lung biopsy sample and useful to the pathologist in establishing the diagnosis?

  a. Interstitial fibrosis
  b. Perivascular lymphocytic inflammatory infiltrate
  c. Bronchiolitis obliterans
  d. Pulmonary hemorrhage and intra-alveolar siderophages
  e. Hyaline membranes and type 2 alveolar epithelial hyperplasia

Solutions to Case Studies and Practice Problems

CASE 26.1 The most correct answer is d, decreased oncotic pressure.

Though each of the options can be involved in the development of pulmonary edema, nephrotic syndrome can result in a reduction of plasma oncotic pressure, which normally serves as a force that moves fluid from the interstitium into the vascular system, counteracting the hydrostatic force of blood pressure. Lymphatic obstruction (*answer a*) can cause pulmonary edema but is unlikely in this patient. Liquid aspiration (*answer b*) and shock (*answer c*) can cause pulmonary edema through microvascular/alveolar injury, but both are unlikely in this patient. Pulmonary vein

obstruction (*answer e*) can cause pulmonary edema due to an increase in hydrostatic pressure but is unlikely in this patient.

CASE 26.2 The most correct answer is a, pulmonary hypertension.

In pulmonary hypertension, large arteries develop atheromata, mimicking systemic arteries in the setting of hypertension-related atherosclerosis. The presence of atherosclerosis in pulmonary arteries is nearly pathognomonic of pulmonary hypertension. Idiopathic pulmonary hemosiderosis (*answer b*), Wegener's granulomatosis (*answer c*), and Goodpasture syndrome (*answer d*) are all hemorrhagic lung diseases and would likely not be distinguishable on gross examination, especially in the absence of clinical information. Lower extremity deep vein thrombosis (*answer e*) is a risk factor for pulmonary thromboembolism, not pulmonary arterial atheromata.

CASE 26.3 The most correct answer is e, hyaline membranes and type 2 alveolar epithelial hyperplasia.

The morphology of acute radiation pneumonitis is diffuse alveolar damage often with type II pneumocyte hyperplasia and atypia; hyaline membranes are the hallmark of diffuse alveolar damage (Chap. 23). Interstitial fibrosis (*answer a*) typifies *chronic* radiation pneumonitis and is unlikely this soon following irradiation. Perivascular lymphocytic inflammatory infiltration (*answer b*) and bronchiolitis obliterans (*answer c*) are typical of acute and chronic (respectively) rejection of a pulmonary allograft. Pulmonary hemorrhage and intra-alveolar siderophages (*answer d*) are nonspecific findings and can be seen in any disorder with ongoing hemorrhage; such findings are not typical of acute radiation pneumonitis, and, even if present, would not help establish the diagnosis.

Chapter 27

Pulmonary Embolism

ASHUTOSH SACHDEVA, MD AND
GEORGE M. MATUSCHAK, MD

Learning Objectives

- The student will be able to describe the clinical symptoms and signs of patients presenting with pulmonary embolism (PE).

- The student will be able to define the pathophysiology of PE and the risk stratification of patients diagnosed with thromboembolism.

- The student will be able to evaluate shock and right ventricular dysfunction as a discriminator of outcome during or after PE.

- The student will be able to provide a stepwise approach to the treatment of patients diagnosed with acute PE.

Introduction

The anatomical structure of the pulmonary vasculature predisposes to its ability to filter intravascular substances that develop within, or gain access to, the venous circulation. With respect to this filtering function, several clinical syndromes may occur depending upon the nature and quantity of the filtered intravascular materials as well as the physiological reserve of the individual. Although diverse substances including **fat, air, amniotic fluid, tumor cells,** and **septic material** can embolize to the lungs, acute **pulmonary thromboembolism** is the focus of this chapter because of its overwhelmingly predominant frequency and clinical importance.

Etiology and Epidemiology of Pulmonary Embolism

Pulmonary embolism and **deep venous thrombosis (DVT)** represent a continuum of the same underlying disorder of **venous thromboembolism (VTE)**, the abnormal intravascular clotting within the venous system. Pulmonary thromboemboli originate from large thrombi in the deep veins of the lower extremities including the iliac, femoral, superficial femoral, and pelvic veins in 75%-90% of cases. The remaining pulmonary thromboemboli arise from venous thromboses of the upper extremities that are commonly associated with central venous or dialysis catheters, cardiac pacing wires, and other devices. Rates of VTE rise with increasing age, with an approximate doubling of risk over each 10-year interval. The estimated annual incidence of PE in the United States exceeds 600,000 cases, causing or contributing to death in up to 200,000 cases each year (Fig. 27.1). Overall, PE is the third most common cause of death in hospitalized patients. Approximately 10% of patients with acute PE die within the first hour. Subjects presenting with hemodynamic instability defined as right ventricular dysfunction and shock have a worse prognosis (Chaps. 28 and 29), and manifest an in-hospital mortality rate as high as 30%, primarily as a result of recurrent embolism. However, accurate diagnosis and effective treatment significantly reduce the mortality rate to 2%-8%.

Risk Factors for Pulmonary Emboli #87

As described by the German pathologist Rudolf Virchow in 1856, the major events that predispose to the development of VTE are summarized by **Virchow's triad**: **venous stasis** as occurs after prolonged immobilization; **endothelial injury** of the vessel wall; and **hypercoagulability** with activation of the clotting system. Because most clinically significant PE emanate from the deep veins of the lower extremities, the major risk factors for VTE are those processes that predispose a patient to the development of DVT. Accordingly, the likelihood of developing VTE is collectively increased by a postoperative state with prolonged bed rest or immobilization, trauma to the blood vessel wall, and acquired or hereditary risk factors for hypercoagulability.

Orthopedic surgery of the lower extremity has long been recognized as one of the strong risk factors for VTE. Thus, DVT may develop in >50% of patients who do not receive prophylactic anticoagulant therapy while undergoing elective hip or knee replacement surgery. In such cases, >90% of proximal thrombi in hip replacement patients occur ipsilaterally to the operated site. Other acquired risk factors include major trauma, abdominal surgery requiring >30 minutes of anesthesia, spinal cord injury with associated paralysis of the lower extremities, the antiphospholipid antibody syndrome, advanced malignancy, and the post-partum state (Table 27.1).

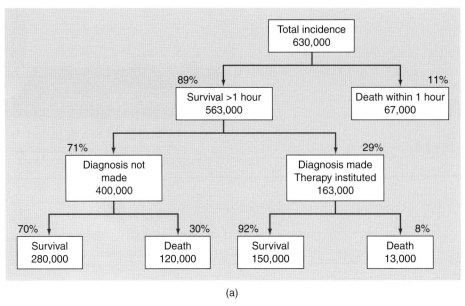

(a)

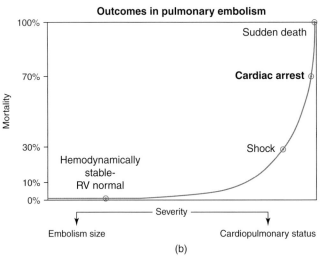

(b)

FIGURE 27.1 (a) Of the ~200,000 deaths/yr from PE in the United States, 13,000 occur in patients who received treatment, while 94% of patients who die of PE do not receive treatment because the diagnosis is not made. (b) The relationship of severity and mortality in patients with multiple or severe PE. *Adapted from Wood et al.* Major pulmonary embolism: review of a pathophysiological approach to the golden hour of hemodynamically significant pulmonary embolism. Chest. *2002;121:877-905.*

▶▶ CLINICAL CORRELATION 27.1

There is nearly an **eightfold increased risk** for acute VTE in patients with a history of VTE who undergo major surgery, who experience periods of immobility, or who are hospitalized for medical illnesses, compared with patients without such a history. These patients, and others with risk factors, must be aggressively targeted for prophylactic therapy.

Hereditary abnormalities of coagulation termed **thrombophilias** further constitute recognized risk factors for VTE and PE (Table 27.2). These hereditary thrombophilias by themselves not only predispose to VTE, but interact synergistically with acquired surgical, medical, obstetric, and other risk factors (Table 27.1) to amplify the likelihood of developing VTE.

Such inherited thrombophilias should be suspected when a patient has recurrent or life-threatening VTE and PE, has a family history of VTE, is younger than 45 years of age, and has few or no medical or surgical risk factors. Female patients with inherited thrombophilias may furthermore give a history of multiple spontaneous abortions, stillbirths, or both. The most clinically important hereditary thrombophilia associated with VTE in up to 40% of cases is the **Factor V Leiden mutation**. In such patients, the mutated **activated Factor V (Factor Va)** is resistant to the anticoagulant effects of protein C, or in other words is responsible for protein C resistance. Heterozygosity for the Factor V mutation increases the risk of VTE by 5- to 10-fold, whereas homozygosity increases risk by approximately 80-fold.

Table **27.1** Risk factors for venous thromboembolism

Strong Risk Factors	Moderate Risk Factors
Fracture of hip, pelvis, or leg	Prior VTE
Knee or hip replacement surgery	Postpartum period
Major traumatic injury	Malignancy
Spinal cord injury	Estrogen therapy, oral contraceptives
Antiphospholipid antibody syndrome	Congestive heart failure
Weak Risk Factors	Stroke
Advanced age >60 years	Respiratory failure
Obesity	Indwelling central venous catheter
Antepartum period	Arthroscopic knee surgery
Varicose veins	

Clinical Vignette

A 68-year-old obese male presented to the emergency department with lightheadedness progressing to near-syncope and progressive shortness of breath of three days' duration. His symptoms started a week ago when he first experienced pleuritic chest pain that radiated to his right side. He had undergone sinus surgery 3 weeks prior to presentation. His past medical history was significant for hypertension, obstructive sleep apnea, and diastolic heart failure; a DVT following knee surgery had occurred 15 years previously. He quit smoking 20 years ago and did not report alcohol use. Physical exam revealed tachypnea, sinus tachycardia at a HR = 118 beats/min, BP = 98/62 mm Hg, and S_aO_2 = 90% while on 6 L/min of supplemental inspired O_2. Auscultation of the chest showed scattered wheezes and left basilar crackles (Chap. 14). No calf tenderness was present. Given the high clinical suspicion for acute PE, a CT angiogram of the chest was performed that revealed multiple filling defects (Fig. 27.2) (see Chap. 15). The patient was thereafter anticoagulated with **low-molecular-weight heparin (LMWH)**.

Table **27.2** Hereditary risk factors for venous thromboembolism

Factor V Leiden mutation	Prothrombin gene mutation 20210A
Protein S or C deficiency	Antithrombin III deficiency
Hyperhomocysteinemia	

Clinical Presentation of Pulmonary Embolism

Acute PE may variably present with symptoms ranging from mild acute, unexplained dyspnea to sustained shock. On occasion, the patient may be asymptomatic or have relatively nonspecific symptoms and be diagnosed only by imaging procedures performed for other purposes. In the **Prospective Investigation of Pulmonary Embolism Diagnosis (PIOPED)** study of patients with documented PE, dyspnea was present in 73% of cases and pleuritic chest pain in 66%, whereas hemoptysis occurred in only 13% of patients. Thus, the classic triad of the sudden onset of dyspnea, pleuritic chest pain, and hemoptysis actually occurs in a minority of cases. Dyspnea is thought to result from reflex bronchoconstriction secondary to release of endogenous mediators as well as increased pulmonary artery pressure, reduced pulmonary compliance because of surfactant depletion, and stimulation of pulmonary C-fibers (Chaps. 5, 6, 10, and 11). In patients with large thromboemboli or preexisting pulmonary comorbidities, right ventricular strain may furthermore be contributory to the sensation of dyspnea. **Hemoptysis** is more typically noted with pulmonary infarction but may also result from transmission of systemic arterial pressure to the pulmonary microvasculature via bronchopulmonary anastomoses, with subsequent capillary disruption. Alternatively, hemoptysis may reflect hemorrhagic pulmonary edema from surfactant depletion or neutrophil-associated capillary injury (Chaps. 10 and 28).

Regarding signs in acute PE, tachypnea that is characterized by a respiratory f >20 breaths/min is observed in 70% of patients, with crackles noted in 51% (Chap. 14). Cardiovascular manifestations are less common, with tachycardia characterized by a HR >100 beats/min observed in 30%, an S_4 gallop rhythm in 24%, and an accentuated pulmonic

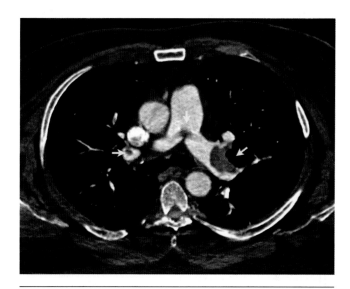

FIGURE 27.2 Contrast CT angiogram of the chest showing multiple intravascular filling defects (yellow arrows) in the left and right pulmonary artery branches secondary to obstruction by thromboembolic material.

component of the second heart sound in 23%. At least 70% of patients with PE do not have leg symptoms or signs at the time of diagnosis, as noted in the clinical vignette above. On the other hand, asymptomatic PE occurs in up to one-half of patients with leg DVT. Overall, the important point to be noted is that these discussed symptoms and signs are neither sensitive nor specific, and thus can be found both in patients with PE and without PE in conjunction with other cardiopulmonary conditions. Therefore, an imaging evaluation is always necessary to diagnose or exclude PE.

Differential Diagnosis

Considering that symptoms and signs in PE are frequently nonspecific, other diagnoses must be evaluated (Table 27.3). Chest radiography is useful in diagnosing pneumonia, pleural effusions, pneumothorax, or pulmonary edema of cardiogenic or noncardiogenic origin, all of which can present with dyspnea or chest pain. Myocardial ischemia may present with acute chest pain or pressure associated with dyspnea. Also, based on prior clinical history, exacerbations of asthma or COPD, gastroesophageal reflux disease, and esophageal dysmotility are differential diagnostic possibilities.

Natural History of Venous Thromboemboli

As noted earlier, the lungs are the most common target organ for intravascular emboli because the entire cardiac output passes through the pulmonary vasculature each minute. In **massive pulmonary thromboembolism** that causes **sudden death**, the pulmonary artery trunk and often the main pulmonary arteries are blocked by large thromboemboli. Even so, obstruction of a single pulmonary artery may still be fatal when recurrent previous bouts of VTE have occluded multiple pulmonary arterial branches. In shape and size, thromboemboli conform to their veins of origin in the form of **intravascular casts**. In many instances, they are V-shaped or Y-shaped when their source was confluent deep veins. This may be one reason that in massive PE, large emboli do not always completely occlude pulmonary blood flow. Moreover, intravascular thromboemboli are often retained at the bifurcation

of the pulmonary trunk or at more distal points of ramification within the pulmonary vasculature. Often by impacting at a bifurcation, a **saddle thromboembolus** is prevented from completely occluding the vessels involved, thereby avoiding sudden death (Chap. 26).

If a patient survives the acute thromboembolic episode associated with PE, many clots will be removed by thrombolysis, such that 60%-80% of these clots disappear within weeks or months. Remaining thromboemboli become adherent to the pulmonary arterial wall, undergo organization, and are converted into fibrous masses which may occupy much of the lumen of the main pulmonary arteries and its branches. Clot retraction and/or recanalization of the vessels occur subsequently. Remnants of the original thromboembolus may manifest as fibrous septa or networks, with so-called bands and webs visible within the affected pulmonary vessels (Chap. 26).

Infarction of lung tissue following an acute PE is more likely to occur when insufficiency develops in the **bronchial arterial circulation** in addition to the peripheral pulmonary arterial thromboembolic obstruction. This scenario may result from pulmonary vascular congestion of the lungs, particularly in association with reductions in Q̇ accompanying congestive heart failure (Chap. 28). Importantly, thromboembolic damage to the pulmonary endothelium may produce lung hemorrhage with or without infarction. Hemorrhagic pulmonary infarctions often occur in multiple pulmonary vascular segments, and these like thromboemboli themselves, are seen more often in lower than in upper lobes. Such hemorrhagic pulmonary infarctions are classically wedge-shaped and bordering the pleura, with their apices directionally adjacent to the thromboembolic obstruction. The **pleuritic chest pain** that typically accompanies pulmonary infarction is caused by inflammation of the visceral and parietal pleura, and may occasionally be accompanied by the presence of a **pleural friction rub** (Chap. 14).

Pathophysiology of PE

Life-threatening pulmonary thromboemboli may be caused by a single, massive thromboembolus in a person with otherwise normal cardiopulmonary physiology, or they may result from discrete or recurrent submassive thromboemboli in a subject with abnormal underlying physiology. Acute thromboembolism of the pulmonary circulation has two principal pathophysiological effects, being cardiovascular and pulmonary.

1. **Cardiovascular Effects**

The main pathophysiologic effects of pulmonary thromboembolism depend upon: (a) the magnitude and extent of the embolic obstruction; (b) the preexisting reserve of the patient's pulmonary vasculature; and (c) secondary effects on the pulmonary vasculature caused by the process of embolization. The resulting decrease in total cross-sectional area of the pulmonary arterial tree, coupled with acute increases in the resistance to right ventricular outflow and humoral mediator release, determine the severity of hemodynamic consequences. Notably, patients without prior cardiopulmonary disease can tolerate maximal acute elevations in mean

Table **27.3** **Differential diagnosis of acute pulmonary embolism**

Pneumonia	Pneumothorax	Pleural effusion
Pulmonary edema	Asthma exacerbation	COPD exacerbation
Myocardial infarction	Congestive heart failure	Acute pericarditis
Esophageal dysmotility	Gastroesophageal reflux disease	

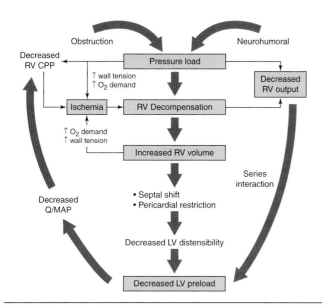

FIGURE 27.3 Pathophysiological interactions during hemodynamically significant PE. Here, CPP represents coronary perfusion pressure. *Adapted from Wood et al.* Major pulmonary embolism: review of a pathophysiological approach to the golden hour of hemodynamically significant pulmonary embolism. Chest. *2002;121:877-905.*

P_{PA} of ~40 mm Hg. This increased resistance to pulmonary blood flow, accompanied by elevated P_{PA} and right systolic ventricular pressure following severe thromboembolism, in turn lead to acute failure of the right ventricular pump. Additionally, **ventricular septal bowing** that alters left ventricular performance decreases cardiac output and thus systemic BP and coronary blood flow that may be lethal (Fig. 27.3). In fact, loss of consciousness (**syncope**) from reduced cerebral blood flow in this setting, with or without accompanying seizures, occurs in approximately 15% of patients with massive PE.

Secondary effects of pulmonary thromboembolism on the pulmonary vasculature may include reflex, humoral, or other reactive forms of vasoconstriction. Following PE, potent pulmonary vasoconstrictive agents like **5-hydroxytryptamine** and **thromboxane A$_2$** may be released during platelet activation, thus further diminishing vascular reserve in the presence of prior cardiac or pulmonary disease. In such circumstances, even relatively small thromboemboli may produce significant increases in PVR that lead to right ventricular failure. Interestingly, emboli of air, amniotic fluid, and fat have been theorized to produce more significant hemodynamic effects than expected based on size alone. It is likely their secondary effects on activation of intravascular coagulation and release of humoral substances potentiate their obstructive effects.

2. **Pulmonary Effects**
   a. **Pulmonary Gas Exchange.** Sudden interruption of the pulmonary artery blood flow to a region of lung acutely leads to ventilated but nonperfused lung units, thereby increasing V_D and the V_D/V_T ratio (Chaps. 6 and 8). Thus, the main abnormalities associated with PE are reductions in P_aO_2 and in P_aCO_2 that reflect the elevated V_D/V_T ratio and ultimately yield a widened $(A - a)P_{O_2}$ gradient (Chaps. 9 and 12).

   b. **Hypoxia.** Although arterial hypoxemia can occur in acute PE, the underlying reasons are unclear. Proposed mechanisms include: (1) $\dot{V}_A/\dot{Q}$ mismatch; (2) ventilation of nonperfused lung units, that is, a rise in $\dot{V}_D$; (3) arteriovenous shunting within the lung or heart; and (4) a reduced $\dot{Q}$. Perfusion of unventilated lung may be due to opening of preexistent pulmonary arteriovenous anastomoses from elevated pulmonary artery pressures. Alternatively, development of areas of atelectasis distal to the embolic obstruction of the pulmonary vascular bed may be induced by loss of surfactant and hemorrhage. Moreover, increases in P_{PA} due to PE may additionally shunt blood from the right atrium directly into the left atrium across a patent foramen ovale (PFO) (Chap. 39). In most cases, such mechanisms are probably acting together, with the relative importance of each dependent on underlying pulmonary disease, the degree of thromboembolic obstruction, the extent of reduced cardiac output, and the development of alveolar collapse, edema, or hemorrhage. Importantly, P_aO_2 is normal in up to 10% of patients diagnosed with PE, and thus a physician should not exclude consideration of PE based upon P_aO_2 alone.

   c. **Hypocapnia.** Arterial hypocapnia and respiratory alkalosis are commonly seen in patients with acute PE due to their hyperventilation. However, these are nonspecific findings in that they can be found in many other forms of respiratory disease as well. In a retrospective study of 78 patients with documented PE, an increased $(A - a) P_{O_2}$ gradient or hypocapnia was found in 77 patients despite no other known cardiopulmonary disease. These data suggest that the combination of a normal $(A - a) P_{O_2}$ gradient and a normal P_aCO_2 make the diagnosis of PE less likely.

Clinical Probability Model

The *a priori* **clinical probability of PE**, determined by evaluating the patient and assessing risk factors, is important in interpreting the results of a **ventilation/perfusion (V/Q)** lung scan. In the PIOPED study, 67% of patients with a high clinical probability of PE based upon underlying risk factors plus a clinical presentation consistent with PE and no apparent alternate diagnoses, were demonstrated to indeed have PE. Unfortunately, many evaluated patients will fall within an **intermediate probability** category. An algorithm to establish the clinical probability of PE is shown in Table 27.4. However, clinical probability alone is insufficient to definitively establish or exclude PE. Rather, diagnostic imaging is always necessary.

Laboratory Evaluation in Patients Suspected of Pulmonary Embolism

As noted earlier, measuring **arterial blood gases (ABGs)** may reveal hypoxemia, hypocapnia, and respiratory alkalosis. Rarely, hypercapnia is observed when massive PE occurs in the setting of respiratory failure or shock. Although an increased

Table **27.4** Determining the clinical probability of PE

High clinical probability (60%-70%)
Clinical presentation is consistent with PE
Known risk factor for PE is present
An alternate diagnosis is not apparent (eg, pneumonia, congestive heart failure)
Low clinical probability (10%)
No identifiable risk factors
Presence of an alternate diagnosis to explain the pulmonary findings
Intermediate probability (20%-30%)
All other patients

(A − a) Po_2 is frequently seen, the prospective PIOPED trial found that 8%-23% of patients with PE that was confirmed by angiography had normal (A − a) Po_2 gradients, and 7% of all patients with confirmed PE had completely normal ABG results.

D-dimer is the proteolytic degradation product of cross-linked fibrin. Circulating levels of D-dimer are typically elevated in patients with acute VTE, but elevated [D-dimer] occurs in many other conditions including liver disease, surgery, malignancy, infections, and increasing age. Even so, the **negative predictive value** of a D-dimer determination is approximately 94% (see Chap. 14). Thus, a positive D-dimer test result is not helpful in establishing a diagnosis of VTE, while a negative D-dimer result is useful in excluding the diagnosis of VTE in patients with low or intermediate pretest

clinical probability (Table 27.4). Furthermore, D-dimer testing is of limited utility in the diagnostic evaluation of patients who have chronic (recurrent) pulmonary thromboembolism.

▶▶ CLINICAL CORRELATION 27.2

The D-dimer assay is of limited value in patients with a high clinical probability of PE. The specificity of an increased D-dimer level is reduced in patients with malignancy, pregnant women, and hospitalized and elderly patients. Thus, in most hospitalized patients obtaining a D-dimer has limited utility when PE is suspected. Conversely, in those hemodynamically stable patients with a low or intermediate clinical probability of PE, a normal [D-dimer] as measured by sensitive ELISA usually avoids unnecessary further investigation.

Elevations of circulating **brain natriuretic peptide** (**BNP**) as a marker of ventricular stretch, and blood levels of cardiac **troponins** indicative of myocyte death, have been shown to correlate with the presence of right ventricular overload. As such they reflect a greater risk of adverse outcomes when elevated in patients with PE, notably including respiratory failure and death.

The standard **electrocardiogram** (ECG) is neither sensitive nor specific for PE. Most often it will show sinus tachycardia accompanied by nonspecific ST segment and T wave changes. Other findings may include an incomplete right bundle branch block, and a S1, Q3, T3 pattern (ie, a deep "S" wave in lead I, "Q" wave in lead III accompanied by "T" wave inversion) representing an electrocardiographic right ventricular strain pattern or cor pulmonale (Fig. 27.4).

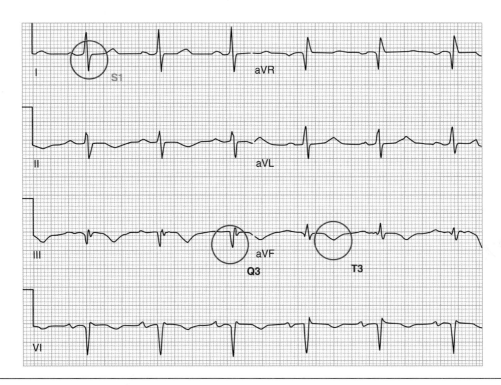

FIGURE 27.4 ECG depicting a S1, Q3, T3 pattern in a patient with PE that is suggestive of right ventricular strain.

Chest radiography in patients with PE may reveal unilateral atelectasis, abnormalities of lung parenchyma, and/or pleural effusions (Chap. 15). Less frequent abnormalities on the AP x-ray include **Westermark sign**, which is asymmetry of lung markings due to absence of perfusion distal to a clot, and a **Hampton hump** describing a pleural-based wedge-shaped opacity due to pulmonary infarction. Unfortunately, these findings on chest x-ray are not diagnostic solely of PE, while chest CT angiography has superior sensitivity for these findings (Chap. 15).

Diagnostic Imaging for Acute and Chronic Pulmonary Embolism

Helical Computed Tomographic Angiography

Technical advancements have led to the growing use of helical (spiral) CT angiograms for evaluating patients with suspected PE. The recent PIOPED-II study examined **four-detector CT angiography** in 824 patients who were suspected of having PE. Among 773 patients in this cohort with interpretable CT angiograms, the overall sensitivity and specificity of this technique were 83% and 96%, respectively. In addition to the technique's ability to directly visualize intravascular thromboemboli (Fig. 27.5), lung parenchymal abnormalities can be detected that might otherwise account for a patient's dyspnea and other cardiopulmonary symptoms if no thromboemboli are visualized.

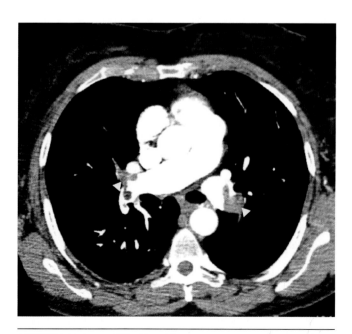

FIGURE 27.5 A contrast CT angiogram of the chest showing multiple filing defects (arrowheads) in the left and the right pulmonary arteries secondary to obstruction by thromboembolic material.

Despite this diagnostic utility, there are drawbacks to the use of helical CT angiography in establishing or excluding PE. First, it requires the use of intravenous contrast material that is problematic to administer in patients with renal dysfunction or to those with contrast allergy. Second, the procedure carries a higher radiation exposure than a V/Q scan, and may miss subsegmental PE, whose incidence varies between 5% and 30% across different studies. Third, such a CT scan requires the patient to perform a breath-hold for 15-25 seconds, and any motion artifact due to a patient's inability to hold their breath causes suboptimal visualization of segmental arteries. Importantly, a negative helical CT angiographic study does not definitively exclude PE in those patients with high clinical probability (Table 27.4) since ~5% of this cohort will still have a PE. Likewise, there remains a 10% chance that high-probability patients have underlying PE when a "technically unsatisfactory" CT has been achieved.

Ventilation/Perfusion Scan

Owing to the improving performance of routine spiral CT at detecting an acute PE, ventilation/perfusion (V/Q) lung scanning is being performed less often but remains a valuable diagnostic test. The perfusion scan utilizes human albumin macroaggregates or microspheres labeled with ^{99}Tc. Once injected intravenously, the aggregates or microspheres lodge in pulmonary arterioles and capillaries and give a map of the pulmonary circulation. For the ventilation scan, a single deep inhalation of ^{133}Xe to TLC is followed by a 20-second breath hold and then by 45 seconds of tidal breathing, followed by a washout period. Several images are taken during the V/Q scan, with the rationale that only the ventilation is normal in nonperfused areas, and thus a visual V/Q mismatch is diagnostic of PE (Fig. 27.6).

In this sense, a normal V/Q scan virtually excludes the diagnosis of PE, while a high probability V/Q scan is diagnostic of PE (>90%) in the presence of an intermediate-to-high clinical pretest probability. Conversely, additional diagnostic workup is still indicated in the presence of a low clinical pretest probability, since the V/Q scan can be falsely positive (45%-66%) in this clinical scenario. In any case, the results of most V/Q scans are graded as low (16%) or intermediate (41%) probabilities, and consequently most patients will need further workup to make a definitive clinical diagnosis.

Duplex Venous Ultrasonographic Studies of Lower Extremities

The non-invasive assessment by duplex venous ultrasonography with **Doppler flow studies** for DVT may be helpful in evaluating the many patients who will remain with intermediate clinical and V/Q scan probabilities for PE. This imaging modality carries a sensitivity and specificity of 89% and 100%, respectively. However, it is less sensitive (38%) in high-risk but asymptomatic patients. The rationale for performing venous Doppler studies of the lower extremities is that if a proximal DVT is diagnosed, anticoagulation is indicated just as if the

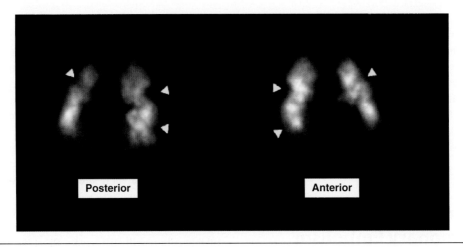

FIGURE 27.6 Perfusion images from a V/Q scan. Arrowheads point to mismatched perfusion defects that are consistent with subsegmental emboli.

patient had a documented PE. Given this situation, a single negative leg duplex venous ultrasonographic study does not rule out the possibility of a subsequent DVT, and consequently a repeat study in 1 week is recommended for high-risk patients.

Pulmonary Angiography

Pulmonary angiography remains the gold standard for the diagnosis of PE, and represents an important test for the evaluation of chronic thromboembolic disease. A properly performed pulmonary angiogram has a sensitivity and specificity for acute PE of >95%. The diagnosis is based on visually confirmed pulmonary artery occlusion or presence of intraluminal filing defects (Fig. 27.7). Other suggestive findings include

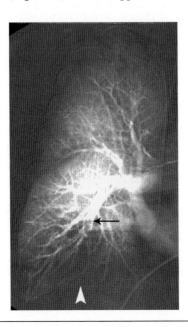

FIGURE 27.7 Pulmonary angiogram of the right lung showing an acute pulmonary embolism in a 78-year-old woman (arrow). The arrowhead points to the oligemic lung fields. *Adapted from Wittram et al: Acute and chronic pulmonary emboli: angiography-CT correlation Am J Roentgenol. Jun;186(6 Suppl 2):S421-9, 2006.*

asymmetrical blood flow, slow filling of the artery, and abrupt arterial cutoff.

A negative pulmonary angiogram with magnification excludes clinically relevant PE. Properly performed, the mortality of the procedure is extremely low (<0.5%) and morbidity occurs in about 5% of patients. Those events relate primarily to complications from catheter insertion, arrhythmias, hypotension, and reaction to contrast materials, among other factors.

Risk Stratification in Patients with Known or Suspected PE

Risk stratification should be performed promptly in patients with suspected acute PE according to the risk of adverse outcomes. In this context, sustained shock identifies patients at high risk for such an adverse outcome (Fig. 27.8). Likewise, echo findings of RV dysfunction, hypokinesis, and dilatation in hemodynamically stable patients, ventricular septal bowing, and CT evidence of RV dysfunction, have all been associated with increased short-term mortality. Furthermore, plasma biomarkers of myocardial dysfunction or injury including elevated [BNP] and [troponin] may be useful for risk stratification. Markers of RV dysfunction and injury have a high negative predictive value; therefore, the absence of RV dysfunction plus a normal [troponin] help to identify patients who may be eligible for early hospital discharge.

Treatment of Patients with PE

The clinical aims of current therapies for PE are six-fold: (1) reduction of mortality; (2) improvement in pulmonary gas exchange; (3) stabilization of circulatory abnormalities; (4) decrease in obstruction of the pulmonary vascular bed; (5) inhibition of thrombus extension; and (6) prevention of recurrences. An acute PE requires initial short-term therapy with a rapid-onset anticoagulant, followed by therapy with a

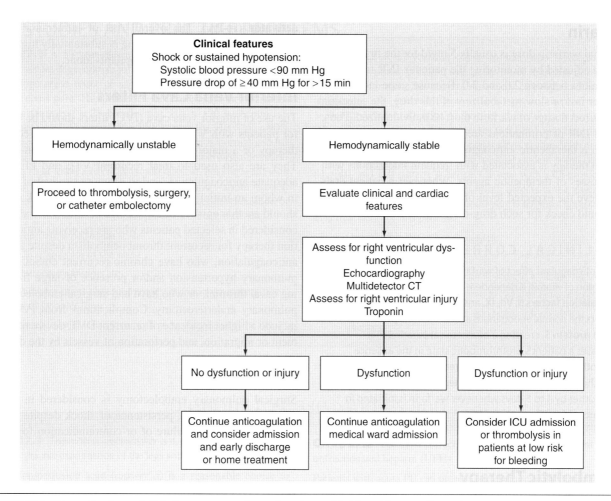

FIGURE 27.8 Risk stratification and clinical management of a confirmed acute PE. *Adapted from Agnelli G and Becattini C:* Acute Pulmonary Embolism, *N Engl J Med. Jul;363(3):266-274, 2010.*

vitamin K antagonist for at least 3 months. In patients at high risk for recurrence, a more extended duration of therapy is warranted. The patient should be risk-stratified promptly at presentation to determine optimal pharmacological therapy. As shown in Fig. 27.8, hemodynamic stability is central to determining the treatment algorithm for each patient.

Anticoagulation Therapies in Treating PE

Therapy is usually begun with IV administration of **unfractionated heparin (UFH)** or subcutaneous dosing with **low molecular weight heparin (LMWH)**. Co-administration overlap of either of these two agents with an oral vitamin K antagonist such as **warfarin** over a period of 5 days is recommended. The overall goal is to keep an appropriate level of anticoagulation at all times.

Low Molecular Weight Heparins

Treatment with LMWH has several advantages over unfractionated heparin: (1) convenient once or twice daily dosing;

(2) a fixed dose is administered; (3) laboratory monitoring is not usually necessary; (4) it is less likely to induce thrombocytopenia; and (5) it can be used instead of heparin in DVT and stable patients with PE. The only LMWH formulation approved in the United States is **enoxaparin**. As noted above, LMWH should be overlapped with warfarin for at least 5 days, and until the patient's **international normalized ratio (INR)** for the **prothrombin time (PT)** is within the therapeutic range of 2.0-3.0 for two consecutive days.

Unfractionated Heparin

Heparin is given according to a weight-based nomogram as an initial IV bolus of 80 U/kg followed by a continuous IV infusion of 18 U/kg/h. The patient's aPTT should be monitored every 6 hours and should be kept at 1.5-2.5 times that of the laboratory's control value. It is essential that the patient be well anticoagulated within the first 24 hours of presentation. The main side effects of UFH therapy include bleeding, thrombocytopenia, and osteoporosis. In any patient who develops thrombocytopenia while on heparin, **heparin-induced thrombocytopenia (HIT)** should be considered.

Chapter **28**

Acute Lung Injury and the Acute Respiratory Distress Syndrome: Pathophysiology and Treatment

GEORGE M. MATUSCHAK, MD AND
ANDREW J. LECHNER, PhD

Learning Objectives

- The student will be able to describe the definition, prevalence, and impact of ALI and ARDS in multidisciplinary critical care medicine.

- The student will be able to list and define the direct and indirect risk factors for ALI/ARDS, and distinguish the clinical features of ALI and ARDS.

- The student will be able to summarize the initiating pathophysiology of ALI/ARDS, and factors that perpetuate or are associated with its nonresolution, especially ventilator-associated lung injury.

- The student will be able to explain and defend current guidelines for the treatment and supportive care of patients with ALI/ARDS.

Introduction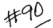

Acute lung injury (**ALI**) and the **acute respiratory distress syndrome** (**ARDS**) represent a spectrum of respiratory failure of rapid onset characterized by diffuse, bilateral lung injury and severe hypoxemia that are caused by **noncardiogenic pulmonary edema**. ALI/ARDS can affect patients of any age or preexisting condition, although both predispose to worse outcomes. Respiratory failure may be initiated by pulmonary or extrapulmonary insults that increase alveolar epithelial and endothelial permeability, flood alveoli, and reduce lung compliance in a pattern reflecting an acute restrictive lung disease. Despite numerous prospective, double-blind clinical trials in patients with ALI/ARDS, the only treatment that improves survival is mechanical ventilation using a **lung protective strategy** in which tidal volume V_T is carefully titrated to ~6 mL/kg of predicted body weight. **Positive end-expiratory pressure** (**PEEP**) ventilation is useful for **alveolar recruitment** in lungs that will be prone to **atelectasis**. Clinical vigilance must be comprehensive and anticipatory to guard against development of ventilator-associated pneumonia or worsened ALI. Although mortality can exceed 50%, survivors have a good prognosis for recovery of lung function.

General Features of ALI/ARDS

ALI and ARDS affect over 190,000 patients annually in the United States and cause 75,000 deaths. They occur rapidly and show diffuse, bilateral lung injury readily evident by x-ray or CT. Patients exhibit severe hypoxemia despite use of supplemental O_2, and are considered emblematic of a noncardiogenic pulmonary edema with low alveolar ventilation/perfusion ratios $(\dot{V}_A/\dot{Q})$ and abnormal physiological shunting of O_2. Such acute respiratory failure usually occurs with neutrophil (PMN)-mediated lung inflammation. Pathological increases in the permeability of alveolar epithelial and endothelial cells lead to dyspnea, tachypnea, and arterial hypoxemia. These permeability defects increase efflux of proteins and fluids from blood into the alveolar interstitium and airspaces, while alveolar liquid clearance mechanisms are impaired that normally would resolve the edema. Consequently, alveolar O_2 exchange deteriorates.

ALI/ARDS is complex and multiphasic. The initiating factors that may cause early lung dysfunction may differ from those that perpetuate, complicate, or delay its resolution. ALI/ARDS can be caused by **pulmonary-specific mechanisms**, notably severe pneumonia, aspiration of gastric contents, embolism of fat, air, or amniotic fluid, chest trauma, near-drowning, and inhalation of noxious gases. ALI/ARDS can also occur due to **systemic conditions**, notably bacteremic sepsis, peritonitis, pancreatitis, hemorrhagic shock, burns, massive transfusions, and drug overdoses. Such indirect factors reflect pulmonary manifestations of acute systemic inflammation and generalized endothelial injury that may involve many organ systems. Approximately 15% of deaths from ALI/ARDS are due to progressive respiratory failure with intractable hypoxemia, increased dead space ventilation, and hypercarbia. The main cause underlying death in ALI/ARDS (~75% patients) is the **multiple organ dysfunction syndrome** (**MODS**) involving the heart, kidneys, coagulation system, and liver as well as lung.

Clinical Definitions of ALI/ARDS

In 1994, the American-European Consensus Conference on ARDS issued definitions that have been widely adopted by clinicians and researchers. These include:

1. **Acute lung injury**. A syndrome of acute and persistent lung inflammation with increased vascular permeability characterized by:
   a. *acute onset* (within days of exposure to predisposing direct or indirect causes);
   b. *diffuse bilateral infiltrates* on x-ray consistent with noncardiogenic edema;
   c. $\mathbf{P_aO_2/F_IO_2}$ ≤*300 mm Hg*, regardless of the level of PEEP during mechanical ventilation. The ratio P_aO_2/F_IO_2 estimates lung oxygenation efficiency across the range of supplemental O_2 provided to patients. P_aO_2 is measured in mm Hg and F_IO_2 is a decimal between 0.00 and 1.00. For example, in a subject with $P_aO_2 = 100$ mm Hg on room air ($F_IO_2 = 0.21$), the $P_aO_2/F_IO_2 = 100/0.21 = 476$ mm Hg;
   d. *no clinical evidence of left-sided heart failure or elevated left atrial pressure*, that is, an elevated P_{PW} if a **pulmonary artery catheter (PAC)** had been placed, as in congestive heart failure (Fig. 28.1). A relatively normal heart size by x-ray supports the clinical absence of left ventricular failure as the explanation for pulmonary edema. If a PAC is in use, the wedge pressure is ≤18 mm Hg. Clinical evidence of left heart failure includes systolic left ventricular (LV) dysfunction, plus appropriate physical findings, such as LV S_3 gallop and peripheral edema, especially when supported by LV dilation or reduced ejection fraction by echocardiography or catheterization, or enlarged cardiac silhouette plus pleural effusions.

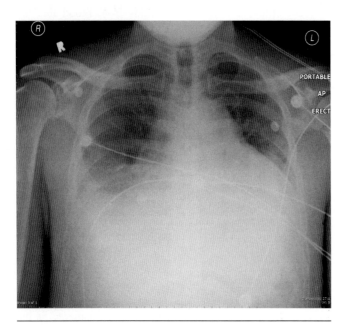

FIGURE 28.1 A chest radiograph showing cardiomegaly and bilateral pleural effusions, findings that are compatible with elevated left atrial pressure, interstitial cardiogenic edema, and LV systolic dysfunction as seen in congestive heart failure.

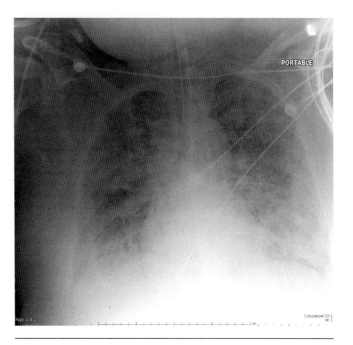

FIGURE 28.2 A chest x-ray showing diffuse, bilateral pulmonary infiltrates in all lung quadrants (acute air-space disease) typical of ALI/ARDS. The costophrenic angles are relatively clear, indicating the absence of pleural effusions.

2. **Acute respiratory distress syndrome**. A more severe physiological expression of ALI, at the further end of a spectrum of evolving lung injury characterized by:
   a. *acute onset*;
   b. *diffuse bilateral infiltrates* on x-ray consistent with pulmonary edema;
   c. $\mathbf{P_aO_2/F_IO_2}$ ≤*200 mm Hg*;
   d. *no evidence of left-sided heart failure*, including normal heart size on x-ray (Fig. 28.2). If a PAC is used, the measured P_{PW} is ≤18 mm Hg.

Pathophysiology of ALI/ARDS

Normal lung function requires dry, open alveoli overlying perfused capillaries with intact gas exchange and a normal work of breathing. It requires coordinated interaction of several key physiological processes plus appropriate lung immune and inflammatory responses. Three interrelated pathophysiologic abnormalities typify events that cause or precipitate ALI/ARDS.

1. **Increased microvascular permeability (noncardiogenic pulmonary edema)**

Normal pulmonary capillaries are selectively permeable, with serum proteins confined to intravascular spaces, while smaller molecules and water cross endothelial membranes by hydrostatic and osmotic forces. As discussed in Chap. 7, the **Starling's equation** describes forces directing fluid movement between the vessels and the interstitium:

$$F = K \cdot [(P_{MV} - P_{PMV}) - \sigma\,(\pi_{MV} - \pi_{PMV})]$$

where: F = net transvascular fluid movement

K = filtration coefficient for permeability of the capillary endothelium

P_{MV} = hydrostatic pressure within microvessels

P_{PMV} = hydrostatic pressure in the perimicrovascular space

σ = protein reflection coefficient, normally 1.0 (arbitrary units)

π_{MV} = protein colloid osmotic pressure in the circulation

π_{PMV} = protein colloid osmotic pressure in the perimicrovascular space

At least four mechanisms promote fluid retention in capillaries to prevent interstitial edema and alveolar flooding. First, airspace liquid is cleared by apical Na^+ transporters in alveolar epithelial cells. Second, larger plasma proteins like albumin maintain osmotic gradients favoring water reabsorption. Third, tight junctions between pulmonary endothelial cells prevent leakage. Fourth, interstitial lymphatics return alveolar fluid to the circulation. Abnormalities in Starling's forces during ALI/ARDS include:

a. Decreased σ during sepsis, causing larger proteins like albumin to enter the interstitium, so that protein-rich edema floods alveoli.

b. Reduced π_{MV} from excessive IV infusions and/or reduced acute phase protein synthesis, favoring increased transvascular fluid flux into distal airspaces.

c. Increased P_{MV} from IV fluids to treat hypovolemia, or decreased venous return due to increased intrathoracic pressures during positive-pressure ventilation.

d. Increased π_{PMV} from plasma proteins entering alveolar interstitium, or from loss of alveolar epithelial Na^+ transport, both retarding alveolar liquid clearance.

These cause gravitationally dependent alveolar edema, first evident in inferior lung zones of supine patients (Fig. 28.3), worsening $\dot{V}_A/\dot{Q}$ mismatch and reducing P_aO_2.

2. Alveolar instability and de-recruitment with decreased lung compliance: pathophysiology and potential for ventilator-associated lung injury

As described in Chap. 5, compliance quantifies changes in lung volumes (ΔV) that are caused by distending airway or intrapleural pressures (ΔP) as occur during spontaneous respiration. Compliance ($\Delta V/\Delta P$) is often reduced in ALI/ARDS, leading to alveolar instability and collapse when approaching end-expiratory pressures. This **de-recruitment** of formerly functioning alveoli results from several factors:

a. *Alveolar edema inactivates surfactant* as plasma proteins leak into airspaces.

b. *Edematous alveoli show increased surface tension*, and are prone to collapse (ie, they undergo **atelectasis**) during end-expiratory pauses in patients with ALI/ARDS. Such distal airspaces fail to expand cyclically during inspiration due to excessively high alveolar opening pressures (see Chaps. 5 and 6).

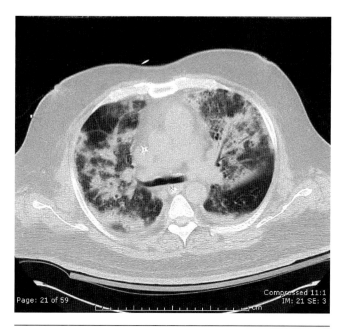

FIGURE 28.3 Computed tomographic (CT) scan of the chest (lung attenuation window) in a patient with severe ARDS due to bilateral *S. pneumoniae* pneumonia. Note extensive opacification of alveolar units and prominent air bronchograms, compared with the small residual area of normal, radiolucent (black)-appearing lung in the right upper and left lower portions of this image.

c. *Functional residual capacity (FRC) declines* in ALI/ARDS patients, who often breathe rapidly and shallowly to maximize their $\dot{V}_E$ while minimizing the work of breathing that would be required to expand their noncompliant or "stiff" lungs.

d. Superimposed mechanical **ventilation-associated lung injury** (**VALI**) may occur, especially at V_T's exceeding 10 mL/kg of predicted body weight (PBW) that were historically used to ventilate adults with ALI/ARDS.

When previously normal alveoli become atelectatic due to alveolar flooding and inflammatory exudates, mechanical ventilation of patients with high V_T's to sustain $\dot{V}_E$ is equivalent to forcing each positive-pressure inspiration into infant-sized lungs. At the same time, alveoli that are not yet edematous receive excessive ventilation that is redirected toward the open lung and away from atelectatic regions (Figs. 28.3 and 28.4). This dilemma sets the stage for three forms of VALI that are not mutually exclusive:

a. **barotrauma**: pressure-related lung injury

b. **volutrauma**: alveolar over-distention injury

c. **cyclical shear stress** from excessive tidal swings in alveolar diameters

3. Dysregulated and excessive acute lung inflammatory responses

ALI/ARDS reflects excessive inflammation in the alveolar interstitium and airspaces (Fig. 28.5), involving massive neutrophil influx due to upregulated adhesion molecules on PMNs and vascular endothelia. The inflammation is sustained

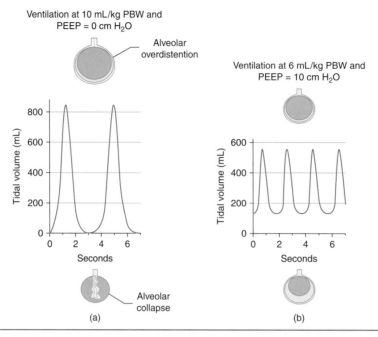

FIGURE 28.4 Effects on achieved tidal volumes in sedated patients using a conventional ventilation strategy of 10 mL/kg PBW without PEEP (a) versus the protective lung ventilation strategy of 6 mL/kg PBW and carefully adjusted PEEP (b).

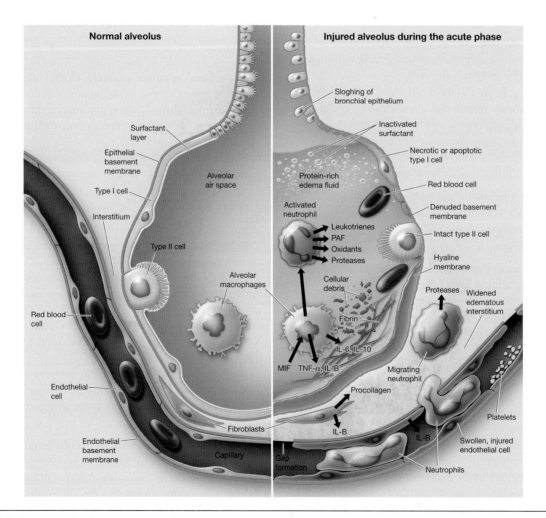

FIGURE 28.5 The normal alveolus versus the acutely injured alveolus in ALI/ARDS.

by additional chemotactic signals and host-derived mediators. As a result, PMNs in **bronchoalveolar lavage fluid** (**BALF**) may approach 50% of all cells recovered, versus ≤3% PMNs in BALF from healthy volunteers. Major inflammatory mediators in this acute phase include:

a. **cytokines**, notably TNF-α, IL-1β, IL-6, IL-8, IL-10, G-CSF, and GM-CSF;

b. **chemokines**, such as macrophage inhibitory factor and chemoattractant protein;

c. **arachidonic acid metabolites**, including prostanoids and leukotrienes;

d. **oxyradicals/oxidants**, including superoxide anion and peroxynitrite;

e. **proteases** that degrade alveolar structures and enhance inflammation;

f. **fibrin**, following activation of tissue factor and the coagulation system.

Together, these processes cause acute lung dysfunction, tachypnea with distress, declining P_aO_2 by blood gases or declining S_aO_2 by pulse oximetry, and chest radiographs or CT scans showing bilateral infiltrates. Of note, such infiltrates may be asymmetric in patients with coexisting chronic obstructive pulmonary disease. Thus progressively impaired gas exchange occurs, with $\dot{V}_A/\dot{Q}$ mismatch and physiological shunt causing hypoxemia. Additionally, physiological dead space may increase despite a constant $\dot{V}_E$, retarding CO_2 elimination. Ventilator-induced rises in intrathoracic pressure also inhibit venous return, with fewer alveoli perfused despite ongoing ventilation. In advanced cases of ALI/ARDS, CO_2 excretion falls and P_aCO_2 rises.

#91

▶▶CLINICAL CORRELATION 28.1

Transfusion-related acute lung injury (**TRALI**) is an important form of ALI/ARDS with similar clinical features but is temporally related to transfusion of blood products. TRALI is the leading cause of transfusion-related death in the United States. Patients affected with TRALI typically develop fever with cough, dyspnea, and hypoxemia within 6 hours of receiving red cells, platelets, or fresh frozen plasma.

Typical Presentation and Progression of ALI/ARDS

Despite these diverse precipitating factors, most ALI/ARDS patients follow similar clinical courses that are characterized initially by severe hypoxemia requiring prolonged mechanical ventilatory support (days to weeks). Patients generally progress through three pathologic stages (see Chap. 26). An initial **exudative stage** with diffuse alveolar damage gives way over the first week to a **proliferative stage** with resolving pulmonary edema, proliferating type II cells, squamous metaplasia, interstitial infiltration by myofibroblasts, and deposition of collagen. For unclear reasons, some patients progress to a third **fibrotic stage** with accelerated collagen deposition,

obliteration of normal lung architecture, diffuse fibrosis, and parenchymal cyst formation. This last subgroup accounts for most patients who die "of" ALI/ARDS with intractable hypoxemia and increasing dead space ventilation that require progressively higher F_IO_2 and the associated risk of lung O_2 toxicity. Prolonged ventilation with $F_IO_2 \geq 0.60$ is associated with increased inflammation and fibrosis.

The bedside **physical exam** usually reveals tachycardia, tachypnea, diffuse crackles over the chest, increased work of breathing, and frequent dependence on the accessory respiratory muscles (trapezius, scalene, sternocleidomastoid, and pectoralis). Typical **laboratory findings** in ALI/ARDS are nonspecific and may include **leukocytosis**, evidence of **disseminated intravascular coagulation** (**DIC**), and **lactic acidosis**. Arterial blood gases usually show acute respiratory alkalosis, reduced S_aO_2 (<90%), decreased P_aO_2/F_IO_2 ratio, and severe hypoxemia that collectively reflect right-to-left shunt physiology. **Chest radiographic findings**, while distinctive, are also seen in diffuse lung hemorrhage and acute interstitial edema. Importantly, ALI/ARDS is a clinical syndrome, not a specific disease. It is always caused by underlying conditions that must be diagnosed and treated, in addition to the respiratory failure.

As to the subsequent course in such patients, oxygenation may improve over the first few days as edema resolves. Nevertheless, patients can remain ventilator-dependent due to continued hypoxemia, high $\dot{V}_E$ requirements, and poor lung compliance. Lung radiographic densities become less opaque as edema resolves, but interstitial infiltrates may persist. In the exudative and proliferative phases, lung flooding may resolve but patients continue to exhibit increased dead space ventilation seen as an increased $\dot{V}_E$ with normal or elevated P_aCO_2. Oxygenation may respond favorably to PEEP by reversing atelectasis (Fig. 28.4), or remain problematic because of surfactant dysfunction. Organizing fibrosis may occur in the proliferative phase, causing increased airway pressures, pulmonary hypertension, and honeycomb appearances on x-ray.

Complications in ALI/ARDS Patients

Serious complications can occur daily in ICU patients, and those with ALI/ARDS and coexisting MODS are particularly prone to deep venous thrombosis, pulmonary thromboembolism, gastrointestinal bleeding, malnutrition, untoward effects from sedative and neuromuscular blocking medications, and superimposed catheter-related infections. In addition, several lung-specific complications may develop, most especially ventilation-related trauma, shear stress injury, and VALI already described.

In addition, nosocomial **ventilator-associated pneumonia** (**VAP**) in mechanically ventilated patients is a feared complication, with mortality rates of up to 50%. The "attributable mortality" for VAP is 33%-50%, despite aggressive supportive care and targeted antimicrobial therapy in affected patients. VAP develops in 9%-27% of ventilated patients, and the risk of VAP increases 1%-3% per day of intubation. Late-onset VAP, developing after ≥5 days of intubation and ventilation, is frequently caused by multiple drug resistant (MDR) organisms such as methicillin-resistant *Staphylococcus aureus*, *Pseudomonas aeruginosa*, or *Acinetobacter baumannii*. VAP is clinically diagnosed by the development of new fever, increased purulent secretions from the endotracheal tube, and new or worsening infiltrates seen on chest x-rays.

The manner in which ALI/ARDS patients are mechanically ventilated has immediate consequences on oxygenation, but also impacts acute inflammatory responses within alveoli. Thus, how such diffusely injured lungs are ventilated by positive-pressure ventilation may: (1) augment inflammatory injury by superimposing additive pressure- or volume-related trauma; (2) delay resolution of lung injury; or (3) enhance recovery of pulmonary gas exchange, lung cell function, and non-pulmonary organ homeostasis.

> ▶▶ CLINICAL CORRELATION 28.2

The hypoxemia, hypotension, and deteriorating lung compliance of many ALI/ARDS patients may not be immediately apparent. In such a setting, **pneumothorax** can be difficult to visualize on bedside chest films obtained in the supine patient. Such occult pneumothoraces may enlarge in patients on positive pressure ventilation, compressing central veins and causing cardiogenic shock from diminished ventricular preload. Emergent needle decompression and tube thoracostomy are required when pneumothorax is detected in such a ventilated patient.

Definitive Treatment of ALI/ARDS

The first priority in patients with ALI/ARDS is to stabilize their abnormal gas exchange and hemodynamics, ideally to prevent hypoxic organ damage, respiratory muscle fatigue, increased work of breathing, and cardiopulmonary arrest. Rapid clinical assessment followed by transfer to an ICU is important. Most patients will require intubation and mechanical ventilation with a high initial F_IO_2 (commonly 1.00) to relieve hypoxemia, and application of PEEP to increase their FRC. Diagnosing the underlying causes of ALI/ARDS also is critically important. For septic patients, aggressively seeking the cause is indicated (eg, pneumonia, catheter-related bacteremic sepsis, postsurgical abdominal abscess), since infections and purulence within closed spaces must be drained, and empiric broad-spectrum antimicrobial therapy begun quickly.

Given the increased vascular permeability in ALI/ARDS, the appropriate goals for fluid administration, volume status, and hemodynamic management will differ across patient categories. Administering sufficient IV fluids to perfuse nonpulmonary organs may aggravate alveolar edema and cause life-threatening hypoxemia. Similarly, aggressive diuresis may improve pulmonary gas exchange by lowering left atrial pressure and thus the gradient for alveolar flooding from leaky capillaries. Early initiation of supplemental nutrition within 72 hours of ICU admission, preferably by enteral route, is indicated and has been associated with improved outcomes in limited trials.

The Lung Protective Mechanical Ventilation Strategy

Historically, a tidal volume (V_T) of 12-15 mL/kg PBW was recommended in ALI/ARDS. However, it is now clear that a **low V_T lung protective strategy** reduces mortality and is the single most important evidence-based therapy that should be initiated in mechanically ventilated patients with ALI/ARDS. In 2000, the NIH ARDS Network published results of a randomized, controlled multicenter clinical trial in 861 patients. The trial compared a low V_T strategy (6 mL/kg and a plateau pressure <30 cm H_2O) with a higher V_T cohort (12 mL/kg, plateau pressure <50 cm H_2O). Plateau pressure, P_{PLAT} in vivo is that airway pressure during the brief pause after a mechanical inspiration ends and before the subsequent expiration begins (see Chap. 30). Measured P_{PLAT} in ventilated patients reflects the static distending pressure in the lungs when airflow (and thus, frictional resistance to airflow) is zero. As such, P_{PLAT} reflects lung compliance measured during a 0.5 second inspiratory hold in a relaxed, sedated patient. The chief therapeutic goal of minimizing VALI is achieved when P_{PLAT} is <30 cm H_2O.

In this ARDS Net Trial, in-hospital mortality was 40% among the 12 mL/kg group versus 31% in the 6 mL/kg group. This highly significant 22% reduction in mortality necessitated stopping the trial early for ethical reasons. With an absolute risk reduction of 9% using low V_T ventilation, one life is saved for every eleven ALI/ARDS patients treated by this modality. There were also more ventilator-free days, thereby decreasing the likelihood of VAP, as well as more organ failure-free days in patients in the low V_T group. The prescribed steps in the lung protective strategy to establish initial ventilator V_T and frequency (*f*) adjustments are the following:

a. Calculate the patient's **predicted body weight** (PBW);
b. Set initial V_T to 8 mL/kg PBW and ventilator mode to "Volume Assist-Control";
c. Decrease V_T to 7 mL/kg after 1-2 hours, then to 6 mL/kg PBW after another 1-2 hours;
d. Set *f* to maintain adequate V_E but <35 breaths/min to reduce VALI even if P_aCO_2 increases slightly reflecting mild hypoventilation (**permissive hypercapnia**);
e. Establish a P_{PLAT} goal of <30 cm H_2O;
f. Check P_{PLAT} with a 0.5 second inspiratory pause every 4 hours and after each change in PEEP or V_T.

> ▶▶ CLINICAL CORRELATION 28.3

Other Evidence-Based Approaches for Treating ALI/ARDS. Pulmonary artery catheters provide significant physiological data in ALI/ARDS patients, including wedge pressure, cardiac output, pulmonary arterial and right atrial pressures, **mixed-venous O_2 saturation, $S_{\bar{v}}O_2$,** and RV preload. However, a recent NIH trial comparing management guided by PAC versus a central venous catheter found no improvement in 60-day mortality or days until ventilator weaning. Furthermore, although ALI/ARDS is an inflammatory process and steroid medications have powerful anti-inflammatory properties, no clinical trial has shown significant benefit using methylprednisolone or other steroids to prevent or treat the lung inflammation of ALI/ARDS. Indeed, high dose methylprednisolone during the fibroproliferative stage of ARDS increased mortality at 60 and 180 days if begun >2 weeks after diagnosis.

Prognosis

Survival has improved for patients with ALI/ARDS, particularly since widespread institution of the lung protective strategy for mechanical ventilation. Overall mortality from ARDS uncomplicated by MODS remains 25%-35% despite improved ICU management, availability of new antimicrobial therapies, nutritional support, and other factors. However, mortality in patients with ALI/ARDS and MODS increases proportionately with the number of dysfunctional nonpulmonary organs, reaching 50%-75% with concurrent septic shock plus MODS. Thus, severe sepsis, septic shock, and MODS are more powerful predictors of survival than respiratory parameters per se.

Advanced age and preexisting liver dysfunction also connote a poor outcome.

It is difficult to predict outcome in a specific patient with ALI/ARDS based on initial severity of physiological impairments including oxygenation. Such findings do not reliably distinguish survivors from nonsurvivors, nor do the patient's initial respiratory compliance, radiographic findings, or required PEEP. However, failure to improve clinically over the first several days, particularly regarding oxygenation, predicts a complicated course and greater mortality risk. Long-term prognosis for recovery of lung function following ALI/ARDS is reasonably good with respect to lung function. Within six months after hospital discharge, spirometric lung volumes largely return to premorbid or predicted values, except in patients with preexisting lung disease. At one year after discharge, the commonest pulmonary physiological finding is mild to moderate reduction in the single-breath diffusion capacity for carbon monoxide, DL_{CO} (see Chap. 16). Exertional O_2 deoxygenation remains in perhaps 6% of survivors, reflecting persistent fibrotic remodeling that retards diffusive gas exchange in the distal airways and alveoli.

Suggested Readings

1. Bernard GR, Artigas A, Brigham KL, et al. for the American-European Consensus Conference on ARDS. Definitions, mechanisms, relevant outcomes, and clinical trial coordination. *Am J Respir Crit Care Med.* 1994;149:818-824. *As the title and publication date suggest, this landmark paper established workable and international guidelines for the recognition of ALI/ARDS that have stood the test of time.*

2. Ware LB, Matthay MA. The acute respiratory distress syndrome. *N Engl J Med.* 2000;342:1334-1349. *Among the many reviews of the subject, this one provides excellent overviews and anticipated the findings of several subsequent clinical trials.*

3. Rubenfeld GD, Herridge MS. Epidemiology and outcomes of acute lung injury. *Chest.* 2007;131:554-562. *A succinct update* on predisposing factors that worsen ALI and worsen 28-day mortality figures.

4. The ARDS Network. Ventilation with lower tidal volumes as compared with traditional tidal volumes for acute lung injury and the acute respiratory distress syndrome. *N Engl J Med.* 2000;342:1301-1308. *This paper reported the first, and still the only, evidence-based trial of an intervention that significantly improved outcome from ARDS.*

5. Tobin MJ. Advances in mechanical ventilation. *N Engl J Med.* 2001;344:1986-1996. *An excellent primer on the innovative strategies that work best in managing patients with intractable hypoxemia, including the role of permissive hypercapnia.*

CASE STUDIES AND PRACTICE PROBLEMS

CASE 28.1 A 59-year-old woman presents with shortness of breath that worsened in the past 24 hours. She is severely dyspneic and cannot complete a full sentence. Vitals include radial pulse = 116 beats/min and respiratory f = 40 breaths/min. Diffuse bilateral crackles are heard on posterior exam; a chest x-ray shows diffuse airspace disease. Which criteria would best distinguish between ARDS and congestive heart failure in this patient?

a. The subacute onset of her symptoms

b. A calculated P_aO_2/F_IO_2 ratio ≥250 in this woman

c. Bilateral infiltrates and a pulmonary wedge pressure of ≤18 mm Hg

d. An improved clinical profile following intubation and PEEP ventilation

e. Responsiveness to antibiotics against community-acquired pathogens

CASE 28.2 A 41-year-old man is hospitalized after attempting to synthesize methamphetamine. He was found unconscious in a room with strong ammonia fumes. A chest x-ray shows left upper lobe and right middle lobes infiltrates. Blood gases on 100% O_2 show $pH_a = 7.31$, $P_aCO_2 = 50$ mm Hg, $P_aO_2 = 180$ mm Hg. His status does not improve, and 72 hours later a repeat chest x-ray shows infiltrates in the left upper, left lower, right upper, and right middle lobes. What underlying lung pathophysiology is most likely involved?

a. Ammonia-enhanced reabsorption of alveolar fluid and protein

b. Excessive surfactant release with resultant alveolar instability

c. CNS depression, insufficient ventilation, and reduced P_AO_2

d. Alveolar overdistention causing increased functional residual capacity

e. Sloughed epithelium, endothelial cell injury, and surfactant inactivation

Solutions to Case Studies and Practice Problems

CASE 28.1 The most correct answer is c.

Regardless of how this patient's pulmonary complaint arose, the presence of bilateral infiltrates in the absence of a significantly elevated wedge pressure would be definitive of ARDS, while a $P_aO_2/F_IO_2 >250$ mm Hg in itself (*answer b*) would tend to exclude ARDS. She might indeed have community-acquired pneumonia that worsened overnight (*answer a*) and that would respond to antibiotics (*answer e*), but those issues do not in themselves rule out congestive heart failure (CHF). Since both ARDS and CHF patients can have pulmonary edema, each could develop atelectasis and thus respond favorably to mechanical ventilation with PEEP (*answer d*).

CASE 28.2 The most correct answer is e.

ALI and ARDS can originate from insults to either side of alveolar septa. In this case, ammonia fumes damaged first the delicate squamous epithelium covering most alveolar surfaces, and then the capillary endothelium as well. With such septal injury, plasma extravasating from the pulmonary capillaries will enter the airspaces. Such alveolar fluid is not easily reabsorbed if the epithelium is injured (*answer a*), and will degrade surfactant rather than enhance its secretion (*answer b*). Surfactant inactivation in turn will cause alveolar instability and not overdistention (*answer d*), with the resulting atelectasis spreading to even previously uninjured lung lobes. The systemic hypoxemia of ALI/ARDS certainly compromises non-pulmonary organs, including the central nervous system and/or respiratory muscle groups. Those failures would lead eventually to respiratory muscle fatigue and alveolar hypoventilation (*answer c*).

Chapter 29

Pathophysiology and Diseases of the Pleural Space

GEORGE M. MATUSCHAK, MD AND
ANDREW J. LECHNER, PhD

Introduction

Diseases of the pleural space are common in clinical medicine. One of the most frequent manifestations of pleural disease is a pleural effusion. Consequently, knowledge of the pathophysiological basis for disorders that culminate in pleural effusions is important for their timely diagnosis and proper treatment. Additional information regarding the laboratory evaluation of various types of pleural effusions is presented in Chap. 19.

Physiology of the Pleural Space

The pleural space is a low-pressure environment between the parietal pleura that covers the inner surface of the ribs and thoracic musculature, and the visceral pleura covering the lungs' external regions. These have a combined surface area of about 4,000 cm^2. The forces regulating pleural fluid formation by the parietal and visceral pleura are summarized by the **Starling's equation** (as established in Chaps. 7 and 19):

$$F = K \left[(P_{MV} - P_{PL}) - \sigma (\pi_{MV} - \pi_{PL}) \right]$$

where: F = pleural fluid flow
K = filtration coefficient, a function of the surface area and permeability of pleural microvessels
P_{MV} = pleural microvascular hydrostatic pressure
P_{PL} = pleural pressure
σ = the reflection coefficient for protein movement across the pleura
π_{MV} = colloid osmotic pressure in pleural microvessels
π_{PL} = colloid osmotic pressure in the pleural space

Notably, the protein reflection coefficient σ defines the barrier function of the pleural membranes, such that decreases in σ typified by inflammatory conditions correlate with increased permeability to protein (see also Chap. 28). The intravascular concentration of albumin (MW ≈ 65 KDa) is the primary determinant of serum colloid osmotic pressure.

The normal entry rate of pleural fluid into the pleural space in humans is considered to be approximately 0.5 mL/h or 12 mL/day, and this pleural fluid derives from microvascular filtration governed by Starling's forces across both the parietal pleura and visceral pleura. Although a degree of fluid reabsorption occurs within both the parietal and visceral pleura membranes, actual pleural fluid reabsorption from the pleural space itself occurs via **lymphatic stomata** in the parietal pleura (Fig. 29.1). Thus, at any time the total volume of pleural fluid in normal individuals is 0.1-0.2 mL/kg, or approximately 10-20 mL in a 70 kg subject. These parietal pleural lymphatic stomata are fenestrated openings in the mesothelial cell layer that average 10-12 μm in diameter, and are especially prevalent in dependent regions of the pleural space, especially on the diaphragmatic surface and in the mediastinal regions (Fig. 29.2).

Pathophysiology of Pleural Effusions

There are seven general mechanisms by which pleural effusions can develop (Table 29.1). Students should be aware that these can occur singly or in combination.

Clinical Manifestations of Pleural Effusions

A comprehensive medical history and physical exam of the chest are critical elements in guiding the diagnostic workup of a patient with a pleural effusion. Symptoms related to a pleural effusion depend on its size and the state of underlying lung function. Shortness of breath at rest and on exertion, as well as cough are the main symptoms. However, the clinical

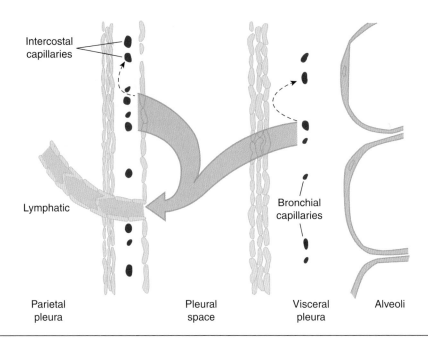

FIGURE 29.1 Representation of normal pleural fluid formation and reabsorption. Microvascular filtrate from microvessels in the parietal and visceral pleura is partly reabsorbed within each membrane (*dashed arrows*), whereas the remaining low-protein interstitial fluid traverses the pleural mesothelia by bulk flow into the pleural space. Pleural fluid exits the pleural space via lymphatic stomata in the parietal pleura. *Redrawn from Chretien et al. The Pleura in Health and Disease. Marcel Dekker; 1985.*

presentation can be dominated by other respiratory symptoms if there is coexisting asthma, COPD, or pneumonia. The primary physical findings in patients with a pleural effusion are dullness to percussion over the affected area, decreased tactile fremitus, diminished breath sounds, and occasionally egophony at the upper level of large effusions (Chap. 14). Very large pleural effusions can be associated with bulging of the intercostal spaces or contralateral shift of the mediastinum.

Radiographic evaluation is important in confirming the presence of a pleural effusion, as well as in formulating the most likely differential diagnostic possibilities. On upright chest radiographic frontal views, larger pleural effusions usually manifest as a **meniscus-shaped density** in the **costophrenic sulcus** (Fig. 29.3); smaller effusions may appear only as blunting of the costophrenic sulcus in upright views. Generally, at least 300-500 mL of fluid in the pleural space is required for visualization on x-ray. Accordingly, lateral views are useful for confirmation, as are supine portable AP films that can disclose free-flowing effusions as unilateral increases in radiographic density because of gravitational layering of the fluid over the involved hemithorax.

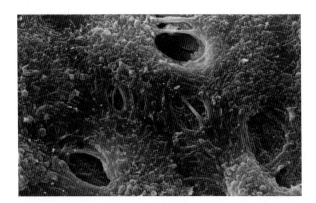

FIGURE 29.2 Scanning electron micrograph of monkey parietal pleura demonstrating lymphatic stomata interposed between the smaller cuboidal mesothelial cells. *From Miura T et al: Lymphatic drainage of carbon particles injected into the pleural cavity of the monkey, as studied by video-assisted thoracoscopy and electron microscopy, J Thorac Cardiovasc surg Sep; 120(3):437-447, 2000.*

Table **29.1** **Mechanisms for development of pleural effusions**

Mechanism	Clinical Examples
Increased P_{mv} in parietal pleural microvessels	Congestive heart failure
Decreased π_{mv} in blood	Cirrhosis, nephrotic syndrome
Increased permeability of pleural microvessels	Inflammation, infection, tumor
Decreased lymphatic drainage	Lymphoma, yellow nail syndrome
Decreased peri-microvascular pressure	Atelectasis, trapped lung
Transdiaphragmatic flow of peritoneal fluid	Hepatic hydrothorax
Iatrogenic fluid instillation	Misdirected central venous catheters

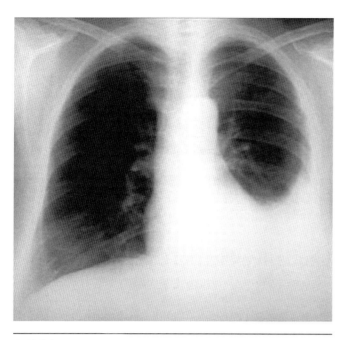

FIGURE 29.3 Meniscus-shaped density in the region of the left costophrenic sulcus on frontal chest radiography indicative of a moderate-sized pleural effusion.

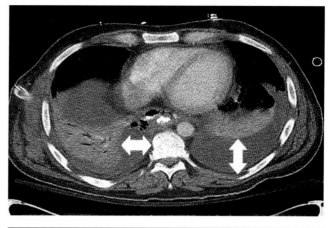

FIGURE 29.4 Chest CT scan at the mid-chest level (mediastinal window) demonstrating large bilateral pleural effusions (*white double-headed arrows*) with adjacent lung compression.

In such situations, pleural effusions are manifest as a diffuse, generalized haziness over the ipsilateral lung field with visible underlying lung vascular markings, together with absence of other signs of pulmonary consolidation such as air bronchograms (Chap. 15). The main value of **lateral decubitus films** is to confirm the presence of a pleural effusion as well as to evaluate the possibility of a loculated fluid collection. Fluid that is free-flowing will layer to a thickness of at least 10 mm on such decubitus views, in contrast to loculated fluid collections that have a similar appearance and shape regardless of the patient's position. Chest CT imaging is the most sensitive method to detect pleural fluid collections and pleural disease (Chap. 15). Pleural effusions can easily be identified by their homogeneous lower density with variable degrees of lung compression (Fig. 29.4).

Diagnosis of Pleural Effusions

The main indication for thoracentesis (Fig. 19.6) is a clinically significant pleural effusion of unknown or unclear etiology by medical history, physical exam, and chest imaging studies. Not all effusions require diagnostic thoracentesis. For example, in a patient with bilateral pleural effusions and overt clinical evidence of CHF without fever, chest pain, or dyspnea out of proportion to the size of the effusion, transudative effusions are most likely, especially if they regress during the first several days of diuretic therapy and other cardiac-targeted treatments. In this setting, the lack of at least a partial resolution of the pleural effusion, or the finding of unilateral effusions, or the presence of fever and/or chest pain are indications for thoracentesis.

Transudative Pleural Effusions

Transudative pleural effusions are caused by two primary mechanisms: (1) increases in the hydrostatic pressure (eg, P_{MV}) of pleural membrane microvessels; and (2) decreases in serum colloid osmotic pressure (eg, π_{MV}). In other words, the pleural membranes themselves are not diseased in a subject with a simple transudative pleural effusion. Accordingly, transudative effusions are characterized by low pleural fluid concentrations of constituent plasma proteins (principally albumin), as well as other plasma biomarkers such as lactate dehydrogenase (LDH) and cholesterol when pleural fluid is sampled by diagnostic thoracentesis. By extension, pleural fluid/serum ratios for these substances are also low, in contradistinction to exudative effusions (Table 29.2).

The most common cause of a transudative pleural effusion is **congestive heart failure** (**CHF**), with approximately 500,000 effusions from this condition diagnosed annually in the United States. Effusions in CHF are principally due to elevations in the microvascular hydrostatic pressure within pleural microvessels, and they are bilateral with the right side fluid volume greater than the left side in 85% of patients.

Table **29.2** Features differentiating transudative and exudative pleural effusions

Transudative Effusions	Exudative Effusions
Pleural fluid/serum protein ratio ≤0.5	Pleural fluid/serum protein ratio >0.5
Pleural fluid/serum LDH ratio ≤0.6 or ≤2/3 normal upper limit for serum	Pleural fluid/serum LDH ratio >0.6 or >2/3 normal upper limit for serum
Pleural fluid cholesterol ≤60 mg/dL	Pleural fluid cholesterol >60 mg/dL
(Serum-pleural) albumin gradient >1.2 g/dL	(Serum-pleural) albumin gradient ≤1.2 g/dL

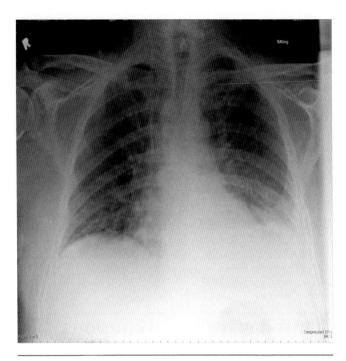

FIGURE 29.5 A small-to-moderate pleural effusion on the left side in a patient with **nephrotic syndrome**.

These effusions are usually accompanied by clinically overt symptoms and signs of left ventricular dysfunction, including bilateral inspiratory lung crackles. In ~5% of patients, isolated left side transudative pleural effusions occur. The **nephrotic syndrome** is associated with small to moderate pleural effusions in about 20% of patients (Fig. 29.5). The primary cause of effusions in nephrotic syndrome is a decrease in serum colloid osmotic pressure, particularly when serum albumin concentrations are <1.5 g dL.

▶▶CLINICAL CORRELATION 29.1

Hepatic hydrothorax is observed in 5%-10% of patients with cirrhotic liver disease and portal venous hypertension. Such effusions are typically transudative, owing to trans-diaphragmatic movement of abdominal ascitic fluid from the peritoneal compartment to the pleural space via diaphragmatic openings. Thus they are generally, but not uniformly, associated with clinically detectable ascites. Hepatic hydrothorax is unilateral and right-sided in approximately 50%-80% of patients; bilateral and isolated left-sided effusions occur in approximately 15% of patients. Patients with hepatic hydrothorax usually have other stigmata of chronic liver disease, such as jaundice and liver function test abnormalities. The diagnosis of hepatic hydrothorax can be confirmed if necessary by a **radionuclide scan** in which tracer that is injected into the peritoneal compartment appears within 2 hours in the pleural space. Treatment is directed toward the underlying cirrhotic condition with sodium restriction, diuretic

therapy, and other adjunctive measures. Refractory hepatic hydrothorax occurs in approximately 10% of patients. This condition generally improves after a **transjugular intrahepatic portosystemic shunt (TIPS)** that lowers portal venous pressure and hence, the rate of peritoneal ascites formation.

Pulmonary thromboembolism (Chap. 27) can cause either transudative or exudative pleural effusions. Pulmonary infarction and its associated pleural inflammation generally cause an exudative effusion. Common causes of transudative as well as exudative effusions are depicted in Table 29.3.

Exudative Pleural Effusions

Exudative pleural effusions primarily result from increased permeability of microvessels in the pleural membranes (ie, an increased value of σ). Accordingly, pleural fluid concentrations of protein and other plasma biomarkers are elevated, as are their ratios (Table 29.2). The most frequent cause of an exudative fluid is a **parapneumonic effusion**, which occurs in about 40%-50% of bacterial pneumonias (Chaps. 34 and 35). Annually, between 250,000 and 500,000 parapneumonic effusions develop in hospitalized patients in the United States. Parapneumonic pleural effusions are categorized into three main groups: (1) uncomplicated parapneumonic effusions; (2) complicated parapneumonic effusions; and (3) thoracic empyema. Each of these is briefly reviewed below.

An **uncomplicated parapneumonic effusion** is an exudative, free-flowing pleural effusion that develops in conjunction with infectious pneumonia (Chaps. 34-36). These effusions are generally small and resolve completely following appropriate

Table 29.3 Common causes of transudative vs exudative pleural effusions

Transudative Effusions	Exudative Effusions
Congestive heart failure	Pneumonia
Cirrhosis Hepatic hydrothorax	Complicated parapneumonic effusion
Pulmonary thromboembolism	Empyema
Nephrotic syndrome	Malignancy
Hypothyroidism	Pulmonary thromboembolism
Peritoneal dialysis fluid	Benign asbestos pleural effusion
	Connective tissue disease
	Postpericardial injury syndrome
	Pancreatitis
	Tuberculous pleurisy
	Esophageal rupture
	Drug reaction
	Yellow nail syndrome

antimicrobial therapy directed at the pneumonia. Consequently the majority of parapneumonic pleural effusions are uncomplicated. However, approximately 10%-15% do evolve into **complicated parapneumonic effusions** that are operationally defined as those that require pleural space drainage for resolution. These are associated with significant morbidity and mortality if not managed appropriately, because of the development of intrapleural adhesions, persistently trapped loculated fluids, and development of **trapped lung**. The latter situation refers to a restriction of normal lung expansion because of fibrous thickening of the visceral pleura. Clinical features that predispose to, or are indicative of a complicated parapneumonic effusion include protracted respiratory symptoms (eg, 7-10 days to several weeks) despite antimicrobial therapy. Complicated parapneumonic effusions are also associated clinically with large effusions that occupy >40%-50% of a hemithorax, with those that contain loculated or multiloculated fluid collections on chest CT scan with a thickened or enhancing visceral pleura, where intrapleural air-fluid levels are discernible, or when anaerobic pulmonary infections are accompanied by pleural effusion (Fig. 29.6). Pleural fluid analyses showing a pH <7.3, an [LDH] >1,000 U/L, and a pleural fluid glucose <40 mg/dL also support the diagnosis of a complicated parapneumonic effusion. **Thoracic empyema** represents overt pus in the pleural space and is most often the end result of a complicated parapneumonic effusion.

There are three recognized stages in the development of complicated parapneumonic effusions, and these carry important patient care implications. In the early **exudative** or **capillary leak stage** lasting 2-5 days following the onset of the pleural effusion, the effusion is usually amenable to simple drainage by **tube thoracostomy** (Chap. 19). The **fibrinopurulent** or **bacterial invasion stage** extends for 3-14 days from onset, and the **organizational** or **empyema stage** from 10 to 21 days. Because of the rapid conversion from a free-flowing effusion

during the exudative phase of a complicated parapneumonic effusion to the loculated, infected fluids of the fibrinopurulent phase, it is strongly recommended that all patients with parapneumonic pleural effusions undergo diagnostic thoracentesis. This procedure both evaluates the patient for the possibility of a complicated parapneumonic effusion and documents the need for drainage of the pleural space, in addition to prompt initiation of antimicrobial therapy.

Pleural effusions associated with extension of neoplastic disease to the pleural space are typically exudative in nature because of pleural inflammation that increases pleural membrane permeability, as well as fibrin deposition that limits the rate of egress of fluid out of the pleural space via lymphatic drainage. However, patients with neoplastic disease may have multiple reasons to have a pleural effusion of both exudative and transudative causes. Thus, diagnostic thoracentesis is always indicated to help distinguish among these possibilities (Table 29.4).

Benign asbestos pleural effusion (BAPE) is an exudative fluid collection resulting from prior exposure to asbestos. It is characterized by a long latency period averaging 20-25 years and is initiated by inhalational exposure and deposition of asbestos fibers within the respiratory bronchioles and alveolar ducts. Because of their straight, linear structure and peripheral lung deposition, amphibole asbestos fibers are most associated with BAPE. Following fiber inhalation, an ensuing macrophage-driven inflammatory reaction extends outward to the pleural space, where cytokines including TNF-α are released along with growth factors, proteases, and reactive nitrogen and oxygen species, culminating in oxidative DNA damage and pleural inflammation. Because there are no unique diagnostic features of BAPE on pleural fluid and cellular analyses, it remains a diagnosis of exclusion. However, previous asbestosis exposure suggesting the possibility of BAPE is commonly manifested as calcific or noncalcific parietal plaques in the mid-thoracic regions or involving the diaphragmatic pleura (Chap. 23). Asbestos-related parenchymal abnormalities may coexist, such as nodular or reticular opacities. Finally, yellow nail syndrome is a rare disorder of lymphatic vessels characterized by recurrent exudative pleural effusions, lymphedema and yellowish discoloration of the nails.

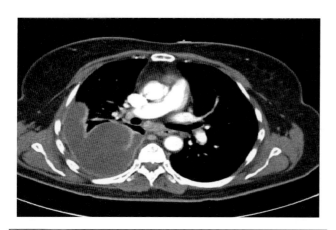

FIGURE 29.6 Chest CT scan demonstrating a typical appearance of a right-sided complicated parapneumonic effusion, featuring a loculated, septated pleural fluid collection with contrast enhancement of the visceral pleura. Thoracentesis yielded pus confirming empyema. *From Limsukon et al.* Parapneumonic pleural effusions and empyema thoracis: differential diagnosis and workup. Medscape.com, 2011. Available at: http://emedicine.medscape.com/article/298485-overview.

Table **29.4** **Potential causes of pleural effusion associated with malignancy**

Pleural inflammation from metastatic tumor involvement
Atelectasis from central bronchial obstruction in lung cancer
Postobstructive pneumonia (eg, parapneumonic effusion)
Decreased serum colloid osmotic pressure from malnutrition and hypoalbuminemia
Pulmonary thromboembolism
Cardiotoxic effects of chemotherapy or underlying congestive heart failure

Solutions to Case Studies and Practice Problems

CASE 29.1 The most correct answer is d, order antibiotic therapy and perform emergent diagnostic thoracentesis.

Despite this patient's history of congestive heart failure, the presentation including productive cough, dyspnea and fever is typical for an infectious pneumonia, presumably bacterial in etiology. Indeed, the presence of air bronchograms on chest x-ray is indicative of alveolar consolidation. In the setting of suspected bacterial pneumonia in a patient with fever and a moderately large unilateral pleural effusion, a parapneumonic effusion is likely, and performing a diagnostic thoracentesis as soon as possible is indicated. Antimicrobial therapy alone is inadequate treatment for a potentially complicated parapneumonic effusion. Obtaining a chest CT scan for better visualization of the right pleural space (*answer a*) is not indicated at the present time, since the effusion is already large enough to safely perform thoracentesis, which is important to properly stratify the effusion as uncomplicated, complicated, or possibly an empyema. Since time is of the essence in diagnosing a parapneumonic effusion in a febrile, symptomatic patient because of the possible need for chest tube drainage to avert fibrinous loculations, ordering antibiotic therapy and a repeat chest radiograph in 48 hours (*answer b*), or ordering antibiotic therapy and a diagnostic thoracentesis in 48 hours (*answer c*) if symptoms persist are inappropriate management. By the same token, evaluating the patient for pulmonary thromboembolism (*answer e*) is incorrect because the presentation is not suggestive of this disorder. Furthermore, non-invasive thoracic imaging studies still will not enable one to categorize the effusion as transudative versus exudative and if the latter, whether a complicated parapneumonic effusion is present that demands additional focused management.

CASE 29.2 The correct answer is a, a parapneumonic effusion is a diagnostic possibility.

This patient in all likelihood has cancer in the left lung and either lymphangitic spread of tumor or alternatively, a distal post-obstructive pneumonia from the tumor mass. Because of the latter possibility, a pleural effusion in this setting should not automatically be equated with a malignant pleural effusion, especially inasmuch as no pleural fluid cytological results are reported. Congestive heart failure (*answer b*) remains a potential cause for the effusion but is incorrect since the pleural fluid chemistry values clearly demonstrate an exudative effusion, whereas a transudative effusion would be anticipated were congestive heart failure the predominant mechanism. Pulmonary thromboembolism (*answer c*) has been excluded by the pleural fluid chemistry values and is incorrect, since nearly 50% of effusions associated with thromboembolism are exudative. *Answer d* is not the right choice, because elevations in microvascular hydrostatic pressure within the pleura are typically observed in transudative, not exudative effusions. Likewise, *answer e* is incorrect in this case because serum colloid osmotic pressure (largely determined by the serum albumin concentration) is not a central operative mechanism for exudative pleural effusions.

Chapter **30**

Principles and Goals of Mechanical Ventilation

DAYTON DMELLO, MD AND
GEORGE M. MATUSCHAK, MD

Learning Objectives

- The student will be able to list the indications for mechanical ventilation (MV).
- The student will be able to describe common modes of MV, frequently used ventilator settings, and waveform monitoring of airway pressures during MV.
- The student will be able to describe the process of ventilator weaning and eventual liberation of patients from MV.
- The student will be able to distinguish alternative modes of MV and the basic principles of non-invasive ventilation.

Introduction

The Greek physician and philosopher Claudius Galen (129-199 CE) was the first to artificially reproduce the process of ventilation. He inflated the lungs of a dead animal with bellows during one of his numerous experiments, subsequently described in his iconic text, *On the Parts of the Human Body*. It was not until more than 1,500 years later that the paradigm of artificial respiration was used for human resuscitation. The first seemingly authentic report was by Tossach in 1744 concerning the resuscitation of a suffocated miner by mouth-to-mouth technique. Again, it was not until the dreaded poliomyelitis epidemics of the 1940s and 1950s in Europe and the United States that **mechanical ventilation (MV)** was developed as a major therapeutic strategy. Since then, the science of MV has rapidly expanded to encompass a variety of modalities that ensure adequate ventilation and gas exchange by a diverse array of mechanical and physiologic processes. Simultaneously, there has been increasing awareness that unregulated inflation of the lungs may lead to deleterious consequences. Those include excessive stretch and shear forces at the alveolar level that cause physiologically harmful effects on both the respiratory and cardiovascular systems (Chap. 28).

Indications for Mechanical Ventilation

Mechanical ventilation is indicated in any clinical situation where hypoxemia or hypercarbia secondary to underlying abnormal or dysfunctional lung pathophysiology cannot be corrected by spontaneous respiration. Often MV is initiated when lung gas exchange is normal but protection of the anatomical airway by a **cuffed endotracheal tube** is necessary, to prevent aspiration of oropharyngeal or gastrointestinal contents. This commonly occurs in the setting of a decreased consciousness with depressed protective laryngeal reflexes and incomplete glottic inlet closure (Chap. 11). Finally, MV may be necessary when the work of breathing, while sufficient to eliminate CO_2 in cases of severe metabolic acidosis, leads to

tachypnea and respiratory muscle fatigue. A prime example of such a scenario is severe sepsis, wherein endotracheal intubation and MV are initiated to avoid impending **respiratory failure** secondary to excessively high work of breathing. Used in this way, MV decreases both respiratory muscle fatigue and myocardial O_2 requirements and thereby promotes clinical recovery. Other indications for initiating MV are to regulate P_aCO_2 in patients with increased intracranial pressure, or to provide an air splint in patients with massive chest injury and **flail chest**.

Review of the Mechanics of Ventilation

Normal respiration involves the active process of inspiration, created by the generation of negative intrapleural pressure caused by caudal diaphragmatic movement. Expiration is ordinarily a passive process, whereby the diaphragm returns to its baseline position. This differential pressure gradient between the pleural space and the alveolar airspaces causing normal inspiration and expiration is schematically represented in Fig. 30.1.

In general, mechanical ventilation includes two basic designs or subtypes:

1. **Negative pressure ventilation:** Historically the chest or the entire body below the neck was surrounded by a device capable of creating a cyclical partial vacuum that enhanced the normally negative gradient between P_{IP} and P_{AW}. Inspiration was initiated by this partial vacuum, and expiration occurred when the negative pressure was released. Primary examples of negative pressure ventilation included the **iron lung** and **cuirass shell** ventilators (Fig. 30.2). Such forms of ventilation are rarely used today.

283

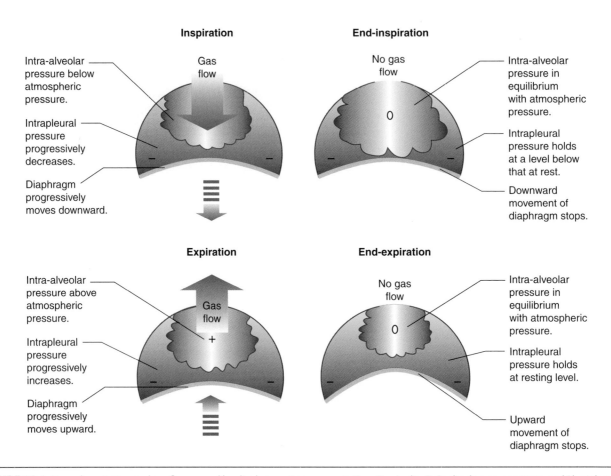

FIGURE 30.1 Normal respiration and gas flow caused by diaphragmatic movement. *From Des Jardins T:* Cardipulmonary anatomy and Physiology: Essentials of Respiratory Care, *5th ed. Thomas Delmar Learning, 2008.*

2. **Positive pressure ventilation:** A piston-based system of valves controlled by a microprocessor creates positive P_{AW} relative to P_B during inspiration, while expiration is a passive process caused by lung and chest wall recoil. This is the current standard of all modern mechanical ventilators, with the exception of some forms of high-frequency ventilation in which expiration is an active process. Components of a simple ventilation system are diagrammed in Fig. 30.3.

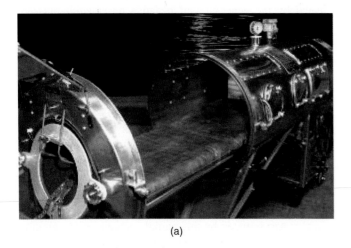

(a)

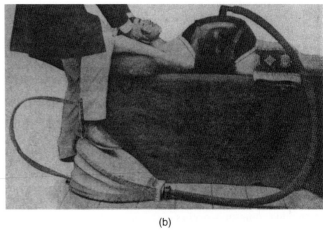

(b)

FIGURE 30.2 (a) The Emerson iron lung, circa 1950. The patient lies within the chamber with only his/her head outside, which when sealed provides an effectively oscillating atmospheric pressure. (b) The cuirass shell ventilator, circa 1905, which applied negative pressure to the thorax by means of a foot-operated bellows.

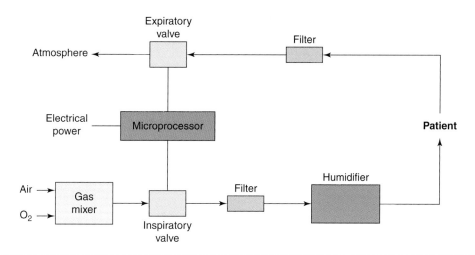

FIGURE 30.3 Block diagram of a simple ventilator circuit. *Adapted from Hess DR.* Essentials of Mechanical Ventilation. *2nd ed. McGraw-Hill, 2002.*

Modes of Positive Pressure Mechanical Ventilation

Conventional ventilator modes typically involve limiting either the maximal or **peak airway pressure** (P_{PEAK}) or the maximal inspired tidal volume (V_T) that the patient receives. Newer ventilators have expanded on this traditional approach by creating hybrid modes, wherein both P_{PEAK} and V_T can be regulated to some degree. This chapter will focus on the more established modes of each.

1. **Volume-controlled ventilation:** Also known as **volume-limited ventilation** or **volume-targeted ventilation**, this mode involves setting V_T, respiratory f, and the inspiratory flow rate to specific values, while P_{PEAK} is allowed to vary on a breath-to-breath basis. Thus the ventilator delivers a consistent V_T, either at the set rate (**controlled breath**) or when inspiratory effort is initiated by the patient (**assisted breath**). In the latter, the inspiratory time interval and thereby the **inspiratory time/expiratory time ratio (I:E ratio)** will vary based upon the patient's spontaneous f. Although V_T had been conventionally set at 10-12 mL/kg of predicted body weight (PBW) for patients without lung injury, recent trials have validated the use of lower V_T that are closer to 6 mL/kg of PBW in patients with ALI or ARDS (Chap. 28). When V_T, P_{AW}, and flow rates are plotted versus time in this ventilator mode, the waveforms for each resemble those in Fig. 30.4. *(#94)*

2. **Pressure-controlled ventilation:** Also referred to as **pressure-limited ventilation** or **pressure-targeted ventilation**, this mode involves setting an upper limit on P_{PEAK} during inspiration, while manipulating f and thus the I:E ratio. As a result, V_T fluctuates on a breath-to-breath basis, based upon the patient's dynamic lung and chest wall compliance. The ventilator is limited by the set inspiratory P_{PEAK}, and again will either ventilate the patient at a set rate (controlled breath) or whenever breathing is initiated or attempted by the patient (assisted breath). In the

latter variation, the flow rate at which V_T is delivered also remains variable, based upon a patient's effort and demand. Presetting inspiratory time to exceed the expiratory time is termed **inverse-ratio pressure control ventilation**. It is less commonly used in clinical practice, except in severe ARDS for salvage therapy or to reduce **ventilator-induced lung injury** (**VALI**) (Chap. 28). Typical waveforms for P_{AW}, flow rate, and delivered V_T during pressure-controlled ventilation are depicted in Fig. 30.5.

▶▶CLINICAL CORRELATION 30.1

Both volume-controlled and pressure-controlled ventilation are examples of **assist-control ventilation (A/C).** The machine-delivered A/C breaths on both modes may be assisted (spontaneously initiated) or controlled (ventilator initiated). The older term **continuous mandatory ventilation (CMV)** has been used when all delivered breaths are ventilator initiated, and no patient-initiated breaths are machine-assisted. CMV as a stand-alone mode is largely nonexistent on modern ventilators. Instead, A/C ventilation has emerged and remains the standard.

3. **Pressure support ventilation (PSV):** The PSV mode involves assisting a patient's spontaneous respiratory effort by the ventilator, up to a preset level of inspiratory pressure. Since the patient must initiate a spontaneous breath before assistance is delivered, setting an inspiratory support pressure is all that is required. Therefore, patient effort decides the respiratory rate, flow rate and V_T on a breath-to-breath basis. This is a commonly used mode during the process of weaning a patient off MV (see below), since all breaths are spontaneous and the level of pressure support can be sequentially decreased to impose a near-normal workload on the respiratory breathing apparatus prior to extubation. Pressure, flow and V_T waveforms during this mode are depicted in Fig. 30.6.

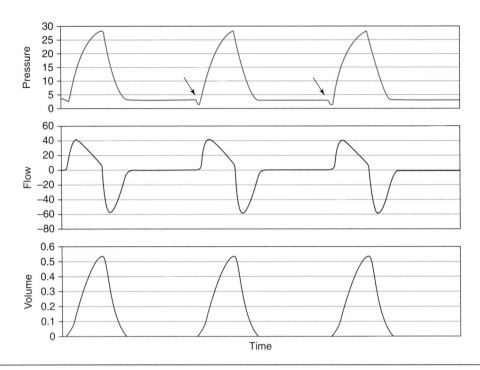

FIGURE 30.4 Waveforms in volume-controlled ventilation. Here the first breath is ventilator-initiated, while the second and third are patient-initiated as seen by the small negative deflections due to patient effort at breath initiation (arrows). *Adapted from MacIntyre NR, Branson RD. Mechanical Ventilation, © Saunders; 2009.*

4. **Synchronized intermittent mandatory ventilation (SIMV):** The SIMV mode represents a blend between either volume-control or pressure-control ventilation, plus pressure support ventilation, that is, either volume-control SIMV or pressure-control SIMV. Again, the delivered breaths are of two types: a **mandatory delivered breath** based on a minimum preset f (with preset V_T during VC-SIMV or preset inspiratory pressure during PC-SIMV); and a **spontaneous patient-initiated breath** that is pressure supported (by preset support pressure), as in PSV. The

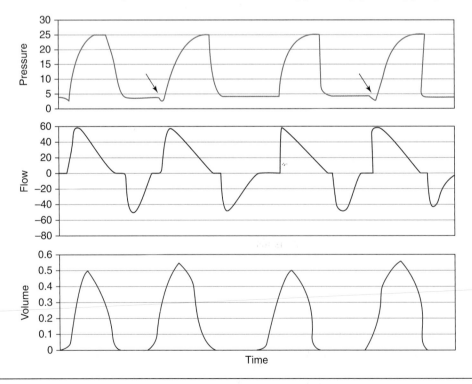

FIGURE 30.5 Waveforms in pressure-controlled ventilation. Patient-initiated breaths are denoted by arrows. Note breath-to-breath variations in V_T. *Adapted from MacIntyre NR, Branson RD. Mechanical Ventilation, © Saunders; 2009.*

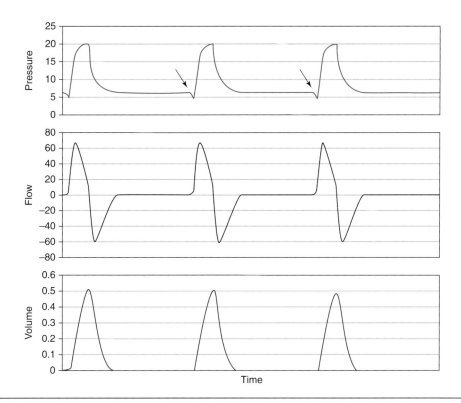

FIGURE 30.6 Waveforms in pressure support ventilation (PSV). All breaths are patient-initiated (arrows). Note the small breath-to-breath variations in V_T. *Adapted from MacIntyre NR, Branson RD.* Mechanical Ventilation. *© Saunders; 2009.*

important point is that mandatory breaths may be either controlled or assisted. There are different ventilator algorithms in use to determine whether the delivered breath will be controlled or assisted. With either, the goal remains to maximally synchronize the ventilator breaths with a patient's spontaneous breathing pattern. Simply stated, this mode encourages spontaneous breathing by the patient, but provides a predetermined minimum level of MV that is set by the clinician. Pressure, flow and V_T waveforms during this mode are depicted in Fig. 30.7.

Distinguishing between Peak and Plateau Airway Pressures   #95

As introduced earlier, P_{PEAK} is the maximum P_{AW} achieved during an MV inspiration, and when displayed is principally used to measure total resistance in the proximal larger airways plus the ventilator circuit, although its absolute value is also affected by the elastic recoil force of the chest wall and lungs. Therefore, when the inspiratory V_T is constant, a rising P_{PEAK} is most often indicative of increasing airway resistance, for example, acute bronchospasm with airway narrowing from any cause, presuming no change in compliance of the lungs plus thoracic cage. Conversely, P_{PLAT} represents the required distending pressure to balance elastic recoil at the level of terminal bronchioles and alveoli when airflow is zero (Chap. 6). This P_{PLAT} is best measured by creating an **inspiratory pause** at the end of an MV inspiration, commonly 0.5-second, to allow

equilibration between inspiratory and alveolar pressures, after which it is measured and/or displayed (Fig. 30.8). Conceptually, P_{PEAK} always exceeds P_{PLAT} since airway resistance is never zero, while P_{PLAT} may be nearly equal to P_{PEAK} but can never exceed it. Thus, an absolute increase in P_{PLAT} when a mechanically delivered V_T is constant indicates decreased compliance of the lungs plus chest wall, as in pneumonia, ARDS, pneumothorax, and some other restrictive lung diseases (Chap. 23 and 28).

> ►►CLINICAL CORRELATION 30.2
>
> Common causes of increased P_{PEAK} include acute bronchoconstriction and secretion buildup within the ventilator circuit. Therefore, an isolated elevation in P_{PEAK} without a concomitant elevation of P_{PLAT} is often treated with bronchodilators and endotracheal or tracheostomy tube suctioning. Additionally, kinks in the ventilator tubing or an excessively narrow endotracheal tube or tracheostomy tube may also increase P_{PEAK} by virtue of their effects on total system resistance to air flow. Elevations of both P_{PEAK} and P_{PLAT} usually reflect alveolar disease or dysfunction from various etiologies. In this context, an increased P_{PLAT} is causally associated with VALI and pneumothorax. A central goal of the ARDS Network recommendation to treat ARDS patients using $V_T = 6$ mL/kg of PBW is to maintain P_{PLAT} <30 cm H_2O, even at the expense of low V_T and **permissive hypercapnia**, that is, a controlled elevation of P_aCO_2.

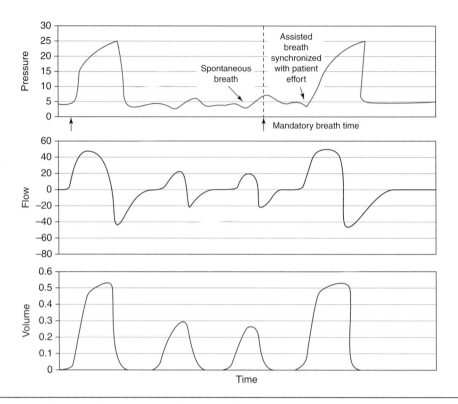

FIGURE 30.7 Waveforms during SIMV ventilation. Breaths 1 and 4 are mandatory while breaths 2 and 3 are supported. Note variations in V_T between mandatory and supported breaths. Mandatory breaths are either controlled (breath 1) or assisted (breath 4). *Adapted from MacIntyre NR, Branson RD. Mechanical Ventilation. © Saunders; 2009.*

PEEP and Auto-PEEP Mechanical Ventilation

Ordinarily, there is no airflow at the end of a normal expiration since P_{AW} and alveolar pressure (P_A) are equal. During spontaneous breathing, the small negative P_{IP} present at the end of expiration creates a normal FRC (Chap. 4). Patients with respiratory compromise that requires MV tend to lose FRC volume due to surfactant abnormalities and alveolar instability that cause alveolar de-recruitment, atelectasis, and hypoxemia. Therefore, mechanically ventilated patients typically require a small amount of PEEP to maintain alveolar volume at end-expiration, increase P_{AW}, and sustain or improve S_aO_2. Using a preset ventilator for this purpose is termed **extrinsic PEEP**.

However, if these ventilated alveolar airspaces are incompletely emptied at the end of the expiratory phase, then P_A will exceed P_{AW} as expected with continued outward air flow. In this situation where $P_A > P_B$ at end-expiration, an iatrogenic form of PEEP is induced that has been variously termed **auto-PEEP**, **intrinsic PEEP**, or **occult PEEP**. In a clinical setting employing volume-controlled ventilation, the presence of auto-PEEP is assessed by performing an **end-expiratory hold maneuver**. Analogous to measuring P_{PLAT} at end-inspiration as described earlier, the hold maneuver creates a 0.5-second pause at the end of expiration by occluding the expiratory circuit. This pause allows P_{AW} and P_A to equilibrate, and the resulting rise in P_{AW} equals the auto-PEEP present (Fig. 30.9). Likewise, a failure of the flow waveform to return to baseline at the end of expiration and before the next inspiratory phase provides a visual clue that auto-PEEP is occurring. Alternatively, if the application of new or greater PEEP during MV fails to increase P_{PEAK}, then a commensurate level of auto-PEEP already exists that is being negated by the application of extrinsic PEEP. Like PEEP

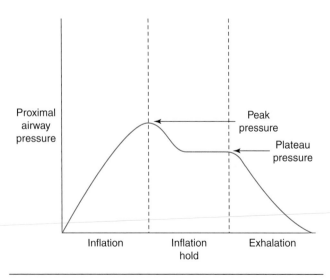

FIGURE 30.8 Pressure-time curve demonstrating peak pressure and plateau pressure after an inspiratory hold maneuver. *Adapted from Marino PL. The ICU Book, 2nd ed. © Lippincott, Williams & Wilkins; 1998.*

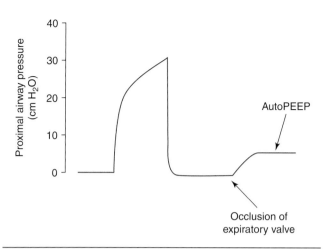

FIGURE 30.9 Pressure-time curve demonstrating the presence of auto-PEEP after an expiratory hold maneuver. *Adapted from MacIntyre NR, Branson RD. Mechanical Ventilation. © Saunders; 2009.*

Table **30.1** Suggested parameters for initiation of ventilator weaning

Weaning Parameter	Threshold Value
P_aO_2/F_IO_2	>200
Vital capacity	>10 mL/kg of PBW
$\dot{V}_E$	<10 L/min
Airway occlusion pressure at 1 sec	<3.5-6 cm H_2O
Maximal negative inspiratory pressure	< −25 cm H_2O
Ratio of f/V_T	<100

itself, any excessive auto-PEEP has deleterious cardiovascular and pulmonary effects, including hypotension secondary to decreased venous return (Chaps. 7, 8, and 9).

▶▶**CLINICAL CORRELATION 30.3**

An excessively high *f* during volume-controlled MV in the A/C mode is a very common cause of rapidly generated auto-PEEP due to incomplete alveolar emptying, and causes desaturation and hemodynamic collapse. Careful attention should be paid to reducing the ventilator rate, especially in scenarios that predispose to air trapping, such as those patients with bronchospastic COPD.

Liberation from Mechanical Ventilation

Liberation from MV involves weaning patients from ventilator support and ultimately removing their endotracheal or tracheostomy tube so that spontaneous breathing resumes. It is not necessary to await complete resolution of an underlying disease prior to initiating ventilator weaning. Rather weaning should proceed in concert with management of underlying disease processes, provided there are no contraindications to doing so. In that sense, a number of physiological and clinical parameters have been suggested as indicators of initiating the weaning process (Table 30.1), although their predictive value remains uncertain when applied to individual patients. Therefore, ventilator weaning should be initiated and trialed on a daily basis according to clinical judgment when the underlying etiology necessitating MV is controlled or is improving.

Weaning from MV typically commences with switching from an assisted or controlled ventilator mode to a supported mode such as PSV or SIMV. Subsequent monitoring of V_T is of paramount importance in determining an individual patient's suitability for extubation. In this context, a commonly used clinical formula is the **Rapid Shallow Breathing**

Index (**RSBI**), obtained by dividing the respiratory *f* (per minute) by V_T in liters when the patient is placed on minimal pressure support. Early clinical studies suggested that an RSBI >105 predicted a 95% likelihood of the need for reintubation. Currently, an RSBI <100 is frequently used as evidence of a patient's readiness for weaning and subsequent extubation.

▶▶**CLINICAL CORRELATION 30.4**

To date, numerous clinical trials have failed to demonstrate the superiority of one particular weaning technique over another, and additional trials are needed to establish a true evidence-based weaning paradigm. Currently, a daily **spontaneous breathing trial** (**SBT**) is attempted by placing the ventilated patient on a minimal level of pressure support. This strategy ensures that evaluation for weaning is part of the ongoing daily therapeutic plan. The ability of the ventilated patient to tolerate an SBT for 30-120 minutes is good evidence for possible extubation if other clinical prerequisites are met, including an adequate cough reflex and an appropriate level of responsiveness.

Non-Invasive Ventilation

Non-invasive ventilation, or **non-invasive positive pressure ventilation** (**NIPPV**), is the process of providing assisted ventilation without the use of an indwelling endotracheal tube or tracheostomy tube. Typically, NIPPV is achieved using a nasal or full-face mask that provides a tight seal, so that positive pressure can be delivered without significant air leak. Its advantages mainly relate to the absence of an indwelling endotracheal tube and thus the complications of longstanding endotracheal intubation. Those complications include vocal chord injury and often the need for sedation or neuromuscular paralysis. Although there are numerous modes of NIPPV, a common delivery system applies **inspiratory positive airway pressure** (**IPAP**) to unload and assist the inspiratory muscles as during invasive ventilation. An alternative NIPPV mode applies continuous **positive pressure during expiration** (**EPAP**) that resembles PEEP during invasive ventilation.

The indications for NIPPV are as diverse as those for invasive ventilation. Notably, the best clinical evidence for utilizing NIPPV to treat acute respiratory failure exists for acute exacerbations of COPD (Chap. 22), cardiogenic or noncardiogenic pulmonary edema, and respiratory muscle weakness secondary to neuromuscular disease. Importantly, little evidence supports the use of NIPPV in conditions characterized by acute hypoxemia without a concomitant increase in the work of breathing, such as pulmonary embolism. Additionally, the patient being considered for NIPPV needs a reasonably preserved cough reflex, and should be alert enough to expel secretions during the use of NIPPV. The failure to do so may result in inspissation of pulmonary secretions and clinical decompensation during a trial of NIPPV. In this sense, the inherent delay involved in intubating patients who have failed an NIPPV trial has been shown to adversely affect clinical outcomes. Therefore, sound clinical judgment should be exercised when determining suitable candidacy for NIPPV, and the known contraindications to NIPPV should be carefully evaluated (Table 30.2).

Conclusions

Mechanical ventilation of the critically ill patient remains a dynamic and continuously evolving process, characterized by a paucity of evidence and absence of large-scale clinical trials.

Table **30.2** Contraindications for non-invasive positive pressure ventilation

Absolute Contraindications	Relative Contraindications
Comatose state	Shock
Cardiorespiratory arrest	Altered sensorium
Uncontrollable upper GI bleeding	Decreased ability to clear oropharyngeal secretions
Potential for upper airway obstruction, eg, airway compression or tumors	Recent gastrointestinal tract surgery
	High risk for aspiration
Any disease state or condition requiring endotracheal intubation or airway stabilization	Mask intolerance or patient noncooperation

Additionally, there is a lack of consensus in the standardization of ventilator terminologies, thus creating a dizzying choice of ventilator modes that may be promoted as unique by a device manufacturer despite clinically proven rigorous scientific data. Ultimately, a thorough understanding of the basic principles of patient-ventilator physiology must be coupled with proficient clinical judgment to navigate this complex and challenging maze of information. Students are directed to the **Suggested Readings** for advanced bibliographic materials in this area.

Suggested Readings

1. Marino PL. *The ICU Book*, 3rd ed. Philadelphia, PA: Lippincott, Williams & Wilkins; 2008. *Essential reading for any physician-in-training with an interest in pulmonary and/or critical care medicine specialties.*

2. Hess DR, Kacmarek RM. *Essentials of Mechanical Ventilation*, 2nd ed. New York, NY: McGraw-Hill; 2002; Tobin MJ. *Principles & Practice of Mechanical Ventilation*, 2nd ed. New York, NY: McGraw-Hill; 2006. *Both texts, now revised since* their first appearances 20 years ago, offer in-depth training and clear operational diagrams of all major ventilatory strategies.

3. Fink MP, Abraham E, Vincent J, Kochanek PM. *Textbook of Critical Care*, 5th ed. Philadelphia, PA: Elsevier Saunders; 2005. *The continued popularity of this text is derived from the extraordinary expertise of its editors as practitioners of intensive care medicine at the highest levels in the United States and Europe.*

CASE STUDIES AND PRACTICE PROBLEMS

CASE 30.1 A 70-year-old man is receiving mechanical ventilation for acute respiratory failure secondary to an exacerbation of underlying COPD. He is sedated and paralyzed on volume assist-control ventilation, at initial settings of: $V_T = 560$ mL (8 mL/kg); $f = 20$ breaths/min; PEEP = 5 cm H_2O; and $F_1O_2 = 0.40$. Within 2 minutes, his $S_aO_2\% = 94\%$, BP = 140/100 mm Hg, HR = 90 b/min, and P_{PEAK} and P_{PLAT} are 24 and 21 cm H_2O, respectively. One hour later, the patient has become hemodynamically unstable, with PB = 90/70 mm Hg, HR = 126 b/min, $S_aO_2 = 85\%$, $P_{PEAK} = 34$ cm H_2O, and $P_{PLAT} = 32$ cm H_2O. Results of a portable chest x-ray and arterial blood gas analysis are pending. What should be the next intervention in treating this patient?

a. Increase V_T to 700 mL (10 mL/kg) to improve patient's lung expansion.

b. Increase f to 24/min to increase $\dot{V}_E$, given that the patient is sedated and paralyzed.

c. Decrease f to 12/min and then recheck airway pressures in 5 minutes.

d. Perform aggressive endotracheal suctioning and chest percussion.

CASE 30.2 A 34-year-old male is admitted to the ICU for a ruptured appendix. He has never smoked and his past medical history is unremarkable. On day 2 in the unit, his peritonitis worsens and he exhibits respiratory failure necessitating intubation and mechanical ventilation. His attending physician decides to implement a $V_T = 500$ mL and orders that ventilator f be modified only as needed to maintain stable arterial blood gases, and "a little hypercapnia is OK." Which of the following events occurring within the next 4 hours would alert the ICU staff that the patient's suspected acute lung injury has abruptly and significantly worsened?

a. The patient's P_{PEAK} decreases by 6 cm H_2O pressure.

b. His shunt fraction calculated at bedside decreases from 45% to 28%.

c. His calculated plasma [HCO_3^-] increases from 17 mM to 20 mM.

d. The patient's S_aO_2 decreases from 92% to 89% by pulse oximetry.

e. His P_{PEAK} and P_{PLAT} both increase by 8 cm H_2O pressure.

CASE 30.3 A 44-year-old man weighing 90 kg is in the intensive care unit for the past 4 days due to severe head and abdominal trauma from a motor vehicle accident. He has been on IV lipid emulsion throughout this period. Worsening neurological deficits now necessitate intubation and mechanical ventilation (MV). Current ventilator settings are delivering 400 mL room air/breath at 14 breaths/min. Blood gas analyses 10 minutes ago reveal a $pH_a = 7.31$, $P_aCO_2 = 56$ mm Hg, and $P_aO_2 = 60$ mm Hg; pulse oximetry shows $S_aO_2 = 72\%$. Which of the following is the most appropriate next step in managing this patient?

a. Switch his IV feeding solution to 5% dextrose.

b. Add 15 cm H_2O of positive end-expiratory pressure.

c. Convert him from room air to an $F_IO_2 = 0.50$.

d. Double his breathing frequency on MV.

e. Increase his V_T on MV by 150 mL/breath.

Solutions to Case Studies and Practice Problems

CASE 30.1 The most correct answer is c, decrease respiratory frequency and recheck P_{AW}.

This patient demonstrates the classic clinical scenario of increased auto-PEEP. Given his underlying exacerbation of COPD with accompanying alveolar distention and air-trapping, the initial f of 20/min is too rapid to permit complete alveolar emptying and causes further alveolar hyperinflation with hemodynamic compromise. This is reflected in the increased peak pressure commensurate with an increased plateau pressure. Decreasing the ventilator rate will facilitate alveolar emptying by increasing the duration of expiration, thereby reversing the air-trapping and auto-PEEP pathophysiology, with a resultant drop in both peak and plateau pressures. Increasing either V_T (*answer a*) or ventilator rate (*answer b*) will worsen the auto-PEEP. Although tracheobronchial suctioning would help clear mucus plugging and airway secretions (*answer d*), it would not alter the underlying auto-PEEP process.

CASE 30.2 The most correct answer is e.

P_{PEAK} and P_{PLAT} increase in parallel as would be expected in a patient with an acute onset or worsening of a restrictive parenchymal process, in this instance caused by edema. Either a decrease in P_{PEAK} (*answer a*) or in shunt fraction (*answer b*) over a 4-hour period would be interpreted as welcome signs that the patient's acute lung injury has stabilized and that MV was appropriate. Likewise, a modest increase in [HCO_3^-] (*answer c*) would be considered an acceptable side effect of MV, particularly in a patient likely to have metabolic acidosis that consumes body bicarbonate stores. Although his $S_aO_2 = 89\%$ is approaching a critical value (*answer d*), a 3% change would not be the most troubling development in such a patient.

CASE 30.3 The most correct answer is e, increase the patient's V_T by 150 mL/breath.

The current ventilator setting is delivering <5 mL/kg and is inducing respiratory acidosis with an excessively high V_D/V_T ratio, which will not be corrected simply by increasing ventilator f (*answer d*). By Dalton's law, his low P_aO_2 is caused by alveolar hypoventilation and supplemental oxygen is probably unnecessary (*answer c*). Likewise, changing the feeding solution to 5% dextrose will only increase the patient's P_aCO_2 because of the increased respiratory quotient that occurs with carbohydrate catabolism (*answer a*). Consideration of using PEEP is premature at this point (*answer b*).

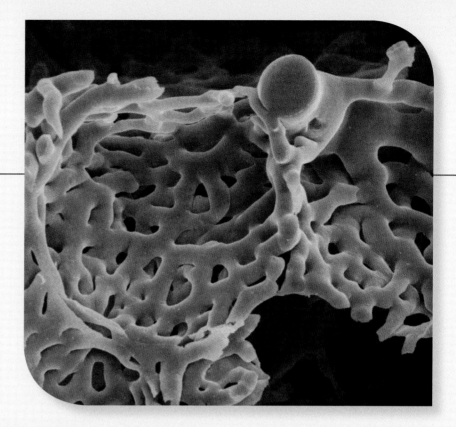

CANCER AND RELATED LUNG MASSES

Pathology of Lung Tumors

DAVID S. BRINK, MD

Introduction

Although some use the term "tumor" as a synonym of neoplasm, its core meaning is swelling or mass. Using this broader definition of "tumor," lung tumors include non-neoplastic masses, as well as benign and malignant neoplasms. (#97)

The most common benign lung tumor is a **pulmonary hamartoma**, typically a popcorn-shaped mass of cartilage, fat, fibrous tissue, and blood vessels (Fig. 31.1). A hamartoma is a non-neoplastic mass of tissue in a normal anatomic location but with abnormal architecture. Despite its name, cytogenetic evidence suggests that the pulmonary hamartoma is neoplastic. Benign neoplasms of the lung include **fibroma** (a proliferation of spindle cells resembling mature fibroblasts), **leiomyoma** (a proliferation of spindle cells resembling mature smooth muscle cells), **hemangioma** (a proliferation of mature endothelial cells forming blood vessels of variable size), **chondroma** (a proliferation of cells resembling mature chondrocytes admixed with chondroid extracellular matrix), and **inflammatory pseudotumor** (a myofibroblastic proliferation).

The most common malignant neoplasm in the lung is a metastasis. Among primary malignant neoplasms of the lung, 90%-95% of these are derived from bronchial epithelium and are collectively referred to as bronchogenic carcinoma; the remaining 5%-10% of primary malignant pulmonary neoplasms comprise a heterogeneous group of cancers. Unless otherwise specified, the term "lung cancer" typically refers to bronchogenic carcinoma rather than metastasis or non-bronchogenic malignancies.

Bronchogenic Carcinoma

Excluding non-melanoma skin cancers (squamous cell carcinoma of the skin and basal cell carcinoma of the skin), **bronchogenic carcinoma** represents the second most common cancer in the United States (see Fig. 32.1) and the most common cause of cancer-related death in men and women. The development of bronchogenic carcinoma is a multistep process in which numerous specific mutations accumulate in a temporal sequence. Common oncogenes involved in the pathogenesis of bronchogenic carcinomata include *c-MYC*, *k-RAS*, *EGFR*, *c-MET*, and *c-KIT*. Tumor suppressor genes that are commonly deleted or inactivated in the pathogenesis of bronchogenic carcinoma include *p53*, *RB*, *p16*, and unknown genes on the short arm of chromosome 3. Risk factors for the development of bronchogenic carcinoma are discussed in Chap. 32 and include tobacco smoking. Of note, tobacco smoking also increases the risk of the development of cancer of the lip, tongue, floor of the mouth, pharynx, larynx, esophagus, urinary bladder, pancreas, and kidney.

Bronchogenic carcinoma is further subclassified by microscopic morphologic criteria. Broadly speaking, there are four major types of bronchogenic carcinoma, and each can be further subtyped. All types are associated with cigarette smoking and are aggressive, locally invasive, and frequently are already widely metastatic at the time of diagnosis. Furthermore, all types are associated with paraneoplastic syndromes (Chap. 32). The four major types of bronchogenic carcinoma are **squamous cell carcinoma (SCCA)**, **adenocarcinoma**, **large cell carcinoma**, and **small cell carcinoma** (Fig. 31.2).

Squamous cell carcinoma is more common in men and generally is a central disease (Fig. 31.3), often with central necrosis, cavitation, and hilar lymph node involvement. However, the incidence of SCCA in more peripheral lung locations is increasing. Microscopically, SCCA is characterized by production of keratin and/or by the presence of intercellular bridges between malignant epithelial cells. In well-differentiated SCCAs, keratin and/or intercellular bridges may be easily identified; in more poorly differentiated SCCA, mitotic activity is typically increased, and keratin and intercellular bridges are more difficult to identify. Variants of SCCA include papillary, clear cell, small cell (not to be confused with small cell carcinoma, see below), and basaloid. Common genes implicated in the pathogenesis of SCCA include *p53*, *RB*, *p16*, and many others.

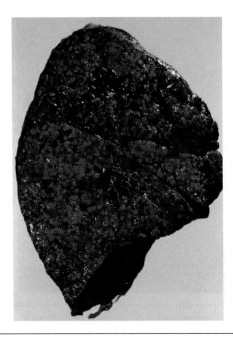

FIGURE 31.6 Bronchioloalveolar carcinoma is frequently multinodular, especially if it is nonmucinous. Note the numerous nodules spread throughout the cut surface of the lung. *Courtesy of Dr. R.A. Cooke, Brisbane, Australia.*

Large cell carcinoma is an anaplastic carcinoma in which the large malignant cells are so poorly differentiated as to defy further classification. Since many show minimal squamous or glandular differentiation at the ultrastructural level, most large cell carcinomata likely represent very poorly differentiated examples of SCCA or adenocarcinoma (Fig. 31.7). However, neuroendocrine differentiation is present in some examples of large cell carcinoma with genetic features similar to small cell carcinoma. Such large cell carcinomata with neuroendocrine differentiation can be thought of as a large cell variant of small cell carcinoma, a somewhat paradoxic designation. Subtypes of large cell carcinoma include **giant cell carcinoma**, **clear cell carcinoma**, and **spindle cell carcinoma**.

Small cell carcinoma, like SCCA, is generally a central disease (Fig. 31.8) and is very strongly associated with smoking. Small cell carcinoma is a neuroendocrine lesion that almost invariably has metastasized by the time of diagnosis. It is named for its characteristic malignant cells that are smaller than malignant cells in other types of bronchogenic carcinoma. The malignant cells do not show squamous or glandular morphology, and small cell carcinoma is universally considered high-grade. Reflecting their neuroendocrine differentiation, immuno-histochemical staining will typically be positive for neural markers, for example, neurofilament, chromogranin, synaptophysin, and neuron-specific enolase (NSE). Ultrastructural analysis shows dense-core, membrane-bound neurosecretory granules. Common genes implicated in the pathogenesis of small cell carcinoma include *p53* and *RB*.

Approximately 10% of cases of bronchogenic carcinoma show a combined pattern, usually of SCCA and adenocarcinoma, or of SCCA and small cell carcinoma.

▶▶ CLINICAL CORRELATION 31.1

Cytologic analysis of sputum and/or bronchial brushings (Chaps. 18 and 19) can establish a diagnosis of bronchogenic carcinoma in 80%-90% of cases, potentially eliminating the need for diagnostic biopsy. However, false-positive diagnoses can be made, typically in the setting of pulmonary infarct, bronchiectasis, fungal/viral infection, lipid pneumonia, or following irradiation. With regard to the specific subtype of bronchogenic carcinoma, cytologic diagnosis agreement with histologic diagnosis (the "gold standard") is 70%-90%. The best

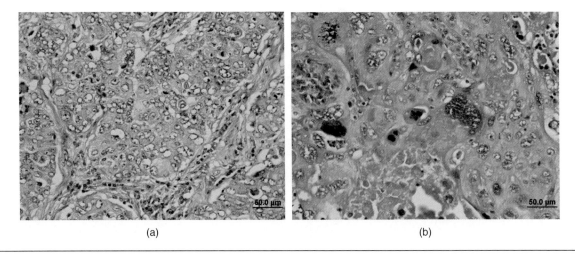

(a)   (b)

FIGURE 31.7 Large cell carcinoma. Most large cell carcinomas are thought of as very poorly differentiated squamous cell carcinomas or adenocarcinomas. (a) The neoplastic cells are very large with marked pleomorphism and show no definitive squamous or glandular differentiation. (b) At the same magnification, even larger neoplastic cells are noted in an example of the giant cell variant of large cell carcinoma.

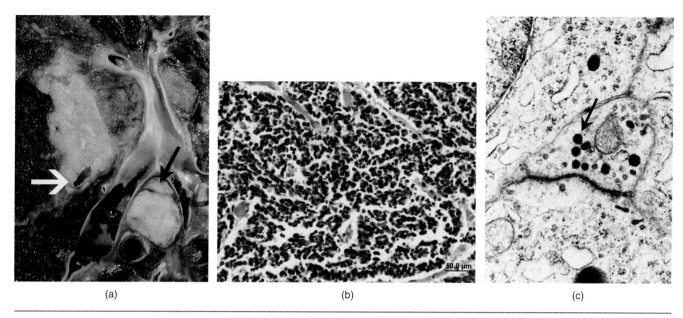

(a)   (b)   (c)

FIGURE 31.8 (a) **Small cell carcinoma**, like squamous cell carcinoma, is typically located near the hilum; the white arrow indicates a bronchial lumen, and the tumor is the off-white lesion surrounding the lumen. The black arrow indicates a lymph node with apparent metastatic disease. (b) Microscopically, the malignant cells of small cell carcinoma show a very high nuclear/cytoplasmic ratio and characteristically show nuclear "molding," a term used to describe the appearance of nuclei being indented by neighboring cells. (c) Ultrastructurally, the neuroendocrine nature of the neoplasm is manifest by the presence of dense-core neurosecretory granules (arrow). (a): *From Kemp et al.* Pathology: the Big Picture, *McGraw-Hill; 2008.* (c): *From Rosai and Ackerman's Surgical Pathology, 9th ed., Mosby-Elsevier, 2004.*

agreement by such assays is for small cell carcinoma and for well-differentiated squamous cell carcinomas and adenocarcinomas.

Bronchogenic carcinoma begins as a focus of epithelial atypia progressing to a lumpy excrescence that elevates or erodes the epithelium. As the neoplasm grows, it can extend into the bronchial lumen to cause obstruction, penetrate the bronchial wall to invade peribronchial tissue, or grow within the parenchyma displacing other structures. Depending on the location within the respiratory tract, bronchogenic carcinoma can involve the pleural surface and spread through the pleural cavity or into the pericardium. In addition to metastasis through pleural fluid, bronchogenic carcinoma can metastasize via lymphatic and blood vessels. Most cases of bronchogenic carcinoma show lymph node metastases at the time of diagnosis; typical lymph nodes involved include tracheal, bronchial, and mediastinal. The most common sites of distant metastasis of bronchogenic carcinoma include the adrenals, liver, brain, and bone. The presentation of bronchogenic carcinoma is markedly variable and is discussed, along with staging of disease, in Chap. 32.

Bronchial Carcinoid

Carcinoids (or **carcinoid tumors**) are neuroendocrine neoplasms with malignant potential and represent 1%-5% of all primary pulmonary neoplasms. They show equal incidence in men and women and typically present in a patient less than

40 years old. The development of bronchial carcinoid tumor has no known relationship to smoking or to other environmental factors.

Grossly, bronchial carcinoids [Fig. 31.9(a)] are typically in a mainstem bronchus as a polypoid spherical intraluminal mass or as a mucosal plaque (a "collar button lesion"). They are typically yellow, in contrast to bronchogenic carcinoma, which is typically white or off-white unless discolored by hemorrhage. Microscopically [Fig. 31.9(b)], the neoplastic cells of carcinoid tumor are monotonous with uniform, round nuclei and are arranged in nests, cords, and islands separated by a delicate fibrous stroma. Similar to small cell carcinoma, cells of bronchial carcinoids contain dense core granules (typical of neuroendocrine differentiation) that are visible on electron microscopic analysis. Many of the neuroendocrine immunohistochemical stains that are positive in small cell carcinoma are likewise positive in bronchial carcinoids (Fig. 31.10). Bronchial carcinoids are subdivided into two subtypes: typical and atypical. **Typical carcinoids** have no necrosis, have fewer than two mitotic figures per high-power field, and have 5- and 10-year survival rates of 87%. **Atypical carcinoids** show focal necrosis and/or two or more mitotic figures per high-power field and have 5- and 10-year survival rates of 56% and 35%, respectively.

Carcinoid tumors are not unique to the respiratory tract and occur elsewhere, notably the alimentary tract. **Carcinoid syndrome** features intermittent attacks of diarrhea, flushing, and cyanosis when such alimentary tract carcinoid tumors metastasize to the liver. Patients with bronchial carcinoids only rarely develop carcinoid syndrome.

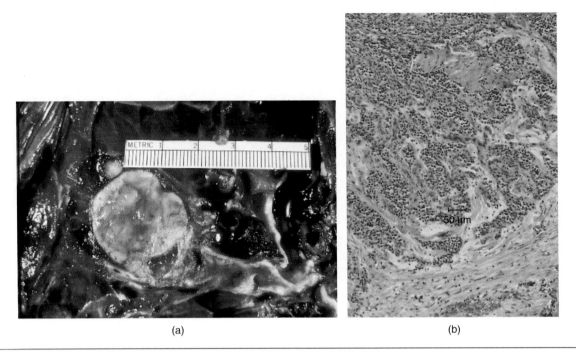

(a)

(b)

FIGURE 31.9 (a) **Carcinoid tumor** grossly is typically well-circumscribed and more yellow than most neoplasms. (b) Histologically, the cells of bronchial carcinoid are arranged in nests, cords, and islands. (a): *From* Rosai and Ackerman's Surgical Pathology, *9th ed., Mosby-Elsevier 2004.*

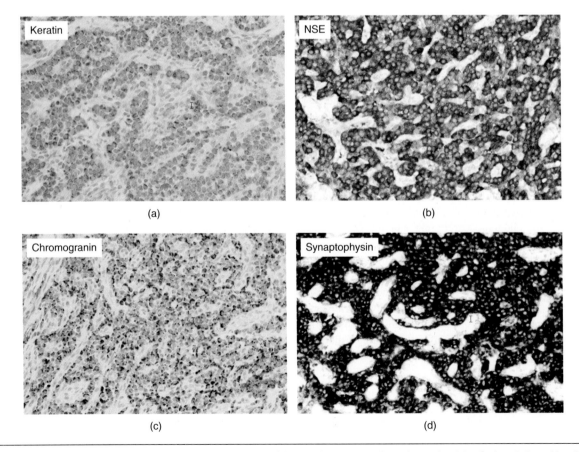

(a)

(b)

(c)

(d)

FIGURE 31.10 (a) **Carcinoid tumor**. Reflecting the epithelial nature of the neoplasm, immunohistochemical staining for keratin is positive. Reflective of the neuroendocrine nature of carcinoid tumor, various neuroendocrine markers will be positive: shown are neuron-specific enolase (NSE) (b), chromogranin (c), and synaptophysin (d). Small cell carcinoma, also a neuroendocrine neoplasm, frequently stains with these markers as well.

▶▶CLINICAL CORRELATION 31.2

A 15-year-old boy presented with a >1-year history of cough, intermittent hemoptysis, and a right lower lobe infiltrate, during which time he had been treated with antibiotics. Months later, he was admitted with cough, marked fatigue, dyspnea, fever, and right-sided chest pain; during his hospital stay, he was treated with ceftriaxone. Subsequently, his intermittent cough continued, especially when running for football, basketball, and baseball. He then had a recurrence of hemoptysis, was diagnosed with streptococcal pharyngitis ("strep throat"), and treated with azithromycin and clindamycin. Over a 17-month period, several chest x-rays and CT showed persistence of a right lower lobe infiltrate (Fig. 31.11).

Bronchoscopy was performed, demonstrating obstruction of a bronchial lumen. Biopsy of the intraluminal mass was performed for a frozen section analysis, in which tissue is frozen and sectioned in "real time," while the patient remained in the operating room. The frozen section (Fig. 31.11) showed morphologic findings suspicious for carcinoid tumor, a diagnosis confirmed on subsequent paraffin-embedded sections [see Figs. 31.9(b) and 31.10)]. The patient's recurrent hemoptysis was due to spontaneous hemorrhage of the bronchial carcinoid, a highly vascular neoplasm, biopsy of which is frequently complicated by hemorrhage that is difficult to control. Because of its luminal obstruction, the boy was at risk of developing lipid pneumonia and recurrent bacterial pneumonia distal to the obstruction, which were responsible for the persistent right lower lobe infiltrate seen by x-ray and CT.

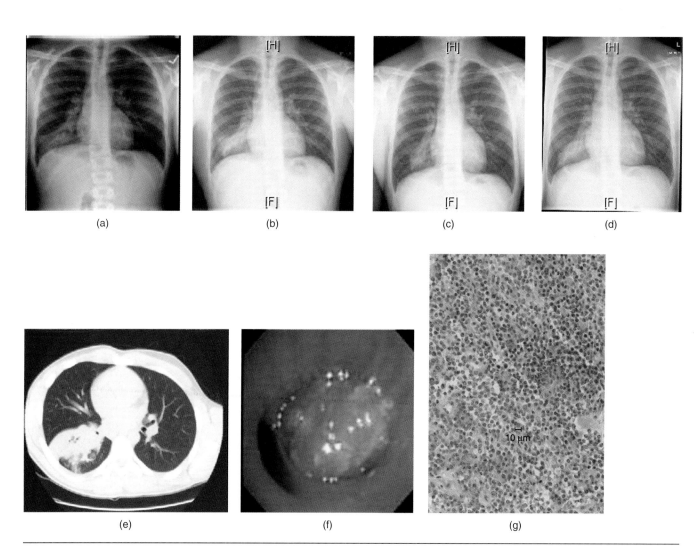

(a) (b) (c) (d)

(e) (f) (g)

FIGURE 31.11 Shown in (a), (b), (c), and (d) are four x-rays obtained over 17 months, each showing a right lower lobe infiltrate. (e) A subsequent CT highlighted the RLL infiltrate. (f) Bronchoscopy showed luminal obstruction. (g) Frozen section analysis of the endobronchial mass showed monotonous cells arranged in cords and nests, suspicious for endobronchial carcinoid tumor, a diagnosis confirmed on analysis of fixed tissue with immunohistochemical staining [see Figs. 31.9(b) and 31.10].

Non-Bronchogenic Malignancies of the Pulmonary Tract

The most common lung malignancy is a metastasis. Of primary lung malignancies, approximately 5% are not bronchogenic carcinoma. Examples include **fibrosarcoma** (malignant proliferation of cells resembling fibroblasts), **leiomyosarcoma** (malignant proliferation of cells resembling smooth muscle cells), **hemangiopericytoma** (malignant proliferation of cells resembling pericytes), **Hodgkin disease** (a malignant proliferation of **Reed-Sternberg cells**, the original nature of which is arguably lymphoid or histiocytoid), and **non-Hodgkin lymphoma** (malignant proliferation of cells with lymphoid differentiation). **Pseudolymphoma** and **lymphocytic interstitial pneumonia** are not frank malignancies but likely represent an early stage of lymphoproliferative disorder and are sometimes referred to as **borderline lesions**.

Pleural Tumors

The most common pleural tumor is a metastasis. Pleural metastasis is common among carcinoma of the lung, breast, and ovary and is often accompanied by pleural effusion (Chaps. 19, 26, and 29) that is typically serous or serosanguineous in composition.

Solitary fibrous tumor (**pleural fibroma**, benign **mesothelioma**) is a localized growth of fibrous connective tissue, typically attached to the pleura by a pedicle (Fig. 31.12). The vast majority of solitary fibrous tumors are benign, though malignant versions exist.

Malignant mesothelioma usually arises in parietal or visceral pleura but can occur in the peritoneal cavity. The most important risk factor for development of malignant mesothelioma is asbestos exposure (Chap. 23), which increases the risk >1,000-fold. With heavy asbestos exposure, the lifetime risk of malignant mesothelioma is 7%-10%. In contrast to the synergy of asbestos and smoking in development of bronchogenic carcinoma, smoking does not significantly increase the risk of malignant mesothelioma.

Grossly, malignant mesothelioma typically ensheathes the lung and is soft, gelatinous, and variably gray to pink. It is frequently associated with extensive pleural effusion (Chaps. 19, 26, and 29) and direct invasion of adjacent chest structures (Fig. 31.13). Microscopically, malignant mesothelioma is subdivided into a sarcomatoid variant (composed of spindle cells), an epitheliod variant (with papillary architecture and often resembling adenocarcinoma), and a biphasic variant showing features of both. Ultrastructural analysis can be helpful in distinguishing the epithelioid variant of malignant mesothelioma from adenocarcinoma: In mesothelioma, the neoplastic cells will show prominent microvilli. Immunohistochemical staining has largely replaced ultrastructural analysis in establishing the diagnosis (see Clinical Correlation 31.3).

▶▶ CLINICAL CORRELATION 31.3

In the setting of a pleural malignancy with epithelioid, papillary architecture, the pathologist can be faced with a diagnostic dilemma: is the lesion adenocarcinoma of

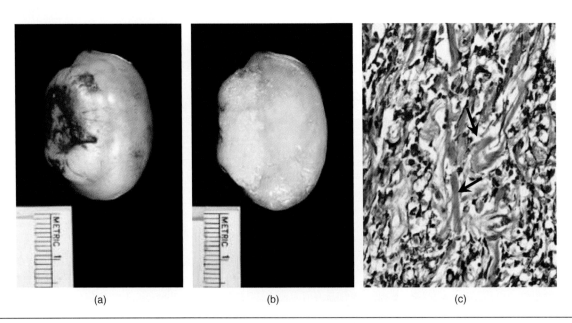

(a)   (b)   (c)

FIGURE 31.12 Solitary fibrous tumor of the pleura. (a) Grossly, a solitary fibrous tumor is typically polypoid; the hemorrhagic portion at left side of the image represents the pedicle that attached the tumor to the pleural surface. (b) The cut surface shows pale rubbery connective tissue. (c) Histologically, broad bands of collagen (arrows) are separated by spindle cells. This lesion, like most solitary fibrous tumors, is benign; however, malignant versions exist. *From* Rosai and Ackerman's Surgical Pathology, *9th ed., Mosby-Elsevier, 2004.*

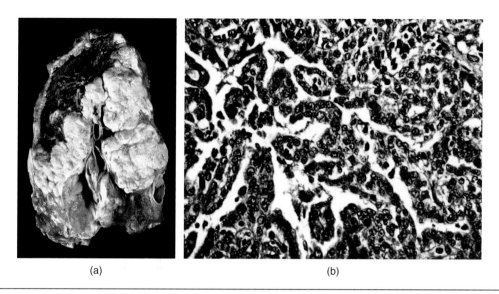

(a)   (b)

FIGURE 31.13 Malignant mesothelioma. (a) Grossly, advanced malignant mesothelioma typically ensheathes the lung, as seen here. (b) Histologically, malignant mesothelioma can show an epithelioid, papillary morphology; alternatively, the microscopic appearance can be sarcomatoid or biphasic (not shown). *From* Rosai and Ackerman's Surgical Pathology, *9th ed., Mosby-Elsevier, 2004.*

the lung metastatic to the pleura or a primary pleural malignant mesothelioma? Making the correct diagnosis is important for proper clinical management; in the setting of historical occupational asbestos exposure, the diagnosis often has significant legal implications. Historically, ultrastructural analysis was of great value in separating the two neoplasms (Fig. 31.14).

However, the role of ultrastructural analysis has largely been replaced by immunohistochemical analysis, for which the pathologist has a large armamentarium of stains that can aid diagnostic accuracy. Table 31.1 provides an example

of the many immunohistochemical stains applicable to the distinction of malignant mesothelioma from adenocarcinoma. Of note, items marked as "+" or "–" are *usually* positive or negative, respectively; 100% specificity seldom is achieved with immunohistochemical analysis. Due to the vast number of potential stains available, pathologists often consult references before ordering particular stains, including books (eg, Dabbs DJ, *Diagnostic Immunohistochemistry*, 3rd ed. Philadelphia, PA : Elsevier-Saunders; 2010) and online references (eg, PathIQ Immunoquery 2.8 at https:// immunoquery.pathiq.com/PathIQ/Login.do).

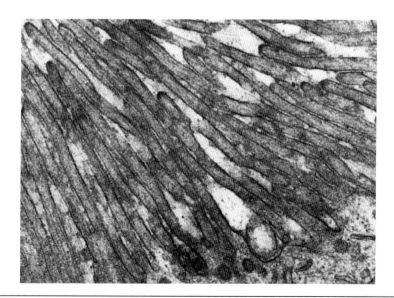

FIGURE 31.14 Ultrastructural analysis of malignant mesothelioma shows prominent, elongated microvilli, a feature that can help differentiate the lesion from adenocarcinoma in cases with equivocal light microscopic morphology. *From* Rosai and Ackerman's Surgical Pathology, *9th ed., Mosby-Elsevier, 2004.*

Table **31.1** Potential immunohistochemical stains to distinguish pulmonary adenocarcinoma from malignant mesothelioma

Immunostain	Pulmonary Adenocarcinoma	Malignant Mesothelioma
Pankeratin	+	+
Epithelial membrane antigen	+	+
S-100	+	+
Carcinoembryonic antigen	+	–
CD15B72.3	+	–
Ber-Ep4	+	–
Bg8	+	–
MOC-31	+	–
TTF-1	+	–
Calretinin	–	+
WT-1	–	+
Keratin 5/6	–	+
Thrombomodulin	–	+
Vimentin	–	+

Clinically, malignant mesothelioma presents with chest pain, dyspnea, and recurrent pleural effusion. Concurrent pulmonary asbestosis (Chap. 23) is present in approximately 20% of patients with pleural malignant mesothelioma and approximately one-half of patients with peritoneal malignant mesothelioma. Malignant mesothelioma is a particularly morbid disease, with a 1-year survival rate of approximately 50% and a 2-year survival rate approaching 0%.

Suggested Readings

1. Kumar V, Abbas AK, Fausto N. *Robbins and Cotran Pathologic Basis of Disease*, 8th ed. Philadelphia, PA: Elsevier; 2007. *Throughout its many editions, this reference work is the most definitive and approachable compendium of pathology images available to students.*

2. *Rosai J. Rosai and Ackerman's Surgical Pathology:* 9th ed. New York, NY: Mosby-Elsevier; 2004. A classic surgical

pathology two-volume text, with far more morphologic detail than in a general pathology text like *Robbins and Cotran's Pathologic Basis of Disease*, and a standard reference text for pathologists working in a clinical setting interpreting surgical pathology specimens.

CASE STUDIES AND PRACTICE PROBLEMS

CASE 31.1 Smokers are at increased risk for which of the following?

a. Bronchogenic carcinoma, small cell carcinoma variant
b. Bronchogenic carcinoma, bronchioloalveolar carcinoma variant
c. Malignant mesothelioma
d. Bronchial carcinoid tumor
e. Pulmonary hamartoma

CASE 31.2 Which of the following findings adversely affects the prognosis of bronchial carcinoid tumor?

a. Growth pattern obstructing bronchial lumen
b. Growth pattern as mucosal plaque
c. Two or more mitotic figures per high-power field
d. History of smoking
e. History of asbestos exposure

CASE 31.3 Which of the following is a finding that would be most useful in distinguishing carcinoid tumor from small cell carcinoma?

    a. The presence of cytoplasmic dense core granules in neoplastic cells

    b. Immunohistochemical positivity for keratin

    c. Immunohistochemical positivity for synaptophysin

    d. Immunohistochemical positivity for chromogranin

    e. Monotonous cells with round nuclei growing in cords and trabeculae separated by delicate fibrous connective tissue septa

Solutions to Case Studies and Practice Problems

CASE 31.1 The most correct answer is a, small cell carcinoma variant of bronchogenic carcinoma.

None of the other possible answers (*b*, *c*, *d*, or *e*) shows a significant association with smoking.

CASE 31.2 The most correct answer is c, two or more mitotic figures per high-power field.

Increased mitotic activity distinguishes atypical from typical carcinoid tumor. The prognosis of atypical carcinoid tumor is worse than that of typical carcinoid tumor. The pattern of growth (*answers a* and *b*) does not significantly alter prognosis directly; however,

there could be an indirect influence by a growth pattern that makes excision difficult. Smoking and asbestos exposure have no significant relationship to the development of or prognosis of carcinoid tumor.

CASE 31.3 The most correct answer is e, monotonous cells with round nuclei growing in cords and trabeculae separated by delicate fibrous connective tissue septa.

Answers a, b, c, and *d* are features that small cell carcinoma shares with carcinoid tumor, reflecting the epithelial (*answer b*) and neuroendocrine (*answers a, c,* and *d*) nature of both neoplasms.

Chapter 32

Lung Cancer

DAVID A. STOECKEL, MD AND
GEORGE M. MATUSCHAK, MD

Learning Objectives

- The student will be able to describe the epidemiology and risk factors for lung cancer.

- The student will be able to enumerate the major histologic types of lung cancer and differentiate how cell types affect tumor growth and behavior.

- The student will be able to recognize the common symptoms and signs of thoracic and extrathoracic lung cancer, and the common paraneoplastic syndromes associated with lung cancer.

- The student will be able to summarize the general principles of lung cancer staging and describe how tumor stages affect treatment options and outcomes.

Epidemiology and Risk Factors

Lung cancer is the leading cause of cancer-related mortality in the United States. In 2009, over 200,000 new cases of lung cancer were diagnosed and, unfortunately, nearly 160,000 deaths occurred as a result of lung cancer (Fig. 32.1). In a sobering testament to its lethality, lung cancer accounts for only 15% of all cancers diagnosed (excluding non-melanomas of the skin), but accounts for 28% of those cancer deaths. Lung cancer has been the leading cause of cancer death in men in the United States since the mid-1950s, and in women since the late 1980s. This is especially striking given that lung cancer was a rare occurrence at the turn of the 20th century (Fig. 32.2).

The incidence of lung cancer increases steadily with age. Over a lifetime, 1 in 13 American men and 1 in 16 American women will be diagnosed with lung cancer. Thankfully, the lung cancer death rate has been declining in men and seems to have reached a plateau in women. African-American men are disproportionally affected compared to other races and ethnicities.

Exposure to tobacco smoke is by far the most substantial risk factor for development of lung cancer, and is at least partially avoidable. Approximately 80%-90% of all patients diagnosed with lung cancer are either current or former smokers. The association between tobacco smoke and lung cancer was postulated a century ago and clearly demonstrated by epidemiologic studies in the 1950s (Fig. 32.3). In the United States, the lifetime risk of lung cancer for a nonsmoker is <1% and increases to 15%-30% with long-term tobacco use. The risk of lung cancer increases with the amount and duration of tobacco exposure, and conversely the risk declines with abstinence. A decrease in risk can be demonstrated within 5 years of quitting smoking, and by 15 years there is an 80%-90% reduction in the risk of developing lung cancer, although that risk remains higher than for a never-smoker. Cigarettes seem to confer a higher risk of lung cancer than the use of pipes and cigars. Passive or "second-hand" exposure to tobacco smoke also increases the risk of lung cancer, but to a much lesser degree than active smoking. Never-smoking women married to husbands who smoke have up to a two-fold increase in the risk of lung cancer compared to never-smoking women with non-smoking spouses.

Exposure to radon, a radioactive gas released by the decay of naturally occurring ^{238}uranium, is the second leading cause

of lung cancer in the United States and accounts for up to 10% of all lung cancer cases. Radon gas collects in poorly ventilated portions of some homes and buildings. Air pollution may account for 2% of lung cancer cases in the United States, but is a more significant factor worldwide, notably where **biomass fuels** are used for residential heating and cooking. Asbestos exposure alone modestly increases the risk of lung cancer, but when combined with tobacco use the risk increases dramatically by 50- to 60-fold (Fig. 32.4). Other risk factors for lung cancer include COPD, interstitial lung disease, and a family history of lung cancer. Finally, the risk of lung cancer is inversely proportional to intake of fruits and vegetables, although prospective trials involving such dietary supplementation have not shown a clear benefit.

Pathogenesis of Lung Cancers

The pathogenesis of lung cancer involves a multistep process that is not completely understood. In most cases, lung cancer is initiated by adverse interactions between carcinogens and the respiratory epithelium that lead to genetic alterations. These alterations can be found in histologically normal tissue from smoker's lungs. New DNA sequencing technologies have uncovered multiple and varied genetic abnormalities that reveal the heterogeneous nature of lung cancer even within a single cell type. Common genetic and molecular alterations include **p53 tumor suppressor gene** mutations, **K-ras proto-oncogene** mutations, and **epidermal growth factor (EGF)** and EGF receptor abnormalities. Genetic evidence of **human papilloma virus (HPV)** infection also suggests a role for viruses in lung cancer pathogenesis. The genetic and molecular

Estimated New Cases

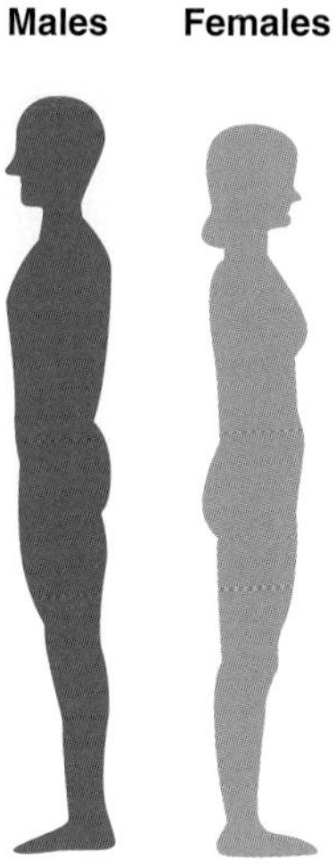

			Males	**Females**			
Prostate	217,730	28%			Breast	207,090	28%
Lung & bronchus	116,750	15%			Lung & bronchus	105,770	14%
Colon & rectum	72,090	9%			Colon & rectum	70,480	10%
Urinary bladder	52,760	7%			Uterine corpus	43,470	6%
Melanoma of the skin	38,870	5%			Thyroid	33,930	5%
Non-Hodgkin lymphoma	35,380	4%			Non-Hodgkin lymphoma	30,160	4%
Kidney & renal pelvis	35,370	4%			Melanoma of the skin	29,260	4%
Oral cavity & pharynx	25,420	3%			Kidney & renal pelvis	22,870	3%
Leukemia	24,690	3%			Ovary	21,880	3%
Pancreas	21,370	3%			Pancreas	21,770	3%
All sites	**789,620**	**100%**			**All sites**	**739,940**	**100%**

Estimated Deaths

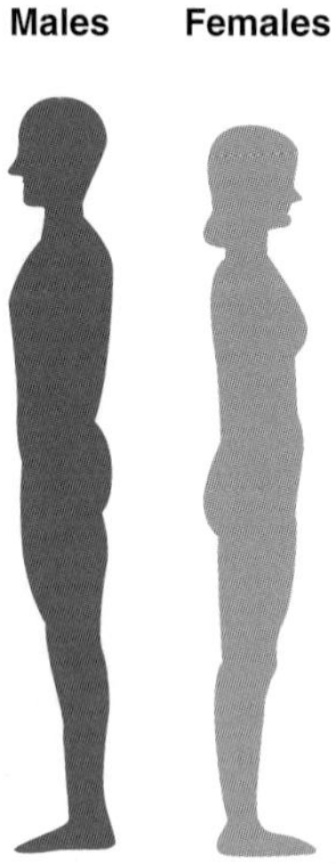

			Males	**Females**			
Lung & bronchus	86,220	29%			Lung & bronchus	71,080	26%
Prostate	32,050	11%			Breast	39,840	15%
Colon & rectum	26,580	9%			Colon & rectum	24,790	9%
Pancreas	18,770	6%			Pancreas	18,030	7%
Liver & intrahepatic bile duct	12,720	4%			Ovary	13,850	5%
Leukemia	12,660	4%			Non-Hodgkin lymphoma	9,500	4%
Esophagus	11,650	4%			Leukemia	9,180	3%
Non-Hodgkin lymphoma	10,710	4%			Uterine corpus	7,950	3%
Urinary bladder	10,410	3%			Liver & intrahepatic bile duct	6,190	2%
Kidney & renal pelvis	8,210	3%			Brain & other nervous system	5,720	2%
All sites	**299,200**	**100%**			**All sites**	**270,290**	**100%**

FIGURE 32.1 Ten leading cancer types for estimated new cancer cases and deaths in the United States for 2010. *From Jemal A et al:* Cancer statistics, 2010, *CA Cancer J. Clin Sep-Oct;60(5): 277-300, 2010.*

characteristics of a cancer affect its promotion, progression, invasion, and metastasis. Although the heterogeneity of lung cancer might frustrate hopes of a single effective treatment, knowledge of the varied abnormalities allows for an individualized approach to treatment and prognostication. In some cases, certain genetic mutations suggest a likelihood of a dramatic response to very specific chemotherapeutic agents.

Review of Lung Cancer Histopathology

Classification of lung cancer by the World Health Organization in 2004 is based upon the appearance of the tumor cells by light microscopy (Table 32.1; see Chap. 31). Diagnostic immunohistochemical staining can corroborate and refine the classification based upon routine stains and light microscopy. In the aggregate, adenocarcinoma, squamous cell carcinoma, and small cell carcinoma account for ~85% of lung cancers.

Adenocarcinoma is the most common histologic type of lung cancer accounting for up to 35% of all lung cancers, and this proportion seems to be increasing as compared to other cell types. It is more common in women and is the lung cancer type found in nearly all nonsmokers. Grossly, adenocarcinoma is irregularly lobulated, grey-white in color, and commonly shows entrapped anthracotic pigment. Histologically, adenocarcinomas are glandular in appearance and may show mucin in the cytoplasm (Fig. 32.5).

Clinically, adenocarcinomas tend to occur in the lung periphery (Fig. 32.6) either synchronously with more than one primary tumor at the same time, or metachronously with multiple

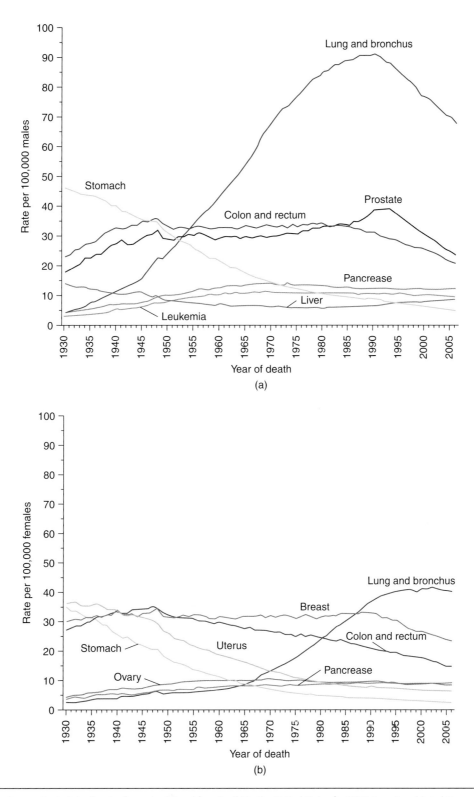

FIGURE 32.2 Annual age-adjusted death rates for males (a) and females (b) in the United States for 2010. *From Jemal A et al: Cancer statistics, 2010, CA Cancer J. Clin Sep-Oct;60(5): 277-300, 2010.*

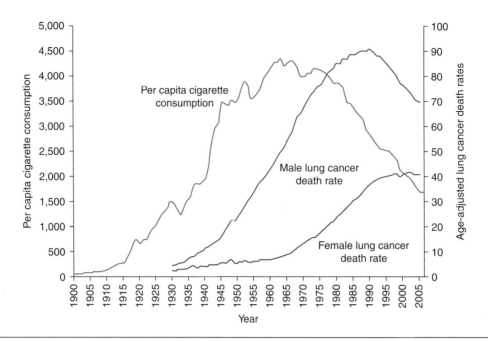

FIGURE 32.3 Relationship between cigarette consumption and lung cancer death rates. *From* Cancer Statistics 2009. © *American Cancer Society.*

primary tumors developing at different times. **Bronchioloalveolar carcinoma** is a subtype of adenocarcinoma requiring special attention as it can mimic pneumonia radiographically as a focal opacity or as more diffuse opacities. Histologically, bronchioloalveolar carcinoma is a well-differentiated tumor that grows along intact alveolar septa in a so-called **lepidic pattern** (Fig. 32.7).

Squamous cell carcinoma is the second most common histologic type of lung cancer. Although declining in occurrence, squamous cell cancer currently stands at ~30% of new cases. This decline may relate to increased preference for low-tar and filtered cigarettes; it is uncommon among nonsmokers. Grossly, squamous cell cancers have irregular and friable grey-to-white surfaces, and necrosis with central cavitation is common (Chap. 31). Histologic features include keratin production and intercellular bridges (Fig. 32.8). Clinically, squamous cell carcinoma often involves the large central airways, and initial symptoms may include cough and hemoptysis. Imaging may reveal obstructive collapse of a portion of the lung or a **cavitary lesion** (Fig. 32.8).

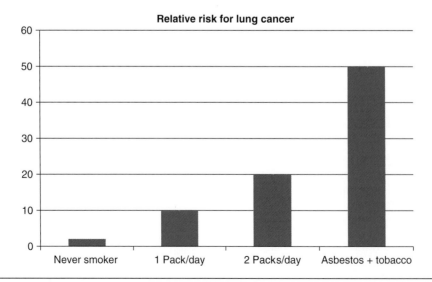

FIGURE 32.4 Relative risks for development of lung cancer from tobacco smoking and asbestos exposure. *Adapted from Albert R. et al.* Clinical Respiratory Medicine, *3rd ed. 2008.*

Table 32.1 WHO classification of invasive malignant epithelial lung tumors

Squamous Cell Carcinoma	Variants: papillary, clear cell, small cell, basaloid
Small Cell Carcinoma	Variants: combined small cell carcinoma
Adenocarcinoma • Mixed Subtype • Acinar • Papillary • Bronchioloalveolar • Solid	Variants: mucinous, non-mucinous, mixed Variants: fetal, mucinous, mucinous cystadenocarcinoma, signet ring, clear cell
Large Cell Carcinoma	Variants: large cell neuroendocrine, combined, basiloid, lymphoepithelioma-like, clear cell, rhaboid
Adenosquamous Carcinoma	
Sarcomatoid Carcinoma	Variants: pleomorphic, spindle cell, giant cell, carcinosarcoma, pulmonary blastoma
Carcinoid Tumor	Variants: typical, atypical
Salivary Gland Tumors	Variants: mucoepidermoid, adenoid cystic, epithelial-myoepithelial

Data from Travis et al., eds: Pathology and genetics of tumours of the lung, pleura, thymus, and heart, IARC Press, 2004.

Small cell carcinoma accounts for up to 25% of all lung cancers, and of all histologic types it is the most strongly associated with smoking. Grossly, small cell tumors are typically grey or tan and fleshy in texture. Histologic findings vary, but the cells are generally small with hyperchromatic nuclei and are fragile, crushing easily upon biopsy (Fig. 32.9). Clinically, these tumors usually present as central masses with marked lymphadenopathy on chest imaging (Fig. 32.9). Small cell

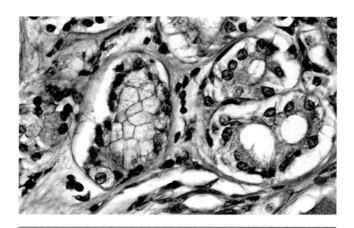

FIGURE 32.5 Adenocarcinoma of the lung. *From* www.microscopyu.com.

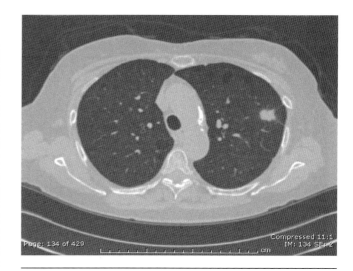

FIGURE 32.6 "Coin lesion" appearance of a left upper lobe adenocarcinoma. Emphysematous blebs are incidentally noted in the left and right upper lobes.

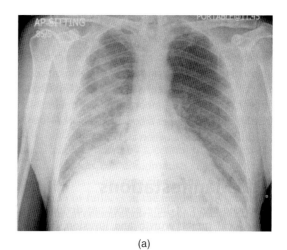

(a)

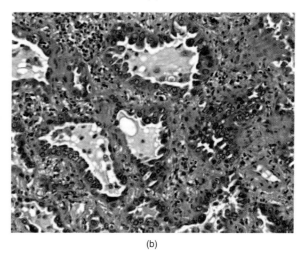

(b)

FIGURE 32.7 (a) Bronchioloalveolar carcinoma on chest x-ray. (b) Lepidic growth pattern of bronchioloalveolar carcinoma. (a): *From* www.radiopaedia.org. (b): *From Yousem and Beasley,* Archives of Pathology & Laboratory Medicine, *vol. 131, pp. 1027-1032; 2007.*

Table **32.3** **Paraneoplastic syndromes associated with lung cancer**

Skeletal and Systemic		Hematologic
Hypertrophic osteoarthropathy	Anorexia, cachexia	Anemia
Clubbing	Fever, malaise	Leukocytosis
Renal, nephrotic syndromes	Collagen-vascular syndromes	Leukemoid reactions
Glomerulonephritis	Dermatomyositis	Thrombocytosis, TTP
Hypouricemia	Polymyositis	Coagulopathies, DIC
Metabolic syndromes	Vasculitis	Thrombophlebitis
Lactic acidosis	Systemic lupus erythematosus	Eosinophilia
Cutaneous	**Endocrine**	**Neurologic**
Acquired hypertrichosis lanuginosa	SIADH production	Sensory neuropathy
Erythema gyratum repens	Nonmetastatic hypercalcemia	Mononeuritis multiplex
Erythema multiforme	Cushing syndrome	Intestinal pseudo-obstruction
Tylosis	Gynecomastia	Lambert-Eaton myasthenia
Erythroderma	Hypercalcitonemia	Encephalomyelitis
Exfoliative dermatitis	Elevated [LSH], [FSH]	Necrotizing myelopathy
Acanthosis nigricans	Hypoglycemia	Cancer-associated retinopathy
Sweet syndrome	Hyperthyroidism	
Pruritus and urticaria	Carcinoid syndrome	

Finally, symptoms and signs of lung cancer may be a result of paraneoplastic phenomena, that is, disorders mediated by secretory products of tumor cells or by anti-tumor antibodies that cross-react with other tissues (Table 32.3). Paraneoplastic syndromes occur in up to 20% of patients with lung cancer, with hypercalcemia leading to constipation, dehydration, lethargy, and confusion being common. Unlike most paraneoplastic syndromes that are associated with small cell lung cancers, hypercalcemia is most common among patients with squamous cell lung cancer.

The **syndrome of inappropriate antidiuretic hormone hypersecretion (SIADH)** is another common paraneoplastic entity. SIADH results in hyponatremia which may lead to confusion, seizures, and coma. **Cushing syndrome** due to tumor cell production of ACTH can lead to hypertension, hypokalemia, and hyperglycemia. Clubbing and hypertrophic pulmonary osteoarthropathy are paraneoplastic syndromes with skeletal manifestations (Fig. 32.12). Hypertrophic osteoarthropathy is characterized by painful proliferative periostitis most commonly involving the wrists, elbows, ankles, or knees. Neurologic paraneoplastic syndromes include **Lambert-Eaton myasthenic syndrome (LEMS)** characterized by limb weakness, autonomic dysfunction, and cranial nerve deficits. This syndrome displays a characteristic improvement in muscular response to repetitive nerve stimulation during neurophysiologic testing. A hypercoagulable state, thrombocytosis, cachexia, and malaise are all common paraneoplastic syndromes. Treatment of the underlying lung cancer is paramount in the treatment of the paraneoplastic syndromes, as many of these will improve if not completely resolved with effective treatment of the malignancy.

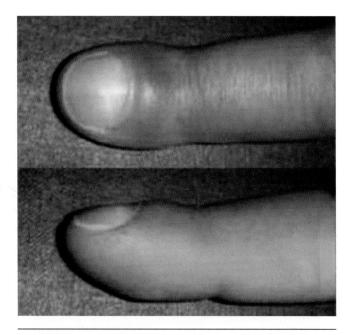

FIGURE 32.12 Representative example of clubbing of the fingers. *Image courtesy of the University of Leeds. From* www.sciencedaily.com

Diagnosis and Staging

Symptoms consistent with lung cancer with or without results of imaging procedures may suggest lung cancer, but histologic or cytologic analysis is required to make the diagnosis. The least invasive means to obtain a specimen for analysis is sputum collection. Although not particularly sensitive, sputum cytology may be helpful with larger central tumors with endobronchial involvement (Chap. 19). Cytologic analysis of needle aspirates of the primary tumor, the involved lymph nodes, or distant metastases is an increasingly common means of establishing the diagnosis. Very occasionally, needle aspirates can be obtained from superficial structures without the use of imaging or endoscopy. More commonly, CT or ultrasound imaging, bronchoscopy, or a combination of these such as endobronchial ultrasound, can be used to guide the aspiration needle to the correct location. Bronchoscopy can also be used to obtain brushings and lavage for cytologic analysis (Chap. 18). In addition, bronchoscopy can provide direct tissue biopsy for histologic analysis if there is large airway endobronchial involvement. Finally, more invasive surgical procedures such as mediastinoscopy, thoracoscopy, or thoracotomy are occasionally required to obtain tissue for diagnosis.

Accompanying such diagnosis is the process of clinical staging that takes into account characteristics of the primary tumor and of nodal or distant metastasis to allow for accurate survival predictions and worthwhile treatment options. The preferred staging at present uses the **International Association of Lung Cancer (IASLC) TNM System** (7th ed.) (Table 32.4). This staging process for a patient with known or suspected lung cancer starts with a thorough but focused history and physical exam, followed by a CT scan of the chest that includes the liver and adrenal glands. In most cases, the patient will undergo whole body PET scanning or integrated PET-CT scanning as an evaluation for metastatic disease.

Table **32.4** **Overview of the TNM staging system for lung and other cancers***

Descriptors	Definitions
T	**Primary tumor**
T0	No primary tumor
T1	Tumor ≤3 cm,[†] surrounded by lung or visceral pleura, not more proximal than the lobar bronchus
T1a	Tumor ≤2 cm[†]
T1b	Tumor >2 but ≤3 cm[†]
T2	Tumor >3 but ≤7 cm[†] or tumor with any of the following[†]: Invades visceral pleura, involves main bronchus ≥ 2 cm distal to the carina, atelectasis/obstructive pneumonia extending to hilum but not involving the entire lung
T2a	Tumor >3 but ≤5 cm[†]
T2b	Tumor >5 but ≤7 cm[†]
T3	Tumor >7 cm; or directly invading chest wall, diaphragm, phrenic nerve, mediastinal pleura, or parietal pericardium; or tumor in the main bronchus <2 cm distal to the carina; or atelectasis/obstructive pneumonitis of entire lung; or separate tumor nodules in the same lobe
T4	Tumor of any size with invasion of heart, great vessels, trachea, recurrent laryngeal nerve, esophagus, vertebral body, or carina; or separate tumor nodules in a different ipsilateral lobe
N	**Regional lymph nodes**
N0	No regional node metastasis
N1	Metastasis in ipsilateral peribronchial and/or perihilar lymph nodes and intrapulmonary nodes, including involvement by direct extension
N2	Metastasis in ipsilateral mediastinal and/or subcarinal lymph nodes
N3	Metastasis in contralateral mediastinal, contralateral hilar, ipsilateral or contralateral scalene, or supraclavicular lymph nodes
M	**Distant metastasis**
M0	No distant metastasis
M1a	Separate tumor nodules in a contralateral lobe; or tumor with pleural nodules or malignant pleural dissemination
M1b	Distant metastasis
Special situations	
TX, NX, MX	T, N, or M status not able to be assessed
Tis	Focus of *in situ* cancer
T1	Superficial spreading tumor of any size but confined to the wall of the trachea or mainstem bronchus

*Table adapted from Detterbeck F. et al: The new lung cancer staging system, Chest Jul;136(1):260-271, 2010.
[†]In its greatest dimension.

In general, imaging alone should not be used to determine stage. The suspected site that would provide for the highest stage, such as a distant metastasis if present, should be biopsied to confirm the suspected stage.

The **T descriptor** in the TNM system is based on characteristics of the primary tumor, and ranges from T1 for small peripheral tumors that do not involve vital structures to T4 for tumors that involve vital, unresectable structures. The T descriptor also increases with size of the primary tumor; a 'T0' indicates that no primary tumor has been found. The **N descriptor** increases from N1 to N3 as progressively more distant hilar and mediastinal lymph nodes are involved; 'N0' indicates no lymph nodes are involved with the cancer. Finally, the **M descriptor** indicates the absence or presence of distant metastases; an 'M0' indicates that no distant metastasis have been found, while M1 indicates the presence of distant metastasis or a malignant pleural effusion.

Although TNM staging can be used for both small cell and non-small cell lung cancers, clinicians frequently distinguish among small cell lung cancer patients with limited versus extensive disease. Patients with **limited disease** include those with no evidence of disease outside of one hemithorax. All others would have **extensive disease**.

Treatment

Treatment of lung cancer depends on the cell type and stage of disease. For stage I, stage II, and selected stage III non-small cell lung cancers (Fig. 32.13), surgical resection is favored as this approach offers a chance of cure and better survival. Left untreated, stage I non-small cell lung cancer has a median survival of ~13 months, whereas >50% of treated patients are alive at 5 years. **Lobectomy** is the treatment of choice with more extensive **pneumonectomy** reserved for patients with disease in locations not amenable to lobectomy. More limited **wedge resections** are an option for patients with poor lung function, advanced age, or very small tumors. Preoperative pulmonary function testing is essential to predict how much lung can be removed without undue postoperative morbidity (Chap. 16). Radiation therapy, including precisely targeted high dose radiation called **radiosurgery**, is an option for patients with early stage non-small cell lung cancer who are unable or unwilling to undergo surgery. Patients with stage II and stage III disease who undergo surgery should receive postoperative or adjuvant chemotherapy if they can tolerate the chemotherapeutic agents.

Surgical resection is not an option for patients with more advanced stage IV non-small cell lung cancer, or for many patients with stage III non-small cell lung cancer. For patients without distant metastasis, concurrent radiation therapy with chemotherapy offers the best survival. For patients with metastatic disease, chemotherapy offers a survival advantage over supportive care alone. Chemotherapy for non-small cell lung cancer usually consists of a platinum-based agent plus one other drug.

Small cell lung cancer is usually considered a disseminated disease at presentation, and thus surgical resection with curative intent is usually not an option. For patients with limited disease, concurrent chemoradiation therapy offers the best overall survival and a chance for long-term survival. For patients with extensive disease, chemotherapy alone is used. Like chemotherapy for non-small cell lung cancer, a platinum-based agent plus a second drug is the usual regimen for small cell lung cancer.

With increasing knowledge of the pathobiology of lung cancer, agents that can be targeted to cancers with specific genetic signatures or other molecular alterations are being developed and successfully used. These agents require a more thorough diagnostic evaluation of an individual tumor, such as genetic mutation analysis, but allow for greater efficacy and possibly less toxicity with treatment.

T/M	Subgroup	N0	N1	N2	N3
T1	T1a	Ia	IIa	IIIa	IIIb
	T1b	Ia	IIa	IIIa	IIIb
T2	T2a	Ib	IIa	IIIa	IIIb
	T2b	IIa	IIb	IIIa	IIIb
T3	T3 >7	IIb	IIIa	IIIa	IIIb
	T3 Inv	IIb	IIIa	IIIa	IIIb
	T3 Satell	IIb	IIIa	IIIa	IIIb
T4	T4 Inv	IIIa	IIIa	IIIb	IIIb
	T4 Ipsi nod	IIIa	IIIa	IIIb	IIIb
M1	M1a Contra nod				
	M1a Pl disem				
	M1b				

FIGURE 32.13 Stage groups based on TNM descriptors from the IASLC TNM staging system (7th ed). *From Detterbeck F. et al: The new lung cancer staging system, Chest Jul;136(1):260-271, 2010.*

Suggested Readings

1. Albert A, Spiro S, Jett J. "Lung Tumors" in: *Clinical Respiratory Medicine* 2nd ed. Philadelphia, PA: Mosby; 2004. *A complete and readable overview of all clinical aspects of lung cancer. Contains many fine photographs and illustrations.*

2. Pelosof LC, Gerber DE. Paraneoplastic syndromes: an approach to diagnosis and treatment. *Mayo Clin Proc.* 2010;85:838-854. *An in-depth yet succinct overview of paraneoplastic syndromes, including those associated with lung cancer.*

CASE STUDIES AND PRACTICE PROBLEMS

CASE 32.1 A 75-year-old woman presents with confusion, dehydration, and constipation. She is found to have hypercalcemia and is admitted for observation and further testing. A new chest x-ray reveals a right hilar mass. A whole body PET-CT scan reveals no evidence of mediastinal lymph node involvement or distant metastasis. What is the most likely explanation for hypercalcemia in this patient?

a. Hypertrophic pulmonary osteoarthropathy secondary to adenocarcinoma of the lung

b. Paraneoplastic syndrome secondary to small cell lung carcinoma

c. Paraneoplastic syndrome secondary to squamous cell lung carcinoma

d. Osteolytic bony lesions secondary to adenocarcinoma of the lung

e. Recent emergence of Cushing syndrome

CASE 32.2 A 75-year-old man with a 60-pack year history of tobacco abuse presents with progressive dyspnea of 4 weeks. He has a history of nonproductive cough, anorexia, and 8 kg weight loss, but denies fever, chills, or night sweats. On physical exam, he has normal vital signs; jugular venous pressure is normal. There is no lymphadenopathy. Cardiac exam shows decreased heart sounds but no other abnormality. On pulmonary exam, the patient has dullness over the left lower lung field, decreased tactile fremitus, and decreased breath sounds. The right lung examination is normal. Chest x-ray shows consolidation in the left lung with moderate pleural effusion. What is the most appropriate management of this patient at this point?

a. Bronchoscopy

b. CT guided needle biopsy

c. Inhaled bronchodilators

d. Intravenous antibiotics

e. Thoracentesis

CASE 32.3 A 50-year-old woman presents to her oncologist for evaluation prior to treatment of a recently diagnosed adenocarcinoma of the lung that is unresectable due to contralateral mediastinal lymph node involvement. She complains of difficulty opening her car door while in the driver's seat, but no problem opening the car door when in the passenger's seat. She denies headaches, visual changes, nausea, vomiting, arthralgias, rashes, sensory changes, or weakness involving other extremities. On exam, she has subtle left upper extremity weakness manifested by a pronator drift on the left. Muscular tone and reflexes seem normal. What is the most likely cause of her symptoms?

a. Hypertrophic pulmonary osteoarthropathy secondary to her lung cancer

b. Lambert-Eaton myasthenic syndrome secondary to her lung cancer

c. Polymyositis secondary to her lung cancer

d. Hypercalcemia secondary to her lung cancer

e. Brain metastasis secondary to her lung cancer

Solutions to Case Studies and Practice Problems

CASE 32.1 The most correct answer is c, paraneoplastic syndrome secondary to squamous cell carcinoma of the lung.

Answer a is incorrect, inasmuch as hypertrophic pulmonary osteoarthropathy secondary to adenocarcinoma of the lung is generally not associated with hypercalcemia even though osseous structures are involved by periostitis and digital clubbing. *Answer b* is unlikely because unlike most paraneoplastic syndromes that are associated with small cell lung carcinomas, hypercalcemia is most common among patients with squamous cell lung cancer. *Answer d* is incorrect here because metastatic disease to the bones has already been excluded by the PET-CT scan findings. *Answer e* is not applicable here because the spectrum of laboratory abnormalities in Cushing syndrome generally does not include hypercalcemia.

CASE 32.2 The most correct answer is e, thoracentesis.

This patient with a long-standing history of exposure to tobacco products and thereby at risk for pulmonary malignancy is symptomatic with shortness of breath and physical findings consistent with his radiographically demonstrable left-sided pleural effusion. *Answer a*, bronchoscopy, is not the recommended initial diagnostic procedure because thoracentesis may both improve the patient's dyspnea even while providing diagnostic material to help establish whether the pleural effusion is due to a malignant cause, which if the case, would represent M1a disease. *Answer b*, CT guided needle biopsy is not appropriate here considering the presence of readily obtainable pleural fluid by thoracentesis. *Answer c*, inhaled bronchodilators is not the most appropriate management at this point in view of the lack of wheezing on physical examination. Similarly, *answer d* represents empiric treatment for pneumonia. Yet, the patient is without fever or chills to support that diagnosis; such treatment is also unlikely to improve the patient's symptoms acutely and will not furnish diagnostic material for additional study.

CASE 32.3 The most correct answer is e, brain metastasis.

Answer a would be an unlikely explanation of the patient's focal neurological deficit that is limited to the left upper extremity, inasmuch as the chief features of hypertrophic pulmonary osteoarthropathy are symmetrical, painful, proliferative periostitis in association with digital clubbing. Similarly, *answer b* is incorrect, considering that Lambert-Eaton myasthenic syndrome presents in a generally symmetric manner with associated autonomic dysfunction and cranial nerve deficits, rather than isolated weakness of an extremity. Again, *answer c*, polymyositis, is not an appropriate response here because of the focal nature of the patient's symptoms and lack of muscular tenderness. *Answer d*, hypercalcemia is incorrect in this instance considering the lack of associated symptoms of confusion or constipation and the physical examination which is not remarkable for signs of dehydration.

Chapter 33

Diseases of the Upper Airways and Sinuses

DAVID S. BRINK, MD AND ANDREW J. LECHNER, PhD

Learning Objectives

- The student will be able to distinguish the acute and chronic forms of rhinitis and sinusitis in terms of their etiologies, histologic appearance, and resolution.

- The student will be able to enumerate the common neoplastic diseases of the sinuses and nasopharynx and the frequency of benign versus malignant growth.

- The student will be able to describe the range of disease types and severities that may involve the larynx, including the vocal chords and upper trachea, and when neoplastic, the likelihood of their progression to malignancy and metastasis.

Introduction

Given their proximity to the environment, it is not surprising that the nasal cavities, sinuses, oropharynx, and trachea are all sites for infectious, inflammatory, and neoplastic diseases. As detailed in Chaps. 2 and 10, much of the lung's conducting zone is well constructed to warm, humidify, and cleanse the inspiratory gas stream while maintaining physical barriers to aspiration events during eating, drinking, and speech. This chapter will focus on diseases that bear directly on respiratory function and pulmonary medicine rather than provide a compendium of all illnesses that might properly be considered the clinical domain of otolaryngology. Students are encouraged to consult adjoining chapters in this book for more specific details regarding anatomical landmarks, histologic configurations, and regional host defense mechanisms.

Diseases of the Nose, Sinuses, and Nasopharynx
Infections and Inflammatory Processes (#102)

Inflammatory diseases are the most common disorders of the nose and its accessory paranasal sinuses. **Rhinitis**, or inflammation of the nasal mucosa, may be either infectious or allergic in its etiology. Nasal and sinus infections are usually viral in origin, particularly with **adenoviruses**, **echoviruses**, and **rhinoviruses**. Macroscopically, the affected areas appear red and swollen and may express copious watery exudates, all of which narrow or occlude nasal air passages and increase dynamic upper airway resistance. The histologic presentation is of respiratory mucosal edema, often with inflammatory cell infiltrates. Secondary bacterial infections are common in this setting, in which case neutrophilic influx and purulence are prominent. Uncomplicated cases of acute rhinitis normally resolve in 5-7 days in the immunocompetent host, although sequential infection of deeper airways can occur. As for viral and bacterial infections of the lung parenchyma, treatment options for rhinitis vary from curative to palliative depending upon the pathogen.

Allergic rhinitis, or **hay fever**, is caused by IgE-mediated reactions to any of the numerous allergens that are known to affect specific individuals. As many as 20% of the American public is affected by such seasonal disease, with the most common irritants as in asthma being plant pollens, fungi, animal dander, and insect droppings (Chap. 21). In such settings, there is also marked mucosal edema and redness of the affected nasal passages, while histologically the inflammatory infiltrates are often distinctly eosinophilic in composition. **Nasal polyps** are focal, usually non-neoplastic protrusions that commonly arise in the setting of such chronic rhinitis; they may be up to 3-4 cm in greatest dimension. Polyps are often asymptomatic and only found during routine physical exam. Alternatively, they may present with complaints of persistent **rhinorrhea** (runny nose), noisy breathing, and snoring. Histologically, the polyp is often covered by an intact respiratory epithelium that overlies a markedly edematous connective tissue stroma, usually with mucoid hyperplasia and cyst formation visible, as well as chronic inflammatory cell infiltrates (Fig. 33.1). Persistent polyps can become infected, even as they encroach upon airway lumens and impair sinus drainage. Medical treatment is primarily with nasal or oral corticosteroids, with surgical excision the best option for patients in whom such medical interventions fail.

Acute sinusitis usually results from normal oropharyngeal flora causing inflammation and edema of the sinus mucosa. Obstruction of sinus outflow may cause **empyema** or lead to formation of a **mucocele**, a localized mucus accumulation in the absence of bacterial colonization. Indeed, diabetics can develop **mucormycosis**, often a life-threatening fungal sinusitis. The progression of acute sinusitis to **chronic sinusitis** is common, particularly with repeated exposure to a causative agent, in the immunosuppressed population, and in

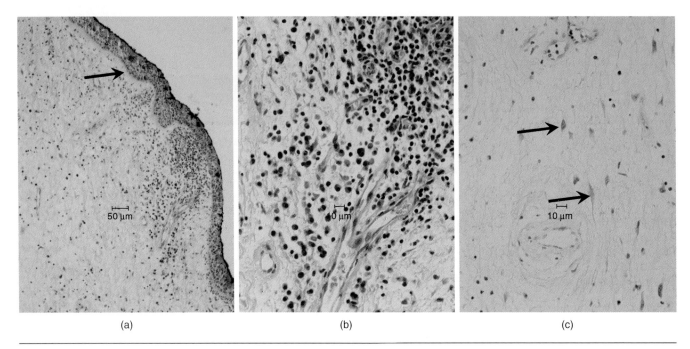

(a)   (b)   (c)

FIGURE 33.1 Nasal inflammatory polyp. (a) At low power, the polyp shows respiratory epithelium overlying a thickened basement membrane (arrow) and edematous stroma with an inflammatory infiltrate. (b) At high power, the inflammatory infiltrate is seen to be composed of lymphocytes, plasma cells, and scattered eosinophils. (c) Deeper in the polyp, inflammation is less severe, and edema dominates the morphology; some inflammatory polyps show fibroblast atypia (arrows), occasionally mimicking the appearance of neurons.

#103

patients with anatomical anomalies like deviated nasal septa that block sinus drainage. Such chronic sinusitis (Fig. 33.2) may become superimposed with bacterial infection or become complicated by **meningitis**, **osteomyelitis**, **orbital cellulitis**, or **cavernous vein thrombosis**. Patients with **Wegener's granulomatosis** often show nasal as well as intrapulmonary disease, in which there are microscopic findings of vasculitis, geographic necrosis, histiocyte accumulation, granulomatous inflammation, and epithelial ulceration. Chronic sinusitis is a presenting symptom in **Kartagener syndrome** due to defective ciliary clearance mechanisms, along with bronchiectasis and **situs inversus**.

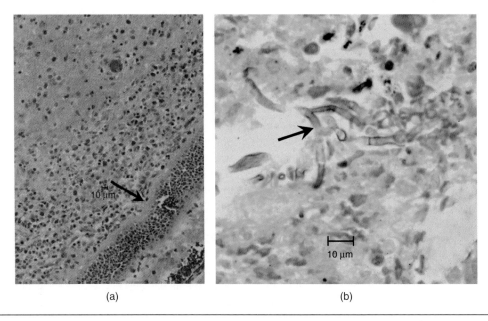

(a)   (b)

FIGURE 33.2 Sinusitis. (a) In this example of sinusitis, thickening of the basement membrane is apparent (arrow) typical of many chronic inflammatory processes involving mucosa. Here, the dominance of eosinophils in the inflammatory infiltrate is suspicious for allergic fungal sinusitis. (b) GMS staining identifies septate hyphae (arrow), morphologically consistent with *Aspergillus* species.

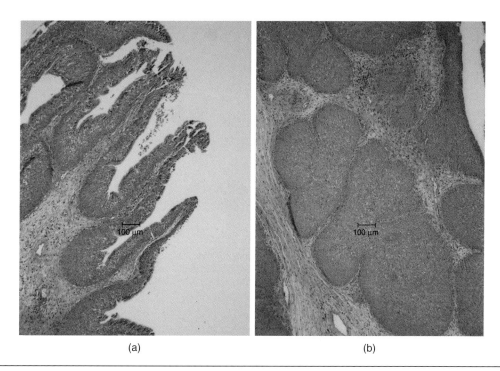

(a)   (b)

FIGURE 33.3 In sinonasal papilloma, the epithelium is stratified squamous. (a) In the everted/exophytic pattern, the epithelium covers finger-like projections of loose connective tissue. (b) Papillomata arising from the lateral wall typically show an inverted/endophytic growth pattern, with inward growth of the epithelium into the stroma, occasionally mimicking invasive carcinoma.

Necrotizing lesions of the nasal passages and sinuses may arise from several of the etiologies described above, notably those that reflect actual or potential systemic diseases, like mucormycosis and Wegener's granulomatosis. Focal necrosis of these regions can also occur as a consequence of adjacent superimposed bacterial infection, tumor-related granulomatous inflammation, and some neoplastic processes involving other leukocytes, including natural killer cells.

Inflammation of the oropharynx and its associated lymphoid tissues causes **pharyngitis** and **tonsillitis**, respectively. As mentioned above, these often follow chronologically and anatomically from antecedent upper respiratory infections with rhinoviruses, adenoviruses, influenza, and **respiratory syncytial virus** (**RSV**). As for the nasal passages and sinuses, the pharynx becomes red and swollen with edematous mucosa and pseudomembranous exudates. **Follicular tonsillitis** is common and painful, with physical exam showing enlarged reddened tonsils covered with pinpoint exudates that adhere to or appear to be emerging from tonsillar crypts. Superinfection is common with β-hemolytic *Streptococci* and *Staphylococcus aureus*, whose late sequelae can produce **rheumatic fever** and **glomerulonephritis** (Chaps. 26 and 40).

Tumors of the Nose, Sinuses, and Nasopharynx

Sinonasal papillomas are benign neoplasms that arise from the sinonasal mucosa and most commonly present in adult men whose primary complaint is nasal obstruction. Histologically, they consist of proliferating squamous epithelium among other mucin- positive cells. As such, their cytologic atypia is not impressive, and the cells as a group are usually mature and well-differentiated. The presence of **human papilloma virus** (**HPV**) types 6 and 11 is detected in many sinonasal papillomas. Papillomas that originate in the nasal septum are most common; most often these have an **exophytic growth** pattern, emerging mushroom-shaped from the mucosa with a core of connective tissue [Fig. 33.3(a)]. Papillomas that originate from the middle meatus or middle or inferior turbinates are of an **inverted type** with an **endophytic growth** pattern that resembles plant root tubercles penetrating the underlying stroma [Fig. 33.3(b)]. Such inverted papillomas recur at a high rate if not completed excised surgically, and they are also the type most often associated with coexisting or subsequent carcinomas, in 3%-10% of patients.

Nasopharyngeal angiofibromas are relatively uncommon and benign growths that occur almost exclusively in adolescent males, presumably reflecting androgen dependence of the tumor. They arise principally from the posterolateral wall of the nasopharynx, from where they may grow to completely occlude the nares (Fig. 33.4). Histologically, these tumors appear composed mostly of an intricate blend of microvasculature and fibrotic stroma. As a result of this vascular composition, they often bleed profusely during surgical excision.

Olfactory neuroblastomas or **esthesioneuroblastomas** are uncommon but highly malignant small-cell tumors of neuroendocrine origin. Electron microscopic analysis shows neurosecretory granules, and sections for light microscopy can be stained immunohistochemically for **neuron-specific enolase**

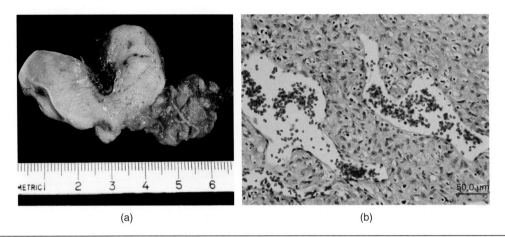

(a)   (b)

FIGURE 33.4 Nasopharyngeal angiofibroma. (a) The gross appearance of nasopharyngeal angiofibroma is that of a well-circumscribed, pale, spongy lesion, occupying the left portion of the image. (b) Histologically the angiofibroma shows numerous thin-walled vessels separated by dense fibrous stroma, the morphology of erectile tissue, similar to that in the penis and clitoris. (a): *From Rosai.* Rosai and Ackerman's Surgical Pathology, *9th ed. New York, NY: Mosby-Elsevier; 2004.*

(**NSE**), **neurofilaments**, and **chromogranin** (Fig. 33.5). They arise superiorly and laterally in the nose, where they are often locally invasive and cause distant metastases in ~20% of patients. Overall 5-year survival is relatively poor, although most olfactory neuroblastomas are radiosensitive if treated early or in combination with surgery.

Nasopharyngeal carcinomas are malignant epithelial tumors that are rare in the United States but very common in southeast Asia and parts of Africa. Epidemiological evidence indicates that they most often result from the combined effects of a person's genetic predisposition, local environmental factors, and **Epstein-Barr virus** (**EBV**) infection. Histologically, they

resemble other squamous cell carcinomas with large cells, prominent nucleoli, and indistinct cell borders. These tumors have a strong tendency to spread to regional lymph nodes, such that **cervical lymphadenopathy** is a common presenting symptom. By growing silently, these carcinomas often present when already unresectable. In many countries, they are the most common pediatric cancer. Radiotherapy is currently considered the treatment of choice, and 3-year survival ranges from 50% to 70%.

Three major subtypes of nasopharyngeal carcinoma are recognized. **Keratinizing squamous cell carcinoma** is the most common form in the United States and is not associated

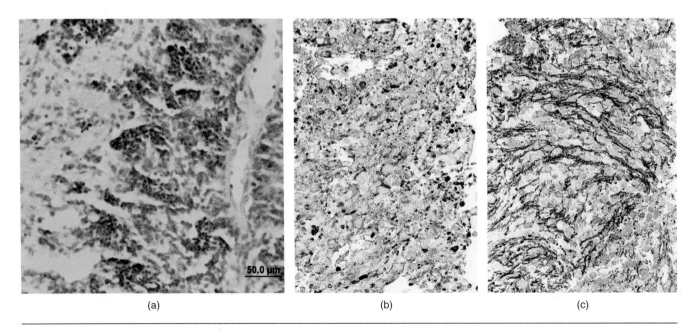

(a)   (b)   (c)

FIGURE 33.5 **Olfactory neuroblastoma** (esthesioneuroblastoma). (a) The "small blue cells" dominating the right portion of the image typify neuroblastoma; the pale pink neurofibrillary background, apparent to the left, offers a clue to the nature of the otherwise undifferentiated "small blue cells." Immunohistochemical staining can assist in the recognition of the "small blue cells" as neuroendocrine. Shown are immunohistochemical stains for chromogranin (b) and neurofilament (c). (b) and (c): *From Rosai.* Rosai and Ackerman's Surgical Pathology, *9th ed. New York, NY: Mosby-Elsevier; 2004.*

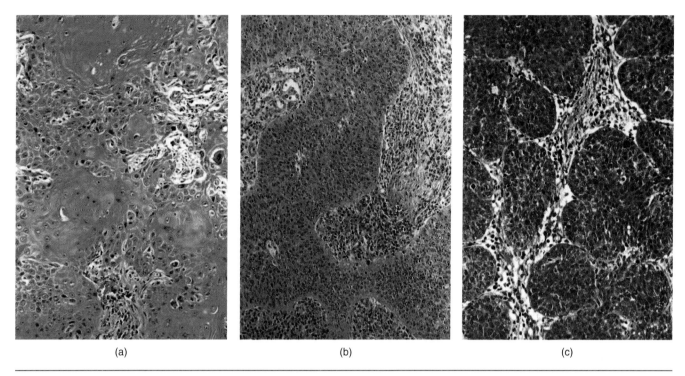

(a)   (b)   (c)

FIGURE 33.6 Nasopharyngeal carcinomas. Keratinizing squamous cell carcinoma (a) is not typically associated with EBV infection, in contrast to nonkeratinizing squamous cell carcinoma, which is divided into differentiated (b) and undifferentiated (c) subtypes. *From Shanmugaratumk Sobin LH:* Histological typing of upper respiratory tract tumors. *Geneva, 1978. World Health Organization.*

with EBV infection [Fig. 33.6 (a)]. It also has the worst prognosis, presumably because it is the least radiosensitive variant. **Nonkeratinizing squamous cell carcinoma** [Fig. 33.6 (b)] is probably the most common form, at least in the eastern hemisphere. It is clearly associated with EBV infection and shows intermediate radiosensitivity. Finally, the **undifferentiated carcinomas** [Fig. 33.6 (c)] are also common worldwide, likewise showing association with EBV infection, and are considered the most radiosensitive. Because this variant is often found with an accompanying lymphocytic infiltrate, they are occasionally referred to as **lymphoepitheliomas**.

A wide variety of other tumors may occur in the sinuses and nasopharynx, and in most cases these resemble histologically their counterparts found at other sites. Notable among these are **plasmacytomas** that arise in lymphoid structures adjacent to the nose and sinuses; these occasionally can exhibit polypoid growth that resemble polyps described above. In addition, patients may present less commonly with **adenocarcinoma**, **sarcomatoid carcinoma**, **basaloid carcinoma**, **malignant lymphoma**, **malignant melanoma**, and some salivary gland tumors including **adenoid cystic carcinoma**.

Diseases of the Larynx and Trachea
Infections and Inflammatory Processes

Like the nasopharynx, the larynx is exposed to a variety of inflammatory and infectious conditions. Collectively these cause **laryngitis**, the most common laryngeal disorder.

Chronic nonspecific laryngitis can result from infection or persistent exposure to tobacco, alcohol, gastric acid, or other toxins. Histologically, the laryngeal wall shows a typical submucosal inflammatory infiltrate with lymphocytes, histiocytes, and plasma cells. The epithelium itself may appear hyperplastic over the affected mucosa. In heavy smokers, such chronic laryngitis is considered an important predisposing condition for squamous epithelial changes and possibly carcinoma. Among the systemic infections that can cause laryngitis, fungi are particularly common and include *Histoplasma*, *Aspergillus*, *Blastomyces*, *Candida*, and *Cryptococcus* spp. *Mycobacterium tuberculosis* may involve the larynx as well. Certain systemic granulomatous diseases, notably sarcoidosis, are rarer but presumably causal agents.

Acute laryngoepiglottitis presents as marked swelling and edema of the epiglottis that can involve the vocal chords sufficiently to produce a medical emergency. It is common in children and can be caused by *Haemophilus influenzae* or, less often, by some strains of β-**hemolytic** *Streptococcus*. Infections with RSV or parainfluenza viruses are common causes of **laryngotracheobronchitis** or **croup**. Again, more commonly in children, patients with laryngotracheobronchitis often present with marked respiratory stridor due to significant inflammation and edema in the upper airways (Chaps. 14 and 40). Incidence continues to decline among infants with use of the *H. influenzae* **type B** (**HIB**) **vaccine**.

Laryngeal nodules, or **singer's nodules/polyps**, represent a noninflammatory condition that arises from overuse/abuse of the voice. For the most part, these small (usually

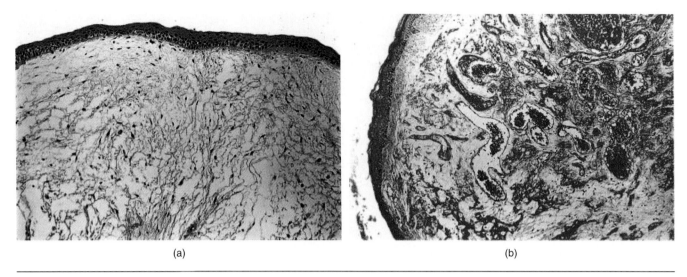

(a)   (b)

FIGURE 33.7 Laryngeal nodule. (a) The example shows stratified squamous mucosa overlying loose connective tissue with a fibromyxoid quality. (b) The example has become extensively vascularized. *From Rosai.* Rosai and Ackerman's Surgical Pathology, *9th ed. New York, NY: Mosby-Elsevier; 2004.*

<5 mm), smoothly rounded, and benign lesions occur on the anterior third of the true vocal chords and are most common in adult males (Fig. 33.7). Histologically, laryngeal nodules are covered by squamous epithelium overlying a core of loose connective tissue that features edema and fibroblast proliferation. Over time the nodules become vascularized and contain hyaline tissue that is the source of one misnomer for these nodules, **amyloid tumor**. Although laryngeal nodules can lead to progressive hoarseness, they have no known association with cancer. True amyloid deposition can occur in the larynx, but it is not a component of classic laryngeal nodules.

Non-neoplastic conditions that involve the trachea include **amyloidosis**, **rheumatoid nodules**, and *tracheopathia osteoplastica*. The latter is idiopathic and consists of numerous small nodules composed of bone and cartilage that arise in the tracheal submucosa. Of course the trachea can become infected and/or inflamed due to the same types of pathogens and environmental insults that have been described above for the nasopharyngeal regions. However, there is no particular propensity for the trachea to be more sensitive to these conditions than is the remainder of the conducting zone. Serious injuries to the trachea's respiratory mucosa during the course of mechanical ventilation or bronchoscopy are fortunately rare. Like the accidental aspirations of foreign objects, most involve simple abrasions of the tracheal epithelium that heal without incident. Catastrophic hemorrhage into the distal airways is usually attributable to the rupture of blood vessels serving intratracheal masses as these are being inspected or excised. While some of these injuries are clearly medical emergencies, they too resolve spontaneously in most instances.

Precancerous Lesions and Tumors of the Larynx and Trachea

Laryngeal papillomas are benign squamous neoplasms usually found on the true vocal chords, are associated with HPV infection (types 6 and 11), and have differing clinical presentations in the pediatric and adult populations. In children they are often multiple and recur frequently, yielding **juvenile laryngeal papillomatosis**. These may spread from the child's vocal chords to adjacent regions of the larynx, where they have a small chance of malignant transformation and can occasionally cause airway obstruction and rarely death. In adults, a laryngeal papilloma is usually solitary, rarely spreads or recurs once excised, and has virtually no malignant potential. Grossly, laryngeal papillomas are soft, raspberry-like nodules <1 cm in diameter [Fig. 33.8 (a)]. Histologically, the papilloma in cross section appears with finger-like projections composed of fibrovascular cores, all covered by squamous epithelium (Fig. 33.8). **Tracheal papillomas** are likewise the most common benign neoplasms in this central airway. These also differ in their complexity and recurrence with patient age and can present as **tracheal papillomatosis**.

Laryngeal keratosis is a benign epithelial or squamous cell hyperplasia that occurs in smokers and in those who overuse or abuse their voices (Clinical Correlation 33.1). By laryngoscopy, keratosis presents as a thickened white mucosal surface. Microscopically these lesions show **hyperkeratosis** (excessive keratin synthesis) and **acanthosis** (thickened hyperplastic epithelium).

▶▶CLINICAL CORRELATION 33.1

Many approaches to vocal training for the stage consider rather heretical the idea that *overuse* of the voice leads to hoarseness, laryngeal nodules, or any other laryngeal disease. Indeed, many voice teachers stress to their pupils that voice-related laryngeal disease is a result of *abuse* of the voice rather than its overuse. In this context, new parents soon realize that an infant is capable of prolonged sound production at high volume, yet the infant seldom becomes hoarse from crying in the absence of an upper respiratory

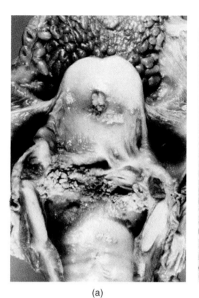 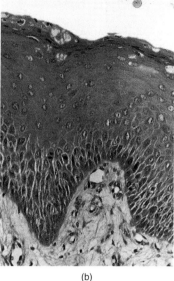

(a)   (b)

FIGURE 33.8 Laryngeal papillomatosis. (a) The larynx of an 18-year-old boy who died of suffocation due to extensive laryngeal papillomatosis. The organ has been opened posteriorly. Beginning at age 7, he had nearly 50 resections of laryngeal papillomata. (b) Microscopically, the epithelium of a papilloma shows orderly maturation, with cuboidal cells at the basal layer transitioning to flattened cells toward the surface. *From Rosai.* Rosai and Ackerman's Surgical Pathology, *9th ed. New York, NY: Mosby-Elsevier; 2004.*

viral infection or comparable comorbidity. In contrast, otherwise healthy adult sports fans often experience several days of voice impairment after attending an exciting event. Perhaps the infant has not learned yet to abuse the voice in the same manner as its parents.

Laryngeal dysplasia may occur with keratosis or independently and features cellular atypia and disordered maturation over a wide range of appearances. Dysplasia is graded as mild, moderate, or severe depending on the degree of atypia and extent of involvement through the epithelial layer. Full-thickness atypia (with an intact basal lamina) that does not invade the submucosal layer is termed a **carcinoma in situ** (**CIS**). Most CIS forms of dysplasia are considered precursor lesions to **invasive carcinoma**; the risk of developing malignancy is estimated to be 23%-28% when a biopsy shows both keratosis and severe atypia. More than 75% of patients with invasive carcinomas have CIS in their history. Most CIS cases are found only on the true vocal chords, since they evoke an early symptom of non-resolving hoarseness.

At least 95% of laryngeal malignancies are **laryngeal squamous cell carcinomas** that are typically graded as well, moderately, or poorly differentiated. Overall, these laryngeal malignancies account for ~2% of all cancers in men and ~0.5% of all cancers in women. As for cancers deeper in the lung (Chaps. 31 and 32), the most important risk factor is tobacco use, followed distantly by alcohol consumption, HPV infection, previous irradiation, metastasis, and laryngeal dysplasia (see above). The laryngeal carcinomas follow

distinct patterns of longitudinal spread across specific glottic structures (Fig. 33.9). The occurrence frequencies at each site influence both the likelihood of lymph node metastasis and the expected 5-year survival rate (Table 33.1). Not surprisingly, the most common malignant tumor in the trachea is **tracheal squamous cell carcinoma**. Most of these malignancies occur in the distal third of the trachea and/or adjacent to the hilum and carry a poor prognosis.

Important considerations regarding laryngeal carcinoma include both the limited lymphatic circulation and the paucity of mucoserous glands in the vicinity of the vocal chords. As a result, glottic carcinomas tend to remain localized for extended periods of time and so are curable if detected and resected early in their course. Nevertheless, invasive glottic carcinomas require a total laryngectomy. Supraglottic tumors may be treatable with a more limited supraglottic laryngectomy, sparing the vocal chords. However, such patients require good pulmonary reserves and intact reflexes to avoid subsequent aspiration events. Infraglottic tumors often will produce a symptom of dyspnea that becomes severe enough to require emergent tracheostomy. In at least 30% of laryngeal carcinoma patients, the lesion crosses the midline (by direct extension or through contralateral lymph node metastasis), which worsens the prognosis. Laryngeal and tracheal carcinomas can be staged using the same **International Association of Lung Cancer (IASLC) TNM System** as for lung cancer itself (Chap. 32). However, the precise categorizations of laryngeal and tracheal carcinomas into TNM staging subclasses go beyond the intended scope of this book.

There are many rarer and histologically distinguishable laryngeal and tracheal tumors. Clinically, the most aggressive

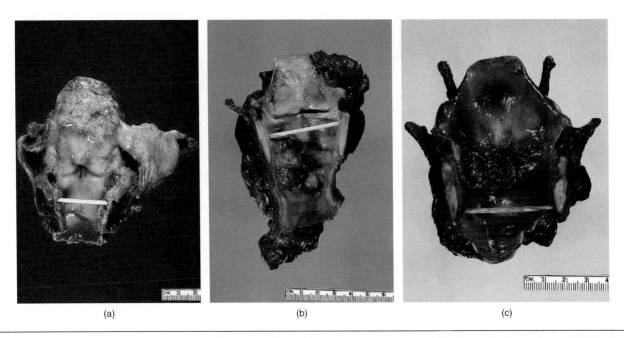

(a) (b) (c)

FIGURE 33.9 Laryngeal carcinoma. The anatomic relationship of laryngeal carcinoma to the true vocal chord is a major determinant of likelihood of lymph node metastasis, survival rate, and, if small, the extent of excision. Shown are three laryngectomy specimens, each opened posteriorly with toothpicks holding open the thyroid cartilage to allow visibility of the anterior mucosal surface. (a) A supraglottic tumor has replaced much of the epiglottis. (b) An infraglottic carcinoma is visible as multiple polypoid masses. (c) A transglottic carcinoma on the left side involves the false and true vocal chords and crosses the midline. *From Rosai. Rosai and Ackerman's Surgical Pathology, 9th ed. New York, NY: Mosby-Elsevier; 2004.*

among these in the larynx include **small cell carcinoma**, **basaloid squamous carcinoma**, and **sarcomatoid (or spindle cell) carcinomas**. **Verrucous carcinoma** is an extremely well-differentiated polypoid type of squamous carcinoma that can show marked local invasion of the larynx but rarely metastasizes. **Adenoid cystic carcinoma** may involve the larynx or the trachea and is the second most common tracheal malignancy. Larynx and trachea can develop adenocarcinomas, carcinoid tumors, and sarcomas, but collectively these represent a very small percentage of all cases.

Table **33.1** **Effect of location on outcome for laryngeal squamous cell carcinoma**

Anatomic Site	%Total Case	Rate of Lymph Node Metastasis	5-year Survival
Glottic	60%-65%	<1%	80%
Supraglottic	30%-35%	30%-40%	65%
Transglottic[a]	<5%	50%-60%	50%
Infraglottic	<5%	50%	40%

[a]Transglottic tumors cross the laryngeal ventricles to involve the supraglottis and infraglottis.

Suggested Readings

1. Kumar V, Abbas AK, Fausto N. *Robbins and Cotran's Pathologic Basis of Disease*, 7th ed. Philadelphia, PA: Elsevier; 2005. *An excellent text that offers more detail and many images of this group of diseases.*

2. Rosai J. *Rosai and Ackerman's Surgical Pathology*, 9th ed. New York, NY: Mosby-Elsevier; 2004. *A classic surgical pathology two-volume text, with far more morphologic detail than in a general pathology text like Robbins and Cotran's Pathologic Basis of Disease, and a standard reference text for pathologists working in a clinical setting interpreting surgical pathology specimens.*

CASE STUDIES AND PRACTICE PROBLEMS

CASE 33.1 A 55-year-old man presents to his physician with hoarseness for 3 weeks. He has not had a recent episode of straining his voice. After a thorough history and physical exam, the most appropriate next step would be which of the following?

a. CT scan of the neck
b. Direct laryngoscopy
c. Laryngeal biopsy
d. Radiograph of the neck
e. Reassurance of the patient

CASE 33.2 A 35-year-old woman presents to her primary care physician with hoarseness of 7 days' duration. Physical examination of the patient reveals a solitary soft berry-shaped nodule in the larynx on the true vocal chord. Which of the following is the most accurate prognosis for this woman's complaint?

a. The lesion will likely recur regardless of treatment.
b. This carcinoma often spreads from the true chords to other laryngeal sites.
c. The nodule shows no correlation with human papilloma virus infection.

d. Biopsy will show that the nodule is covered with respiratory mucosa.
e. This nodule is benign with virtually no malignant potential.

CASE 33.3 A 12-year-old boy who emigrated with his paternal uncle from sub-Saharan Africa 6 weeks earlier presents today with a mass in his nasopharynx. Biopsy shows an undifferentiated tumor with large epithelial cells admixed with lymphocytes; nucleoli are prominent, but cell borders are indistinct. Which of the following most accurately describes this boy's tumor?

a. It has no known association with Epstein-Barr virus infection.
b. This tumor subtype is highly sensitive to radiation therapy.
c. Such malignancies are strongly keratin-negative by immunohistochemistry.
d. Left untreated, this subtype uniformly has a very poor outcome.
e. This tumor type grows very rapidly and occurs only in North America.

Solutions to Case Studies and Practice Problems

CASE 33.1 The most correct answer is b, direct laryngoscopy.

The differential diagnosis for hoarseness is lengthy when there is laryngeal involvement. These range from simple self-resolving infectious processes causing laryngitis through nodules, papillomas, carcinoma in situ, and then laryngeal carcinoma. The vigilant clinician will want to inspect the area directly before deciding whether antibiotics, standard or advanced imaging, bronchoscopy, an invasive biopsy procedure, or pain palliation with reassurance is appropriate.

CASE 33.2 The most correct answer is e, benign without malignant potential.

This woman's laryngeal papilloma is characteristically solitary and positioned to produce hoarseness but its likelihood for regrowth after excision and its metastatic potential are both very low. If biopsied it would show squamous epithelium overlying fibrovascular cores. If not already established, the woman should

be tested for papilloma virus infection, since this papilloma has a high association rate with HPV types 6 and 11.

CASE 33.3 The most correct answer is b, highly sensitive to radiation therapy.

Undifferentiated nasopharyngeal carcinomas of the type in this youth lack the striking keratin outer layer that is the dominant histological finding among the well-differentiated tumors in the U.S. population; despite the lack of a keratin layer, the cells make keratin and would show positive immunohistochemical staining for keratin, as is typical of squamous cell carcinomas in general. They do show strong association with EBV infection and are the predominant tumor subtype among individuals who have grown up in Asia or Africa. With radiation treatment, to which undifferentiated carcinomas are susceptible, the prognosis for non-recurrence in this young man is quite good.

INFECTIONS OF THE LUNG

Chapter 34

Pathology of Lung Infections

DAVID S. BRINK, MD

Learning Objectives

- The student will be able to describe the three main inflammatory responses to pulmonary infection (intra-alveolar suppurative, interstitial mononuclear, and granulomatous) and identify characteristic microbiological etiologies for each.

- The student will be able to distinguish bronchopneumonia from lobar pneumonia and identify specific etiologies of each.

- The student will be able to describe the clinical settings in which a lung abscess can develop and identify microorganisms that can cause abscess formation.

- The student will be able to distinguish primary tuberculosis from secondary (reactivation) tuberculosis, based on morphologic as well as clinical features.

- The student will be able to recognize common fungi causing pulmonary infection.

- The student will be able to describe *Pneumocystis jiroveci* pneumonia and recognize the causative microorganism.

Introduction

As summarized in Chap. 10, the respiratory system has many defenses against infectious disease. The vibrissae in the nose and the mucociliary covering of the mucosa in the conducting portion of the respiratory system trap particles and microorganisms, moving them cephalad to the pharynx to be expectorated or swallowed. Macrophages within the respiratory parenchyma phagocytize small particles and microorganisms and, if overwhelmed, recruit neutrophils from alveolar septal capillaries. Finally, immunoglobulin A in the mucosal secretions supports humoral immunity. In general, suboptimal humoral immunity and/or suboptimal nonimmune defense systems increase the risk for pyogenic bacterial infection, whereas suboptimal cell-mediated immunity increases the risk of infection by intracellular and low-virulence organisms, typically viruses and some bacteria. Other risk factors for the development of respiratory tract infection include decreased/absent cough reflex, reduced phagocytic/bactericidal activity of alveolar macrophages (eg, by alcohol, smoking, anoxia, oxygen intoxication), pulmonary congestion/edema, accumulation of airway secretions (eg, cystic fibrosis or distal to an obstruction), and mucociliary dysfunction, both congenital (eg, **immotile cilia syndrome**, **Kartagener syndrome**) and acquired (eg, viral illness, toxic effects of inhaled smoke).

This chapter will focus on the pathology of infectious disease and is organized by general morphologic similarities. There are three major morphologic patterns in infections of the respiratory tract: intra-alveolar accumulation of neutrophils, with or without abscess formation; interstitial expansion by mononuclear inflammatory cells; and granulomatous inflammation. Lung infections can also be organized based on their clinical settings rather than by their morphologic patterns (Table 34.1).

▶▶ CLINICAL CORRELATION 34.1

It is worth considering the term "pneumonia." Some authors use the word when referring to **pneumonitis** (lung inflammation) due to a bacterial infection. Others use pneumonia to refer to any infectious pneumonitis, and others use it synonymously with "pneumonitis"

without qualifiers. Whether a disease is more commonly referred to as pneumonia or as pneumonitis largely reflects traditional clinical usage rather than rational differentiation of the terms.

Suppurative Bacterial Pneumonia (#104)

In suppurative bacterial pneumonia, there is **consolidation** (ie, solidification) of lung parenchyma due to the accumulation of neutrophil-rich intra-alveolar exudate (Fig. 34.1). The consolidation of bacterial pneumonia is classically subclassified into two patterns: **lobar pneumonia** and **bronchopneumonia** (or **lobular pneumonia**).

In lobar pneumonia, there is consolidation of contiguous airspaces, typically an entire lobe (Fig. 34.2). Lobar pneumonia is identifiable on an x-ray by a well-circumscribed radiopacity correlating to the affected lobe. Lobar pneumonia evolves through phases of **congestion**, **red hepatization**, **gray hepatization**, and **resolution** (Fig. 34.3).

During the congestion phase, the affected lobe is heavy, red, and boggy; histologically, there is vascular congestion,

331

Table **34.1** The pneumonia syndromes organized by clinical setting (#105)

Community-Acquired Acute Pneumonia	Community-Acquired Atypical Pneumonias
Streptococcus pneumoniae	Mycoplasma pneumoniae
Haemophilus influenzae	Chlamydia spp.
Moraxella catarrhalis	Coxiella burnetii (Q fever)
Staphylococcus aureus	Respiratory syncytial virus
Legionella pneumophila	Parainfluenza virus (children)
Klebsiella pneumoniae	Influenza A & B viruses (adults)
Pseudomonas spp.	Adenovirus, SARS virus
Hospital-Acquired Pneumonia	**Aspiration Pneumonia (usually mixed flora)**
Klebsiella spp.	Bacteroides spp. Prevotella spp.
Serratia marcescens	Fusobacterium spp. S. pneumoniae
Escherichia coli	Peptostreptococcus spp.
S. aureus	S. aureus H. influenzae
Pseudomonas spp.	Pseudomonas aeruginosa
Chronic Pneumonia	**Necrotizing Pneumonia and Lung Abscess**
Nocardia asteroides	Anaerobic bacteria
Actinomyces israelii	S. aureus
Mycobacterium tuberculosis	Klebsiella pneumoniae
Atypical Mycobacteria spp.	Streptococcus pyogenes
Histoplasma capsulatum	S. pneumoniae type 3
Blastomyces dermatitidis	
Pneumonia in the Immunocompromised Patient Setting	
Cytomegalovirus	Pneumocystis jiroveci
Aspergillus spp.	Candida spp.
Mycobacterium avium-intracellulare	Usual bacteria, viruses, and fungi listed above

Adapted from Husain AN. The Lung. In: Kumar V., et al. Robbins and Cotran Pathologic Basis of Disease, 8th ed. Philadelphia, PA: Saunders-Elsevier; 2010.

accumulation of intra-alveolar neutrophils, and pulmonary edema. Eventually, the lungs develop the consistency of liver (hepatization). Early in hepatization, the gross appearance is red, and the microscopic morphology comprises alveoli packed with neutrophils, erythrocytes, and fibrin; fibrous or fibrin-opurulent pleural exudates are common in this phase. Later in the hepatization phase, the color of the lobe becomes gray as the fibrinous inflammatory exudate persists but becomes devoid of erythrocytes. As the inflammatory reaction resolves, the consolidated exudate is digested, leaving a granular semi-solid fluid to be resorbed. Due to the availability and efficacy of antibiotic therapy, lobar pneumonia is now rare.

In bronchopneumonia, the pattern of consolidation is of noncontiguous airspaces and typically involves more than one lobe with a **bronchiolocentric** distribution. Grossly, the patches of consolidation are gray-red to yellow with a surrounding rim of hyperemia and edema (Fig. 34.4). Histologically, broncho-pneumonia progresses through stages similar to lobar pneumonia (Fig. 34.3). Pleural involvement in bronchopneumonia is less common than in lobar pneumonia. Radiographically, broncho-pneumonia is typified by multiple foci of radiopacity.

The clinical presentation of lobar pneumonia and of bronchopneumonia includes malaise, fever, and a productive cough, occasionally with pleurisy and pleural friction rub. Appropriate antibiotic therapy (Chap. 35) usually results in restoration of lung structure and function. Complications include **abscess** formation (see below) due to tissue destruction and necrosis, empyema (Chaps. 26 and 29), organization of the

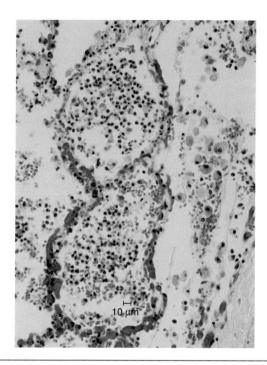

FIGURE 34.1 In **suppurative bacterial pneumonia**, alveoli are filled with a neutrophil-rich inflammatory exudate. Although this image was taken from a case of bronchopneumonia, at high magnification distinguishing bronchopneumonia from lobar pneumonia is not possible.

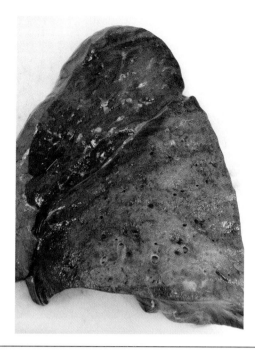

FIGURE 34.2 Lobar pneumonia. Shown is the cut surface of a left lung with lobar pneumonia affecting the lower lobe. The lower lobe is markedly paler than the upper lobe. On palpation, the lower lobe would be consolidated with markedly reduced or absent crepitus. *From Kemp et al.* Pathology: the Big Picture, *McGraw-Hill; 2008.*

intra-alveolar exudate into solid fibrous tissue [Fig. 34.3(c)], and dissemination of the infectious organism, possibly leading to meningitis, arthritis, endocarditis, or sepsis. The mortality of patients hospitalized for bacterial pneumonia is less than 10%, with death typically related to the development of one of the aforementioned complications or due to the presence of a

significant predisposition like debilitation or chronic alcoholism. There are numerous etiologies for suppurative bacterial pneumonia, many of which are briefly discussed below.

Streptococcus pneumoniae (previously *Pneumococcus pneumoniae*) is a gram-positive coccus; its cocci are typically paired. It is the most common cause of lobar pneumonia

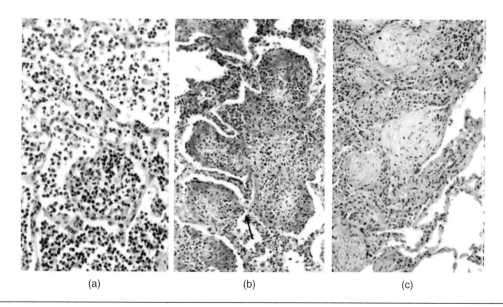

(a) (b) (c)

FIGURE 34.3 Phases of acute pneumonia. (a) Following the congestion phase (with few neutrophils), acute pneumonia enters the red hepatization stage, with alveoli filled with neutrophils and erythrocytes. (b) Subsequently, as the gray hepatization stage evolves, neutrophils and fibrin fill the alveolar spaces. (c) Following gray hepatization, the pneumonia can resolve or, alternatively, the intra-alveolar exudate can undergo organization, in which alveoli are filled by nodules of fibroblasts, collagen, and macrophages. *From Kumar et al.* Robbins and Cotran Pathologic Basis of Disease, *8th ed. Saunders-Elsevier, 2010.*

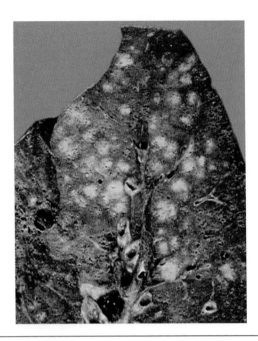

FIGURE 34.4 Bronchopneumonia. The cut surface of the lung shows numerous pale patches of consolidation. *From Travis et al. Non-Neoplastic Disorders of the Lower Respiratory Tract. © American Registry of Pathology; 2002.*

(>90% of cases) and is the most common cause of community-acquired acute pneumonia (15%-25% of cases). The most common microbiologic isolates are types 1, 2, 3, and 7. Of note, *S. pneumoniae* type 7 also causes lung abscess (see below). *Staphylococcus aureus* is another gram-positive coccus, but in contrast to the paired cocci of *S. pneumoniae*, the cocci of *S. aureus* are typically in "grapelike" clusters (Fig. 34.5). *S. aureus* typically causes bronchopneumonia with multiple abscesses (see below) but can cause lobar pneumonia. Risk factors for *S. aureus* pneumonia include recent measles

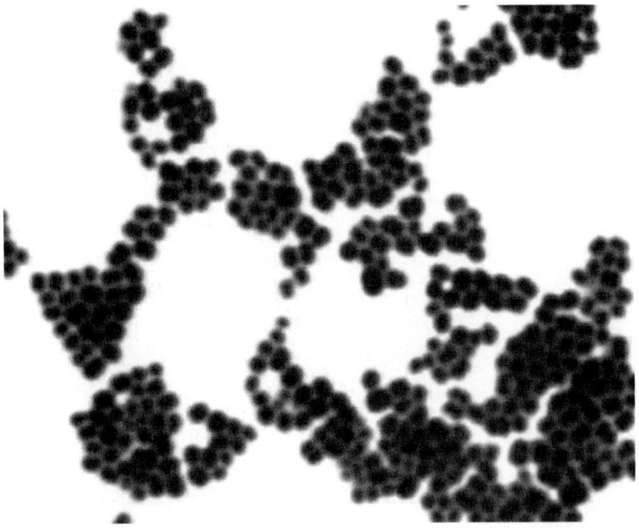

FIGURE 34.5 *Staphylococcus aureus.* Shown is a Gram stain of *S. aureus* in culture. The cocci are arranged in grapelike clusters.

infection in children, recent influenza infection in adults, and intravenous drug abuse.

Haemophilus influenzae is a gram-negative coccobacillus that generally causes bronchopneumonia that notably in children can be complicated by empyema (Chaps. 26 and 29) and extrapulmonary infection. Risk factors for *H. influenzae* pneumonia include recent viral infection, cystic fibrosis, chronic bronchitis, and bronchiectasis (Chaps. 20, 22, and 38). *Moraxella catarrhalis* is another gram-negative coccobacillus that generally causes bronchopneumonia. Risk factors for *M. catarrhalis* pneumonia include old age and chronic obstructive pulmonary disease (Chaps. 20 and 22).

Klebsiella pneumoniae is the most common gram-negative bacillus (rod) causing bacterial pneumonia. The morphology is that of bronchopneumonia or lobar pneumonia as well as lung abscess formation (see below). Clinically, *K. pneumoniae* pneumonia has an abrupt onset with a cough productive of gelatinous sputum. Risk factors for *K. pneumoniae* pneumonia include debilitation, malnourishment, and alcoholism. Recovery is often complicated by abscess formation, fibrosis, and/or bronchiectasis (Chap. 20), and *K. pneumoniae* pneumonia has a significant mortality rate, even with therapy. *Pseudomonas aeruginosa*, another gram-negative bacillus, typically causes bronchopneumonia with abscess formation (see below) and, frequently, empyema (Chaps. 26 and 29). *P. aeruginosa* pneumonia is commonly nosocomial, and risk factors include neutropenia, extensive burn injuries, cystic fibrosis, and mechanical ventilation. *Legionella pneumophila*, the cause of **Legionnaire disease**, is a gram-negative bacillus that lives in warm water. Morphologically, Legionnaire disease is bronchopneumonia. Risk factors include old age, organ transplantation, and cardiac, renal, immunologic, or hematologic disease. Legionnaire disease is fatal in approximately 15% of cases.

Nocardia asteroides is a gram-positive, aerobic, partially acid-fast, thin, branching, filamentous bacterium (Fig. 34.6). It causes bronchopneumonia with abscess formation (see below), typically in the setting of an immunocompromised host.

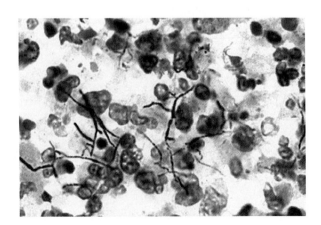

FIGURE 34.6 The partially acid-fast nature of the thin, branching, filamentous bacterium *Nocardia asteroides* is shown in this image. *From Travis et al. Non-Neoplastic Disorders of the Lower Respiratory Tract. © American Registry of Pathology; 2002.*

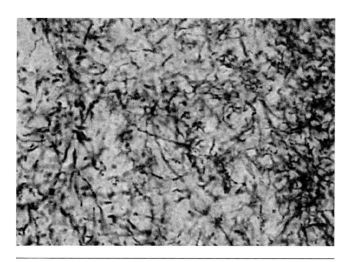

FIGURE 34.7 *Actinomyces*, shown in a tissue Gram stain, illustrates the gram-positive, filamentous, branching nature of this bacterium. *From Travis et al.* Non-Neoplastic Disorders of the Lower Respiratory Tract. *© American Registry of Pathology; 2002.*

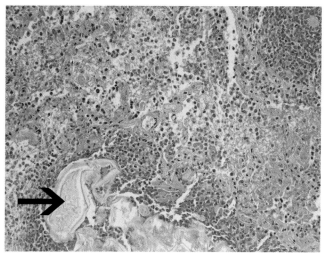

FIGURE 34.8 Aspiration pneumonia. While neutrophils dominate the inflammatory response, a clue that aspiration is the etiology is the presence of foreign material (arrow) within the parenchyma. *From Kemp et al.* Pathology: the Big Picture, *McGraw-Hill; 2008.*

Actinomyces israelii, like *N. asteroides*, is a gram-positive, thin, branching, filamentous bacterium (Fig. 34.7) that causes bronchopneumonia with abscess formation (see below). Unlike *N. asteroides*, however, *A. israelii* is anaerobic and is not partially acidfast. A common risk factor for *A. israelii* pneumonia is chronic obstructive lung disease. *Actinomyces* colonies are yellow, malodorous, and commonly referred to as **sulfur granules**, due to their morphologic similarities with elemental sulfur.

▶▶ C L I N I C A L   C O R R E L A T I O N   3 4 . 2

Sulfur granules are commonly seen within tonsillar crypts in tonsillectomy specimens. Their presence in tonsillar crypts is responsible in part for persistent malodorous breath despite teeth brushing and mouthwash usage.

The final form of acute bacterial pneumonia to be considered is **aspiration pneumonia** (Fig. 34.8). It differs from other forms of bacterial pneumonia in that the pneumonitis is partly chemical (due to gastric acid injury) and partly bacterial (typically mixed flora of oral cavity residents). Focal necrosis with subsequent abscess formation (see below) is common in aspiration pneumonia. Risk factors include acute alcohol intoxication, coma, anesthesia, sinusitis, gingivo-dental sepsis, and decreased or absent cough reflex.

As alluded to above, many of the causes of bacterial pneumonia can also result in the formation of a **lung abscess** (Fig. 34.9). Microorganisms typically cultivated from lung abscess fluid include aerobic and anaerobic streptococci, *Staphylococcus aureus*, many gram-negative microorganisms, and oral cavity anaerobes (eg, *Bacteroides, Fusobacterium, Peptococcus*). The most common cause of lung abscess is aspiration, but lung abscess can also complicate acute bacterial pneumonia due to *S. aureus, K. pneumoniae*, and *S. pneumoniae* type 3. **Septic embolism**, resulting from thrombophlebitis with

subsequent embolism or right-sided bacterial endocarditis, can result in abscess formation, as can traumatic lung injury. Other settings in which a lung abscess may develop include spread of an infection from nearby tissue, bronchiectasis (Chap. 20), and hematogenous seeding; 10%-15% of abscesses are related to carcinoma (Chap. 31) obstructing an airway. Abscesses can be single or multiple and can affect any part of the lung, although the specific pattern of involvement offers a clue to the etiology. Aspiration-induced abscesses are usually single and on the right; abscesses following acute bronchopneumonia or in the setting of bronchiectasis are usually multiple and basal; and abscesses secondary to septic embolization or hematogenous seeding are usually multiple with a haphazard distribution. Lung abscesses range from a few millimeters in diameter to several centimeters in greatest dimension. Because of anatomic drains (ie, the airways) in the lung, abscesses may only be partially filled with pus, the remainder being air-filled. Symptoms/signs of lung abscess include cough, fever, copious and malodorous (purulent or sanguineous) sputum, fever, weight loss, and digital clubbing. Complications of lung abscess include empyema (Chaps. 26 and 29), hemorrhage, septic embolization (which can lead to brain abscess or meningitis), and **reactive amyloidosis**. —#106 —

In the setting of immunocompromise, a few fungi can infect the lung and induce a suppurative inflammatory reaction. *Candida* species occasionally infect the lung, although esophageal, vaginal, and cutaneous infections are more common. The morphology of *Candida* is budding yeast, frequently with **pseudohyphae** (Fig. 34.10). The inflammatory reaction is typically suppurative, but occasionally it can be granulomatous.

Aspergillus species are **angioinvasive molds** that frequently induce thrombosis and infarction with subsequent suppuration. Morphologically, their hyphae are 5-10 μm wide, with a rather stiff appearance and a tendency toward 45-degree branching, a commonly quoted criterion that in reality has

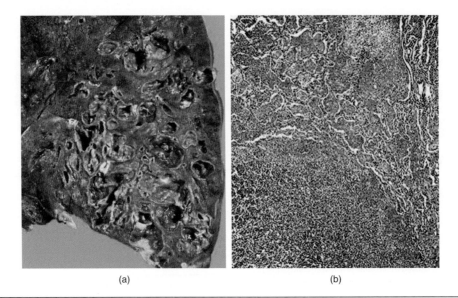

(a)   (b)

FIGURE 34.9 Lung abscess. (a) Grossly, the cut surface of the lung shows numerous abscess cavities in this example of *Staphylococcus* pneumonia. While the pus within a lung abscess can drain through airways, it does not always do so, as seen in the bottom left portion of (b), an example of *Klebsiella* pneumonia. *From Travis et al.* Non-Neoplastic Disorders of the Lower Respiratory Tract. © *American Registry of Pathology; 2002.*

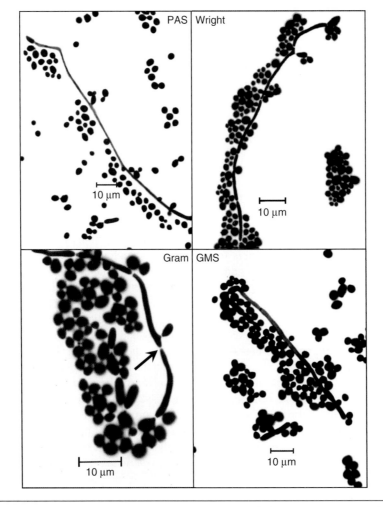

FIGURE 34.10 *Candida albicans.* Shown is *C. albicans* in culture using a variety of stains. The long structures are pseudohyphae. The key to distinguishing pseudohyphae from true hyphae is the "pinched" appearance connecting them (arrow).

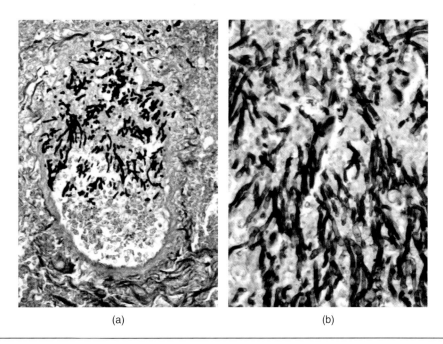

(a)   (b)

FIGURE 34.11 *Aspergillus* spp. are angioinvasive molds that typically cause thrombosis. (a) Numerous black-stained hyphae are within the lumen of a blood vessel and extend through its wall (top of image). (b) Hyphal morphology is apparent with stiff hyphae, easily identified septa, and a tendency toward 45-degree branching.

little diagnostic value (Fig. 34.11). **Hematogenous spread** is common, with involvement of heart valves and brain.

A less common fungal infection, **mucormycosis (zygomycosis)**, is a clinical mimic of **aspergillosis**. Mucormycosis can be caused by a number of molds in the **Zygomycetes** class including *Rhizopus* (most common cause), *Mucor*, *Rhizomucor*, *Absidia*, and *Cunninghamella*. Like *Aspergillus*, these

fungi are angioinvasive, resulting in thrombosis and infarction [Fig. 34.12(a), (b)] with subsequent suppurative inflammation. The hyphae of the Zygomycetes have few septa (although they are commonly described as aseptate), are of widely variable width with a ribbon-like appearance, and have a tendency toward 90° branching, again, a commonly quoted criterion that in reality has little diagnostic value [Fig. 34.12(c)].

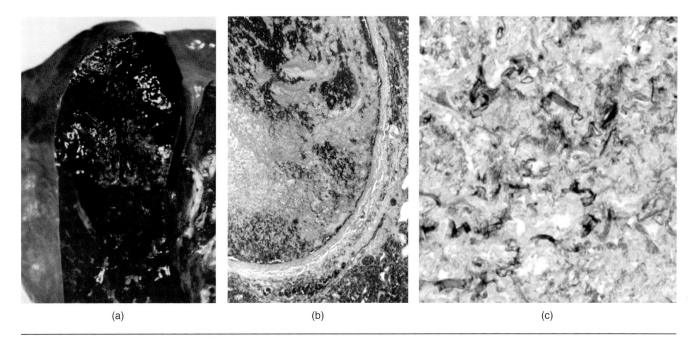

(a)   (b)   (c)

FIGURE 34.12 **Mucormycosis**. (a) Grossly, the cut surface of the lung shows a wedge-shaped deep red lesion, a pulmonary infarct. (b) Associated with the infarct is thrombosis of a pulmonary arterial branch. (c) GMS staining shows hyphae consistent with molds of the class Zygomycetes. The hyphae show more variable width than *Aspergillus* and have a more ribbon-like appearance with rarer septa.

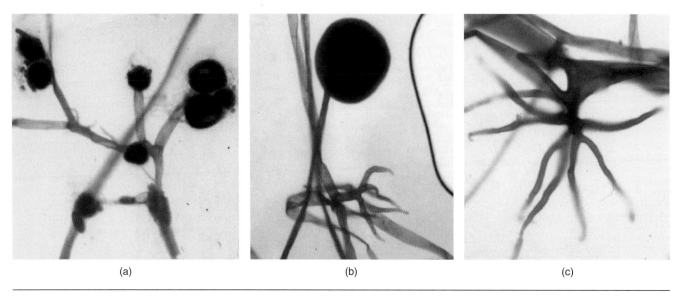

(a)   (b)   (c)

FIGURE 34.13 Fungi grown in culture. (a) *Mucor*. (b) and (c) Photos of *Rhizopus*; note the rootlike rhizoids in both images. Structures such as these assist in the morphologic identification of fungi.

▶▶ **CLINICAL CORRELATION 34.3**

Fungi can be identified by microscopic analysis of cultures. Whereas many yeasts and molds have similar appearances in tissues, there are specific morphologic features best seen in culture that can be identified. Shown in Fig. 34.13 are cultures of *Mucor* and *Rhizopus*. *Rhizopus* has rootlike structures (rhizoids), whereas *Mucor* does not.

Infectious Interstitial Pneumonitis

Many viral and a few bacterial pneumonias show an inflammatory infiltrate dominated by interstitial mononuclear cells rather than the intra-alveolar polymorphonuclear cells that typify acute bacterial pneumonia. Grossly, infectious interstitial pneumonitis appears red-blue, congested, and **hypocrepitant**. In severe cases, diffuse alveolar damage (Chaps. 23 and 28) may develop. The pathogenesis of infectious interstitial pneumonitis begins with entry of the microorganism into the alveolus, where type 1 pneumocytes become infected and lose their integrity as a membrane, resulting in pulmonary edema (Chaps. 7 and 26). The proteinaceous edema fluid and necrotic cell debris form **hyaline membranes**, and there is type 2 pneumocyte hyperplasia. Again, the inflammatory infiltrate is predominantly interstitial and mononuclear, comprising lymphocytes, plasma cells, and macrophages.

Clinically, infectious interstitial pneumonitis is often referred to as **atypical pneumonia**, the most common cause being *Mycoplasma pneumoniae*. Risk factors for *M. pneumoniae* pneumonia include childhood, adolescence, and life in closed communities like a school, military camp, or prison. Other microbes that can cause infectious interstitial pneumonitis include the bacterium *Chlamydia pneumoniae*, and numerous

viruses (influenza, parainfluenza, RSV, adenovirus, rubeola or measles, varicella-zoster, and rhinovirus). Most also cause upper respiratory tract infection with **coryza**, pharyngitis, laryngitis, and tracheobronchitis (Chap. 33). In the immunocompromised, cytomegalovirus can cause a life-threatening pneumonitis with interstitial mononuclear inflammation, focal necrosis, and cells with characteristic viral inclusions (Fig. 34.14).

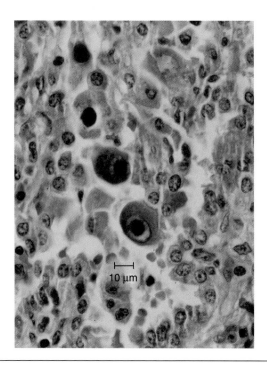

FIGURE 34.14 Cytomegalovirus (CMV). The cytopathic changes of CMV infection include cytomegaly, small basophilic cytoplasmic inclusions, and large basophilic nuclear inclusions.

Granulomatous Infectious Pneumonitis

Tuberculosis (**TB**) is a communicable granulomatous disease caused by *Mycobacterium tuberculosis* (**MTB**), an **acid-fast bacillus** (**AFB**) (Fig. 34.15), and, though it usually involves the lung, can affect any organ. Morphologically, the hallmark of tuberculosis is caseating granulomatous inflammation (Fig. 34.16). A granuloma is a circumscribed collection of **epithelioid histiocytes**. The term "epithelioid" describes an increase in cytoplasm, imparting an appearance resembling squamous epithelial cells. The granulomata in tuberculosis typically show central necrosis that, at the gross level, has a cheese-like consistency, referred to as **caseous**. The virulence of tuberculosis is largely due to tissue destruction by a host-mediated, type IV (delayed, cell-mediated) hypersensitivity reaction. This hypersensitivity is exploited in the **purified protein derivative** (**PPD**) screening test. The clinical course of tuberculosis is variable and is covered in more detail elsewhere in this book (Chap. 36).

Approximately 5% of people newly infected with MTB develop disease, termed **primary tuberculosis**. The inhaled microorganisms implant in distal airspaces of the lower upper or upper lower lobes; subsequently, a 1-1.5 cm focus of granulomatous consolidation develops, the **Ghon focus**. Involvement of an ipsilateral hilar lymph node follows, and the combination of the Ghon focus and the involved lymph node is called the **Ghon complex**. Primary TB is usually asymptomatic, with lesions eventually undergoing fibrosis and calcification (Fig. 34.17). However, approximately 5% of cases of primary TB, principally among the immunocompromised, show dissemination to other sites. The lesions in disseminated disease are often small, the size of millet seeds, a fact that gave rise to the term **miliary tuberculosis**. Approximately 5%-10% of cases of primary TB progress to secondary tuberculosis.

Secondary TB describes reactivation of a dormant primary infection in a previously infected host. Classically, the

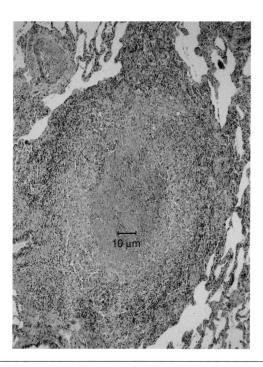

FIGURE 34.16 A **necrotizing granuloma** is shown with central necrosis. The term **caseous** refers to the gross morphology of the necrotic tissue, which has the consistency of soft cheese.

lesions in secondary TB are localized to the apex of one or both lungs, and cavitation of lesions is typical; the lesions are usually less than 2 cm in greatest dimension and are typically within 2 cm of the visceral pleura (Fig. 34.18). Lymph node involvement in secondary TB is less common than in primary TB. Other forms of secondary TB include **progressive pulmonary TB** (**fibrocaseous TB**), in which the apical lesions cavitate and there is pleural involvement, leading to serous pleural effusion, tuberculous empyema, and obliterative fibrous pleuritis. **Miliary pulmonary TB** describes diffuse involvement of the lung by small (~2 mm) foci of granulomatous inflammation with pleural effusion, empyema, or pleuritis. **Endobronchial, endotracheal,** and/or **laryngeal TB** can also occur. **Systemic miliary TB** most commonly involves liver, bone marrow, spleen, adrenals, meninges, kidneys, fallopian tubes, and epididymis. **Isolated organ TB** has also been described. In contrast to primary TB, secondary TB typically is symptomatic, with insidious gradual systemic signs/symptoms of malaise, anorexia, weight loss, low-grade fever, night sweats, and localized symptoms of productive cough, hemoptysis, and/or pleuritic pain.

Infections with atypical *Mycobacteria* also cause a granulomatous inflammatory response and are further discussed in Chap. 36. Several fungal pneumonias show the granulomatous inflammatory response and are briefly discussed below.

Histoplasmosis mimics TB clinically and morphologically (Fig. 34.19). The etiologic agent, *Histoplasma capsulatum*, is a dimorphic, nonencapsulated fungus (despite its name) that is endemic to the Mississippi River Valley and southeastern United States. The fungus lives as a mold in

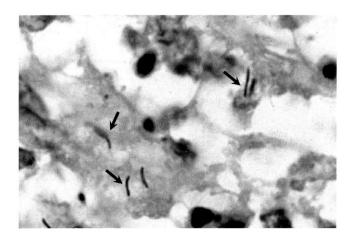

FIGURE 34.15 **Acid-fast bacilli** (**AFB**) are shown at the arrows. Pathologists often colloquially refer to the organisms as **red snappers**.

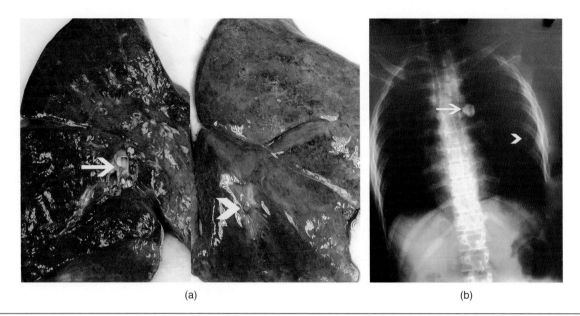

(a)   (b)

FIGURE 34.17 **Healed primary TB**. Upon healing, the Ghon complex often calcifies. (a) A lung cut in two with its hilum shown by the white arrow. On the right side, the visceral pleural surface is shown. Calcified lymph nodes in the hilum (white arrow) and the pleural surface near the calcified **Ghon focus** (white arrowhead) are shown. (b) healed primary tuberculosis is evident in this x-ray as a calcified lymph node (white arrow) and a barely visible calcification in the lung (white arrowhead). *From Kemp et al.* Pathology: the Big Picture, *McGraw-Hill; 2008.*

warm, moist soils enriched by bird or bat droppings. Inhalation of the spores leads to germination. In contrast to the mold morphology in the environment, its form at 37°C is that of a yeast that is 2-5 μm in diameter.

Blastomycosis is caused by *Blastomyces dermatitis*, another dimorphic fungus endemic to the Mississippi River Valley and southeastern United States. Like *H. capsulatum*, *B. dermatitis* exists as a mold in the environment and as a yeast at body temperature [Fig. 34.20 (b)]. However, its yeast form

is larger (up to 25 μm) than that of *Histoplasma*. Morphologically, a clue that a yeast is in fact *Blastomyces* is the presence of **broad-based budding** [Fig. 34.20 (c)]. The granulomatous inflammation of blastomycosis is a bit different than that of previously mentioned granulomatous pneumonias in that the granulomata here typically are admixed with a neutrophilic inflammatory infiltrate, referred to as **suppurative granulomatous inflammation** [Fig. 34.20 (a)]. When a focus of blastomycosis is near an epithelium, that surface may undergo

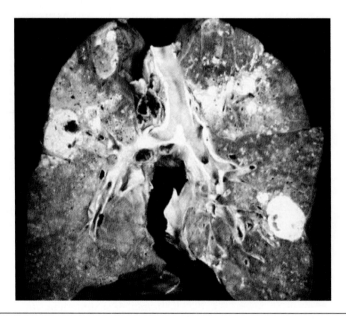

FIGURE 34.18 **Secondary tuberculosis**, where the foci of granulomatous inflammation are typically within 2 cm of the pleural surface and not infrequently undergo cavitation. *From Travis et al.* Non-Neoplastic Disorders of the Lower Respiratory Tract. © *American Registry of Pathology; 2002.*

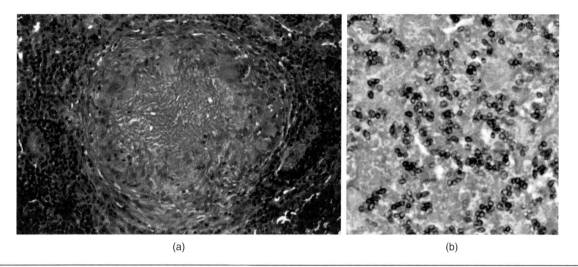

(a)   (b)

FIGURE 34.19 Histoplasmosis. (a) A pulmonary necrotizing granuloma in the setting of histoplasmosis. (b) GMS staining shows 2-5 μm yeast, morphologically consistent with *Histoplasma capsulatum*. Subsequent culture analysis confirmed the diagnosis.

pseudoepitheliomatous hyperplasia, so named because of its morphologic similarity to squamous cell carcinoma (previously called squamous cell epithelioma); it can be misdiagnosed as cancer.

The third dimorphic fungus that can cause granulomatous pneumonia is *Coccidioides immitis*, the etiology of **coccidiomycosis** and endemic to the Southwestern and far Western USA. The granulomatous inflammation resembles that of histoplasmosis and contains 20-60 μm nonbudding spherules often filled with endospores (Fig. 34.21).

In the immunocompromised host, *Cryptococcus neoformans* can infect the lung and produce a granulomatous inflammatory reaction that is typically asymptomatic. Virulence of

C. neoformans is primarily related to involvement of the central nervous system. Morphologically, *C. neoformans* is a 5-10 μm yeast with a thick halo due to its gelatinous capsule (Fig. 34.22).

Severe Acute Respiratory Syndrome

Severe acute respiratory syndrome (SARS) first appeared in China in 2002 and subsequently spread to other continents. Its etiology is a newly discovered **coronavirus** that infects the lower respiratory tract (in contrast to most other

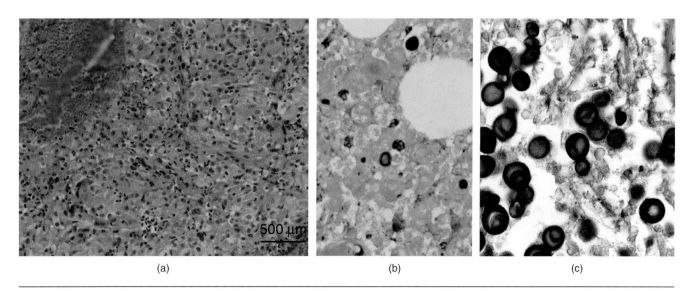

(a)   (b)   (c)

FIGURE 34.20 Blastomycosis. (a) The granulomata of blastomycosis typically show neutrophils admixed with the epithelioid histiocytes, a combination referred to as suppurative granulomatous inflammation. (b) By GMS stain *Blastomyces dermatitis* is a yeast at body temperature, typically somewhat larger than *Histoplasma capsulatum*. (c) Broad-based budding is a morphologic clue that distinguishes *Blastomyces* from other yeast. (c) *From Travis et al.* Non-Neoplastic Disorders of the Lower Respiratory Tract. © *American Registry of Pathology; 2002.*

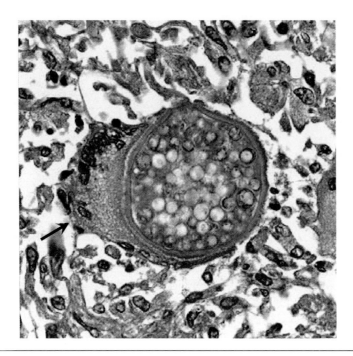

FIGURE 34.21 *Coccidioides.* A multi-nucleated giant cell (arrow) is attempting to phagocytose this mature spherule of *Coccidioides. From Travis et al.* Non-Neoplastic Disorders of the Lower Respiratory Tract. © *American Registry of Pathology; 2002.*

coronaviruses, which cause approximately one-third of *upper* respiratory infections) and subsequently spreads throughout the body. Following an incubation of 2-10 days, the infected person develops dry cough, malaise, myalgia, fever, and chills with less common upper respiratory symptoms. Its pathogenesis is not well understood. A third of SARS patients improve

and resolve the infection; the remainder progress to severe respiratory distress with dyspnea, tachypnea, and pleurisy. Therapy is largely supportive, and mortality is approximately 10%. In fatal cases, the morphology of lung involvement is diffuse alveolar damage (Chaps. 23 and 28) with multinucleated giant cells.

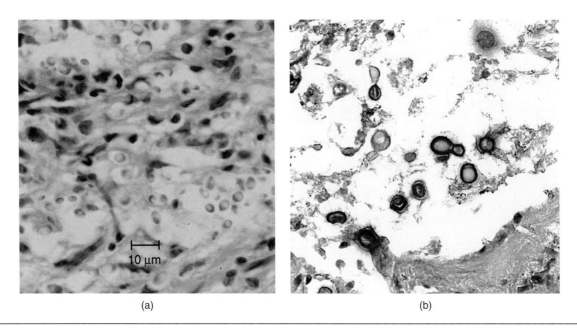

(a)

(b)

FIGURE 34.22 (a) With H&E staining, *Cryptococcus* yeasts are surrounded by a pale halo (the capsule). (b) Mucicarmine staining highlights the capsule. (b): *From Travis et al.* Non-Neoplastic Disorders of the Lower Respiratory Tract. © *American Registry of Pathology; 2002.*

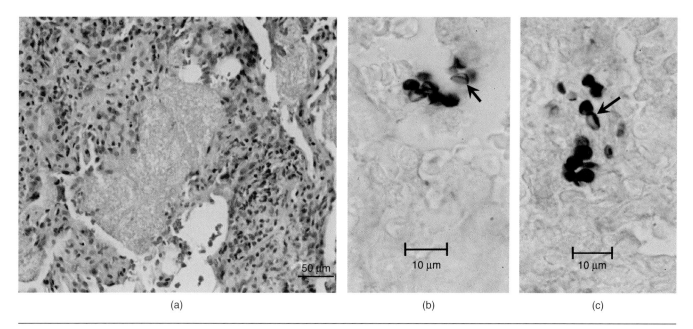

(a)   (b)   (c)

FIGURE 34.23 *Pneumocystis jiroveci.* (a) The dominant finding in *P. jiroveci* pneumonia is a foamy intra-alveolar exudate. (b) and (c) GMS staining highlights *P. jiroveci* organisms. When viewed from the correct angle, the organism's cup-like shape is apparent (arrows).

Pneumocystis Pneumonia

Among the many other microorganisms that can infect the lung, one additional infection that is common in the setting of the immunocompromised patient will be considered. *Pneumocystis jiroveci* (formerly *Pneumocystis carinii*) is a microorganism with features of a protozoan and of a fungus, although it is currently considered a fungus. While *P. jiroveci* induces interstitial mononuclear inflammation, the more impressive morphologic finding is a foamy, pale eosinophilic intra-alveolar exudate. When stained for fungus, this exudate is seen to contain cup-shaped microorganisms, often within macrophage cytoplasm (Fig. 34.23).

▶▶**CLINICAL CORRELATION 34.4**

The common clinical term, PCP, originally stood for *Pneumocystis carinii* pneumonia. Despite this taxonomic change in the microorganism's name, the term PCP persists, and defenders of its use say the abbreviation now stands for *Pneumocystis* pneumonia.

Suggested Readings

1. Travis WD, Colby TV, Koss MN, Rosado-de-Christenson ML, Müller NL, King TE. *Atlas of Nontumor Pathology: Volume 2: Non-Neoplastic Disorders of the Lower Respiratory Tract.* American Registry of Pathology; 2002. *For many years, the Armed Forces Institute of Pathology (AFIP) was responsible for the publication of numerous tumor atlases, frequently referred to as "The Fascicles." Later, the AFIP expanded its atlas publication to include non-neoplastic disease. This text offers well-organized and exceedingly well-illustrated discussions of pulmonary disease with a focus on morphology but with generous clinical and radiographic coverage. In accordance with the 2005 Defense Base Realignment and Closure (BRAC) law, the AFIP is on track to disestablish and permanently close by September 15, 2011.*

2. Katzenstein AL. *Katzenstein and Askin's Surgical Pathology of Non-Neoplastic Lung Disease,* 4th ed. Philadelphia, PA: Saunders; 2006. *Prior to the publication of the AFIP nontumor "fascicles," previous editions of this book served surgical pathologists as a sort of "gold standard" for the interpretation of non-neoplastic lung pathology.*

3. Kumar V, Abbas AK, Fausto N. *Robbins and Cotran Pathologic Basis of Disease,* 8th ed. Philadelphia, PA: Elsevier; 2009. *Throughout its many editions, this reference work is the most definitive and approachable compendium of pathology images available to students.*

CASE STUDIES AND PRACTICE PROBLEMS

CASE 34.1 A 75-year-old man with diabetes mellitus, chronic obstructive pulmonary disease, and congestive heart failure presents with malaise, fever, and a productive cough. A chest radiograph shows well-circumscribed radiopacity of the entire left lower lobe. Gram stain of sputum is most likely to show which of the following?

   a. Gram-negative bacilli

   b. Gram-negative coccobacilli

   c. Gram-positive cocci in pairs

   d. Gram-positive cocci in grapelike clusters

   e. Acid-fast bacilli

CASE 34.2 A 40-year-old man presents to the emergency room, having fallen down some steps and sustained traumatic injury to his back. A chest radiograph is obtained and is negative for bone fractures; however, there is a focus of calcification in what appears to be the lower portion of the left upper lobe and a second focus of calcification in the left hilum. Which of the following is most likely the correct diagnosis?

   a. Primary tuberculosis at present

   b. Primary tuberculosis in the past

   c. Secondary (reactivation) tuberculosis

   d. Miliary tuberculosis

CASE 34.3 A child being treated for leukemia develops a pulmonary infarct and subsequently dies of a stroke. At autopsy, the infarct is seen to be associated with a thrombus. Histologically, the infarct is infiltrated by neutrophils, and the thrombus contains hyphae that are 5-10 μm wide and have easily identified septa. Which of the following is the best diagnosis?

   a. Aspergillosis

   b. Mucormycosis

   c. Candidiasis

   d. Blastomycosis

   e. Histoplasmosis

Solutions to Case Studies and Practice Problems

CASE 34.1 The most correct answer is c, gram-positive cocci in pairs.

The patient has lobar pneumonia. *Streptococcus pneumoniae* (*Pneumococcus*) is the cause of more than 90% of cases of lobar pneumonia, the patient has several risk factors for pneumococcal pneumonia, and the morphology of *S. pneumoniae* is gram-positive cocci in pairs (*answer c*). *Klebsiella pneumoniae* can cause lobar pneumonia less commonly, and its morphology is gram-negative bacilli (*answer a*). *Haemophilus influenzae* and *Moraxella catarrhalis* are both gram-negative coccobacilli (*answer b*) but typically cause bronchopneumonia. *Staphylococcus aureus* generally causes bronchopneumonia, although it can cause lobar pneumonia less commonly than *Pneumococcus*; its morphology is gram-positive cocci in clusters (*answer d*). Acid-fast bacilli (*answer e*) cause granulomatous inflammation (eg, tuberculosis) and would not be visible on a gram stain.

CASE 34.2 The most correct answer is b, primary tuberculosis in the past.

The locations of the calcifications are characteristic of a Ghon complex, typical of primary tuberculosis. Calcification occurs

with healing and would not be present if the patient currently had primary tuberculosis (*answer a*). The lesions of secondary (reactivation) tuberculosis (*answer c*) are typically within 2 cm of the pleura of the lung apex. The lesions of miliary tuberculosis (*answer d*) are widely disseminated throughout the lungs and small enough not likely to be visible on a chest radiograph. While the patient may have miliary TB (*answer d*), statistically speaking, it is more likely that he does not.

CASE 34.3 The most correct answer is a, aspergillosis.

Aspergillus species are angioinvasive and typically cause thrombosis and infarction with subsequent suppuration. Mucormycosis (*answer b*) clinically mimics aspergillosis; however, the Zygomycetes hyphae are only sparsely septate. The patient is at risk for candidiasis (*answer c*), but *Candida* morphology is budding yeast with pseudohyphae. The causative organisms of blastomycosis (*answer d*) and histoplasmosis (*answer e*) are yeasts at body temperature; hyphal forms of these microorganisms would only be expected at temperatures lower than body temperature as usually found in soils.

Chapter 35

Management of Pneumonias

DAVID A. STOECKEL, MD AND
GEORGE M. MATUSCHAK, MD

Learning Objectives

- The student will be able to define the categorization of clinical pneumonia into community-acquired versus hospital-acquired pneumonia.

- The student will be to describe the epidemiology of community-acquired versus hospital-acquired pneumonia.

- The student will be able to recognize the common symptoms and signs of infectious pneumonia.

- The student will be able to summarize the general principles of treatment of infectious pneumonia.

Introduction #107

Although the symptoms and signs of infectious pneumonia were known and described by both patients and physicians in ancient times, the pathophysiology of pneumonia has only recently become clear. Consequently, effective treatment for bacterial pneumonia has been available for <100 years. The presence of bacteria in the respiratory tissue of patients with pneumonia was first identified in the latter half of the nineteenth century. However, without effective antimicrobial medications, the morbidity and mortality from pneumonia remained high during the first half of the twentieth century. Thus, prior to the availability of penicillin in the 1940s, 80% of patients in the United States with bacteremic pneumococcal pneumonia died. The mortality rate dropped to approximately 20% after the clinical introduction of penicillin, and the current mortality rate for community-acquired pneumonia is approximately 4%. Even so, pneumonia remains the most common cause of infectious death in the United States. Also of concern, many of the once highly effective antimicrobial medications for the treatment of pneumonia have been rendered ineffective with the emergence of resistant organisms.

In clinical practice, infectious pneumonia is divided into two main categories: (1) **community-acquired pneumonia (CAP)**; and (2) **hospital-acquired pneumonia (HAP)**. Community-acquired pneumonia can be defined as any infectious pneumonia in patients who are not hospitalized, or who have been hospitalized for <48 hours and not admitted to a hospital or extended health care facility in the past 90 days. By contrast, hospital-acquired pneumonia includes pneumonias that develop in patients who have been hospitalized for >48 hours, or who have been admitted to hospitals or extended health care facilities in the previous 90 days. Categorizing pneumonia as either CAP or HAP is useful because the spectrum of likely infectious pathogens differs significantly between the two groups. Management decisions can thereby be tailored to the most likely pathogens in each setting, even before the potential isolation of a specific pathogen. Immunosuppressed persons are at special risk of developing pneumonia due to any of the organisms commonly associated with CAP or HAP, as well as to **opportunistic pathogens** that usually do not cause disease among immunocompetent patients.

Management of Community-Acquired Pneumonia

The first step in management of CAP is prevention. Vaccines against three common CAP pathogens are available: influenza, *Streptococcus pneumonia* (pneumococcus), and *Haemophilus influenzae*. Seasonal influenza vaccination is recommended for children who are 6-23 months old, adults >50 years of age, healthcare providers, and certain other high-risk individuals including those with significant medical comorbidities. Likewise, pneumococcal vaccination is recommended for adults ≥65 years of age and for certain other high risk individuals, again including those with significant medical comorbidities.

Evaluation of a patient with suspected CAP starts with a comprehensive history including the presence or absence of fever, chills, malaise, cough, sputum production, dyspnea, and chest pain among other symptoms. Physical findings compatible with pneumonia include tachypnea, increased tactile fremitus, dullness to percussion, and inspiratory crackles or egophony on chest auscultation (Chap. 14). Opacities or parenchymal consolidation on thoracic imaging studies support the clinical diagnosis (Figs. 35.1, 35.2; see also Chap. 15).

Because CAP by definition involves patients who develop pneumonia outside of a health care setting, one of the first steps in management is to decide the most optimal setting to provide safe treatment for the patient. For example, will outpatient treatment suffice, or does the patient need to be admitted to the hospital and if so, is intensive care unit (ICU) admission warranted? These questions are best answered by the initial assessment of severity of a patient's pneumonia. In this regard, a helpful tool is the **CURB-65 score** which is a refinement of an instrument originally set forth by the British Thoracic Society. CURB-65 is an acronym for the five

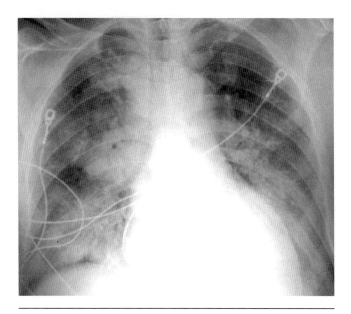

FIGURE 35.1 Chest radiograph of a 53-year-old male patient with severe community-acquired pneumonia and acute respiratory failure demonstrating bilateral patchy airspace opacities, greater on the right side.

components of the score: **C**onfusion, **B**lood **u**rea nitrogen level, **R**espiratory rate, **B**lood pressure, and **age of 65** years or older (Table 35.1).

The risk of mortality increases with increasing values of a CURB-65 score. Thus, patients with a CURB-65 score of 0 or 1 are considered at low risk for complications and can be usually considered for ambulatory treatment. In this context, however, other clinical factors such as the patient's living environment and social support, as well as comorbidities need to be taken into account to assure the safety and efficacy of treatment. Admission to the hospital is recommended when

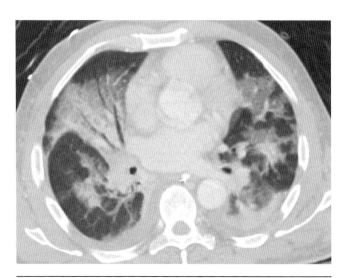

FIGURE 35.2 Chest CT scan of the same patient depicted in Fig. 35.1 at the mid-chest level demonstrating bilateral patchy air space opacities in a patient with CAP. Air bronchograms are notable on the patient's right side. Small bilateral pleural effusions are also present.

Table 35.1 Computing a patient's CURB-65 score

Clinical Factor	Points
Confusion	1
Blood urea nitrogen >19 mg/dL	1
Respiratory rate >30 breaths/min	1
Systolic blood pressure <90 mm Hg or diastolic blood pressure <60 mm Hg	1
Age ≥65 years	+ 1
Maximal total points	5

the patient's CURB-65 score is ≥2 and many patients with scores of ≥3 will require admission to the ICU. The **American Thoracic Society (ATS)** and **Infectious Disease Society of America (IDSA)** have also developed consensus-related criteria for **Severe CAP** (Table 35.2). By these criteria, patients with ≥ one major criteria or ≥ three minor criteria require ICU admission.

Diagnostic tests to determine the specific organism responsible for the patient's CAP who will be treated as outpatients are optional. These tests include blood cultures, sputum Gram stain and culture, and urinary antigen tests for *Legionella* spp. and *S. pneumonia* (Chap. 19). Patients with a history of unusual environmental exposures, international travel within the past 2 weeks, pleural effusion, and severe underlying comorbidities such as active alcohol abuse, chronic liver disease, chronic obstructive lung disease, and asplenia, represent

Table 35.2 Criteria for severe community-acquired pneumonia

Major Criteria
Invasive mechanical ventilation
Septic shock with the need for vasopressors
Minor Criteria
Respiratory rate ≥30 breaths/min
P_aO_2/F_iO_2 ratio ≤250 (see Chap. 28)
Multilobar infiltrates on chest imaging
Confusion/disorientation
Uremia (blood urea nitrogen level ≥20 mg/dL)
Leukopenia (white blood cell count <4000/μL)
Thrombocytopenia (platelet count <100,000/μL)
Hypothermia (core temperature <36°C)
Hypotension requiring aggressive fluid resuscitation

From Mandell LA et al. Infectious Disease Society of America/American Thoracic Society consensus guidelines on the management of community-acquired pneumonia in adults. *Clin Infect Dis. Mar 1;44 Suppl 2:S27-72, 2007.*

Table 35.3 Most common causes of community-acquired pneumonia

Patient Type	Etiology
Outpatient	Streptococcus pneumoniae
	Mycoplasma pneumoniae
	Haemophilus influenzae
	Respiratory viruses
Inpatient (non-ICU)	Streptococcus pneumoniae
	Mycoplasma pneumoniae
	Chlamydia pneumoniae
	Haemophilus influenzae
	Legionella spp.
	Aspiration (of mixed oropharyngeal flora)
	Respiratory viruses
Inpatient (ICU)	Streptococcus pneumoniae
	Staphylococcus aureus
	Legionella spp.
	Gram-negative bacilli
	Haemophilus influenzae

From Mandell LA et al. Infectious Disease Society of America/American Thoracic Society consensus guidelines on the management of community-acquired pneumonia in adults. *Clin Infect Dis. Mar 1;44 Suppl 2:S27-72, 2007.*

subpopulations in which such further testing for a specific organism is indicated. For patients with CAP who are admitted to the hospital, pretreatment blood cultures and sputum Gram stain and cultures are indicated if the patient has severe CAP or comorbidities. Patients requiring endotracheal intubation should have specimens obtained from the lower respiratory tract in the form of endotracheal aspirates or **bronchoalveolar lavage** (Chap. 18).

The choice of initial antibiotic(s) in CAP is guided by the anticipated susceptibility of the most likely pathogens. In some cases a pathogen will be identified via sputum smears, cultures, serologic or other diagnostic tests. Unfortunately, such results are rarely available when treatment needs to be initiated. At best, the identity of a pathogen is known within the first 24 hours, although the identification process usually takes longer. In many instances, a pathogen will never be identified. Clinically, the likely pathogens are determined by both the severity of the pneumonia and the specific comorbidities of the patient (Table 35.3). Across all severities of CAP, *Streptococcus pneumoniae* is the most commonly identified pathogen, whereas *Mycoplasma pneumoniae*, *Chlamydia pneumoniae*, and respiratory viruses are more common pathogens in patients who are less severely ill. In contrast, *Staphylococcus aureus*, *Legionella* spp., and gram-negative bacilli are more often found in patients with severe pneumonia. Specific comorbidities and the likely pathogens in CAP are shown in Table 35.4. Less common pathogens and associated clinical scenarios are listed in Table 35.5.

Physician task forces within the ATS and IDSA have developed evidence-based guidelines which suggest that initial antibiotic therapy for CAP be based on both the severity of pneumonia and the individual patient's specific comorbidities. In subjects who are to be treated as outpatients, a **macrolide** antibiotic is preferred, unless the patient has significant comorbidities in which case a respiratory **fluoroquinolone** is recommended. A **β-lactam** antibiotic plus a macrolide may be used in place of a respiratory fluoroquinolone. If the severity of pneumonia requires inpatient treatment, the preferred therapy is either a respiratory fluoroquinolone or a combination of a β-lactam antibiotic and a macrolide. Finally, for the severity ill patient with CAP that requires ICU admission, a β-lactam antibiotic or ampicillin-sulbactam in addition to a respiratory fluoroquinolone or macrolide is recommended. If a specific pathogen is identified, the antimicrobial regimen is subsequently tailored to the antimicrobial sensitivity of that organism.

▶▶CLINICAL CORRELATION 35.1

Patients with CAP should be treated with antimicrobial therapy for a minimum of 5 days and should be afebrile for at least 48 hours prior to discontinuing antibiotics. A longer duration of treatment is indicated in patients who are not clinically stable after 5 days. If the patient initially required intravenous antibiotic therapy, then a switch to oral antibiotic treatment is generally done only when there is hemodynamic stability and clinical improvement. A failure to improve, or a deterioration of the patient's condition despite antimicrobial treatment, can occur for a variety of reasons. The clinician must consider both the possibility of infection by a pathogen resistant to the chosen antibiotics, and the spread of intrapulmonary infection beyond the lungs. Thus, development of a **complicated parapneumonic effusion** or frank **empyema** in the pleural space is a common cause of treatment failure (Chap. 29). In addition, the development de novo of superimposed pulmonary infections such as a **ventilator-associated pneumonia** can result in failure of a patient to clinically improve (Chap. 28). The stress of CAP on the patient's systemic inflammatory responses can also exacerbate underlying co-morbidities, or cause the development of other medical problems. Lastly, the clinician must consider whether the initial diagnosis of CAP was correct.

Management of Hospital-Acquired Pneumonia

Hospital-acquired pneumonia (HAP) is defined as a pneumonia that occurs 48 hours or more after admission to the hospital. HAP includes pneumonias that develop after a patient is intubated and placed on mechanical ventilation (ie, **ventilator-associated pneumonia (VAP)**; Chap. 28). It also includes pneumonia which develops in patients who have resided in an extended care facility or hospital in the previous 90 days (eg, a **healthcare-associated pneumonia**). Moreover, pneumonia in patients receiving hemodialysis, chemotherapy, or wound care outside the home is also considered a healthcare-associated pneumonia. This definition encompasses these several groups of patients because each is at risk for infection with a similar spectrum of pathogens including **multidrug-resistant (MDR)** organisms. Current data suggest that HAP occurs in up to 1% of all hospitalized patients and in perhaps one-third of patients who are being mechanically ventilated (Chaps. 28 and 30). The clinical importance of HAP is underscored by the fact that as a disease category it has been shown to have an attributable mortality rate of up to 50%, despite optimal supportive care.

As with CAP, the management of HAP begins with prevention. Avoidance of endotracheal intubation, if possible by utilizing non-invasive mechanical ventilation with a facial mask, reduces the risk for development of HAP, as do processes that tend to reduce the duration of intubation. Maintenance of a semi-recumbent position with the head elevated 30°-45° above the supine position decreases the risk of aspiration of oral or gastric substances into the lungs, thereby reducing the incidence of HAP in ICU patients. Finally, appropriate hand hygiene by all medical staff and appropriate use of antibiotics are important in the prevention of HAP.

The development of fever, leukocytosis or leukopenia, purulent sputum, and respiratory distress generally herald the development of HAP. In addition, new or progressive pulmonary infiltrate(s) on chest imaging studies is generally required for the diagnosis of HAP (Fig. 35.3).

In this setting, a positive culture of sputum or tracheal aspirates corroborates the diagnosis of HAP and provides valuable guidance regarding the initial choice of antimicrobial treatment. In addition to imaging the chest and culturing of the respiratory tract, preferably via endotracheal aspirate or bronchoscopy, patients with suspected HAP require evaluation of their oxygenation via **pulse oximetry** or arterial blood gas sampling (Chaps. 17-19). Blood cultures also should be

Table 35.4 Risk factors for multidrug resistant pathogens causing HAP

Antimicrobial therapy in preceding 90 days
Current hospitalization of ≥5 days or more
High frequency of antibiotic resistance in the community or specific hospital unit
Risk factors for healthcare-related pneumonia
Hospitalization for 2 days or more in the preceding 90 days
Residence in nursing home or extended care facility
Home infusion therapy (including antibiotics)
Home wound care
Family member with multidrug-resistant pathogen
Immunosuppressive disease and/or therapy

From American Thoracic Society; Infectious Disease Society of America: Guidelines for the management of adults with hospital-acquired, ventilator-associated pneumonia, *Am J Respir Crit Care Med Feb 15;171(4):388-416, 2005.*

obtained. It is recommended that cultures of both the lower respiratory tract and blood be collected before starting or changing antibiotics.

Prompt initiation of appropriate antibiotic therapy is indicated in all patients suspected of having HAP, since mortality increases with delay of antibiotic therapy or with the initiation of inappropriate antibiotic therapy. The initial antibiotic regimen is chosen empirically based upon risk factors for specific organisms and local patterns of organism prevalence and antimicrobial resistance. The first consideration when choosing empiric therapy for HAP is to determine the risk of MDR pathogens. Patients are considered to be at low risk for MDR pathogens if HAP develops within the first 4 days of hospitalization and if they do not have other risk factors for MDR pathogens (Table 35.4).

Likely pathogens in these patients include *Streptococcus pneumoniae*, *Hemophilus influenzae*, methicillin-sensitive *Staphylococcus aureus*, and antibiotic-sensitive enteric gram-negative bacilli (Table 35.5). Accordingly, appropriate antibiotic choices include ceftriaxone, ampicillin/sulbactam, ertapenem, and those quinolones that show good activity against *S. pneumoniae*.

If patients are at risk for an MDR pathogen, or if HAP develops on or after the fifth hospital day or with a described risk factor (Table 35.4), then potential pathogens include *Pseudomonas aeruginosa*, **extended spectrum beta-lactamase (ESBL)** producing *Klebsiella pneumoniae*, *Acinetobacter* spp., or **methicillin-resistant *Staphylococcus aureus* (MRSA)**. Correspondingly, appropriate initial antibiotic choices therefore include an anti-pseudomonal cephalosporin, a carbapenem, or a β-lactam/β-lactamase inhibitor combination plus an aminoglycoside or anti-pseudomonal fluoroquinolone plus vancomycin or linezolid (Table 35.6). These

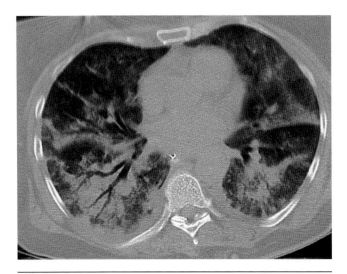

FIGURE 35.3 Hospital-acquired pneumonia due to **methicillin-resistant *S. aureus* (MRSA)** in a 59-year-old female. This HRCT demonstrates diffuse bilateral airspace opacities.

Table **35.5** Initial antibiotic therapy for early-onset HAP in patients without significant risk factors for MDR pathogens

Potential Pathogens		
S. pneumoniae	Escherichia coli	Klebsiella pneumoniae
H. influenzae	Proteus spp.	Enterobacter spp.
Methicillin-sensitive S. aureus	Serratia marcescens	

Recommended Antibiotic Therapy							
ceftriaxone	OR	levofloxacin, moxifloxacin, or ciprofloxacin	OR	ampicillin/ sulbactam	OR	ertapenem

From American Thoracic Society; Infectious Disease Society of America: Guidelines for the management of adults with hospital-acquired, ventilator-associated pneumonia, Am J Respir Crit Care Med Feb 15;171(4):388-416, 2005.

choices include "double antibiotic coverage" of gram-negative organisms and coverage of MRSA. Double gram-negative antibacterial coverage increases the likelihood that the organism will be susceptible to at least one of the antibiotics. Local antimicrobial resistance patterns should further be taken into account when choosing antimicrobial combinations.

After 48-72 hours, it is important that the patient with suspected HAP be clinically reevaluated. If the patient has improved and cultures identify a specific pathogen, the antibiotic regimen may be "de-escalated" to include a single agent to which the pathogen is sensitive. If the patient is clinically improved but cultures are negative, discontinuation of antibiotic coverage for HAP should be considered, especially if blood cultures are negative and the lower respiratory tract specimen is without a significant number of inflammatory cells.

Table **35.6** Initial empiric antibiotic therapy for HAP in patients with late onset disease or risk factors for MDR pathogens

Potential Pathogens	
S. pneumoniae	MDR pathogens:
H. influenzae	Pseudomonas aeruginosa
Antibiotic sensitive gram-negative bacilli	Klebsiella pneumoniae (ESBL)
Legionella pneumophila	Acinetobacter spp.
	Methicillin-resistant S. aureus

Recommended Combination Antibiotic Therapies (3-Tiered Approach)				
1. anti-pseudomonal cephalosporin (cefepime or ceftazidime)	OR	anti-pseudomonal carbapenem (imipenem or meropenem)	OR	β-lactam/β-lactamase inhibitor (piperacillin/ tazobactam)
		PLUS		
2. anti-pseudomonal fluoroquinolone (ciprofloxacin or levofloxacin)		OR		Aminoglycoside (amikacin, gentamicin, tobramycin)
		PLUS		
3. linezolid or vancomycin				

From American Thoracic Society; Infectious Disease Society of America: Guidelines for the management of adults with hospital-acquired, ventilator-associated pneumonia, Am J Respir Crit Care Med Feb 15;171(4):388-416, 2005.

▶▶ CLINICAL CORRELATION 35.2

If the patient with HAP has not improved by 48-72 hours of antibiotic treatment, then evaluation for empyema, lung abscess, remote sites of infection, or other pathologic processes that could mimic pneumonia should start. The recommended total duration of antibiotic therapy for HAP with non-MDR organisms is at least 7 days, whereas duration of antibiotic therapy

for MDR organisms is generally 14 days. An important danger of prolonging antibiotic treatment beyond 14 days is colonization of the patient with antibiotic-resistant bacteria that may thereafter predispose to future episodes of HAP. Empiric double gram-negative bacterial coverage can be discontinued after 5 days in an improving patient who is showing a good clinical response to therapy.

Suggested Readings

1. Mandell LA, Wunderink RG, Anzueto A, et. al. Infectious Disease Society of America/American Thoracic Society consensus guidelines on the management of community-acquired pneumonia in adults. *Clin Infect Dis. 44 (Suppl. 2):S27;2007. A comprehensive, readable reference detailing all aspects of the management of CAP.*

2. Official Statement of the American Thoracic Society and the Infectious Disease Society of America. Guidelines for the management of adults with hospital-acquired, ventilator-associated, and healthcare-associated pneumonia. *Am J Respir Crit Care. 2005;171:388. A comprehensive and well-documented evidence-based guideline detailing the pathogenesis, risk factors, various diagnostic approaches and strategies, as well as the recommended approaches and rationales to antibiotic treatment of all types of HAP.*

CASE STUDIES AND PRACTICE PROBLEMS

CASE 35.1 A 65-year-old man with a past medical history of severe chronic obstructive pulmonary disease (COPD) presents with a 3-day history of fever, decreased appetite, progressive shortness of breath, cough productive of purulent sputum, and pleuritic chest pain. On physical examination, the patient is awake but confused and in moderate respiratory distress with a respiratory frequency of 32 breaths/min. His vital signs include a blood pressure of 120/70 mm Hg, pulse rate of 102/min, and an axillary temperature of 38.7°C (101.5°F). Chest examination shows increased tactile fremitus over the posterior right lung base, as well as dullness to percussion and bronchial breath sounds over this area; inspiratory crackles are evident over the left upper anterior chest. Laboratory findings are significant for a P_aO_2/F_IO_2 ratio of 225, an elevated circulating leukocyte count of 17,000/μL, and a blood urea nitrogen level of 30 mg/dL. A chest x-ray today reveals consolidation in the right lower lung as well as infiltrates in the left upper lobe. Blood and sputum samples for Gram stain and cultures are obtained but results are pending. The most appropriate management of this patient now includes which of the following actions?

a. Admission to the medical floor of the hospital and treatment with a macrolide antibiotic

b. Admission to the intensive care unit (ICU) and observation

c. Admission to the medical floor of the hospital and treatment with a respiratory fluoroquinolone

d. Admission to the ICU and treatment with a β-lactam antibiotic

e. Admission to the ICU and treatment with a β-lactam antibiotic plus a macrolide

CASE 35.2 A 26-year-old man is involved in a motor vehicle accident and suffers a closed head injury with a subdural hematoma, splenic laceration, and bilateral femur fractures. The patient is intubated in the emergency department for airway protection and subsequently undergoes surgical drainage of the subdural hematoma and operative reduction and fixation of the femur fractures. The splenic laceration does not require surgical intervention. One week after admission, the patient develops fever, leukocytosis, and increased purulent secretions from the endotracheal tube. A portable chest radiograph reveals a right lower lobe infiltrate and a pleural effusion. A ventilator-associated pneumonia is suspected and a tracheal aspirate and blood cultures are obtained. The patient is then started on antibiotic therapy with vancomycin, piperacillin/tazobactam, and gentamicin. Over the next 3 days, the patient remains febrile and becomes increasingly tachycardic and hypotensive with a progressively rising leukocyte count. The tracheal aspirate reveals many polymorphonuclear neutrophils and grows methicillin-resistant *Staphylococcus aureus* sensitive to vancomycin. The blood cultures remain negative. A CT scan of the chest is obtained and reveals a right lower lobe infiltrate with a moderate right-sided pleural effusion. Which of the following actions would be the most appropriate next step in the management of this patient?

a. Conduct bronchoscopy to obtain a lavage sample for Gram stain and culture, while continuing his current antibiotic regimen.

b. Discontinue vancomycin and start linezolid while continuing piperacillin/tazobactam and gentamicin.

c. Discontinue vancomycin, piperacillin/tazobactam, and gentamicin and start linezolid, cefepime and levofloxacin.

d. Perform diagnostic thoracentesis and continue the patient's current antibiotic regimen.

e. Continue current antibiotics and order observation without further diagnostic studies at this time.

Solutions to Case Studies and Practice Problems

CASE 35.1 The most correct answer is e, admission to the ICU and treatment with a β-lactam antibiotic plus a macrolide.

This patient is elderly, confused, has multilobar pulmonary infiltrates of presumed infectious origin, and is already manifesting signs of acute hypoxemic respiratory failure as well as renal dysfunction. Moreover, he has a CURB-65 score of 4, placing him at increased risk of death from complications of community-acquired pneumonia. For all of these reasons, it is important that the patient be admitted to an ICU rather to the inpatient medical floors (*answers a, c*). Considering this case presentation, observation in the ICU without antibiotic treatment within 4 hours greatly increases the likelihood of a poor outcome and is never appropriate management for severe CAP (*answer b*). Although treatment with a β-lactam antibiotic is an important aspect of the management of severe CAP (*answer d*), it represents incomplete coverage, particularly for *Legionella* spp. that are not sensitive to this antibiotic class. Thereafter co-treatment with a macrolide antibiotic is indicated for patients requiring ICU treatment.

CASE 35.2 The most correct answer is d, perform diagnostic thoracentesis and continuing the current antibiotic regimen.

This patient has developed a ventilator-associated pneumonia and the tracheal aspirate reveals methicillin-resistant *S. aureus* (MRSA) as the pathogen. Unfortunately, despite appropriate therapy, the patient is not responding after 72 hours of treatment. The most likely reason in this instance is the recent development of an empyema involving the right pleural space. A diagnostic thoracentesis should be obtained and, if the findings are consistent with an empyema, a tube thoracostomy should be performed to allow for drainage and resolution of the empyema. Therefore, ordering bronchoscopy (*answer a*) or doing no additional diagnostic intervention (*answer e*) is incorrect; bronchoscopy would be unlikely to yield any additional information since the tracheal aspirate Gram stain and culture are both consistent with a ventilator-associated pneumonia secondary to MRSA. *Answers b* and *c* also are incorrect for this patient because the MRSA organism has demonstrated sensitivity to vancomycin. Accordingly, a switch to a different antibiotic regimen including linezolid in place of vancomycin would be unlikely to prove beneficial, assuming the vancomycin was being dosed correctly.

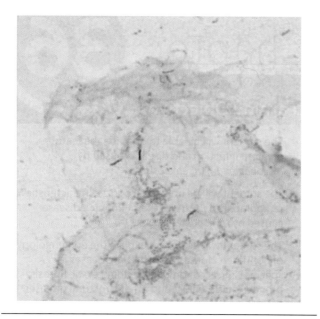

FIGURE 36.1 AFB smear showing *M. tuberculosis*. See also Fig. 34.15 *Courtesy of the CDC, Atlanta.*

to lower regions (lower lobes) in adults. After phagocytosis by alveolar macrophages, MTB organisms undergo intracellular replication. The initial inflammatory response to the MTB infection in the lung is referred to as a **primary** or **Ghon focus**. MTB organisms can thereafter spread, during this early stage, via the lymphatics to the draining lymph nodes and result in hilar or mediastinal lymphadenopathy. Alternatively, the bacilli may enter the bloodstream and spread hematogenously to other organs of the body. Disease presenting at this stage is called **primary tuberculosis** (Fig. 36.2).

However, more commonly the host develops cell-mediated immune reaction involving alveolar macrophages that phagocytize tubercle bacilli, and CD4+ T lymphocytes, which induce protection through the production of cytokines, mainly interferon-γ (IFN-γ). Coincident with the development of immunity, delayed-type hypersensitivity to *M. tuberculosis* develops. This stage is referred to as **latent TB infection** and is the basis of tuberculin skin testing. In most instances, the immune response successfully controls the tuberculosis *infection* although 3%-5% of infected subjects progress to active *disease* within 2 years, termed **progressive primary TB** (Fig. 36.2). Primary tuberculosis

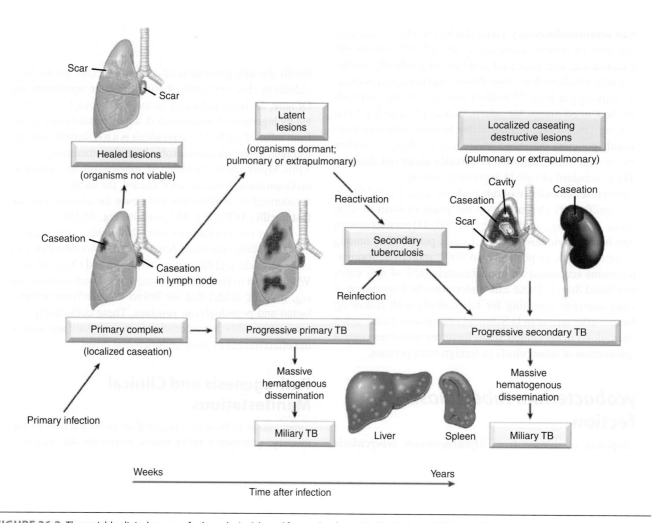

FIGURE 36.2 The variable clinical course of tuberculosis. *Adapted from a sketch provided by Professor R.K. Kumar, Department of Pathology, School of Medical Sciences, the University of New South Wales, Sydney, Australia.*

#110

Table **36.1** Risk factors for progression of tuberculosis disease

HIV infection	Underlying cancer	Silicosis	✓ Chemotherapy
Diabetes mellitus ✓	Malnutrition	Leukemia	Lymphoma
Advanced age	IV drug abuse	Post-gastrectomy	Jejunoileal bypass
Renal failure	Hemodialysis		

✓Immunosuppressive drug therapy (eg, steroids, cytotoxic drugs, TNF-α blockers)

is common among at-risk children up to 4 years of age. Furthermore, among infected individuals, the incidence is highest during late adolescence and early adulthood.

Because the healed primary infected lung foci often contain bacilli that are viable for many years, progression to subsequent *disease* can occur if the immunity wanes, which is referred to as **post-primary** or **reactivation** pulmonary tuberculosis. Overall, individuals infected with MTB have a 5%-10% risk of reactivation during their lives, particularly in the setting of several well-defined **risk factors** culminating in relative degrees of immunosuppression (Table 36.1). In this context, the risk of developing TB disease after infection depends largely on the host's innate susceptibility to the disease and level of function of cell-mediated immune responses. Reactivation disease has a predilection for the upper lobes of the lungs as well as having a propensity for cavitation (Fig. 36.3) without accompanying intrathoracic lymphadenopathy. However, the entire pathogenetic sequence represents a continuum and becomes less distinct in conditions of immune deficiency such as in HIV seropositive individuals. Importantly, the distinction between primary and postprimary tuberculosis has questionable clinical relevance, inasmuch as active tuberculosis should always be treated and pharmacological therapy remains similar.

The development of specific immunity results in activation of macrophages and their accumulation in large numbers at the primary site, leading to hallmark pathologic lesion, the **necrotizing granuloma**. Necrosis results from the tissue damaging effect of delayed-type hypersensitivity. Because the necrotic material resembles soft cheese, it is termed **caseous necrosis** (Fig. 36.4).

Extrapulmonary tuberculosis can involve lymph nodes (lymphadenitis), pleura (empyema and effusions), genitourinary tract, bones and joints (osteomyelitis), meninges (meningitis), peritoneum (peritonitis), pericardium (pericarditis), gastrointestinal tract, and disseminated disease as a result of hematogenous spread especially in immunocompromised hosts such as those with HIV coinfection.

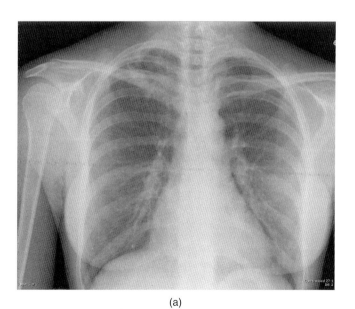
(a)

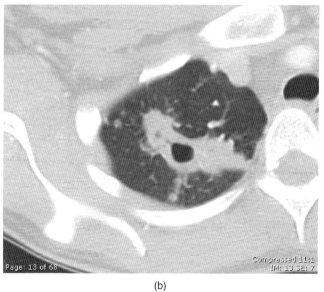
(b)

FIGURE 36.3 (a) The chest x-ray of a patient diagnosed with reactivation tuberculosis. Note the right upper lobe air-space opacities with suggestion of cavitary process. (b) CT scan of the chest (lung attenuation window) of the same patient with reactivation (post-primary) TB. Note extensive cavitation due to necrosis of the lung parenchyma and the satellite nodules. The patient (a resident of Colombia in South America) presented to the hospital with hemoptysis while visiting the United States on a business trip.

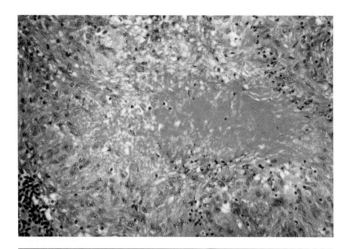

FIGURE 36.4 A photomicrograph of necrotizing granulomatous inflammation with caseation. See also Fig. 34.16. *From* granuloma.homestead.com/tb_microscopic.html.

Table **36.2** Interpretation of tuberculin skin test reactivity indicative of TB infection

5 mm induration
- High probability of infection
- Close contacts of active TB patients
- Chest radiographic evidence of old TB disease
- HIV infection
- Immunocompromised patients
- Organ transplant recipients

10 mm induration
- Medical conditions that increase the risk of progression of active TB
- Immigrants from endemic regions of TB disease
- Residents and staff of institutionalized settings

15 mm induration
- Immunocompetent subjects

▶▶**CLINICAL CORRELATION 36.1**

Tuberculosis is an important opportunistic disease among HIV-infected patients. An individual with skin test-documented latent TB infection that acquires concomitant HIV infection has over a 100-fold increased relative risk of progression to active disease, an increased annual risk if developing active TB disease approximating 8% per year, as well as an accelerated natural history of TB and mortality. The clinical and radiographic manifestations of HIV-related tuberculosis depend on the degree of immunosuppression. When the cell-mediated immunity is only partially compromised (eg, a circulating CD4+ T lymphocyte count >200 cell/µL), pulmonary tuberculosis presents as a typical pattern of upper-lobe opacities and cavitation, without significant lymphadenopathy or pleural effusion (**postprimary disease**). However, as the CD4+ T lymphocyte cell count declines in untreated or advanced HIV infection, the more common manifestation is a primary tuberculosis-like pattern of diffuse interstitial or miliary opacities, airspace opacities with little or no cavitation, and intrathoracic adenopathy. Also of note, extrapulmonary tuberculosis is common among HIV-infected patients, with the most common forms being lymphatic, disseminated, pleural, and pericardial disease, respectively.

Diagnostic Tests for Tuberculosis

A comprehensive medical history should be obtained, exploring TB exposure risks, previous TB infection or disease, and risk factors for progression in an individual with clinical symptoms of productive cough, hemoptysis, or shortness of breath along with systemic symptoms such as fever, chills, night sweats, weight loss, and fatigability. However, objective tests are essential in establishing a secure diagnosis. Culturing *M. tuberculosis*

from sputum or other respiratory specimens confirms diagnosis of pulmonary TB, and from other affected body tissues or fluids for extrapulmonary TB (Chap. 19). On an average, it takes about 2 weeks to culture and identify *M. tuberculosis* in the laboratory, even with rapid culture techniques. Even so, a preliminary diagnosis can be made when acid-fast bacilli are seen on a sputum smear or from other body tissues or fluids in the appropriate clinical setting. With respect to pulmonary TB, three sputum specimens for smear and culture are necessary if initial specimens are negative; if this is not possible because the patient is not expectorating sputum, invasive sampling of the respiratory tract is usually necessary with sputum induction or fiberoptic bronchoscopy.

Tuberculin Skin Test Reactivity

Delayed-type hypersensitivity to *M. tuberculosis* develops with the appearance of immunity and is the basis of **tuberculin skin testing** using an intradermal injection of 0.1 mL of five tuberculin units of **purified protein derivative** (**PPD**), with tests read 48-72 hours afterwards based on the size in millimeters of the resulting induration. Different cut-points with respect to the amount of induration have been established for interpretation of positive tuberculin skin test reactivity, based on risk of *M. tuberculosis* infection and progression to active disease (Table 36.2). The previously sensitized CD4+ T lymphocytes are attracted to the skin-test site and produce cytokines along with cellular proliferation. PPD skin-test positivity, though suggestive of protective immunity, does not assure protection against postprimary disease (reactivation) disease.

Treatment for Tuberculosis

The two overall goals for treatment of tuberculosis are: (1) to cure the individual patient of the disease; and (2) to interrupt transmission by rendering the patient noninfectious. It is imperative that identified or suspected patients be isolated and initiated on proper treatment. Effective isolation of hospitalized patients is achieved by negative pressure rooms with high-level air exchanges. Isolation is discontinued only after either three negative AFB sputum smears (Chap. 19) or clinical improvement on multidrug therapy for at least 2 weeks, and in cases of **multidrug resistant- (MDR-) TB** not until culture-negative. Four major drugs are considered the first-line agents for the treatment of TB: **isoniazid (INH)**, **rifampin (RIF)**, **pyrazinamide**, and **ethambutol**. These agents are recommended on the basis of their bactericidal activity against *M. tuberculosis*; in other words, their ability to rapidly reduce the number of viable organisms and render patients noninfectious. The sterilizing activity of these drugs contributes to their limiting disease relapse, as do their low rates of induction of drug resistance.

The optimum treatment regimen as supported by the results of randomized clinical trials for virtually all forms of tuberculosis in both children and adults consists of a 2-month initial or bactericidal phase of INH, RIF, pyrazinamide, and ethambutol followed by 4-month continuation or sterilization phase with INH and RIF. This regimen can also be administered intermittently by **direct observed therapy (DOT)** given several times a week, which is the standard of therapy by improving completion rates of treatment and thereby limiting development of resistant strains. Treatment of patients with tuberculosis is most successful within a comprehensive framework that addresses both clinical and social issues of relevance to the patient. After initiation of therapy, the treating clinician must monitor its effects on the patient's presenting symptoms and signs, as well as evaluate for possible adverse specific anti-tubercular drugs effects. In this regard, noteworthy are the hepatotoxicity due to INH and RIF, hepatotoxicity and goutlike symptoms of pyrazinamide, optic neuritis due to ethambutol, and peripheral neuritis secondary to B_6 (pyridoxine) deficiency related to INH. For this latter reason all patients receiving INH treatment should also receive 50 mg/d of Vitamin B_6.

In HIV-infected individuals with active TB disease, antiretroviral therapy may paradoxically worsen symptoms and signs via the **immune reconstitution syndrome**, in which fever, new pulmonary lesions, pleural effusions, and other manifestations of TB may become manifest. It is important to recognize this phenomenon in individuals who might otherwise be suspected of therapeutic failure of their TB antimicrobial regimen.

Multidrug Resistant-TB

Special mention of MDR-TB is warranted given its increased prevalence and the new challenge it brings to effective treatment and control of TB. Multidrug resistance is defined when *Mycobacteriae* demonstrate resistance to at least INH and RIF. Median prevalence is >4% worldwide; more than 80% of cases occur in HIV-infected individuals yielding a high mortality rate. In addition to prescribing prolonged courses of combination therapy, patients with MDR-TB and localized disease may benefit from surgical resection. However, complication rates are high in this group of patients.

Latent Tuberculosis Infection

Nearly one-third of the world's population is likely infected with *Mycobacterium tuberculosis*. In most persons, infection with MTB is initially contained by host defenses and the infection remains latent. This **latent tuberculosis infection (LTBI)** has the potential to develop into tuberculosis at any time, especially with reduced immunity. These individuals with active tuberculosis become sources of new infections. Thus, an important priority in countries with low incidence of disease like the United States is to identify and treat persons with LTBI. Treatment of latent infection greatly reduces the likelihood of developing active TB. The diagnosis of LTBI requires not only a positive tuberculin skin test, but also that active TB be ruled out by careful medical history, evaluation of symptoms, and radiographic examination of chest. Medical conditions that increase the risk of developing tuberculosis in the presence of LTBI are noted in Table 36.1.

> ▶▶ CLINICAL CORRELATION 36.2
>
> A 23-year-old medical student born in the United States completed a clinical rotation on medical wards several weeks previously and undergoes yearly tuberculin skin testing. She reports possible exposure to a patient with active TB, although there is uncertainty as to the final diagnosis of that patient. On tuberculin skin testing, the student has an induration of 16 mm compared to a negative reaction the previous year. She has no symptoms and a chest x-ray taken today appears normal. Should this patient receive treatment for LTBI? **Treatment of LTBI** is an important public health initiative toward the elimination of TB in the United States. The goal for treating LTBI is to identify infected patients who will benefit from treatment including the ones at increased risk of recently acquired infection or who have medical conditions that increase their risk of progression to active tuberculosis. Thus, this medical student should be offered daily INH treatment for 9 months, plus 50 mg/d of pyridoxine.

Nontuberculous Mycobacterial Infection

Environmental opportunistic mycobacteria are those that are recovered from natural and human-influenced environments and can infect and cause disease in humans, animals, and birds. The terminology for these mycobacteria is **nontuberculous mycobacteria (NTM)**, even though they cause tuberculous lesions that are referred to as "**atypical**" to distinguish them from typical *M tuberculosis*. NTM are ubiquitous in the environment, including water sources and soil. They are opportunistic pathogens in individuals with cell-mediated immunodeficiency, underlying structural bronchopulmonary disease, or localized cutaneous injury. These NTM encompass many species and have been associated with both pulmonary and extrapulmonary infections and disease. The NTM have variable patterns of susceptibility to antimicrobial agents. Therefore, isolation of the mycobacterium, identification, and susceptibility testing are essential for appropriate and effective treatment.

The epidemiology of pulmonary NTM disease can be challenging, as reporting of this disease to public health authorities is not required. Also, since the organisms are commonly isolated from environmental sources, their growth in culture may raise the question of specimen contamination. There is evidence that the frequency of NTM pulmonary disease is increasing. Unlike infection with *M. tuberculosis*, however, there is no evidence for person-to-person transmission of these environmental opportunistic NTM organisms.

Like *M. tuberculosis*, NTM organisms are **acid-fast bacilli** (**AFB**). They have been conventionally classified according to the time required for clinical specimens to show visible growth on solid media. The so-called rapid growers (within 7 days) include *M. abscessus*, *M. fortuitum*, and *M. chelonae*, while slow growers (within 2-3 weeks) include *M. avium*, *M. kansasii*, *M. ulcerans*, and *M. marinum* among others. Of particular note, *M. avium* and *M. intracellulare* are grouped together as the *M. avium* **complex** (**MAC**). These have become prevalent in HIV-infected subjects, causing not only pulmonary disease but also disseminated disease. MAC-related pulmonary disease is also encountered in individuals with **hairy cell leukemia**, patients with chronic kidney disease undergoing hemodialysis, and increasingly, in individuals with cystic fibrosis.

The **risk factors** for acquiring NTM disease are similar in many respects to those for TB (Table 36.1) since cell-mediated immunity is important in containing the disease. Impairment of immunity and pulmonary defenses as in HIV infection and cystic fibrosis confer a high risk. Preexisting lung diseases including silicosis and other pneumoconioses, bronchiectasis, COPD, and radiographic changes consistent with prior TB have been identified as important risk factors. Diabetes mellitus, alcoholism, malignancy, and smoking have all been associated with NTM.

Diagnosis of NTM Lung Disease

The greatest challenge in diagnosing NTM-related lung diseases is distinguishing between an individual with NTM-related disease versus those who are only "colonized," since NTM are often found in respiratory secretions due to the ubiquitous nature of the organism. The most recent statement by the **American Thoracic Society** (**ATS**) issued in 2007 provides the best guide to the diagnosis and treatment of pulmonary disease caused by NTM (Table 36.3). The cited clinical, radiological, and microbiological criteria are equally important, and all must be met to make a diagnosis of NTM lung disease. These criteria apply to symptomatic patients with radiographic opacities (nodular or cavitary), or an HRCT scan that shows multifocal bronchiectasis with multiple small nodules. Further, these criteria best fit with *Mycobacterium avium* complex (MAC), *M. Kansasii*, and *M. abscessus* infections.

Accordingly, the minimum evaluation of a patient suspected of NTM lung disease should include: (1) performance of a chest radiograph and, in the absence of cavitation, a chest HRCT scan; (2) three or more sputum specimens for acid-fast bacilli; and (3) exclusion of other diagnoses such as TB.

Pulmonary Disease due to NTM Infection in the Immunocompetent Host

Infection with NTM is an increasingly important cause of pulmonary disease in the immunocompetent host. In this population, pulmonary infection occurs following inhalation of aerosolized water droplets. The clinical presentation of disease in such patients is discussed here due to two important species of NTM accounting for the bulk of NTM pulmonary disease. *Mycobacterium avium* complex (**MAC**)-related pulmonary disease is more common than TB as a cause of mycobacterial disease in the United States. The typical MAC pulmonary disease presents either in the nodular/bronchiectatic form, especially as in its primary form, versus the fibrocavitary form as often is the case when it develops as a secondary complication of underlying lung disease. Notably, fibrocavitary features of MAC disease are radiographically indistinguishable from TB.

Table **36.3** Clinical, radiological, and microbiological criteria for NTM infection[a]

1. *Clinical Criteria*
   a. Pulmonary symptoms, nodular or cavitary opacities on chest radiograph, or on HRCT scan that shows multifocal bronchiectasis with multiple small nodules.
   and
   b. Appropriate exclusion of other diagnosis.
2. *Microbiologic Criteria*
   a. Positive culture results from at least two separate expectorated sputum samples.
   or
   b. Positive culture results from at least one bronchial wash or lavage.
   or
   c. Transbronchial or other lung biopsy with mycobacterial histopathologic features (granulomatous inflammation or AFB) and positive culture for NTM or one or more sputum or bronchial washings that are culture positive for NTM.

[a]ATS, Infectious Diseases Society of America, CDC "Treatment of tuberculosis." *Am J Respir Crit care med 167:603, 2003*: CDC. "Control of tuberculosis in the United States: Recommendations from the American Thoracic society, CDC and the Infectious Diseases Society of America." *MMWR 54:RR1, 2005*.

Macrolide antibiotics (eg, **clarithromycin** or **azithromycin**) are the primary drug class for treatment of MAC infection. Thus, MAC isolates from patients with a history of prolonged earlier macrolide exposure or of treatment failure should be tested for susceptibility to clarithromycin.

Hypersensitivity Pneumonitis—"Hot-Tub" Lung Disease

A well-defined manifestation of pulmonary NTM most commonly due to MAC in immunocompetent patients without pre-existing lung disease has been described in association with the use of hot tubs and spas. Thus, this form of NTM is an infectious form of hypersensitivity pneumonitis, and almost all affected patients present with diffuse, bilateral lung opacities consisting of centrilobular nodules or ground-glass opacities in conjunction with cough, dyspnea, and periodic fever. The treatment involves mandatory avoidance of the heated water source, and in some cases of severe disease, adjunctive corticosteroids to suppress the granulomatous inflammatory response.

▶▶ CLINICAL CORRELATION 36.3

Lady Windermere syndrome. There are many atypical presentations of pulmonary MAC. One of these deserves specific mention: the combination of bronchiectasis and small pulmonary nodules that is termed the Lady Windermere syndrome. This is typically associated with MAC infection in patients with no predisposing factors. In its earliest description, six cases were reported of elderly women without typical features of classic pulmonary MAC infection who were found to have isolated lingular or right middle lobe disease (Fig. 36.5). Their physicians hypothesized that habitual, voluntary cough suppression might be responsible for the clinical and radiographic features of this disease. The syndrome was named for Oscar Wilde's comedy, *Lady Windermere's Fan*, because of the fastidious nature of its main character.

M. kansasii is the most pathogenic NTM species affecting the lung. The clinical features of *M. kansasii* resemble those of TB, including upper lobe pulmonary involvement with cavitation (Fig. 36.6). Most patients have predisposing factors, but pulmonary infections without notable risk factors have been reported. Testing of *M. kansasii* isolates for susceptibility to RIF is recommended. Disseminated disease occurs primarily among patients with advanced AIDS and CD4+ T lymphocyte cell counts of <100/μL, as well as in patients with leukemia, lymphoma, or solid-organ transplant recipients.

Nontuberculous Mycobacterial Lung Diseases in Cystic Fibrosis

Cystic fibrosis (CF) is an autosomal recessive disorder resulting in defective or deficient **cystic fibrosis transmembrane conductance regulator (CFTR)** protein resulting in extremely viscous respiratory and gastrointestinal secretion (Chap. 38). CF is considered to be a risk factor for development of NTM pulmonary infection. Sputum cultures from patients with CF often reveal multiple pathogens and with

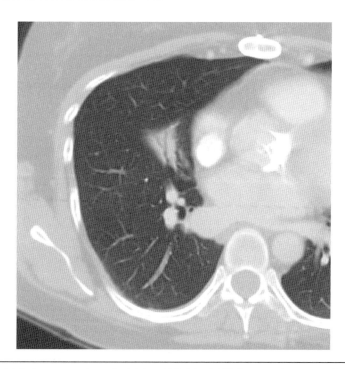

FIGURE 36.5 This patient with Lady Windermere syndrome had right middle lobe (RML) disease with sputum cultures positive for MAC. Note the bronchiectasis with adjacent consolidation and resultant air bronchogram sign. The patient underwent RML lobectomy due to failure of antimicrobial therapy.

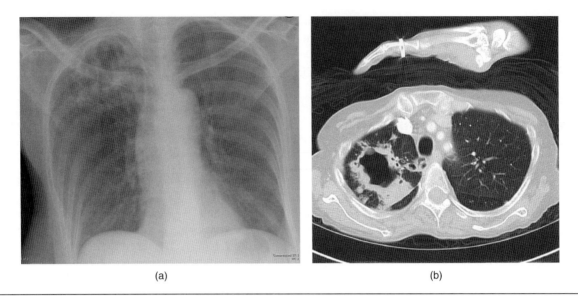

(a)   (b)

FIGURE 36.6 (a) Chest radiograph showing right upper lobe cavitary opacity in a patient with *M. kansasii*. (b) CT scan obtained in the same patient confirms the nature of the lesion, later diagnosed to be *M. kansasii* fibrocavitary lung disease. Note that it is hard to distinguish a nontuberculous mycobacterial (NTM) infection from actual TB on a radiograph or CT alone.

increased patient longevity, more NTM infections are being recognized. It is recommended that all adult patients with CF be screened for the presence of NTM in their pulmonary secretions on a yearly basis.

The most common NTM isolated from sputum of patients with CF is MAC, though *M. kansasii*, *M. abscessus*, *M. fortuitum*, and others have been isolated. The diagnosis of NTM lung disease in patients with CF is particularly challenging, as it can be hard to distinguish colonization from active disease. Persistent presence of organisms in the sputum of CF patients may indicate infection. A patient with CF who repeatedly cultures NTM and has persistent symptoms despite adequate conventional antimicrobial therapy should be evaluated for mycobacterial disease. The characteristic radiographic opacities (Fig. 36.7) include concomitant bronchiectasis and small nodules or associated consolidation, favoring a diagnosis of active infection. The treatment of NTM infection in CF in itself can be challenging given variation and alteration in drug absorption and elimination patterns, the need for longer therapy, and implications for lung transplant candidacy at most centers.

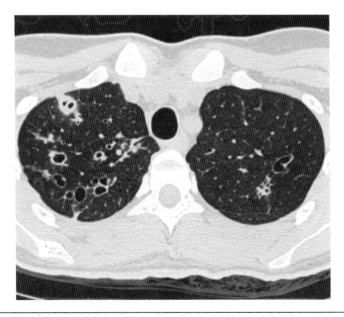

FIGURE 36.7 This patient presented with hemoptysis and grew *M. abscessus* from the bronchoscopic sampling and subsequently diagnosed with cystic fibrosis at age 26. The cystic changes are more pronounced on the right side in this patient.

Suggested Readings

1. ATS, Infectious Diseases Society of America, CDC. "Treatment of tuberculosis." *Am J Respir Crit Care Med.* 2003;167:603; CDC. "Control of tuberculosis in the United States: Recommendations from the American Thoracic Society, CDC, and the Infectious Diseases Society of America." *MMWR* 54:RR1, 2005; and ATS, CDC. "Targeted tuberculin testing and treatment of latent tuberculosis infection." *Am J Respir Crit Care Med.* 2000;161:S221. *These three summary statements served as critical guideposts in treating the resurgence in TB, both in the United States and worldwide, since the HIV epidemic of the early 1980s.*

2. Griffith DE, Aksamit T, Brown-Elliott BA, et al. for the ATS. "An Official ATS/IDSA Statement: Diagnosis, Treatment, and Prevention of Nontuberculous Mycobacterial Diseases." *Am J Respir Crit Care Med.* 2007;175:367. *This equally important policy statement has done much to guide clinical management of the many variants of NTM seen in the past 15 years.*

CASE STUDIES AND PRACTICE PROBLEMS

CASE 36.1 A medical student is participating in her first clinical rotation of Internal Medicine and is asked to conduct a preliminary evaluation on a patient by her chief resident who is busy elsewhere. The floor nurse has just taken vital signs and notices the patient is coughing repeatedly. The nurse reports in passing to the student that the patient is a recent Asian immigrant who speaks no English but family members accompanying the patient had told the nurse that the patient had been coughing up blood for the last week. What should the medical student do at this time before walking into the patient's room?

a. Send the patient for an emergent chest radiograph.

b. Obtain a sputum sample from the patient.

c. Review this patient's previous medical records.

d. Request an N-95 mask for herself and other hospital staff members.

e. Send the patient to the state TB clinic.

CASE 36.2 A 40-year-old woman who was born in India and emigrated to the United States at age 5 presents with a 10-day history of progressive shortness of breath with associated pleuritic chest discomfort, fevers, night sweats, and nonproductive cough. In the past year the patient has traveled to South Africa and India. Her current vital signs include radial pulse = 96 beats/min and respiratory f = 20 breaths/min. Decreased breath sounds are noted on the left posterior exam, as well as a dull note on percussion; a chest x-ray taken today is shown in Fig. 36.8.

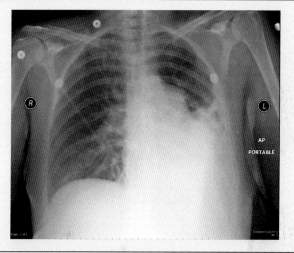

FIGURE 36.8 Chest x-ray for the 40-year-old patient in Case 36.2.

What is the most appropriate next step in evaluating or treating this patient?

a. Conduct fiberoptic bronchoscopy.

b. Perform a thoracoscopic lung biopsy.

c. Order diagnostic thoracentesis.

d. Begin isoniazid (INH) treatment for latent tuberculosis.

e. Start antibiotics for community-acquired pneumonia and order another chest x-ray in 1 week.

Solutions to Case Studies and Practice Problems

CASE 36.1 The most correct answer is d, request N-95 masks.

A physician in training should have a high index of suspicion for tuberculosis especially in patients from regions with high endemic TB activity and who present with hemoptysis. Although other differential diagnoses may explain the patient's symptoms and imaging is required (*answer a*) to further differentiate the processes, it is imperative that preventive steps be taken to minimize transmission to other individuals at risk. Obtaining a sputum sample (*answer b*) will be important to diagnose smear-positive TB, or to help establish another diagnosis, but isolating the patient until three sputum smears are negative is recommended. While reviewing previous medical records is highly desirable in any patient encounter (*answer c*), a more immediate concern is the provision of an N-95 mask to reduce disease transmissibility and risk of infection (*answer d*). Once the diagnosis is established, the patient likely will need referral to the state TB program (*answer e*), as direct observed therapy (DOT) is the standard of care and clearly has contributed to decreased incidence of treatment failure because of improved adherence to therapy.

CASE 36.2 The most correct answer is c, order thoracentesis.

The patient's radiograph demonstrates a homogenous opacity occupying one-half of the left hemithorax that is obscuring the diaphragm, signs that are most consistent with large pleural effusion. Therefore, the next step should be to perform diagnostic thoracentesis in which pleural fluid should be obtained. There is little reason to believe from the history that the patient aspirated a foreign body, and the radiograph does not demonstrate volume loss on the side of opacity, and therefore bronchoscopy is not indicated (*answer a*). The thoracoscopic lung biopsy (*answer b*) is a more invasive procedure and usually would be necessary if thoracentesis is non-diagnostic, specifically to obtain pleural and/or lung biopsies. All patients need to have diagnostic evaluation to exclude active tuberculosis prior to initiation of INH for latent tuberculosis (*answer d*). This is especially important since the monotherapy with INH to a patient with active tuberculosis can lead to the development of INH-resistant tuberculosis. Although antibiotic initiation should be prompt in patients suspected of pneumonia, that step does not preclude diagnostic evaluation of this very significant pleural effusion to exclude a complicated effusion or empyema and thus (*answer e*) is not correct.

PEDIATRIC LUNG DISEASES

Chapter 37

Congenital Anomalies of the Respiratory System

GARY M. ALBERS, MD AND ANDREW J. LECHNER, PhD

Learning Objectives

- The student will be able to describe the anatomical and/or physiological abnormalities underlying major congenital malformations of the lungs.

- The student will be able to identify useful indices of pulmonary function to assess severity of impairment based upon a history and description of the patient.

- The student will be able to tabulate the relative values of the history, physical exam, bronchoscopy, and imaging modalities to establish the likelihood of specific anomalies at different locations within the respiratory system.

Introduction to Abnormal Development of the Respiratory Tract

Accurate and timely identification of congenital anomalies often makes the difference between an infant's survival and death. Such respiratory system defects also illustrate how physicians must carefully choose among many diagnostic modalities available to most effectively and appropriately arrive at a diagnosis and treatment plan. History obtained from caregivers, and a physical exam tailored to the very young patient (Chap. 14), often only point to the need for more advanced diagnostic procedures. While direct visualization is possible with some lesions, diagnostic imaging is often essential. Each diagnostic modality carries with it a unique risk/benefit assessment. Radiography can be helpful, particularly when contrast studies are feasible (Chap. 15), but the latter creates risks of aspiration injuries. Endoscopy or bronchoscopy are often the definitive modalities in specific anatomical regions, notably in the trachea and upper airways (Chap. 18), but these may not be necessary before an operative assessment and intervention. Marked advances in computerized imaging such as CT have led to improved diagnostic accuracy of lesions found at all levels of the respiratory tract. They are most useful in delineating the scope of suspected parenchymal anomalies (Chap. 15), including those in which the traditional boundaries between the conducting and respiratory zones are blurred by the presence of unanticipated structures. Throughout this chapter, the relative values of these diagnostic tests will be emphasized for each type of anatomical deviation from the normal pattern of lung development.

Congenital Defects of the Larynx

Suspicions regarding defective laryngeal anatomy often arise during the physical exam with stridor, chest retractions, and respiratory distress readily visible. Direct visualization may reveal the lesion during attempted intubation to secure the child's airway, whereas imaging modalities often add little unless contrast is used to confirm aspiration events or a paralaryngeal mass is suspected. Use of a rigid endoscope is the preferred means of confirming laryngeal clefts (see below).

Bifid epiglottis is a rare lesion characterized by a midline cleft in the epiglottis. Patients may be asymptomatic or have feeding difficulties with aspiration. Direct visualization of this lesion is the only means of diagnosis. Specific therapy is rarely needed.

Laryngeal atresia is the most catastrophic anomaly of the airways in the newborn. This extremely rare lesion results from failed recanalization of the laryngeal orifice in utero. There is usually no specific cause identified. Depending upon the time of the developmental arrest, both the subglottic and supraglottic structures may be involved. At birth, the neonate has immediate, severe respiratory distress with sternal and costal retractions, and may exhibit extreme respiratory efforts but no detectable airflow. Emergent tracheostomy is required for survival. Diagnosis is most often made at postmortem examination, but may be recognized during attempted laryngeal intubation.

Laryngeal webs result from partial failure of recanalization of the larynx (Fig. 37.1). A web is usually a relatively thin and incomplete membrane, with the posterior aspect of the glottis open. The presentation of a laryngeal web depends upon its extent. Most patients present in the neonatal period with stridor, weak or absent cry, and respiratory distress. However, patients with a larger glottic opening may present much later, with symptoms only seen at exercise or simply with hoarseness. Diagnosis is made by laryngoscopy. Treatment varies with the extent, position, and thickness of the web.

Laryngotracheoesophageal (LTE) clefts are rare lesions in which there is direct communication between the trachea and esophagus starting at the larynx. A type 1 lesion involves only the inter-arytenoid musculature, and presents with weak

365

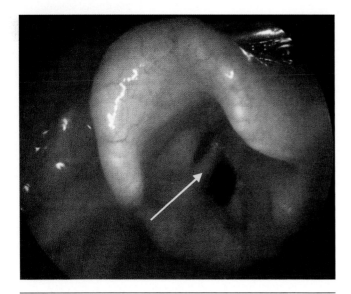

FIGURE 37.1 Photo of a laryngeal web (arrow) at the time of direct laryngoscopy.

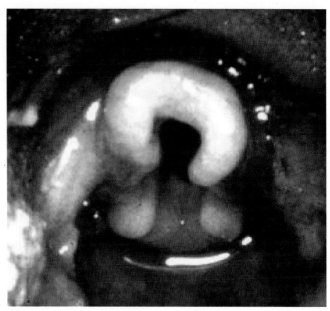

FIGURE 37.2 Laryngomalacia in a neonate, showing an omega-shaped epiglottis. *Image from Wikipedia.*

cry and stridor that may be indistinguishable from laryngomalacia (see below). If the type 1 lesion renders the larynx incompetent, the affected child may aspirate or have feeding difficulties. Type 2 lesions extend through the cricoid cartilage, and type 3 lesions extend into the trachea. The latter render the larynx incompetent, with infants presenting with a weak cry and stridor that are usually accompanied by massive aspiration. Early diagnosis of any LTE cleft is important to prevent the serious respiratory complications of aspiration. The radiological demonstration of a "high" aspiration during a barium swallow exam leads to more specific diagnostic testing. Direct laryngoscopy with the ability to manipulate the arytenoids is the primary diagnostic technique. A cleft may be missed if only a flexible endoscope is used to inspect the larynx, since the cleft may not be readily apparent without separating the arytenoids. Associated anomalies occur in about 60% of cases, usually involving the gastrointestinal tract or other levels of the respiratory tract. The presence of these abnormalities may lead to the evaluation of airway abnormalities, such as in the child with **Opitz G/BBB** syndrome (hypertelorism, prominent occiput and forehead, posteriorly rotated ears, stridor, hoarse cry, and genital anomalies) who should be suspected of having an LTE cleft until proven otherwise. Treatment is surgical and may require temporary tracheostomy. LTE clefts that extend to the carina or beyond are difficult surgical cases but have been successfully repaired when supported by **extracorporeal membrane oxygenation (ECMO)**.

Laryngomalacia (congenital laryngeal stridor) is the most common laryngeal abnormality. It is considered to be more of a functional than an anatomic abnormality of the larynx as supraglottic structures prolapse into the airway during inspiration. The epiglottis often has a characteristic omega shape (Fig. 37.2), or the arytenoids may be large, with short arytenoid-epiglottic folds but are most notable for the tendency to prolapse over the vocal folds. The most common clinical presentation is that of an otherwise healthy child in no respiratory distress making a characteristically harsh inspiratory noise that varies with activity. This noise is often high-pitched with a fluttering character. If severe, laryngomalacia may result in failure to thrive due to feeding difficulties or cyanotic episodes due to airway obstruction. The diagnosis is most often made on clinical grounds, that is, by history and exam, and in the otherwise thriving child this is often sufficient. The natural history of laryngomalacia is variable, but most children outgrow the abnormality in their second year of life. If airway obstruction is severe, surgical therapy may be necessary.

Tracheal Anomalies

As the greatest length of the trachea is intrathoracic, the most common finding on physical exam is wheezing. However, less compliant abnormalities may only become apparent when the child is exertional with crying or a bowel movement. In this situation, airflow may cease and the child becomes cyanotic. Tracheal lesions are seen well by bronchoscopy, which provides useful information about their dynamic properties during breathing. Imaging by CT or MRI with reconstruction of serial airway sections is very useful in assessing the distal extension and caliber of tracheal stenosis and/or the position of surrounding structures that may be impinging on the trachea.

Tracheal agenesis presents as immediately and catastrophically as laryngeal atresia. It is extremely rare, with fewer than 50 cases reported. One may detect the absence of a trachea below the larynx in the neck by palpation, and intubation will be impossible. The etiology of this lesion is unknown but there is a high incidence of associated severe anomalies. At present there is no effective treatment that ensures long-term survival.

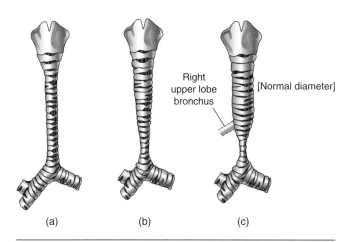

FIGURE 37.3 Various types of tracheal stenosis. (a) Generalized underdevelopment with a uniformly narrow tracheal diameter. (b) A funnel-shaped stenosis that tapers toward the carina. (c) A common variant of segmental stenosis in which an anomalous bronchus emerges above the carina. For visual reference across all three images, the upper one-third to one-half of the trachea in (c) is shown at a normal diameter.

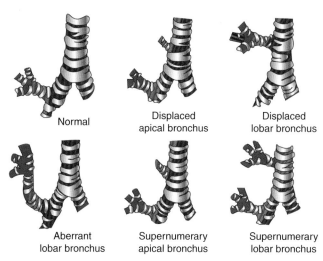

FIGURE 37.4 Observed variations in the anatomical appearance of tracheal bronchus. Those involving the right upper lobe tend to be more common.

Congenital **tracheal stenosis** is an uncommon lesion of intrinsic narrowing of the trachea (Fig. 37.3). It is most often due to the absence of the posterior membranous portion of the trachea, resulting in tracheal walls completely encircled by cartilaginous rings. Stenosis may involve short tracheal segments, or involve the entire extent of the trachea. Its etiology is unknown since there is no period in normal development when complete tracheal rings are present. Patients may present throughout the first years of life, typically with symptoms of recurrent wheezing unresponsive to bronchodilators, depending on the severity of the stenosis. The narrower the stenosis, the younger is the age (hence size) when symptoms present. Symptoms are nonspecific and require a high index of suspicion to proceed to further diagnostic evaluation. The diagnosis may be suggested by plain chest radiograph, with CT and bronchoscopy further defining the abnormality. Short segment stenosis can be successfully treated by excision, but longer stenoses are more problematic. Increasing the tracheal lumen has been attempted by inserting a variety of graft materials to act as stents, including cartilage and pericardial tissue. However, a more recently developed surgical technique called the "slide tracheoplasty" that preserves the native trachea, has become the standard surgical intervention with good success in less extensive lesions.

A **tracheal bronchus** is an abnormal bronchus that arises directly from the trachea, usually in the right upper lobe (Fig. 37.4). Such a bronchus may supply all or part of the lobe affected, or it may comprise an extra airway to the affected lobe. Tracheal bronchi are usually an incidental finding on bronchoscopy, occurring in 2%-5% of the normal population. While tracheal bronchi are generally asymptomatic, they may present with recurrent infection or atelectasis in the involved lobe. Lobectomy is only necessary in patients suffering severe recurrent infections in the affected lobe(s).

#112

Tracheomalacia is a dynamic lesion in which the tracheal lumen collapses during respiration. In contrast to stenosis, tracheomalacia is most commonly the result of misshapen or flattened tracheal rings that do not extend as far around the circumference of the trachea, giving the membranous portion of the trachea greater mobility (Fig. 37.5). Then, when intratracheal pressure (P_{AW}) is less than that of the surrounding tissues, the trachea tends to collapse. During quiet breathing, only severe tracheomalacia may be noted as a harsh, central expiratory wheeze. During forced expiration or cough, the posterior and anterior tracheal walls may touch, producing a characteristic harsh, barking sound. Tracheomalacia in the cervical trachea may result in dynamic inspiratory collapse, with stridor (Chap. 14).

Tracheomalacia is often an isolated lesion in an otherwise normal child, but is almost universally found in children with demonstrated **esophageal atresia** and those with tracheoesophageal fistula (see below), in whom esophageal distention compresses the airway. Secondary tracheomalacia usually is

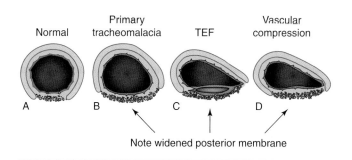

FIGURE 37.5 Various forms of tracheomalacia including both primary congenital defects and those caused by external pressure applied by the esophagus or larger blood vessels. TEF = tracheoesophageal fistula (see below).

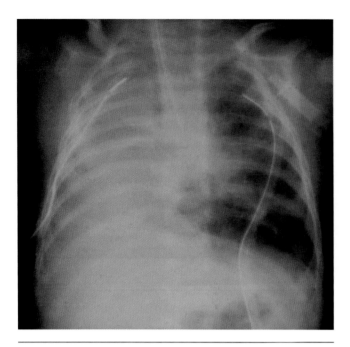

FIGURE 37.8 Chest radiograph of an infant showing congenital absence of the right lung. Note the absence of a normal cardiac shadow in the left chest field, owing to displacement of the heart by the functional, if over-inflated, left lung.

absent airways, vasculature, and lung tissue on the affected side, while aplasia refers to the presence of a rudimentary mainstem bronchus lacking vasculature and lung tissue on the affected side. Most cases present in neonates with respiratory distress, cyanosis, stridor, difficulty feeding, and an abnormal chest exam. However, some affected infants may be asymptomatic. Typically the AP chest x-ray reveals a dense homogeneous infiltrate on the affected side, a marked mediastinal shift toward it, and blurring or loss of the heart border. Pulmonary aplasia may be difficult to differentiate from massive atelectasis on such films alone, while CT imaging can more accurately confirm the presence or absence of pulmonary tissue on that side. Bronchoscopy permits evaluations for endobronchial lesions, compression of airways, and the presence of a bronchial stump, but may not be necessary if the results of the CT scan are conclusive. A barium swallow may be important to evaluate for the presence of a foregut communication that would require early surgical intervention.

There are suggestions that pulmonary agenesis has a significant association with tracheal stenosis. Bilateral pulmonary agenesis does occur, but obviously is a fatal lesion. The prognosis for unilateral pulmonary agenesis varies, having a reported mortality of 30%-50%, with most deaths occurring within the first year of life. Survival longer than 5 years is generally consistent with a normal life span. There may be a worse prognosis with right-sided agenesis, likely due to the increased incidence of cardiovascular lesions seen with anomalies on this side. Longitudinal pulmonary function testing reveals that with age, the patient's FVC will mature to 50%-70% of predicted values. Coincident development of pulmonary hypertension is limited to those patients whose associated cardiovascular anomalies increase pulmonary blood flow as by left-to-right shunts. Most patients are asymptomatic at rest, but not surprisingly they demonstrate obvious pulmonary impairment during exercise testing (Chap. 12).

A **congenital cystic adenomatoid malformation (CCAM)** is a mass of abnormally developed respiratory tissue composed mainly of terminal bronchial elements that lack distal alveolar structures. Such CCAMs are classified by one of two systems: (1) as macrocystic versus microcystic; and (2) as type 1 (several large cysts), type 2 (multiple small cysts), and type 3 (a largely homogeneous, nearly solid mass). Histologically, these CCAM types correlate with the stage of development when the abnormality arose: larger cysts begin later in gestation. Because CCAM is often associated with polyhydramnios, it may be noted by fetal ultrasound, allowing subsequent prenatal planning to optimize lung growth. Type 1 and macrocystic CCAMs present most commonly within the first several months in term infants exhibiting respiratory distress, cyanosis, and feeding difficulties. Postnatal expansion of a CCAM with air or fluid can create a surgical emergency due to compression of lung and cardiac tissue. Expansion by partial aeration of a thin-walled macrocystic lesion makes it difficult to distinguish on plain x-ray from congenital lobar emphysema, diaphragmatic hernia, or lung abscess. However, CT imaging usually reveals a CCAM's characteristic cystic appearance.

When discovered prenatally and of extensive size, CCAMs are occasionally treated by intrauterine aspiration to decrease cyst size or by fetal surgery to remove the mass (Fig. 37.9).

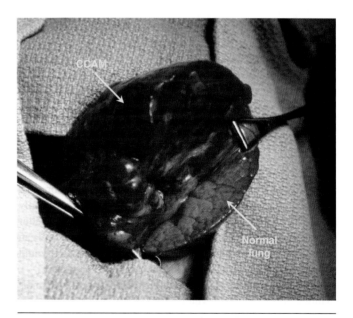

FIGURE 37.9 Surgical excision of a congenital cystic adenomatoid malformation (CCAM). Note its dense fluid-filled appearance in contrast to the healthy aerated lung that is seen below and still attached to the cystic mass.

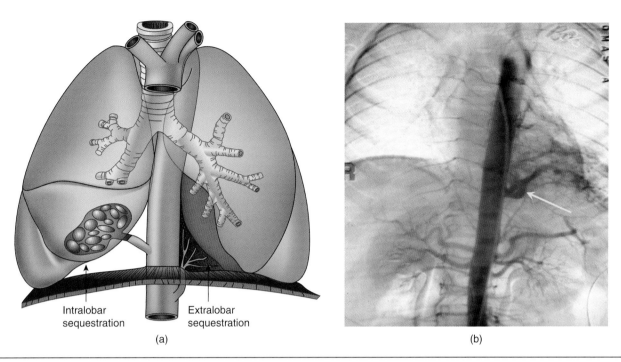

Intralobar
sequestration

Extralobar
sequestration

(a)

(b)

FIGURE 37.10   (a) Extralobar and intralobar pulmonary sequestrations. (b) Aortic angiography, showing an anomalous subdiaphragmatic arterial branch to a left-sided extralobar sequestration (arrow).

Such interventions provide space for normal lung growth to resume. In the absence of **hydrops fetalis**, monitoring CCAM over time is preferred since some resolve spontaneously. Postnatally, surgical resection of CCAM is often done because lesions may become recurrently infected, and their aeration and expansion may further compromise surrounding lung tissue. Lobectomy has become the surgical therapy of choice to avoid post-resection air leaks when smaller tissue volumes are removed, but extensive CCAMs may require pneumonectomy. Type 1 or macrocystic CCAMs generally have good surgical outcomes. Infants with microcystic or types 2 and 3 CCAM often have associated fetal hydrops, pulmonary hypoplasia, or other anomalies that significantly worsen prognosis.

Congenital lobar emphysema is an idiopathic hyperinflation of one or more lobes of the lung, excluding lesions caused by extrinsic compression of the bronchus. Most cases present in the first 6 months of life with symptoms of respiratory distress, tachypnea, or cyanotic spells. On physical exam there are decreased breath sounds on the affected side, as found in other forms of emphysema (Chap. 14). Plain chest x-rays reveal a characteristic hyperinflated lobe with decreased vascular markings. The hyperinflated lobe usually compresses surrounding lung tissue and often causes mediastinal shift. Although any lobe can be involved, the right middle and left upper lobes accounted for 74% of cases in one reported pediatric series. Chest CT imaging may be useful in differentiating difficult cases. Asymptomatic patients may be followed without intervention, while symptomatic patients undergo surgical

resection that is essentially curative. In at least one study, however, surgery offered no significant benefit to long-term pulmonary function over medical management alone.

Pulmonary sequestration describes lung tissue that has lost its communication with the central airways and receives its principal vascular supply from the systemic rather than pulmonary circulation (Fig. 37.10). A sequestered lung segment that is invested by its own pleura is termed extralobar, whereas sequestered lung tissue within the visceral pleura of otherwise normal lung is termed intralobar. A sequestered portion of lung that communicates directly with the gut is termed a **bronchopulmonary foregut malformation.** Because of their abnormal bronchial communication, many lung sequestrations are prone to recurrent infection with poor drainage that often leads to cystic degeneration and possible hemorrhage. The most common presentation is a patient evaluated for recurrent chest infections, although some sequestrations are discovered as densities on routine chest films. Extralobar sequestrations are easily removed in their own pleural investment. Intralobar sequestrations are generally treated by lobectomy or segmental resection. In either situation, careful attention must be paid to termination of the vascular supply as it arises from an abnormal location. Bronchopulmonary foregut malformations are sometimes identified by a barium esophagram that shows communication between the gut and bronchi.

Pulmonary hypoplasia refers to a small lung that has defective or incomplete development disproportionate to gestational or postnatal age (Fig. 37.11). There are often

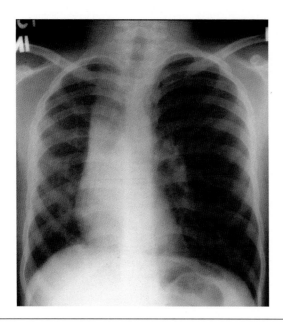

FIGURE 37.11 AP chest x-ray of a young patient with right lung hypoplasia. Note that the normally larger right lung is smaller than the left lung, due to the latter's compensatory hyperinflation that has also displaced the heart silhouette.

fewer airway generations and alveoli, thereby affecting both the conducting and respiratory zone dimensions (Chap. 4). The most common cause of pulmonary hypoplasia is decreased intrathoracic space for lung growth and expansion such as occurs with **diaphragmatic hernia** or **oligohydramnios.** However, its etiology is multifactorial. For example, infants with **Down syndrome** and some other congenital syndromes may develop fewer alveoli and show a relative degree of pulmonary hypoplasia. The diagnosis is suggested by decreased lung size on a chest film in the absence of atelectasis. While promising, the ability of prenatal ultrasound to predict development of pulmonary hypoplasia is still evolving. In the child that presents postnatally, treatment is supportive with the goal of maximizing future lung growth unless there is a space occupying lesion that could be surgically removed or mitigated such as correction of a herniation. Prenatal presentations are just now beginning to see fetal surgical interventions as a viable alternative.

Suggested Readings

1. Geiduschek JM, Inglis AF, O'Rourke PP, et al. Repair of a laryngotracheoesophageal cleft in an infant by means of extracorporeal membrane oxygenation. *Ann Otol Rhinol Laryngol.* 1993;102:827-833. *Papers such as this one illustrate well the need to combine surgical and medical managements of difficult congenital anomalies.*

2. Wood RE. Spelunking in the pediatric airways: explorations with the flexible fiberoptic bronchoscope. *Pediatr Clin North Amer.* 1984;31:785-799. *The author offers a personal and historical perspective on the first uses of bronchoscopy to diagnose and manage neonates and children.*

3. Grillo HC, Wright CD, Vlahakes GJ, et al. Management of congenital tracheal stenosis by means of slide tracheoplasty or resection and reconstruction, with long-term follow-up of growth after slide tracheoplasty. *J Thorac Cardiovasc Surg.* 2002;123:145-152. *These authors present a detailed history of surgical repair of tracheal stenosis with patient outcomes.*

4. Husain AN, Hessel RG. Neonatal pulmonary hypoplasia: an autopsy study of 25 cases. *Pediatr Pathol.* 1993;13:475-484. *These authors presented an important series of patients whose congenitally small lungs could not be restored just 20 years ago.*

CASE STUDIES AND PRACTICE PROBLEMS

CASE 37.1 A term infant shows respiratory distress 0.5 hours after delivery, cyanosis with tachypnea, marked sternal retractions, and decreased breath sounds over the left hemithorax. One examiner hears bowel sounds over the left lower lobe; a chest x-ray shows normal vascular markings, multiple cystic areas on the left, decreased aeration on the right, and right mediastinal shift. What is the most likely diagnosis in this patient?

 a. Severe neonatal bacterial pneumonia

 b. Congenital diaphragmatic hernia

 c. Congenital cystic adenomatoid malformation

 d. Extralobar sequestration

 e. Congenital lobar emphysema

CASE 37.2 A 2-year-old boy has wheezed since early in life and has not responded reliably to asthma therapy. He is described by caregivers as frequently having a congested chest and seems to choke on secretions. He is growing well but recently has developed shortness of breath while playing. A reconstructed CT scan of the boy's chest reveals the image shown at right. Which of the following best describes this patient's diagnosis?

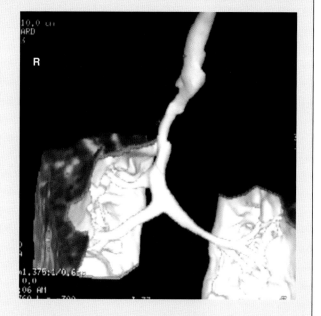

 a. Tracheal stenosis

 b. Extralobar sequestration

 c. Left lung hypoplasia

 d. Bronchogenic cyst

 e. Primary laryngomalacia

Solutions to Case Studies and Practice Problems

CASE 37.1 The most correct answer is b.

Congenital diaphragmatic hernia on the left side displaces or compresses adjacent structures. The early onset of respiratory distress, absence of normal breath sounds but clearly heard bowel sounds on the left, suggest gastric intrusion into the left hemithorax. Pneumonia (*answer a*), CCAM (*answer c*), and lobar sequestration (*answer d*) rarely present as life-threatening at birth and do not explain the bowel sounds. Left lobar emphysema (*answer e*) would be plausible in an older patient in view of the absent breath sounds and mediastinal shift, notably if actual lung hyperinflation had compressed the hilar vasculature.

CASE 37.2 The most correct answer is a.

Tracheal stenosis is evident here as a strikingly tapered airway proximal to the carina. The patient's persistent wheeze that worsens with activity and fails to respond to bronchodilators is consistent with a fixed airway obstruction such as stenosis. The CT image does not provide sufficient detail to assess lung volume (*answer c*), lung sequestration (*answer b*), or impingement on central airways by a bronchogenic cyst (*answer d*). Given the absence of stridor or other more audibly divergent breath sounds and the narrowed tracheal profile make laryngomalacia (*answer e*) much less likely a cause of this child's exertional dyspnea.

Chapter 38

Presentation and Management of Cystic Fibrosis

BLAKESLEE E. NOYES, MD AND
ANDREW J. LECHNER, PhD

Learning Objectives

- The student will be able to describe the genetics, most common gene mutations, and protein abnormalities that characterize cystic fibrosis (CF).

- The student will be able to define the competing hypotheses that have been proposed to cause the clinical manifestations of CF.

- The student will be able to outline the approaches to identify CF patients through newborn screening, and describe the typical presenting signs and symptoms of CF lung and gastrointestinal disease.

- The student will be able to identify the sequence of events that occurs in CF and the rationale for treatment interventions, including for non-pulmonary organs.

Introduction and Historical Background

Cystic fibrosis (CF) was first formally described in 1938 by the pathologist Dorothy Andersen, who recognized a number of patients with characteristic lesions of the pancreas and a clinical syndrome of failure to thrive, diarrhea, and recurrent respiratory infections. However, CF was recognized in European folklore hundreds of years earlier, and anticipated the **sweat electrolyte abnormalities** in CF. An anonymous medieval German source wrote, *"Woe is the child who tastes salty from a kiss on the brow, for he is cursed, and soon must die."* Shortly after Andersen's description, CF was recognized as an **autosomal recessive** disorder. By the mid-1950s, sweat electrolyte abnormalities were identified in CF and the technique to perform a sweat test was described that remains the gold standard to this day. Discovery of the CF gene in 1989 provided a critical advance in understanding the basic defect and pathophysiology in CF, and triggered a number of important advances in treating CF patients. As a direct result, the prognosis for patients with CF continues to improve (see below).

Cystic fibrosis is now recognized as the most common lethal genetic disease in the Caucasian population, with an estimated 30,000 patients in the United States and 27,000 in Europe. CF is most common among Caucasians of northern European descent, with a disease prevalence of ~1 in 3,000 births, and the frequency of being a carrier of a defective CF gene is estimated as 1 in 29. The disease occurs less commonly in other ethnic groups, having approximate incidences of 1 in 4,000-10,000 Latin Americans, 1 in 15,000 African Americans, and 1 in 35,000 Asian Americans.

Etiology and Genetics of Cystic Fibrosis

CF is an autosomal recessive disorder caused by mutations in the gene encoding the **cystic fibrosis transmembrane conductance regulator (CFTR)** protein. The CFTR gene is

#113

located on the long arm of chromosome 7 at position 7q31. Over 2,500 distinct CFTR mutations have been identified, but **deletion of phenylalanine at position 508 (ΔF508)** of the CFTR protein is by far the most common. Between 65% and 75% of CF patients in the United States are homozygous or compound heterozygous for a ΔF508 mutation.

The CFTR protein is expressed primarily on the apical membrane of epithelial cells, where it functions as a regulated **chloride ion (Cl^-) channel.** However, CFTR has other important regulatory roles in ion movement, notably influencing Na^+ transport and water movement across many epithelial cells. CFTR protein is expressed on epithelial cells of many organs, as well as exocrine glands and blood cells, but its most important pathophysiologic consequences involve the respiratory epithelia; the cells lining the ducts of the pancreas; and serous sweat glands. The mature CFTR protein is a 1480-amino acid polypeptide of about 170 kDa (Fig. 38.1).

The CFTR protein is comprised of two hydrophobic **membrane spanning domains (MSD)** and two cytoplasmic **nucleotide binding domains (NBD)** that hydrolyze ATP. CFTR also has a regulatory unit with several **serine residues** that are phosphorylation targets of **cyclic AMP-dependent protein kinase.** The ΔF508 mutation is located within the **NBD1**, and the mechanism by which this type of CFTR dysfunction leads to the clinical manifestations of CF is based upon competing hypotheses. Among those, the **low volume hypothesis** is more generally accepted within the CF research community. It postulates that impaired CFTR function causes

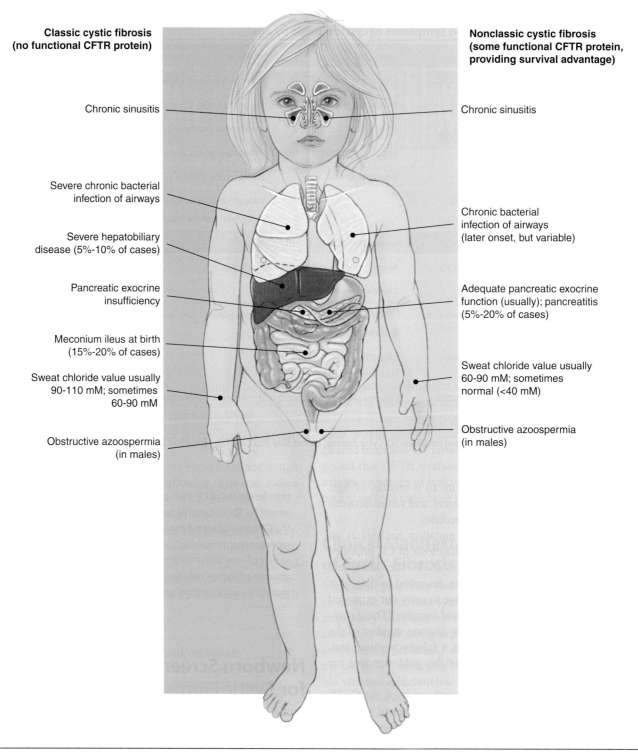

Classic cystic fibrosis
(no functional CFTR protein)

Chronic sinusitis

Severe chronic bacterial
infection of airways

Severe hepatobiliary
disease (5%-10% of cases)

Pancreatic exocrine
insufficiency

Meconium ileus at birth
(15%-20% of cases)

Sweat chloride value usually
90-110 mM; sometimes
60-90 mM

Obstructive azoospermia
(in males)

Nonclassic cystic fibrosis
(some functional CFTR protein,
providing survival advantage)

Chronic sinusitis

Chronic bacterial
infection of airways
(later onset, but variable)

Adequate pancreatic exocrine
function (usually); pancreatitis
(5%-20% of cases)

Sweat chloride value usually
60-90 mM; sometimes
normal (<40 mM)

Obstructive azoospermia
(in males)

FIGURE 38.3 Signs and symptoms of classic versus nonclassic CF, based upon the amount of functional CFTR expressed.

screening program. Patients with persistently elevated IRT values at birth and at 2 weeks (the **IRT/IRT method**) or patients who have an elevated IRT at birth and have either one or two identified CF mutations (the **IRT/DNA method**) are referred to an accredited CF center for diagnostic sweat testing. With the advent of universal newborn screening for CF, the anticipation is that very few patients will be identified through symptomatic disease. Consequently, their early evaluation and treatment at a CF Center is expected to have a substantial impact on pulmonary function results, nutritional status, and survival.

The intent of a newborn screening program for CF is to make a definitive diagnosis of CF (generally by a sweat chloride test) by 1 month of age. Several studies have shown, however, that even with early diagnosis of CF, and even when these patients are followed in a CF Center, abnormal radiographic and clinical features may be apparent in children as young as 6 months of age. This underscores the importance of CF clinicians remaining vigilant and aggressive in their approach to the infant with CF to fully realize the benefits of newborn screening.

Organ System Manifestations of Cystic Fibrosis

Organ-specific symptoms of cystic fibrosis vary substantially in terms of their timing, severity, and sequence of complications. Attempts to correlate onset and severity of respiratory symptoms (phenotype) with the genotype have been notoriously unreliable. On the other hand, gastrointestinal symptoms correlate well with certain genotypes, for example, all patients who are homozygous for ΔF508 are pancreatic insufficient. Principal organs with significant CF-related pathophysiologies are presented individually below.

Pulmonary Disease and CF-Related Respiratory Infections

The lungs of infants with CF are normal at birth, but excessive airway inflammation typically develops shortly thereafter that includes an increase in airway neutrophils and release of proinflammatory cytokines such as IL-8. In conjunction with this process, infants often become infected with a variety of pathogens, most notably *H. influenza* and *S. aureus*. Eventually, most CF patients become infected with *Pseudomonas aeruginosa*. Chronic airway infection ensues with mucus plugging, vicious cycles of inflammation and infection, and airway injury due to the eventual development of bronchiectasis (Chap. 20). Collectively, these events worsen lung function and thereby lead to chronic hypoxemia and hypercarbia.

Thus, the period of indeterminate length when a newborn CF patient is uninfected by bacterial pathogens is followed by a "window of opportunity" during which bacterial infections are transient and amenable to antibiotic eradication. For example, non-mucoid *P. aeruginosa* may be cleared by the host in conjunction with specific antibiotic therapy. Eventually, most CF patients develop chronic infections with mucoid *P. aeruginosa* that form **biofilms**. Such biofilms represent colonies of bacteria that secrete a protective coating and adhere to mucosal surfaces. Once present in the CF airway, biofilms containing mucoid *P. aeruginosa* become resistant to the effects of parenteral, oral, and nebulized antibiotics, thereby eluding both normal host defense and state-of-art antimicrobials.

As this microbial colonization evolves, airway inflammation and destruction progress with inexorable declines in lung function values characteristic of severe obstructive patterns. Recognition that early infection with non-mucoid *P. aeruginosa* is amenable to eradication has led to recommendations for improved surveillance of CF patients and aggressive treatment with nebulized antibiotics when the bacteria are first isolated.

Other pathogens linked to CF lung disease include oxacillin-resistant or **methicillin-resistant *S. aureus* (MRSA)**, *Stenotrophomonas maltophilia*, and *Burkholderia cepacia* (consisting of nine distinct genomic variants or **genomovars**). Evidence has increased that infection in CF patients with MRSA leads to worse pulmonary function values and lower survival rates. Up to 15% of CF patients have *S. maltophilia* isolated from airway cultures, but the impact of this organism on CF outcomes remains poorly defined. Of the members of the *B. cepacia* complex, ***B. cenocepacia* (genomovar III)** is associated with a particularly poor outcome. It is a leading cause of the **cepacia syndrome**, a disease process that is associated with accelerated decline in lung function, fever, bacteremia, and high mortality rates.

Pulmonary infection with **atypical *Mycobacteria*** is an increasingly important issue for CF patients. Routine surveillance of CF patients is in part responsible for greater recognition of this organism's role in serious CF exacerbations. Among the mycobacterial species, ***Mycobacterium avium* complex (MAC)** and *M. abscessus* are most commonly found in CF. The implications of obtaining a definitive diagnosis when mycobacterial disease is suspected are significant, in that the use of triple antibiotic treatment regimens directed against MAC are recommended for up to a year. Infection with *M. abscessus*, even with a variety of treatment regimens, is generally not considered eradicable except when it presents as focal disease.

In addition, CF patients can develop **allergic bronchopulmonary aspergillosis (ABPA)**, a severe response to *Aspergillus fumigatus* characterized by increased circulating [IgE], generally >1,000 IU/mL. Patients with ABPA usually show increased levels of IgG-precipitating and IgE-precipitating antibodies to *A. fumigatus*, as well as cutaneous reactivity to *Aspergillus* extracts. Such patients may have worsening respiratory symptoms that are unresponsive to standard CF therapy, notably severe wheezing, declining PFT results, increased radiographic infiltrates, and central bronchiectasis. Treatment of ABPA entails a combination of **itraconazole** and a prolonged course of systemic corticosteroids.

Gastrointestinal Disease Features of Cystic Fibrosis

As described above, up to 15% of infants with classic CF present with meconium ileus. Roughly 85%-90% of all CF patients have evidence of **exocrine pancreatic insufficiency** that develops variably in the first or second year of life. Symptoms associated with CF pancreatic dysfunction include: large, oily, foul-smelling stools; abdominal distention, discomfort, and flatulence; and increased food and fluid intake. Collectively these symptoms of CF disease in the GI tract lead to poor growth, malnutrition, failure to thrive, and deficiencies of the **fat soluble vitamins** A, D, E, and K. Regular replacement therapy with pancreatic enzymes and provision of supplemental vitamins are essential components of proper nutritional management in CF. The critical link between improved **nutritional status** and better lung function has been recognized clinically for years. Indeed it underscores the importance of a multidisciplinary approach to nutritional management that includes the dietician and gastroenterologist.

Patients with CF are at significant risk for hepatic dysfunction arising from bile duct obstruction, again secondary to serous gland secretion defects and the resulting increase in secretion viscosity. In newborns and infants, this may be noted as transient elevations of **liver transaminases** or in rare cases, as persistent elevations in **conjugated hyperbilirubinemia**. In older CF patients, liver disease may present as focal **biliary cirrhosis** with attendant risks of developing **portal hypertension, splenomegaly,** esophageal varices, multifocal gastrointestinal hemorrhage, and **thrombocytopenia**. In CF patients who have relatively well-preserved lung function, liver transplantation is an option for treating severe liver disease. **Distal intestinal obstruction syndrome** (DIOS) is another potential complication in CF patients, particularly among those who have received inadequate pancreatic enzyme replacement or who have adhered poorly to their treatment programs. Symptoms of DIOS resemble those of the CF infant born with meconium ileus, namely vomiting, abdominal pain, abdominal distention, and absent stools. Treatment approaches include therapeutic barium enemas and regular use of oral products that improve GI transit, such as **polyethylene glycol-electrolyte** solutions.

Common Endocrine Features of Cystic Fibrosis

The obstruction of pancreatic ducts with abnormal CF mucus leads to the characteristic exocrine pancreatic deficiency mentioned above, but also results in **autodigestion** of the pancreas and eventual replacement of pancreatic tissue with fat. As pancreatic islet function declines in the midst of this process, **insulin deficiency** and possibly **insulin resistance** ensue so that a presentation of diabetes develops. About 10% of CF patients develop **cystic fibrosis-related diabetes mellitus** (**CFRDM**) in their second decade of life, with prevalence rates as high as 30%-40% reported among young adults. Although ketosis is not a typical feature of CFRDM per se, the elevated blood sugars in affected CF patients lead to glucosuria and impaired growth. Importantly, CFRDM tends to develop in patients who have more severe disease. It may first come to the physician's attention when problematic hyperglycemia is observed during the early stages of treating a CF patient for a severe pulmonary exacerbation. Oral hypoglycemic agents are generally not helpful in patients with CFRDM, such that insulin injections are required to achieve euglycemia in them.

Reproductive System Defects in CF

In male infants with CF, obstruction of the **vas deferens** is the first pathological abnormality observed, pre-dating any abnormalities within the lungs. Hence, all males with **classic CF** have obstructive **azoospermia**, absence of the vas deferens, and **infertility** (Table 38.1). While females with CF are reported to have abnormal cervical mucus, they are generally fertile and can successfully deliver a normal infant if they receive appropriate perinatal nutrition and have adequate lung function at parturition.

Treatment and Monitoring of CF Pulmonary Disease

The generally recognized cascade of events arising from the abnormal CF gene and protein provides a framework for the approach to CF lung disease (Fig. 38.4). Until recently, many therapies available to CF patients were clustered toward the bottom of the cascade, while experimental approaches targeted its early phases. By example, the possibility of successful gene therapy to correct or replace defective CFTRs generated considerable enthusiasm in the CF community in the early 1990s. For the most part, this approach has not met expectations. Indeed there have been encouraging results from early phase clinical trials of protein therapies with compounds such as **VX809**, **VX770**, and **ataluren** that appear beneficial in patients with specific CFTR aberrant gene products (Clinical Correlation 38.3). Future success of such protein therapies will likely rely upon a tailored approach using compounds that target discrete CF gene mutations.

>> CLINICAL CORRELATION 38.3

The oral agent **VX770** is termed a **CFTR potentiator** since it appears to activate CFTR protein channel activity in those patients with the specific CFTR gene mutation **G551D**. The synthesized CFTR protein in patients with this amino acid substitution is expressed normally on the apices of respiratory epithelial cells, but it functions abnormally. Clinical trials with VX770 have been promising insofar as the sweat [Cl⁻] of G551D patients decreases, and their epithelial Cl⁻ transport normalizes when measured in vitro. Currently it is thought that both a **CFTR corrector** like **VX809** that moves synthesized CFTR channels to their proper apical cellular location, plus a potentiator such as VX770, will be needed in CF patients who are homozygous for ΔF508, the most common gene defect.

Nebulized **hypertonic saline** (a 7% w/v solution of sterile NaCl) has been demonstrated to improve lung function and reduce the frequency of pulmonary exacerbations. Its efficacy supports the low volume hypothesis of CF pathogenesis (Fig. 38.2), in that a hypertonic solution delivered into the airways will draw water to itself by osmosis from the underlying epithelium. This water adds to the aqueous subphase of airway secretions, irrespective of the type of CFTR protein dysfunction.

Pathogenesis of CF lung disease

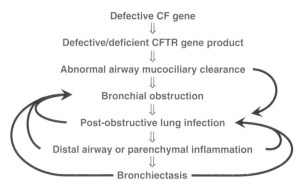

FIGURE 38.4 An overview of the pathogenesis of CF lung disease.

The increased hydration of the periciliary layer (PCL) then allows at least a partial restoration of normal ciliary motion and thus improved clearance of bacteria-laden secretions. Presuming that this is the mechanism of hypertonic saline's actions, it would seem prudent to begin such therapy early in life and perhaps even prior to the onset of pulmonary disease. Hypertonic saline may also relieve bronchial obstruction by improving sputum consolidation and cough clearance.

The sources of airway obstruction in CF are many and include retained mucus, inflammatory debris, microbes and their by-products, and host inflammatory cells recruited to foci of infection. These inflammatory cells include neutrophils that undergo apoptosis, releasing their intracellular constituents including DNA and fragments of DNA. Such DNA appears to contribute to the viscosity of abnormal airway secretions. Nebulized solutions of **recombinant human DNase** (Pulmozyme®) hydrolyze this DNA, reducing mucus viscosity, improving airway clearance, and decreasing the frequency of pulmonary exacerbations. Although more than one-half of CF patients in the United States receive such therapy, there is no consensus as to the severity of PFT findings or the appropriate age that would dictate the start of this treatment.

Airway clearance techniques that improve mucus removal and relieve bronchial obstruction have been a mainstay of CF treatment for decades. Traditionally, airway clearance took the form of **manual chest therapy** and **postural drainage** delivered by a trained caregiver. Newer techniques provide more independence to the patient, including high-frequency chest wall oscillation vests (Fig. 38.5), positive expiratory pressure devices, airway pressure oscillating devices ("flutter valves"), and autogenic drainage. Although the CF community endorses many of these techniques to enhance airway clearance, few randomized controlled studies have documented their efficacy. General recommendations espoused by the **Cystic Fibrosis Foundation** are that some form of airway clearance should be part of every CF patient's daily regimen. A regular exercise program is another important aspect of CF care, improving quality of life and maintaining lung function (Chap. 12). However, there is little evidence that exercise represents an adequate replacement for more standard airway clearance techniques.

Antimicrobial agents, whether parenteral, oral, or aerosolized, remain an integral part of CF care, particularly during an exacerbation of pulmonary symptoms. Statistics from the **CF Foundation Patient Registry** show that CF patients treated more aggressively with antibiotics have improved clinical outcomes versus patients receiving fewer antibiotics. Antibiotic choices are guided by routine surveillance cultures, ideally obtained every 3 months. The need to aggressively treat a first isolation of *P. aeruginosa* in an effort to eradicate this organism was addressed above. For patients with persistent *P. aeruginosa* infection, 28-day on/off cycles with aerosolized **tobramycin** have successfully improved lung function, reduced the log order of *P. aeruginosa* organisms isolated, and decreased the frequency of recurrent infections. The newest anti-*Pseudomonas* agent, **aztreonam lysate for inhalation** via a new nebulizer device shortens administration time to <3 minutes. There are no specific recommendations at present that incorporate this drug into standard therapeutic regimens, but it offers an alternative for patients who have developed **aminoglycoside resistance**.

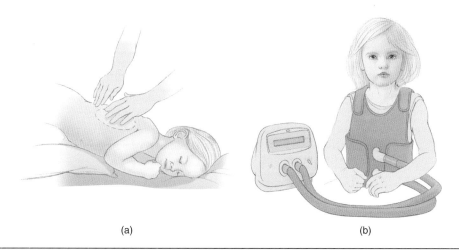

(a)   (b)

FIGURE 38.5 Shown here are the traditional CF airway clearance techniques involving manual chest therapy (a), and a more contemporary approach using an oscillating chest compressor that patients wear like a vest over their regular clothing (b).

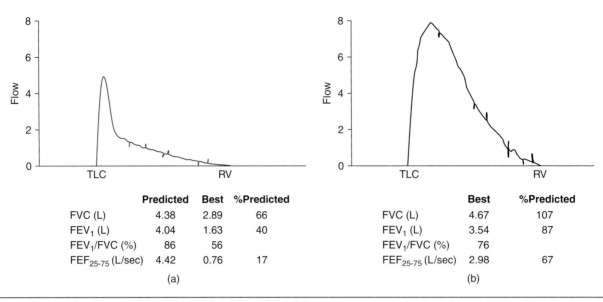

	Predicted	Best	%Predicted
FVC (L)	4.38	2.89	66
FEV$_1$ (L)	4.04	1.63	40
FEV$_1$/FVC (%)	86	56	
FEF$_{25-75}$ (L/sec)	4.42	0.76	17

(a)

	Best	%Predicted
FVC (L)	4.67	107
FEV$_1$ (L)	3.54	87
FEV$_1$/FVC (%)	76	
FEF$_{25-75}$ (L/sec)	2.98	67

(b)

FIGURE 38.6 (a) Spirometry and expiratory flow loops showing severe obstruction in a 15-year-old boy with CF who presented with increased cough and sputum production, dyspnea and new crackles on chest exam. (b) Comparable data for the same youth after completing a 2-week hospital stay that included IV antibiotics and aggressive airway clearance.

Azithromycin may address both the deleterious impact of infection and inflammation in CF, perhaps by inhibiting synthesis of proinflammatory cytokines. The drug's efficacy in CF patients >6 years of age who are infected with *P. aeruginosa* was moderate, showing improvement in FEV$_1$ and fewer respiratory exacerbations. When azithromycin was studied in patients who were not infected with *P. aeruginosa*, their minor clinical improvements were insufficient to recommend its routine use in these patients.

The intense neutrophilic inflammatory response in the lungs of CF patients has led to considerable interest in anti-inflammatory therapies. While oral steroids improve pulmonary function measures, they can cause unacceptable adverse events including cataract formation, hyperglycemia, and persistent growth retardation (noted even 2 years after completing a therapeutic course). Inhaled corticosteroids would seem an attractive alternative but their efficacy has been difficult to document, due in part to obstacles of drug delivery to intermediate and distal airways, and penetration of the thick airway mucus layer. High doses of oral **ibuprofen** have a variety of immunomodulatory effects on neutrophils, including their recruitment, adherence, and release of proinflammatory cytokines. Such high ibuprofen doses also reduced the rate of decline in FEV$_1$ among treated patients over a 4-year period versus controls, while improving their nutritional status when measured by weight gain. Despite such potential benefits, widespread concern regarding ibuprofen's potential side effects has slowed its adoption within the CF community.

Lung Transplantation for Cystic Fibrosis

For CF patients with end-stage pulmonary disease, lung transplantation is the only therapeutic option. Specific criteria for referring a patient for lung transplantation are inexact, but an

FEV$_1$ that is consistently <30% of predicted is generally used as the threshold for referral to a transplant center. In the United States about 150-200 CF patients undergo lung transplantation annually, with many more such patients dying before donor lungs are available. Although selection criteria for potential recipients vary among transplant centers, preexisting infection with certain *B. cepacia* genomovars (particularly *B. cenocepacia*) is an absolute contraindication at most centers. One-year survival after lung transplantation is 85%-90%, but longer term survival is often limited by the development of **bronchiolitis obliterans**, a manifestation of chronic allograft rejection (Chap. 26).

Monitoring CF Lung Disease

Following the course of CF lung disease utilizes clinical symptoms, radiography, PFTs, and in some cases blood gas analysis. Clinical symptoms pointing to worsening lung disease include: increased cough and/or sputum production; anorexia and/or weight loss; reduced exercise tolerance; and chest discomfort or dyspnea. Physical exam may show the presence of new crackles or wheezes, and the presence or worsening of digital clubbing. Chest radiographs or chest CT can show new findings or document progression of underlying lung disease. Pulmonary function testing (Chap. 16) represents the best objective measure of the progression of lung disease as well as the impact of new or more aggressive therapeutic regimens in CF (Fig. 38.6).

Pulmonary function tests to monitor the course of CF lung disease should include determinations of FVC, FEV$_1$, FEV$_1$/FVC, and FEF$_{25-75}$ (Chap. 16). A decrease in any of these values suggests the need for some form of intervention, ranging from a course of oral antibiotics, additional therapies, or even a hospital stay for IV antibiotics and aggressive airway clearance measures (Fig. 38.6). The results of arterial blood

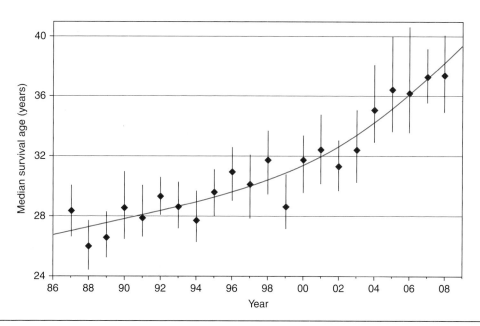

FIGURE 38.7   Median survival data among all identified CF patients in the United States from 1986-2008, as compiled by the National Cystic Fibrosis Foundation Registry.

gas analyses tend to be normal until CF lung disease becomes very severe, limiting their value for routine monitoring.

Survival in Cystic Fibrosis

New basic science knowledge about CFTR function, combined with improved understanding of the basic pathophysiology of CF and advances in translational and clinical research have led to continued increases in median survival among CF patients (Fig. 38.7). Indeed, the latest data available from the CF Foundation Patient Registry show median survival now extends well into the fourth decade. While this survival reflects a highly significant improvement from just 20 years ago, it still lags far behind survival statistics for the general US population. The clear benefits of newborn screening for CF, and continued progress in correcting the basic defects in CF, should lead to marked improvements, perhaps even normalizing survival rates within the reader's lifetime.

Suggested Readings

1. Rowe SM, Miller S, Sorscher EJ. Mechanisms of disease: cystic fibrosis. *N Engl J Med.* 2005;352:1992-2001. *Like so many of the review articles commissioned by the Massachusetts Medical Society, this one provides excellent graphics and numerous relevant references for the reader seeking more depth.*

2. O'Sullivan BP, Freedman SD. Cystic fibrosis. *Lancet.* 2009;373:1891-1904. *The excellent summary of age-related signs of cystic fibrosis found in Table 38.1 reflects the work of these authors, which we gratefully acknowledge.*

3. Mogayzel PJ, Flume PA. Update in cystic fibrosis, 2009. *Am J Respir Crit Care Med.* 2010;181:539-544. *The American Thoracic Society is another professional clinical group which can be relied upon to produce timely, authoritative, and readable reviews on all topics related to the lung.*

CASE STUDIES AND PRACTICE PROBLEMS

CASE 38.1 An 18-year-old cystic fibrosis patient is admitted to a medicine floor with marked increase in coughing, sputum production, and a recent history of fever. Auscultation reveals coarse inspiratory crackles in both bases posteriorly; $S_ao_2 = 90\%$ on room air by earlobe oximetry. A new chest radiograph shows infiltrates in the left lower lobe. The attending physician plans to start IV antibiotic therapy, but sputum cultures are not available yet. In addition to covering for infection with *Pseudomonas aeruginosa*, it will be most important to cover for possible infection by which of the following?

   a. *Klebsiella* spp.

   b. *Haemophilus influenzae*

   c. *Burkholderia cepacia*

   d. *Staphylococcus aureus*

   e. *Streptococcus pneumoniae*

CASE 38.2 A 15-year-old girl with cystic fibrosis complains of new onset nocturia and weight loss. Physical exam reveals mild digital clubbing. Her weight is at the 25th percentile for her age, but until now has always been at the 50th percentile. Her height is at the 50th percentile. Her cardiac, chest, and GI exams today are normal. What is the most likely explanation for nocturia in this patient?

   a. Urinary tract infection

   b. Congestive heart failure

   c. Increased fluid intake

   d. Impaired production of antidiuretic hormone

   e. Onset of diabetes mellitus

CASE 37.3 A 12-year-old boy with CF presents to the emergency room with vomiting and crampy abdominal pain for 24 hours. The emesis is described as bilious and he is not able to tolerate clear liquids. The patient's mother indicates that her son hasn't had a bowel movement for at least 24 hours, and states that he often skips his pancreatic enzyme supplements while at school. What is the most likely explanation for his symptoms?

   a. Viral gastroenteritis

   b. Distal intestinal obstruction syndrome

   c. Appendicitis

   d. Gallstones

   e. Pancreatitis

Solutions to Case Studies and Practice Problems

CASE 38.1 The most correct answer is d, *S. aureus*.

While virtually all of the other listed organisms can cause infections in CF patients, the possibility of this youth developing MRSA carries the greatest potential risk, particularly from nosocomial exposure while in the hospital. *Klebsiella, H. influenzae,* and *B. cepacia,* though potential pathogens in CF, are much less common than *S. aureus*.

CASE 38.2 The most correct answer is e.

The onset of CF-related DM due to endocrine pancreatic insufficiency develops in up to 10% of adolescent CF patients. Patients may present with weight loss (or fall in weight percentiles) and nocturia. A UTI in this girl (*answer a*) is certainly more likely than congestive heart failure (*answer b*) but would not present without pain or fever and would not be accompanied by weight loss.

Fluid accumulation due to excessive intake or reduced ADH levels would likely be evident in both her physical exam and chest film (*answers c* and *d*).

CASE 38.3 The most correct answer is b, distal intestinal obstruction syndrome (DIOS).

The features described are typical for this entity with vomiting, abdominal discomfort, and the cessation of normal stooling patterns. Patients with viral gastroenteritis (*answer a*) typically have a combination of vomiting and diarrhea. Some of the clinical features described may represent appendicitis (*answer c*) but patients generally have high fever and more severe abdominal discomfort. Gallstones (*answer d*) are much less likely, and patients with CF who require pancreatic enzymes do not generally develop pancreatitis (*answer e*).

Chapter 39

Neonatal Respiratory Distress Syndrome and Sudden Infant Death Syndrome

ROBERT E. FLEMING, MD, W. MICHAEL PANNETON, PhD, AND ANDREW J. LECHNER, PhD

Learning Objectives

- The student will be able to describe the clinical features of the neonatal respiratory distress syndrome (RDS) and how those features relate to the physiology of increased alveolar surface tension.

- The student will be able to provide the scientific bases of medical therapies for neonatal RDS including prenatal steroids, continuous positive airway pressure, mechanical ventilation, and exogenous surfactant.

- The student will be able to characterize the diving response and laryngeal chemoreceptor reflex as used to study the sudden infant death syndrome (SIDS).

Neonatal Respiratory Distress Syndrome (RDS)

Introduction to Neonatal RDS

Normal intrauterine lung development is comprised of stages featuring both cellular proliferation to increase total lung size, and cellular differentiation by which the airway and alveolar architectures are elaborated from primordial organ buds (Chaps. 2 and 37). By the time the fetus reaches normal term gestation (~38 weeks), there is ongoing alveolarization and normally the lungs are structurally and biochemically prepared for the transition to extrauterine function in gas exchange. Among the most profound changes in the lung at the time of birth are: (1) the replacement of fluid with gas in the airways, with consequent generation of alveolar surface tension forces that must be overcome; and (2) a fall in pulmonary vascular resistance, with consequent increase in pulmonary blood flow. These changes must occur over a relatively short time frame for normal pulmonary function. As an additional challenge, the newborn's lungs are surrounded by ribs and related thoracic structures that are considerably more compliant than in the adult, owing to their incomplete ossification. This greater thoracic compliance at birth limits the expansive traction that can be exerted by the chest wall on the lungs' visceral pleura, and thus alters the inherent equilibrium that defines FRC and the work of breathing (Chap. 6). Given these challenges, it is no surprise that respiratory failure is a major contributor to newborn morbidity and mortality.

By far, the most common cause of life-threatening respiratory disease in newborns is prematurity. Insufficient development and maturation of the type 2 surfactant-secreting epithelial cells leaves the preterm lung unprepared to overcome surface tension forces at the alveolar gas-fluid interface, as described by the law of Laplace (Chap. 5). The consequences of surfactant insufficiency in the preterm lung and the clinical treatment to overcome these consequences will be discussed in depth here. As these are elaborated below, the student should remember that surfactant dysfunction contributes to the pathogenesis of lung disease beyond the immediate postnatal period, such as ALI and ARDS (Chap. 28), emphasizing the broader implications of the concepts outlined in this chapter.

Historical Perspective: Failure of Oxygen Treatment

Before discussing the pathophysiology of RDS and the current modalities of treatment, it is useful first to consider why the historical mode of treatment, administration of oxygen, was by itself unsuccessful. Doing so will emphasize the particular consequences of diffuse alveolar collapse in the generation of intrapulmonary shunting. It will also emphasize consequences of open fetal cardiovascular channels to the generation of extrapulmonary shunting.

The hypoxemia seen in preterm newborn infants with RDS can be only partially and transiently overcome by placing the infant in high F_IO_2, such as that provided by an oxygen hood (Fig. 39.1). In more severe cases, the situation continues to worsen to a point at which even 100% O_2 cannot maintain normoxemia. The most dramatic example of the failure of O_2 therapy alone was the heroic effort to treat preterm infants in the early 1960s with hyperbaric oxygen. In order to increase O_2 delivery to the disease lungs beyond that supplied at atmospheric pressure, preterm infants with severe RDS were placed in a hyperbaric chamber. One infant treated in

385

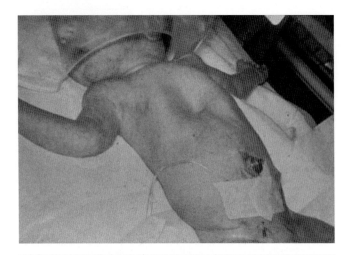

FIGURE 39.1 Archival image of an unknown premature infant who was receiving supplemental O_2 therapy (at ambient P_B) through a plastic hood positioned over the head and neck. Note the extreme sternal concavity associated with the child's inspiratory efforts.

this manner was Patrick Bouvier Kennedy, son of then President John F. Kennedy of the United States. Unfortunately, the benefits of hyperbaric oxygen were transient at best in each of the reported infants (Fig. 39.2). Ultimately all of the reported infants in which hyperbaric oxygen was used, including Patrick Kennedy, died of hypoxemia.

Understanding the Pathophysiology of RDS

Unfortunately, the unstable and deteriorating clinical course of Patrick Kennedy was all too common in an era when methods to intervene successfully in RDS had not yet been developed. In subsequent decades, a vast amount of new information

about the nature of pulmonary surfactant and the developmental biology of the type 2 cell emerged. These included an understanding of the timeline of their maturation and the normal composition of surfactant phospholipids and their associated proteins (Chaps. 5 and 10). The primary abnormality in neonatal RDS is a developmental deficiency in the production or secretion of pulmonary surfactant. The physical, laboratory, radiographic, and pathologic findings in neonatal RDS (Table 39.1) can each be understood based on the pivotal physiologic role of pulmonary surfactant (see Chaps. 5, 15, and 16). It is important to emphasize that neonatal RDS is not the same condition as the **acute lung injury** (**ALI**) and **acute respiratory distress syndrome** (**ARDS**) discussed in Chap. 28. However, abnormalities of the surfactant system can contribute to the pathogenesis of both types of RDS, and there is considerable overlap in the clinical findings.

Presentation of Neonatal RDS

Recall from Chap. 5 that lung inflation and deflation can be modeled as a bubble at the end of a straw, whose expansion and contraction are governed by forces described by the law of Laplace. From this physiological principle, several consequences follow:

1. In the absence of a substance to lower surface tension forces, smaller alveoli collapse into larger ones;
2. Positive airway pressure applied during inspiration inflates such lungs to only small volumes with high **critical opening pressures**, (**P_{CO}**); and
3. Any open lung units are prone to premature collapse toward very low lung volumes during expiration.

Much of what presents as neonatal RDS in a premature infant follows as the predictable consequences of these principles, and can initiate or synergize with defective or suboptimal performances by other organ systems, including the heart.

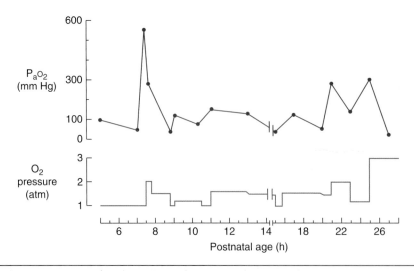

FIGURE 39.2 Response of a neonate's P_aO_2 to exposure to O_2 and to increased atmospheric pressure in a hyperbaric chamber. Note the increasingly aggressive use of multiple atmospheres of pure O_2 and the only transient responses in P_aO_2 that resulted. *Adapted from Cochran WD: A clinical trial of high oxygen pressure for the respiratory distress syndrome, N Engl J Med Feb 18;272:347-51, 1965.*

Table **39.1** Typical findings in infants with neonatal RDS

Physical	Laboratory	Radiographic	Pathologic
Tachypnea	$\downarrow P_aO_2$, and if severe, $\uparrow P_aCO_2$	$\downarrow$ Lung volume	Hyaline membranes
Grunting		"Ground glass" opacities	Atelectatic distal airways
Sternal retractions		Air bronchograms	Underinflation
Nasal flaring			

Risk Factors for Developing #116 Neonatal RDS

A number of specific factors have been identified that increase or decrease the likelihood of an infant developing RDS (Table 39.2). It is important to emphasize that a single risk factor such as prematurity is not 100% predictive, in part because it may be offset by factors like female gender, vaginal delivery, or prenatal glucocorticoids that reduce risk. These will be discussed in subsequent sections of this chapter.

As a cellular and biochemical process, surfactant synthesis is increased by glucocorticoids, thyroid hormone, and thyroid releasing hormone, but is decreased by increased levels of insulin or androgens. Surfactant secretion also is increased by β-adrenergic agonists and by endogenous catecholamines released during the physical stress of labor itself. Due to these and other variables (Table 39.2), not every preterm infant develops RDS while some infants of relatively late gestation do.

Physical Exam in Neonatal RDS

Tachypnea

Because patients with RDS move less air than normal with each inspiratory effort, that is, V_T is less, their respiratory frequency f must increase to maintain $\dot{V}_E$. This extra work of breathing may eventually fatigue neonates, at which point their P_aO_2 falls and P_aCO_2 may rise. Episodic apnea is also common in infants with RDS.

Table **39.2** Relative risk factors for neonatal RDS (#116)

Increased Risk	Decreased Risk
Prematurity	Fetal "stress":
Male gender	Maternal hypertension
Caucasian race	Placental insufficiency
Cesarean section	Prenatal corticosteroids
Maternal diabetes	
Second-born twin	
Family history of neonatal RDS	

Grunting

A patient with RDS reflexively attempts to overcome the tendency for alveoli to collapse during expiration by partially closing the glottis to create an air stent (see Chaps. 25 and 30). The increased P_{AW} generated by expiring against a partially closed glottis stabilizes alveoli. Then as the patient opens the glottis to complete expiration and begin inspiration, the increased P_{AW} is suddenly released and causes an audible grunt. Students may visit Web site http://rale.ca/grunting.htm to hear a recording of grunting.

Chest Wall Retractions

Patients with RDS must generate more negative P_{IP} to move an equivalent volume of air into lungs that are less compliant (see Fig. 5.2). A large negative P_{IP} retracts inwardly the unossified chest wall during inspiration. While sternal and thoracic **retractions** can be seen in many infants, they are particularly prominent among premature ones whose chest walls are excessively compliant (Fig. 39.1).

Nasal Flaring

The nares are prone to inward collapse during inspiration if their patency is not maintained by contraction of the alea nares muscles. The neonate with RDS attempts to minimize nasal resistance to airflow during labored inspiration by reflexively contracting these muscles and thus presents with the clinical finding of nasal flaring.

Laboratory Findings in Neonatal RDS

P_aO_2 and/or S_aO_2 fall in infants with RDS for the same reasons that adults develop hypoxemia (Chaps. 8, 9, and 28). These are summarized in Table 39.3, and as for ARDS can be categorized by their responsiveness to only an increase in F_IO_2.

The neonate unable to maintain $\dot{V}_E$ due to fatigue, or whose functional V_D/V_T increases due to parenchymal hypoplasia, accumulates CO_2 and increases P_aCO_2. By Dalton's law, P_aO_2 declines proportionally (Chaps. 1 and 9). Many babies with RDS do not hypoventilate, but their hypoxemia can arise from **diffusion block**. Such a block may be caused by delayed progression to the alveolar stage (Chap. 2), yielding abnormally thick alveolar septa at birth that impede gas exchange (Chaps. 2 and 9). Diffusion block can also occur from accumulated

Table **39.3** Principal causes of hypoxemia in neonatal RDS

Cause	Effect on $P_a co_2$	Responsive to Increased $F_I O_2$?
Hypoventilation	Increases	Yes
Diffusion block	No change	Yes
$\dot{V}_A/\dot{Q}$ mismatch	No change or decreases	Yes
R to L shunt	No change or decreases	Intrapulmonary: Not without PEEP Extrapulmonary: No

proteinaceous material (**hyaline membranes**) within airways and airspaces, representing in part sluffed epithelial cells of the parenchyma (Chap. 26).

Perhaps an even greater contribution to neonatal hypoxemia is made by $\dot{V}_A/\dot{Q}$ **mismatch**, due to the perfusion of underdeveloped, underventilated, or atelectatic alveoli (Chap. 8). Most significantly, each of these first three causes of hypoxemia can generally be treated by increasing the $F_I O_2$ and thus the $P_A O_2$ to the patient. The fourth cause of neonatal hypoxemia, that of persistent right-to-left shunting cannot be overcome by providing O_2 alone. Oxygen will not be effectively delivered to collapsed unventilated distal airways. If these distal airways remain perfused, there will be an "intrapulmonary" right to left shunt. Such a shunt cannot be overcome by increasing the concentration of inspired oxygen. The alveoli must be "recruited" into participation in gas exchange, for example, by providing distending pressures to overcome their surface tension forces, or providing surfactant to reduce their surface tension forces, to overcome this intrapulmonary shunt.

In addition to such an intrapulmonary right to left shunt, there are in newborn infants two important extrapulmonary sites where shunting can occur. These are the **foramen ovale** and the **ductus arteriosus**. A combination of factors in newborns with RDS, including hypoxemia and acidemia, can cause pulmonary vascular resistance to be elevated. If severe, shunting from right to left across fetal channels can occur. Treating this form of shunting depends upon lowering pulmonary vascular resistance.

As mentioned previously, the infant with RDS must breath rapidly to overcome a small functional V_T. If this response is insufficient, or if the infant tires, then $P_a co_2$ will increase. Thus, hypoventilation can be an additional contributor to the hypoxemia seen in infants with RDS. The resulting respiratory acidosis (Chap. 17) will tend to increase pulmonary vascular resistance and lead to increased right-to-left shunting across fetal channels. In very severe cases, the $C_a O_2$ can become very low, systemic tissues may revert to anaerobic metabolism and an additional metabolic (lactic) acidosis can occur as well. It is this combination of problems that led to the very high mortality and resistance to O_2 therapy in the patient group described earlier.

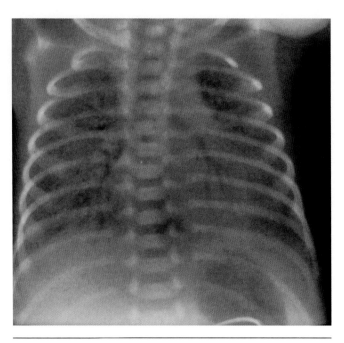

FIGURE 39.3 An AP chest x-ray of a premature infant, in which lengthy air bronchograms are visible as nearly vertical dark streaks against bilateral fields of lung parenchyma that show the characteristic "ground glass" appearance of immaturity.

Radiographic Findings in Neonatal RDS

The diffuse alveolar instability and atelectasis of neonatal RDS decreases TLC to an extent that may be apparent on the AP chest x-ray. In addition, collapsed lung is radiographically denser than normal, increasing the contrast between the parenchyma and conducting airways on film and making **air bronchograms** easily visible (Fig. 39.3; see Fig. 15.8). The contrast between open alveoli and those regions where collapse or consolidation have occurred yield a dark graininess against a lighter background on the chest film, the so-called "ground glass" appearance (compare with images in Chaps. 15, 24, and 28).

Lung Pathology in Neonatal RDS

Macroscopically, the lungs of an infant with neonatal RDS appear smaller than normal. However, they are not hypoplastic but rather underinflated. As expected, they have decreased compliance, that is, they require more gas pressure to inflate to a similar volume, and show a sharply increased P_{CO} compared to normal term lungs. Thus the neonatal RDS lung is also considered "stiff" like those of patients with ALI and ARDS (Chap. 28). The lungs of the patient with RDS can be inflated at normal pressures, however, with fluid rather than air, since surface tension forces are no longer in play and the tissue elastic recoil is normal (Chap. 5).

Microscopically the neonatal RDS lung often appears diffusely atelectatic, but with microscopic areas of overinflation that may be mistaken for emphysematous bullae (Chaps. 26 and 37). Under conventional staining with H&E, such lung sections show both fluid and proteinaceous debris that have

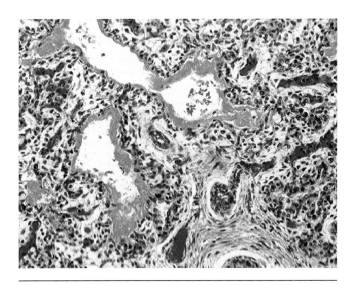

FIGURE 39.4 Diffuse alveolar damage (DAD) and numerous pink-stained hyaline membranes are seen lining the immature airways of this lung from an infant dying of neonatal RDS.

leaked into the alveoli, comprising the hyaline membranes (Fig. 39.4) of **diffuse alveolar damage (DAD)** that are also seen in the lungs of some patients dying of ARDS (Chaps. 26 and 28).

Evolution of Treatments for Neonatal RDS

Oxygen

Supplemental oxygen remains an important modality in treating infants with RDS, as many of the contributors to hypoxemia in this condition respond to oxygen. Much of the blood

that is perfusing the lungs of an infant with RDS does not encounter well-aerated alveoli for the reasons in Table 39.2. This results in a range of $\dot{V}_A/\dot{Q}$ mismatches <1.0 (Chap. 8). When $\dot{V}_A/\dot{Q}$ <1.0 but is less severe than a complete physiological shunt, increasing the P_AO_2 to such underventilated alveoli by raising the F_IO_2 or the total P_B enhances diffusion within them and thereby improves O_2 uptake. Thus O_2 remains an effective treatment for hypoxemia due to hypoventilation, diffusion block, or simple $\dot{V}_A/\dot{Q}$ mismatch (Table 39.2). Using O_2 to augment P_AO_2 also lowers pulmonary vascular resistance by attenuating any **acute hypoxic pressor response (AHPR)** due to alveolar hypoxia (see Fig. 8.3).

Correction of Right-to-Left Shunting

The various shunts that effectively allow blood to bypass the pulmonary microcirculation can occur within the lungs (an **intrapulmonary shunt**) or through the heart and associated large vessels (an **extrapulmonary shunt**) (Fig. 39.5). When such defects can only be corrected by surgical means, they are considered true anatomical shunts in the sense used earlier in this book (Chap. 9). Not unexpectedly, such extrapulmonary shunts represent a significant comorbidity in RDS.

Continuous Positive Airway Pressure

As in adults, anatomical or physiological shunt exceeding 40%-50% in a neonate is unresponsive to only increasing F_IO_2 and requires an **air stent** to recruit underinflated, never-opened, or atelectatic alveoli (Chaps. 9, 28, and 30). As in adults, this is most easily achieved with devices that produce positive airway pressure (P_{AW}) during at least the inspiratory phase and preferably throughout breathing. If intubation is unattainable or undesirable, CPAP appliances suitable for very small patients can increase P_{AW} by at least 5-8 cm H_2O

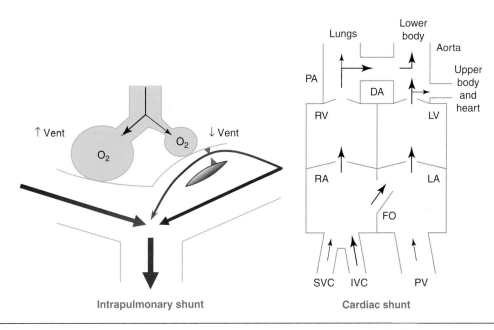

FIGURE 39.5 Diagrammatic representations of intrapulmonary and extrapulmonary shunts. See text for details.

(see Chap. 25). However, intubation permits a more comprehensive approach to mechanical ventilation of the neonate including a weight-appropriate V_T and PEEP. In this manner, an adequate $\dot{V}_E$ may be achieved while minimizing the infant's work of breathing. The staged instillation of exogenous surfactant emulsions over several inspiratory cycles is also facilitated by the availability of a previously positioned endotracheal tube (see below).

Prenatal Steroid Administration

Obstetricians quickly learned to exploit the maturational properties of glucocorticoids on cellular differentiation to accelerate fetal surfactant phospholipid synthesis in utero. Administering even 1-2 doses of **dexamethasone**, **betamethasone**, or related steroids to women at high risk for preterm delivery enhances neonatal survival and reduces RDS incidence by about 50%. Such glucocorticoids rapidly cross the placenta to increase fetal synthesis of surfactant phospholipids. Specific indications for prescribing prenatal steroids include:

1. Threatened premature labor earlier than 33-34 weeks' gestation if pulmonary maturity is unknown, that is, no L/S ratio or other assessment of surfactant system maturity has been made (Chap. 5); or
2. Documented immaturity by L/S ratio or other assessment, and delivery is not anticipated for at least 12 hours to ensure time for benefit to be realized.

Nitric Oxide

Inhaled NO gas relaxes smooth muscle in pulmonary resistance vessels, thereby reducing **pulmonary vascular resistance (PVR)** and normalizing $\dot{V}_A/\dot{Q}$ ratios in lung regions that might contribute to an increased physiological dead space (Chap. 8). Inhaled NO is not routine therapy for neonatal RDS and is only utilized in cases where the patient's PVR is excessive. Once inhaled NO dissolves in blood and tissues, it is rapidly degraded and thus has no appreciable systemic effects.

Surfactant Replacement

One of the most important accomplishments of pediatric pharmacotherapy is development and utilization of exogenous surfactants. While synthetic extracts consisting primarily of DPPC are effective, modified animal lung extracts that include surfactant proteins B and C are more successful (see Chap. 5). These preparations are instilled via an endotracheal tube, from which they rapidly disperse and spread into the peripheral airways. When performed properly, exogenous surfactant administration improves the physical, laboratory, radiographic, and pathologic findings in infants with RDS. Clinical trials also have demonstrated that exogenous surfactant therapy decreases both the morbidity and mortality of infants with RDS.

Prevention of Preterm Delivery

Because prematurity is the most important risk factor for RDS (Table 39.2), delaying preterm delivery is always attractive but not necessarily achievable. Without prenatal glucocorticoids, the incidence of RDS is ~60% in infants <30 weeks' gestation, declining to ~25% if at 30-34 weeks, and <5% among infants >34 weeks' gestation. Preventing preterm delivery is most often attempted with **tocolytic agents**, medications that block or slow intrauterine contractions.

▶▶CLINICAL CORRELATION 39.1

In 1998, one of the authors (Robert E. Fleming) treated a male patient born by uncomplicated C-section at 37 weeks' gestation and weighing 3.51 kg (7.7 lbs). The mother was in good health until premature labor began. Her previous two children were delivered by C-section; the first developed mild neonatal RDS when born at 35 weeks. Those preceding surgical deliveries (involving transverse and vertical incisions) necessitated that subsequent deliveries would also be by C-section to avoid uterine rupture during labor. This male child was tachypneic at birth and was provided "blow-by" supplemental O_2 in the delivery room before transfer to the neonatal ICU. There he exhibited grunting, nasal flaring, and sternal retractions; his AP chest film was read as showing streaky hilar infiltrates and diffuse granular infiltrates. He was placed on CPAP at an estimated $F_{IO_2} = 0.40$, but a capillary blood gas sample taken from a small skin prick showed persistent respiratory acidosis (pH = 7.20, P_{CO_2} = 67 mm Hg). An endotracheal tube was inserted and the infant placed on MV with a peak inspiratory pressure (P_{PEAK}) of 28 cm H_2O to obtain a V_T appropriate for body weight. Once stabilized, he received a single endotracheal dose of synthetic surfactant. Over the next 2 hours, dynamic lung compliance improved such that the same V_T was delivered at a $P_{PEAK} = 20$ cm H_2O. A simultaneous estimate of $S_{aO_2} = 90\%$ by cutaneous oximetry was recorded at an $F_{IO_2} = 0.25$. Aside from mild and transient hypoglycemia, the infant's hospital course was uncomplicated and he was extubated 48 hours later when a P_{PEAK} of 15 cm H_2O was required to attain a normal V_T. He was discharged the next day and has grown into a healthy adolescent. Discharge papers on mother and child read: *"Neonatal RDS due to surfactant deficiency and retained lung liquid; possible maternal gestational diabetes; infant large for gestational age with transient hypoglycemia."*

Prognosis for Infants with Neonatal RDS

For reasons only partially understood, the endogenous surfactant system generally matures sufficiently within 72 hours of birth regardless of gestational age. Thereafter, additional surfactant replacement is rarely necessary or beneficial. However, surfactant deficiency is not the only abnormality of the premature lung. Thus, very premature infants usually require mechanical ventilatory support for a much longer period of time, despite the presence of adequate surfactant in distal

#117 ✓

airways and alveoli. With currently available therapies, the success rate for treating neonatal RDS is very high. Most of the remaining morbidity and mortality in infants with RDS relates to other complications of their prematurity, rather than to surfactant deficiency per se. Even with this caveat, the long-term outcomes of the vast majority of U.S. infants born prematurely are favorable, and continue to show improvement. Survival rates are correspondingly lower in all settings where maternal malnutrition, low socioeconomic status, and limited access to prenatal and postnatal care continue to exert pronounced negative effects.

Sudden Infant Death Syndrome (SIDS)
Introduction

SIDS is defined in the United States as "the sudden death of an infant <1 year of age which remains unexplained after a thorough case investigation, including performance of a complete autopsy, examination of the death scene, and review of the clinical history." Autopsies reveal no infection or other hidden health problems. SIDS is still the leading cause of neonatal death in this country, despite the "Back to Sleep" campaign

that reduced SIDS from 1.2 deaths/1,000 live births in 1992 to 0.51 deaths/1,000 in 2006. The known and suspected risk factors for SIDS are shown in Table 39.4. ✓

Many of these risk factors were addressed in the **"Back to Sleep"** campaign begun in 1992 which recommended that infants be placed in **supine** sleeping positions, in contrast to previous recommendations of prone sleeping positions. The number of SIDS cases has fallen dramatically by over 50% in the United States since that time (Fig. 39.6). Low socioeconomic status, premature birth, maternal smoking, and other factors remain prominent, however, as well as rebreathing asphyxial gases that contain abnormally high levels of carbon dioxide. Several genetic studies also show correlations with SIDS, including heritable arrhythmias (especially **long QT syndrome**), polymorphisms in the serotonin transporter gene, and others associated with development of the autonomic nervous system. It is suspected these genetic variants may interact with other risk factors.

Hypotheses Regarding SIDS Etiology

There have been few new ideas about the etiology of SIDS, and its cause is still completely unknown. Among the many factors that may initiate it, two considered to play pivotal roles

Table **39.4** Risk factors for SIDS

Environmental factors	Putative role in pathogenesis
Prone sleeping	Rebreathing asphyxial gas, reduced heat loss; ↑ sleep consolidation; ↓ arousals
Soft sleep surfaces	Rebreathing asphyxial gas, reduced heat loss
Loose bedding	Rebreathing asphyxial gas, reduced heat loss
Overheating	Prolongation of inhibitory cardiac/respiratory reflexes; reduced gasping
Winter months	↑ Tendency for upper respiratory tract infections and overheating
Maternal factors	**Putative role in pathogenesis**
Smoking	↑ GABA receptor density; ↑ inhibitory activity; ↓ arousal responses
Bed sharing	Rebreathing asphyxial gases and reduced heat loss; overlying
Binge drinking	↑ GABA receptor density; ↑ inhibitory activity
Low socioeconomic	Unknown
Neonatal factors	**Putative role in pathogenesis**
Preterm, ↓ birth wt	Developmental delay and persistence of fetal reflex responses
Male gender	Greater decrease in serotonin receptor binding
Age 2-4 months	Persistent fetal responses before emergent adult excitatory responses
Receptor defects	↓ Excitatory cardiac and respiratory reflexes
Sleep	↓ Excitatory and enhanced inhibitory cardiac and respiratory reflexes
Genetic factors	Autonomic/cardiac instability; neurotransmitter dysfunction; ↓ excitatory responses

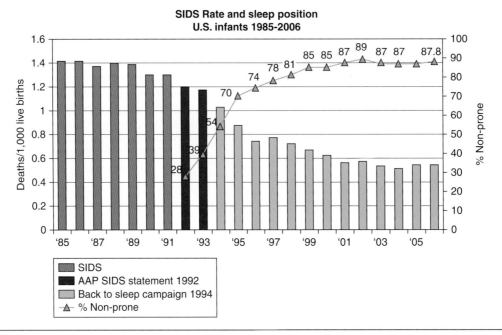

FIGURE 39.6 Survival data among American infants born from 1986 through 2006 before and after introduction of the "Back to Sleep" campaign. The line of triangles represents the paternal self-reported percent of infants routinely bedded in a non-prone position, rising from 28% in 1992 to >87% in 2006. See Suggested Readings.[1,2,3]

involve: (1) central chemoreceptors and the **arcuate nucleus**; and (2) persistent fetal cardiorespiratory reflexes, notably the **diving response** (**DR**) and the **laryngeal chemoreceptor reflex** (**LCR**). These are considered separately below.

Changes in Transmitters/Receptors of the Ventral Medulla

Clinical correlations have been made between: (1) a diminished arcuate nucleus and SIDS, as well as reduced muscarinic (acetylcholine), kainate (glutamate), and lysergic acid (serotonin) receptors in the brainstems of SIDS victims (Fig. 39.7, upper panel); and (2) increased numbers of brainstem serotonergic neurons in SIDS victims (Fig. 39.7, lower panel). However, there is no proof that any of these correlations can explain SIDS-type disruptions in an infant's cardiorespiratory behavior.

Fetal Reflexes

Leiter and Böhm (2007) have suggested that neonates experience changes in the balance between **excitatory adult reflexes** that reduce SIDS risk and **inhibitory fetal patterns** that increase the risk of SIDS. They hypothesize that in some neonates, SIDS vulnerability is heightened and prolonged. The primary responses of the fetus to ambient hypoxia are bradycardia, reduced oxygen consumption, and redistribution of blood flow to essential organs, since respirations are not occurring in utero. Both the DR and the LCR induce bradycardia and sympathetic activation, as well as apnea. Both are considered conservative reflexes since a fetus can only

respond to its environment, not change it. The rationale for these responses during hypoxic situations is that the organism must conserve its intrinsic oxygen stores for the two most essential organs, the heart and the brain.

The DR and LCR Reflexes

Stimulating the mucosa of the upper respiratory tract induces several autonomic adjustments to prevent noxious gases, liquids, or solids from entering the lungs. The DR is a collection of reflexes induced by stimulation of the nasal mucosa that naturally diving mammals utilize very efficiently. It begins with immediate apnea, an abrupt bradycardia, and selective peripheral vasoconstriction. It is present in all mammals including man, and is especially prominent in very young infants (Fig. 39.8). A key feature in relation to SIDS is that diving mammals do not breathe despite being hypercarbic and hypoxemic, and similar cardiorespiratory responses can be induced by nasal stimulation with CO_2. Juvenile rats can be trained to voluntarily submerge to traverse an underwater maze. During their entire underwater excursion, these animals show similar apnea, bradycardia, and increased systemic blood pressure reflecting abrupt peripheral vasoconstriction that reduces blood flow to most tissues (Fig. 39.9).

The LCR is induced by stimulating the mucosa around the glottis with water or acidic fluid (eg, vomitus) that causes cardiorespiratory responses similar to those initiated by the DR (Fig. 39.10). Like the DR, the LCR is most prominent in neonatal animals, is more prolonged in cases of hyperthermia, and is greater in anesthetized humans.

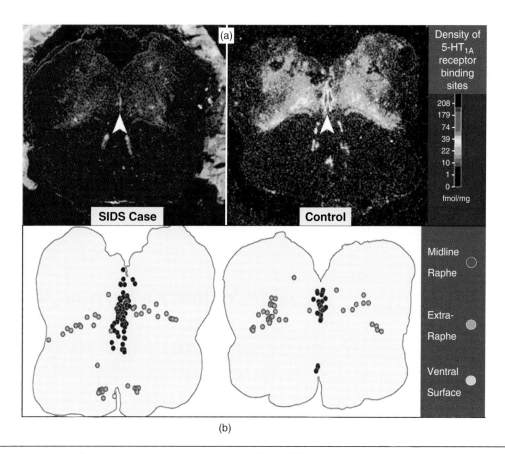

FIGURE 39.7 (a) Autoradiogram illustrating binding to 5-HT$_{1A}$ receptors in the medulla of an SIDS victim (left) and a control brain (right), with less labeling evident in the SIDS case. (b) Distribution of serotonergic neurons in the mid-medulla of an infant who died of SIDS versus their distribution in the brain of a control case, with qualitatively more neurons in the SIDS case. *From Paterson et al:* Multiple serotonergic brainstem abnormalities in sudden infant death syndrome, JAMA Nov 1;*296(17):2124-32, 2006.*

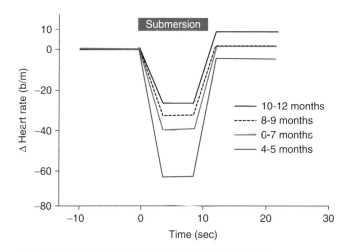

FIGURE 39.8 Mean heart rate (HR) responses during fresh water submersion diving in 21 infants who were 4-5, 6-7, 8-9, or 10-12 months of age at the time of experimentation. Note that the most profound bradycardia is seen in the youngest age group. *From Goskör et al.* Acta Pediatrica. *2002;91:307-312.*

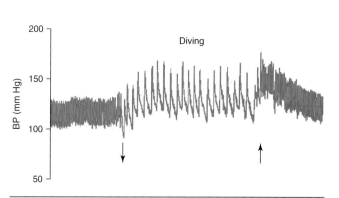

FIGURE 39.9 Note the immediate bradycardia and increase in systemic arterial pressure upon submersion (down arrow) of a Sprague-Dawley rat trained to dive underwater, and their return to normal HR after emersion (up arrow). Apnea also is induced with underwater submersion, but rats fail to breathe despite greatly altered blood gases when submersion is prolonged. *From Panneton et al.* J Appl Physiol. *2010;108:811-820.*

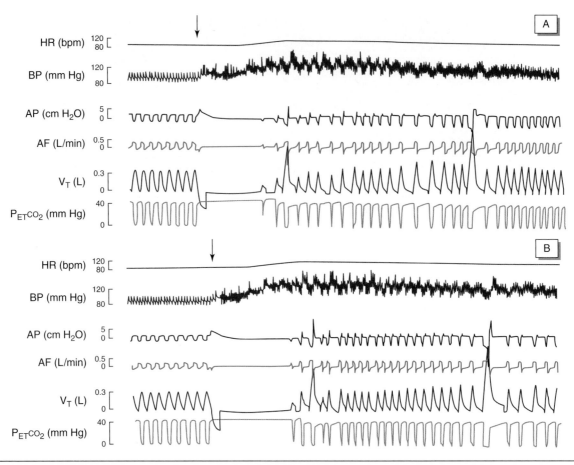

FIGURE 39.10 Respiratory responses to stimulation by distilled water (arrows) at different sites of the respiratory tract in an anesthetized human. AP = airway pressure (P_{AW}); AF = airflow. (A) Stimulation of the larynx causes apnea, cough, and increases in blood pressure and heart rate. (B) Stimulation of the trachea causes similar responses. *Modified from Nishino et al.* Cough and other reflexes on irritation of airway mucosa in man, Pulm Pharmacol Oct-Dec;9(5-6):285-292, 1996.

Suggested Readings

1. Raivio KO, Hallman N, Kouvalainen K, Valimaki I. *Respiratory Distress Syndrome*. London, UK: Harcourt Brace Jovanovich; 1984. *At the time of its publication, this book became the pivotal reference work for past and ongoing studies in neonatal RDS, foreshadowing the emergence of exogenous surfactant as the major medical breakthrough in the field.*

2. Griese M. Surfactant in health and human lung diseases: state of the art. *Eur Respir J.* 1999;13:1455-1476. *An outstanding review for students seeking additional information about neonatal RDS and its etiology.*

3. National Institute of Child Health & Human Development, National Institutes of Health. *The Back to Sleep Public Education Campaign*, available at: http://www.nichd.nih.gov/sids/. 2010. *This is the most updated and authoritative source for clinical trials related to SIDS as sponsored by the NIH and the US Centers for Disease Control and Prevention. It is an excellent resource for both physicians and patient families.*

4. Leiter JC, Böhm I. Mechanisms of pathogenesis in the sudden infant death syndrome. *Respir Physiol Neurobiol.* 2007;159:127-138. *This manuscript reviews potential reflex origins of SIDS and discusses the diving and laryngeal chemoreceptor reflexes. Both are prominent in neonates and induce an abrupt apnea; they are usually overridden by higher neural functions however as we age.*

CASE STUDIES AND PRACTICE PROBLEMS

CASE 39.1 Amniotic fluid from a 30-weeks' gestation fetus shows a lecithin/sphingomyelin ratio of 1.5 and is negative for phosphatidylglycerol. The attending obstetrician had planned to give betamethasone to the mother, but the baby delivers before the drug could be administered. The newborn infant is placed on mechanical ventilation with $F_{I_{O_2}} = 1.00$ and an AP chest x-ray is ordered. Ten minutes later, arterial blood gases show pHa = 7.26, $P_{a_{CO_2}} = 58$ mm Hg, $P_{a_{O_2}} = 65$ mm Hg, $HCO_3^- = 25$ mM. Which of the following statements about this patient is most accurate?

a. The low $P_{a_{O_2}}$ despite breathing 100% O_2 suggests the infant is anemic.

b. The infant has primary metabolic alkalosis with compensatory respiratory acidosis.

c. Placing the endotracheal tube will decrease this infant's $\dot{V}_D$ (L/min).

d. The P_{PEAK} needed to achieve a specific V_T will likely decrease after surfactant is administered.

e. Additional doses of surfactant are required for several weeks.

CASE 39.2 A 5-month-old infant is found dead one early morning in his crib. Physical exam is unremarkable except for the presence of petechial patches, and a diagnosis of SIDS is made. The pathologist speculates that this death could have been the result of a 'fetal inhibitory reflex'. Which of the following statements supports such a conclusion?

a. The diving response utilizes brain receptors shown to induce SIDS.

b. The diving response inhibits the chemoreceptive drive for respiration.

c. The laryngeal chemoreceptor reflex (LCR) stimulates inspiration in neonates.

d. Redistribution of blood flow during a diving response causes brain hypoxia.

e. Inhibitory reflexes cause tachycardia and systemic hypertension, inducing petechia.

CASE 39.3 A newborn girl appears cyanotic at 5 minutes post-delivery, and her $S_{a_{O_2}} = 68\%$ by pulse oximetry on the right foot. After 40 minutes at an ambient $F_{I_{O_2}} = 1.00$ in a nursery tent, the $S_{a_{O_2}} = 70\%$, so the oximetry monitor is moved from the infant's foot to her right hand where $S_{a_{O_2}}$ immediately reads as 97%. Capillary blood gases drawn from a right fingertip show $pH_c = 7.41$ and $P_{c_{CO_2}} = 36$ mm Hg. A new chest x-ray is unremarkable. What is the most appropriate course of action in managing this patient?

a. The $S_{a_{O_2}}$ results from the foot are erroneous and the infant is fine.

b. The infant would benefit from hyperbaric oxygen to increase O_2 delivery.

c. Mechanical ventilation is needed to correct the infant's hypoventilation.

d. The infant requires surgery to close a patent ductus arteriosus.

e. Echocardiography is needed to rule out structural heart defects and measure pulmonary pressures.

Solutions to Case Studies and Practice Problems

CASE 39.1 The most correct answer is d.

The P_{PEAK} required to sustain any given V_T will decline when surfactant dosing has been successful, due to the rapid reduction in alveolar surface tension; additional doses beyond the first or second day are usually unnecessary (*answer e*). Although $C_{a_{O_2}}$ declines in anemia, $P_{a_{O_2}}$ usually does not (*answer a*, Chap. 3). The infant has primarily respiratory acidosis (*answer b*) likely due to diffusion block, and adding only an endotracheal tube will increase V_D rather than decrease it (*answer c*).

CASE 39.2 The most correct answer is b.

The diving response (DR) inhibits chemoreceptor drive to breath, as does the LCR (*answer c*). No brain receptors have been convincingly shown to be involved in SIDS (*answer a*). Both the DR and LCR induce abrupt decreases in cardiac output and increases

in systemic blood pressure, but skin blood flow is reduced dramatically (*answer e*) while the brain is spared (*answer d*).

CASE 39.3 The most correct answer is d, surgical closure of a PDA that has remained open despite exposure to relatively high $P_{A_{O_2}}$.

Careful inspection of the right panel in Fig. 39.5 will remind students that the "venous admixture" of PDA-shunted blood from the RV joins the aortic outflow tract distal to emergence of systemic arteries to the head and upper torso. Thus, the disparate oximetry readings are both correct (*answer a*) and indeed guide the clinician to the diagnosis without requiring additional echo studies (*answer e*). True anatomical shunts like PDA are not appreciably improved by supplemental O_2 alone (*answer b*). There is no evidence from the blood gas values or oximetry data that the infant is hypoventilating (*answer c*).

Chapter 40

Lower Respiratory Tract Infections in Children

BLAKESLEE E. NOYES, MD AND
GEORGE M. MATUSCHAK, MD

#118

Introduction and Epidemiology

Respiratory infections in children, particularly **community-acquired bacterial pneumonias**, are among the most important worldwide public health issues. Pneumonia is the most common cause of death in children <5 years of age and is particularly important in developing countries. It is estimated that 4-5 million children die annually of bacterial pneumonias, with the large majority of those deaths occurring in developing countries. In the United States, about 6 in 1,000 children over the age of 9 years develop pneumonia, while the incidence in children <5 years old is more than 5 times this rate. In less affluent countries, the incidence of pneumonia is an order of greater magnitude, primarily owing to other factors including malnutrition, environmental and indoor air pollution, immunization status, crowding, and coinfection with HIV or measles. Although bacterial pneumonias are an important cause of morbidity and mortality throughout the world, nonbacterial pneumonias and viral lower respiratory tract infections (such as bronchiolitis) are more prevalent in newborns and children. Terms such as **viral pneumonia**, **atypical pneumonia**, and **interstitial pneumonia** are used to describe the clinical presentations and radiographic images of patients presenting with these latter illnesses. This chapter addresses respiratory infections—both "atypical" and bacterial—in newborns and children.

Etiology and Age-Specific Considerations

In determining the possible etiology of pneumonia in a specific child, it is useful to appreciate that certain infectious causes are more or less unique to particular age groups. The most important of these by age cohort are shown in Table 40.1. In the first month of life, most cases of pneumonia are caused by either **group B** *Streptococcus* or **gram-negative pathogens** such as *E. coli*. This chapter will not specifically review pneumonias in neonates, but instead will focus on children beyond the newborn period. Viruses as a group are the most common

causes of pneumonia in younger children. The specific viral pathogens causing such pneumonia, as well as their relative frequencies and usual severities, are depicted in Table 40.2.

Infections with bacterial pathogens become more prevalent in school-aged children and adolescents (though bacterial infections can occur at any age). Organisms such as *C. pneumoniae* and *M. pneumoniae* occur more frequently in adolescents and, to a lesser extent, among children in their elementary school years. It is worth emphasizing that the most common bacterial pathogen causing pneumonia in all children is *Streptococcus pneumoniae*. This is true despite universal administration of the pneumococcal conjugate vaccine which protects against seven serotypes. There is considerable evidence, however, that a number of serotypes not contained in the 7-valent vaccine can cause pneumococcal disease in children. It is unclear at this time as to the impact of the newest pneumococcal conjugate vaccine, which protects against 13 serotypes, on the incidence of bacterial pneumonia due to *S. pneumoniae*.

▶▶ CLINICAL CORRELATION 40.1

Routine immunization with the 7-valent **pneumococcal conjugate vaccine** began in the United States and other countries in 2000. After its widespread use, invasive pneumococcal disease fell by 75% in children under 5 years of age. However, disease caused by serotypes not in the 7-valent vaccine has increased, particularly for serotype 19A, partially offsetting the reduction of invasive disease caused by one of the seven serotypes. The newly licensed 13-valent vaccine contains the same seven serotypes in the

Table **40.1** Lower respiratory tract pathogens in relation to age group[a]

Age Cohort	Pathogens in Order of Frequency Encountered
Neonates (<1 month)	Group B *Streptococci*; *E. coli*; other gram-negative bacteria; *S. pneumoniae*; *Haemophilus influenzae* (type B and nontypable).
1-3 months: febrile	Respiratory syncytial virus (RSV); other viruses (parainfluenza, influenza, adenovirus); *S. pneumoniae*; *H. influenza* (type B and nontypeable).
1-3 months: afebrile	*Chlamydia trachomatis, Mycoplasma hominis, Ureaplasma urealyticum,* cytomegalovirus (CMV).
3-12 months	RSV; other viruses (parainfluenza, influenza, adenovirus); *S. pneumoniae*; *H. influenza* (type B and nontypeable); *C. trachomatis*; *Mycoplasma pneumonia*; Group A *Streptococcus*.
2-5 years	Respiratory viruses (parainfluenza, influenza, adenovirus); *S. pneumonia*; *H. influenza* (type B and nontypeable); *M. pneumonia*; *Chlamydia pneumoniae*; *Staphylococcus aureus*; group A *Streptococcus*.
5-18 years	*M. pneumonia*; *S. pneumoniae*; *C. pneumonia*; *H. influenzae* (type B and nontypeable); *influenza* viruses; adenoviruses; other respiratory viruses.

[a]*Data from Nelson.* Textbook of Pediatrics, *18th ed.*

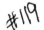

original vaccine and adds an additional 6, including 19A. The CDC found that for 2007, roughly two-thirds of invasive pneumococcal disease cases were caused by serotypes covered in the 13-valent vaccine, raising hope that further reductions in incidence of disease will take place once this vaccine is in general use.

Pathogenesis

The lower respiratory tract is generally sterile as a result of an abundant set of pulmonary host defense mechanisms including mucociliary transport, cough reflexes, components of the complement system, immunoglobulins (particularly secretory IgA), and alveolar macrophages (Chap. 10). Most viral pathogens that cause pneumonia first inoculate and proliferate in the upper respiratory tract. In a subset of patients, viral infection spreads directly to involve more distal portions of the respiratory tract, leading to illnesses such as **bronchiolitis** and **pneumonia**. In the course of the illness, the infected respiratory epithelial cells lose their cilia and are sloughed into the respiratory passages resulting in stasis of mucus and accumulation of cellular debris. An inflammatory response at the sites of tissue damage results in mononuclear cell infiltration, and

Table **40.2** Most common viral and atypical pathogens by age group

Age Cohort	Pathogen	Relative Frequency[a]	Severity of Illness[b]
0-3 months	*C. trachomatis*	++++	+/++
	CMV, RSV	+++	++/+++
	Influenza, parainfluenza	++	++
	Herpes simplex virus (HSV)	++	+++
	Adenoviruses, *Pneumocystis jiroveci*	+	++/+++
4 months-5 years	RSV	++++	++
	Influenza, parainfluenza	+++	++
	Adenoviruses, *P. jiroveci*	++	++/+++
	CMV, HSV	+	++/+++
	M. pneumoniae, C. pneumoniae	+	+/++
6 years-adolescence	*M. pneumoniae*	++++	+/++
	Influenza, *C. pneumoniae*	+++	+/++
	Parainfluenza, adenoviruses	++	++/+++
	CMV, HSV, *P. jiroveci*	+	++/+++

[a]Graded from rare (+) to most common (++++).

[b]Graded from mild (+) to severe (+++) disease.

causes swelling of the submucosa and interstitial structures that further contributes to narrowing of the airways. These pathologic changes are particularly problematic in younger children whose airways are already of a small caliber. Various degrees of obstruction of the airways may lead to areas of **atelectasis**, **interstitial edema**, and **hyperinflation**. The resulting imbalance in $\dot{V}_A/\dot{Q}$ further contributes to underlying alveolar hypoxia. A direct consequence of these multiple airway abnormalities is an enhanced risk of **superinfection** with bacterial pathogens.

The pathogenesis of bacterial infection in the lungs often varies according to the etiological agent. For example, *S. pneumoniae* produces local airway edema allowing proliferation and spread of the organism into adjacent areas of the pulmonary parenchyma. This leads to the typical lobar involvement observed in **pneumococcal pneumonia**. On the other hand, *M. pneumoniae* organisms adhere to the ciliated epithelium and paralyze ciliary function, leading to an intense inflammatory response and cellular necrosis. Much like viral respiratory infections, *Mycoplasma* infection spreads along the bronchial tree. *Staphylococcus aureus* pneumonia is often a unilateral process that is characterized by areas of bronchopneumonia, hemorrhagic necrosis, **pneumatocele** formation, and complicated pleural effusions.

Clinical Manifestations

In children with either viral or bacterial pneumonia, nonspecific upper respiratory tract findings such as rhinitis or cough may be initial symptoms. **Tachypnea** is the most common feature of pneumonia at all ages; this finding along with cough, fever, respiratory distress, and an abnormal chest exam (crackles or wheezes on auscultation) are often present in children with pneumonia. In infants, severe viral or bacterial infections may be accompanied by cyanosis and signs of impending respiratory failure. In older children and adolescents with bacterial pneumonia, symptoms may include shaking chills, high fever, cough, chest pain, and **splinting** (defined here as reduced inspiratory effort due to pleuritic pain). Some children with bacterial pneumonia may present only with fever and chest or abdominal pain, but with cough either absent or a minor feature. Fever is usually present in children with viral pneumonias, although it is often lower than in children with bacterial pneumonia. In reality, there are no sensitive clinical, radiographic, or laboratory findings that reliably distinguish between viral and bacterial pneumonias. In general, x-rays in viral pneumonia show **bilateral interstitial infiltrates**, **hyperinflation**, and **peribronchial thickening** (Fig. 40.1). In contrast, evidence of **lobar consolidation** is typical of bacterial pneumonias such as those caused by *S. pneumoniae* (Fig. 40.2). The peripheral blood leukocyte count in viral pneumonia may be normal, or slightly elevated with a predominance of lymphocytes, while the leukocyte count in bacterial pneumonia tends to be higher with a larger proportion of neutrophils and band forms. Notably, the presence of lobar disease, a large pleural effusion, and high fever are generally and collectively indicative of a bacterial etiology (Fig. 40.3).

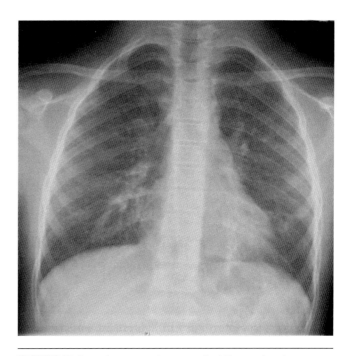

FIGURE 40.1 PA chest x-ray of a 14-month-old boy with tachypnea, cough, and wheeze. His nasopharyngeal culture was positive for respiratory syncytial virus. This film is notable for hyperinflation and central interstitial infiltrates typical of a viral process.

Diagnosis

The chest x-ray confirms the clinical suspicion of pneumonia based on symptoms reported, while demonstrating potential complications such as the presence of a pleural effusion.

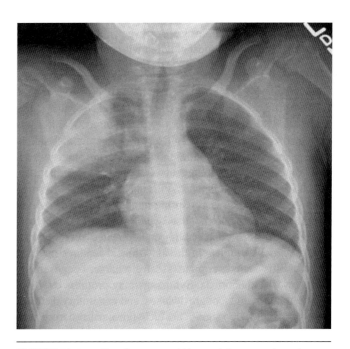

FIGURE 40.2 PA film of a 10-year-old boy with fever, cough, and chest pain. His blood culture was positive for *S. pneumoniae*. This x-ray demonstrates lobar pneumonia in the right upper lobe.

Clinical manifestations of pneumococcal disease are protean, with most children presenting with spiking fevers, cough, an elevated leukocyte count, and lobar or segmental consolidation on chest radiographs. Notably, up to one-fourth of children may have no signs or symptoms attributable to respiratory tract disease and instead present with fever, abdominal pain, or diarrhea. Further, many different radiographic patterns have been described in pneumococcal pneumonia, above and beyond the typical lobar abnormalities (Fig. 40.2). Complications arising from pneumococcal pneumonia are not uncommon in hospitalized children and include **parapneumonic effusions, empyema, abscess formation,** and **necrotizing pneumonia.** Although antibiotic-resistant isolates are not predictive of these morbidities, patients with complicated pneumonias tend to be older, are more likely to be Caucasian, and more likely to present with chest pain. Provided that empiric antibiotic choices are correct, most patients will improve within 2-4 days. Ongoing fever, chills, chest or abdominal pain, or the lack of an improvement in the overall clinical picture should raise concerns for one of the above complications.

Pleural effusions accompanying pneumococcal chest infections are the result of a complicated pathophysiologic process (Chap. 29). Parenchymal lung injury causes an inflammatory response of the pleural surfaces and a subsequent increase in regional capillary permeability. This pleural inflammation also reduces the dynamic process of pleural fluid reabsorption by the parietal pleura. When this is combined with the change in capillary permeability, considerable amounts of fluid can accumulate. Initially, pleural effusions are sterile, free flowing, and contain fluid with few leukocytes. This **exudative phase** (or stage 1) may last for 3-5 days before giving way to the **fibrinopurulent phase** where an increase in leukocytes and a positive Gram stain indicative of infected fluid are observed (Chap. 19). With the development of pus in the pleural space, fibrin deposition between the visceral and parietal pleura ensues. The infected fluid accordingly becomes loculated, fibrin and cellular debris accumulate and more fluid becomes apparent as lymphatic channels become obstructed. The **organizing stage** (stage 3) is characterized by infiltration of fibroblasts, thickening of the pleural membranes and "trapped" lobes (Chap. 26).

In the initial stages of a pleural effusion, fluid removal is amenable to simple needle **thoracentesis** or via chest tube placement. This approach may be both diagnostic and therapeutic (Chap. 19). In the later stages, these approaches may not be successful as the loculated, purulent fluid may be difficult to drain. **Video-assisted thoracoscopic surgery (VATS)** to evacuate pleural fluid and perform **decortications** with debridement of thickened pleural membranes is a surgical option. On the other hand, some clinicians favor an approach of chest tube placement in conjunction with a **fibrinolytic** agent such as **tissue plasminogen activator** instilled into the chest tube (Chap. 27). Less frequently, continuing medical therapy with IV antibiotics alone to manage pneumonias with large effusions is an option. Though *S. pneumoniae* is the most common cause of pneumonias with effusions, other organisms such as **Group A** *Streptococcus, S. aureus, H. influenzae, Pseudomonas*

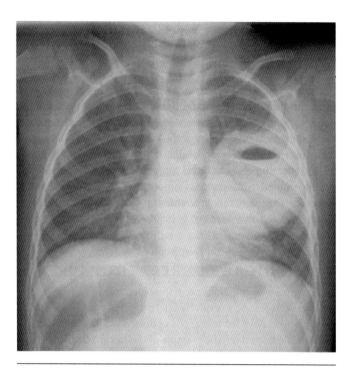

FIGURE 40.4 A PA x-ray of a previously healthy 7-year-old girl with cough, fever, and chest pain. A cavity with an air-fluid level is present in the left lung, indicative of a pulmonary abscess. A culture from a needle aspiration of this cavity was positive for *S. pneumoniae.*

aeruginosa, and *Mycoplasma* spp. can also cause complicated parapneumonic effusions.

The development of a **pulmonary abscess** is another complication of bacterial pneumonias, including those caused by *S. pneumoniae.* A lung abscess is a thick-walled cavity containing pus, leukocytes, and cellular debris. In some circumstances, it is the result of an aspiration event, especially in children with neurodevelopmental deficits. The clinical presentation of a pulmonary abscess mirrors that of children with typical bacterial pneumonias, with fever and cough being the prominent features. The course of illness may be subacute with a slower evolution of signs and symptoms. The chest radiograph shows a typical appearance of a fluid-filled cavity with an air-fluid level (Fig. 40.4). Chest ultrasound or CT scan may be an adjunct to diagnosis and guide possible drainage procedures. Most clinicians recommend IV antibiotics for up to 2 weeks with an additional 2-4 weeks of oral therapy. Newer information suggests that draining abscess fluid or placing a pigtail catheter in the cavity in conjunction with IV antibiotic therapy may shorten the hospital stay.

Other Bacterial Pathogens

H. influenzae **type B** was a frequent cause of significant bacterial disease among children in the past. Invasive diseases caused by *H. influenzae* type B include sepsis, meningitis, epiglottitis, cellulitis, and pneumonia. An effective vaccine to prevent disease caused by this organism became available in the late 1980s and resulted in a dramatic decrease in the incidence of these illnesses. Although *H. influenzae* type B is no longer a significant cause of bacterial pneumonia in affluent countries, the worldwide morbidity and mortality from this organism remains an important problem. Nearly 90% of children who develop infections with this pathogen are <5 years of age, and the majority of these are <2 years old. Pneumonias due to *H. influenzae* cannot be differentiated by clinical criteria from pneumonias caused by other bacteria. Radiographic findings vary, with pleural effusion a common finding. Because of the risk of systemic complications (bacteremia, meningitis) in children <12 months of age in whom *H. influenzae* is considered a likely pathogen, IV antibiotics should be administered. Older children who are at lower risk of developing these complications may be treated with oral therapy.

While not very common, the community-acquired pneumonia caused by **Group A *Streptococcus* (*S. pyogenes*)** is often associated with a particularly protracted and difficult course in some children. Group A *Streptococcus* causes a variety of infections involving the upper respiratory tract and skin, but when it involves the lower respiratory tract, a diffuse infection with interstitial pneumonia may occur. In its severe form, necrosis of the airway mucosa and lung parenchyma takes place accompanied by hemorrhage, exudates, edema, and pleural involvement (Chap. 34). Previous infection with influenza virus, measles, or *Varicella* may place the patient at particular risk of developing severe complications of Group A Streptococcal disease.

In most cases of community-acquired pneumonia caused by ***Staphylococcus aureus***, infection is either by direct inoculation of the organism into the respiratory tree or, less commonly, following bacteremic illness. Exceptions are those patients with indwelling catheters or a recent history of intravenous drug use, where the bacteremic route more commonly causes pneumonia (Chap. 28). Since most clinical protocols for treatment of community-acquired pneumonias do not include therapy directed against *S. aureus*, the clinical picture may be one of ongoing fever, cough, chills, and supplemental oxygen requirement. A subacute or acute deterioration

in clinical status may be observed if this organism is not suspected. Radiographically, unilateral lung involvement is typical with confluent bronchopneumonia and alveolar infiltrates (Chap. 15). As the illness evolves, these areas may coalesce and cavitate, leading to the formation of **pneumatoceles**. In a large proportion of patients whose pneumonia is caused by *S. aureus*, complicated parapneumonic effusions and empyema develop. More severely in some patients, a pyopneumothorax may occur characterized by both pus and air in the pleural space. With the increasing prevalence of **methicillin-resistant *S. aureus* (MRSA)** in the United States and elsewhere, antibiotic therapy may need to be adjusted to account for this organism, depending on local microbiologic surveillance data.

Antimicrobial Treatment Approaches

Since viral pathogens are one of the primary causes of pneumonia, it is not unreasonable to forego antibiotics when the clinical picture appears due to a virus. As noted above however, this may be difficult since the clinical course, radiographic findings, and laboratory tests may not be sufficiently discriminatory. For routine instances of community-acquired pneumonias where a bacterial pathogen is suspected, oral antibiotics are generally sufficient. Macrolides such as **clarithromycin** or **azithromycin** are attractive choices for activity against most causes of pneumonia, including *Mycoplasma* and *Chlamydia* spp. Hospitalization and IV antibiotics should be considered in the following: infants <6 months; those who are more acutely ill with systemic symptoms; patients with S_aO_2 <92% in room air; children with gastric upset; or patients who have not responded to oral therapy. Other complications that occur in the course of a community-acquired pneumonia, including empyema or lung abscess, also would warrant an inpatient stay for IV therapy. The choice of IV antibiotic therapy when a specific etiology is known is shown in Table 40.3. Of course, drug allergies may dictate a change in therapeutic decisions.

Table **40.3** Antibiotic therapy for lower respiratory bacterial pathogens

Pathogen	First Choice	Second Choice
S. pneumoniae (penicillin susceptible or intermediate)	ampicillin, penicillin	cefuroxime, cefdinir, ceftriaxone, azithromycin
S. pneumoniae (penicillin resistant)	2nd or 3rd generation cephalosporin, vancomycin	
S. aureus (methicillin sensitive)	1st generation cephalosporin, oxacillin, amoxicillin/clavulanate	
S. aureus (methicillin resistant)	clindamycin, vancomycin	linezolid
H. influenzae	amoxicillin	amoxicillin/clavulanate, 2nd or 3rd generation cephalosporin
M. catarrhalis	amoxicillin/clavulanate	cefuroxime

Adapted from Kendig's Disorders of the Respiratory Tract, 7th ed.

Antibiotic choices also must take into account the age of the patient and the specific pathogens most likely at that age. For example, in a newborn hospitalized with pneumonia, a combination of ampicillin and gentamicin is preferred for organisms such as Group B *Streptococcus*, *E. coli*, and other gram-negative bacilli.

For children between 3 and 12 weeks of age, where organisms such as *C. trachomatis*, *Bordetella pertussis,* or *Ureaplasma urealyticum* are a consideration, macrolides are the drug of choice. As sensitivity patterns of the organisms causing community-acquired pneumonia have changed over the years, recommendations for oral antimicrobial therapy in the

older child have evolved. When standard doses of amoxicillin fail to improve the clinical picture, high-dose amoxicillin is combined with clavulanate. In the school-aged child or adolescent, an oral macrolide may be added or used as monotherapy. As noted before, complications from bacterial pneumonias require longer courses of both parenteral and oral therapy. A patient's response to antibiotic therapy should take into account clinical signs and symptoms, rather than radiographic findings as the latter may take several weeks to resolve. Reduction in cough or chest pain, the absence of fever, normalization of oxygenation, and the ability to tolerate oral feedings are key indicators that the patient has improved.

Suggested Readings

1. Stein RT, Marostica PJC. Community-acquired pneumonia: A review and recent advances. *Pediatr Pulmonol.* 2007;42: 1095-1103. *Reviews the common etiologies of CAP and explores the impact of lower respiratory tract disease in the developing world. Includes guidelines for treatment approaches as well as numerous references.*

2. Van der Poll T, Opal SM. Pathogenesis, treatment, and prevention of pneumococcal pneumonia. *Lancet.* 2009;374:1543-1556. *An in-depth look at the pathogenesis, clinical, and radiographic picture of the most common pathogen causing*

community acquired pneumonia. An excellent review of the various serotypes causing human disease, and the impact of commercially available vaccines on disease prevalence.

3. Tregoning JS, Schwarze J. Respiratory viral infections in infants: causes, clinical symptoms, virology, and immunology. *Clin Microbiol Rev.* 2010;23:74-98. *An exhaustive review of viral lower respiratory infections in children with 367 references. Discusses the common viral pathogens, treatment approaches, and potential sequelae of early life exposures to these viruses, including the risk of developing asthma.*

CASE STUDIES AND PRACTICE PROBLEMS

CASE 40.1 A 3-month-old infant is seen in the emergency department with copious nasal drainage, cough, fever, wheezing, and respiratory distress. Pulse oximetry in room air shows $S_aO_2 = 88\%$. A nasopharyngeal swab by immunofluorescent technique is positive for RSV. The patient is admitted for further observation. Which of the following treatments is most likely to be beneficial in this patient?

a. Aerosolized albuterol
b. Intravenous ampicillin plus gentamicin
c. Supplemental oxygen
d. Systemic corticosteroids
e. Aerosolized ribavirin

CASE 40.2 A 14-year-old boy is seen in an outpatient setting complaining of fatigue and fever for a week, with a dry cough beginning two days before the visit. On auscultation, crackles are heard over both lung fields. *Mycoplasma* infection is suspected. If true, which of the following would be an unusual coincident finding?

a. Maculopapular rash
b. Close contacts with respiratory illness

c. Positive cold agglutinin titers
d. Diffuse bilateral infiltrates on chest radiograph
e. Lobar pneumonia on chest radiograph

CASE 40.3 An 11-year-old girl is admitted to the hospital with fever, shaking chills, chest pain, and hypoxia. A chest radiograph shows a right lower lobe pneumonia and the chest exam shows decreased breath sounds in the right base. A blood culture obtained on admission is positive for *S. pneumoniae*, sensitive to penicillin. The patient is treated with intravenous ampicillin, but the fever and oxygen requirement continue and the patient continues to complain of chest discomfort. During physical exam on the fourth day of hospitalization, dullness to percussion along most of the right chest is noted with absent breath sounds. The trachea is deviated to the left. What has most likely developed to explain this patient's clinical picture?

a. Empyema
b. Pyopneumothorax
c. Secondary infection with influenza
d. Lung abscess
e. Secondary infection with *S. aureus*

Solutions to Case Studies and Practice Problems

CASE 40.1 The most correct answer is c, supplemental oxygen.

Comfort measures predominate in the treatment of RSV bronchiolitis. Randomized clinical trials and **Cochrane Database Reviews** have not found any evidence for the benefits of bronchodilator therapy, corticosteroids, or nebulized ribavirin in pediatric bronchiolitis. In some circumstances, infants with a history of atopy or a strong family history of asthma or atopy (mother or father) may improve with albuterol. There is no indication for antibiotic therapy in the treatment of viral respiratory infections.

CASE 40.2 The most correct answer is e, lobar pneumonia.

About 10% of patients with *Mycoplasma* disease have a concomitant maculopapular rash in the course of their illness. *Mycoplasma* is highly communicable so that it is often passed from household member to household member or from classmate to classmate. Cold agglutinin titers at >1:32 occur in about one-half of patients with *Mycoplasma* pneumonia. The typical radiographic pattern is one of diffuse pulmonary infiltrates and not lobar consolidation.

CASE 40.3 The most correct answer is a, empyema.

The clinical scenario described is typical of patients developing an empyema when clinical symptoms do not improve in spite of effective antibiotics. A pyopneumothorax, although a possible cause of these symptoms, should cause hyperresonance to percussion and is a less common complication than empyema. Generally, secondary infections are caused by bacteria in the patient with an initial viral syndrome. A pulmonary abscess may also cause the ongoing fever in this situation but some breath sounds would typically be auscultated, the percussion note would not be universally dull, and the trachea would not likely be shifted. Infection with a second bacterial pathogen is distinctly unusual.

Index

Page numbers followed by "f" denote figures; those followed by "t" denote tables.

A

(A − a) Po$_2$, 67
ABC of Acid-Base Chemistry, The, 76
Abdominal muscles, 94
Abscess, lung, 335, 336f, 402, 402f
Absorption atelectasis, 52
Accessory respiratory muscles, 95, 125
Acclimation, 113
Acclimatization, 113, 117
Acetazolamide, 236
Acetone, 65t
Acetylcholine, 193
Acid Bohr effect, 25
Acid-base balance, 74-77
Acid-base disorders
  metabolic acidosis. *See* Metabolic acidosis
  metabolic alkalosis. *See* Metabolic alkalosis
  primary, 151
  respiratory acidosis. *See* Respiratory
    acidosis
  respiratory alkalosis. *See* Respiratory
    alkalosis
Acid-base status, 154
Acid-fast bacilli, 175f, 339, 339f, 354f, 358
Acidosis
  definition of, 151, 152f
  metabolic. *See* Metabolic acidosis
  respiratory. *See* Respiratory acidosis
Acinus, 180f
Acromegaly, 231
Actinomyces spp., 335, 335f
Activated factor V, 256
Acute altitude exposure, 115
Acute eosinophilic pneumonia, 213, 224
Acute hypoxic pressor response, 63, 64f, 115,
    117, 389
Acute interstitial pneumonia, 207-208, 221
Acute laryngo-epiglottitis, 323
Acute lung injury
  air-space opacities with, 137f
  alveoli injury in, 269, 270f
  characteristics of, 268
  chest x-ray findings, 268, 268f
  clinical features of, 267
  complications of, 271-272
  conditions associated with, 208t
  definition of, 267, 268
  description of, 42, 207
  edema associated with, 59
  functional residual capacity declines in, 269
  inflammatory responses in, 269, 271
  laboratory findings, 272

Acute lung injury (*Cont.*):
  mechanical ventilation for
    description of, 267, 271
    lung protective strategy, 272-273
  multiple organ dysfunction syndrome
    secondary to, 267, 273
  noncardiogenic pulmonary edema in,
    268-269
  nondegradable materials as cause of, 89
  pathophysiology of, 268-271
  physical examination findings, 272
  positive end-expiratory pressure for, 267
  presentation of, 272
  prognosis for, 273
  progression of, 272
  pulmonary artery catheter use in, 272
  Starling's forces abnormalities in, 269
  transfusion-related, 271
  treatment of, 272
Acute mountain sickness, 118
Acute radiation pneumonitis, 251
Acute respiratory acidosis, 76
Acute respiratory distress syndrome
  alveoli injury in, 269, 270f
  characteristics of, 268
  chest x-ray findings, 268
  clinical features of, 207, 267
  complications of, 271-272
  conditions associated with, 208t
  definition of, 207, 267, 268
  description of, 42
  edema associated with, 59
  functional residual capacity declines in, 269
  inflammatory responses in, 269, 271
  laboratory findings, 272
  mechanical ventilation for
    description of, 267, 271
    lung protective strategy, 272-273
  mortality rates, 273
  multiple organ dysfunction syndrome
    secondary to, 267, 273
  noncardiogenic pulmonary edema in,
    268-269
  pathophysiology of, 268-271
  physical examination findings, 272
  positive end-expiratory pressure for, 267
  presentation of, 272
  prognosis for, 273
  progression of, 272
  pulmonary artery catheter use in, 272
  Starling's forces abnormalities in, 269
  treatment of, 272

Acute sinusitis, 319
ADAM-33, 183
Adaptation, 113
Adaptive immunity, 82
Adaptive support servoventilation, 237
Adenocarcinoma
  bronchogenic carcinoma, 297, 297f
  histologic appearance of, 308, 311f
  lung cancer, 297, 297f, 308, 310, 311f
Adenoid cystic carcinoma, 326
Adenoidectomy, 234
Adenoviruses, 400
Adventitious breath sounds, 129
Aerobic capacity
  American College of Sports Medicine
    definition of, 103, 104t
  bed rest effects on, 108, 109t
  calculation of, 103
  cold environment effects on, 114
  definition of, 103
  detraining effects on, 108
  exercise benefits for, 109-110
  in females, 104t
  interval training effects on, 110
  in males, 104t
  mortality influenced by, 103-104
  weight-adjusted, 103
Aerobic metabolism, 151
Aerobic training
  Fick equation effects, 106t
  genetic effects on, 108-109
  interval-based, 110
  maximal heart rate affected by, 106-107
  maximal oxygen consumption increases
    secondary to, 107
  $\dot{Q}_{max}$ affected by, 105f
AHPR. *See* Acute hypoxic pressor response
Air bronchograms, 137, 137f, 388, 388f
Air stent, 119, 389
Airborne particles
  impaction clearance of, 82, 83f
  sedimentation clearance of, 82
Air-space opacities, 137, 137f
Airway(s)
  compression of, 143
  defense mechanisms of
    mucociliary clearance, 83-84
    nasal cavity, 81
    oropharynx, 81-83
    respiratory parenchyma, 84-85
    sinuses, 81
  inflammation of, 192

Bronchospasms, 114
Brownian motion, 83
Brush cells, 10, 84, 85f
BTPS, 5
Bullae, 146
Bullectomy, 203
Bullous emphysema, 179, 181f
Bupropion, 201-202
Burkholderia cepacia, 379

C

Cadmium, 89
Caisson, 119
Canalicular stage, of lung development, 18, 19f
Candida albicans, 174f, 335, 336f
C_aO_2. *See* Arterial oxygen content
CAP. *See* Community-acquired pneumonia
Capacity, 32
Capillary transit times, 71
Carbaminohemoglobin, 27
Carbohydrate recognition domains, 86, 87f
Carbon dioxide
    alveoli's role in excretion of, 74-77
    bicarbonate excretion of, 28, 74, 117
    blood transport of, 74
    erythrocytes' role in transport of, 27-28
    solubility of, 5
Carbon dioxide Bohr effect, 26
Carbon dioxide dissociation curve, 74, 75f
Carbon dioxide partial pressure of alveolar
        gas, 3-4
Carbon dioxide plasma buffer line, 76, 76f
Carbon monoxide uptake rate, 73
Carbonic acid, 5, 27
Carbonic anhydrase, 28, 75f
Carbonic anhydrase inhibitors, 236
Carboxyhemoglobin, 27
Carcinoid syndrome, 299
Carcinoids, 299, 300f
Carcinoma
    adenocarcinoma. *See* Adenocarcinoma
    bronchioloalveolar, 297, 297f-298f,
        310, 311f
    bronchogenic. *See* Bronchogenic carcinoma
    large cell, 298, 298f
    squamous cell. *See* Squamous cell
        carcinoma
Carcinoma in situ, 324
Cardiac output
    baseline, 31
    definition of, 55
    description of, 4
    pulmonary capillary responses to, 56-58
Cardiogenic edema, 59
Cardiomegaly, 268f
Cardiopulmonary function
    in cold environments, 113-114
    in hot environments, 114-115
Cardiovascular collapse, 136
Cardiovascular shift, 114
Carina, 162f
Carotid bodies, 96, 97f
Caseous, 339, 340f

Caseous necrosis, 355, 356f
Cavitary lesion, 310, 312f
Cavities, 138, 138f
CCAM. *See* Congenital cystic adenomatoid
        malformation
Centers for Disease Control and Prevention
    exercise recommendations, 109-110, 110t
    influenza vaccination in asthmatics, 196
Central chemoreceptors, 96, 97f
Central hypoventilation syndrome, 99
Central pattern generator, 93
Central sleep apnea
    acetazolamide for, 236
    adaptive support servoventilation for, 237
    bilevel positive airway pressure for, 236-237
    classification of, 236t
    continuous positive airway pressure for, 236
    definition of, 235
    description of, 99, 236
    diagnosis of, 236
    epidemiology of, 235
    pathophysiology of, 236
    theophylline for, 236
    treatment of, 236-237
Central ventral respiratory group, 95
Centriacinar emphysema, 179, 180f
Centrilobular region, 139
Cepacia syndrome, 379
Cerebrospinal fluid, 96
Cervical lymphadenopathy, 322
CF. *See* Cystic fibrosis
C-fibers, 98
Charcot-Leyden crystals, 184, 185f
Charles's law, 4-5
Chemokines, 271
Chemoreceptors, 96, 97f
Chest
    computed tomography of. *See* Computed
        tomography
    magnetic resonance imaging of, 140, 140f
Chest examination
    accessory muscles, 125
    auscultation, 128-130
    chronic obstructive pulmonary disease
        findings, 131
    community-acquired pneumonia findings,
        131
    description of, 125
    inspection, 125-126, 126f
    likelihood ratios in, 130f, 130-131
    palpation, 126-127, 127f
    percussion, 127-128, 128f
    pleural effusion findings, 131
    pulmonary embolism findings, 131
    tracheal position, 126
Chest expansion, 126, 126f
Chest wall retractions, 387
Chest x-rays
    acute lung injury findings, 268, 268f
    acute respiratory distress syndrome findings,
        268
    air-space opacities on, 137, 137f
    anteroposterior, 133, 134f
    asthma evaluations, 192

Chest x-rays (*Cont.*):
    bronchioloalveolar carcinoma findings, 311f
    cavities on, 138, 138f
    chronic obstructive pulmonary disease
        findings, 201
    community-acquired pneumonia findings,
        346f
    cysts on, 138, 138f
    description of, 133
    diffuse alveolar hemorrhage findings,
        225, 225f
    frontal, 133
    interpretation of, 133-134
    interstitial opacities on, 137, 137f
    landmarks on, 134-135
    lateral, 133, 134f, 135
    lower respiratory tract infection findings,
        399f-400f
    lung anatomy application during review of,
        135
    lung disease patterns on, 137f-139f,
        137-139
    lung hypoplasia, 372f
    lymphadenopathy on, 137, 138f
    masses on, 137, 138f
    Mycobacterium kansasii, 360f
    neonatal respiratory distress syndrome
        findings, 388, 388f
    nodules on, 137, 138f
    pleural abnormalities on, 138-139, 139f
    pleural effusion findings, 138, 139f,
        276-277, 277f
    pneumothorax findings, 135-136
    posterior to anterior, 133
    pulmonary disease localization using,
        135-139
    pulmonary embolism findings, 261
    radiographic densities, 133, 134f
    sarcoidosis findings, 222, 223f-224f, 223t
    small cell carcinoma findings, 312f
    subdiaphragmatic gas shadows on,
        136, 137f
    tuberculosis findings, 355, 355f
Cheyne-Stokes respiration, 94, 94f, 100,
        100f, 235, 236f
CHF. *See* Congestive heart failure
Children. *See also* Infants
    community-acquired pneumonia in, 397
    lower respiratory tract infections in.
        See Lower respiratory tract infections
Chlamydia pneumoniae, 397
Chloride shift, 28
"Choke point," 143
Chondroma, 295
Chondromalacia, 368
Chromogranin, 322, 322f
Chronic asthmatic bronchitis, 181
Chronic bronchiolitis, 182
Chronic bronchitis
    definition of, 180, 199
    obstructive, 181
    pathogenesis of, 181, 183f
    pathology of, 180-182
    simple, 181

Chronic eosinophilic pneumonia, 224, 224f
Chronic nonspecific laryngitis, 323
Chronic obstructive pulmonary disease
  airflow limitation in, 201
  alpha$_1$ proteinase inhibitor deficiency as risk
    factor for, 199, 201
  antibiotic therapy for, 203
  arterial blood gas measurements in, 201
  asthma versus, 192, 200t
  bronchial hyperresponsiveness, 200
  bronchodilators for, 202, 203t
  chest examination findings in, 131
  chest x-ray findings in, 201
  chronic respiratory failure secondary to, 202
  cigarette smoking as risk factor for, 200
  cor pulmonale secondary to, 202
  definition of, 199
  diagnosis of, 200-201
  epidemiology of, 199
  exacerbations, 203, 290
  Global Initiative for Obstructive Lung
    Disease Guidelines, 199, 202t
  glucocorticoids for, 202
  immunizations in patients with, 202
  mortality rates for, 199
  non-invasive positive pressure ventilation
    for, 290
  oxygen therapy for, 202
  prevalence of, 199
  prevention of, 201-202
  pulmonary function testing for, 201
  pulmonary rehabilitation for, 203
  risk factors for, 199-200, 200t
  simple chronic bronchitis in, 181
  summary of, 203
  surgical treatment of, 203
  treatment of, 202-203
  wheezing and, 129
Chronic radiation pneumonitis, 251, 252f
Chronic respiratory failure, 202
Chronic restrictive lung diseases. *See also*
    Interstitial lung diseases
  alveolitis associated with, 208
  characteristics of, 208
  hypersensitivity pneumonitis, 211-212, 212t
  idiopathic pulmonary fibrosis, 208-209,
    209f, 221-222, 222f
  interstitial fibrosis associated with, 208
  nonspecific interstitial pneumonia, 209,
    211f, 221, 224
  pulmonary alveolar proteinosis, 214, 215f
  pulmonary amyloidosis, 213, 214f
  pulmonary eosinophilia, 213, 213f
  sarcoidosis. *See* Sarcoidosis
  usual interstitial pneumonia, 209, 210f, 221
Chronic sinusitis, 319-320
Chylothorax, 172, 252
Cicatrization atelectasis, 245
Cigarette smoking
  asthma and, 190
  bupropion for cessation of, 201-202
  cessation of, 201-202
  chronic obstructive pulmonary disease risks,
    200

Cigarette smoking (*Cont.*):
  lung cancer risks associated with, 307, 310f
  nicotine replacement therapies for, 201
  respiratory parenchyma effects, 180
  restrictive lung diseases caused by, 213, 214f
  varenicline for cessation of, 202
Ciliated cells, 9, 83f
Ciliated respiratory epithelium, 81
Circulatory delay time, 236
Clara cell secretory protein, 84
Clara cells, 84
Clarithromycin, 403
Clear cell carcinoma, 298
Clonidine, 202
Clubbing, 314, 314f
CO. *See* Cardiac output
CO$_2$. *See* Carbon dioxide
Coagulation factors, 264
Coagulative necrosis, 247, 248f
Coal worker's pneumoconiosis, 215, 216f, 225t
Coarse crackles, 129
Coccidioides immitis, 341, 342f
Coefficients of diffusivity, 71
Cold environments, 113-114
Collagen vascular diseases, 215
Collectins, 42, 42f
Colloid osmotic pressure
  description of, 58
  pleural fluid accumulation caused by
    elevation in, 171
Community-acquired pneumonia
  antibiotics for, 347
  causes of, 347t, 403
  chest examination findings in, 131
  chest x-ray of, 346f
  in children, 397
  criteria for, 346, 346t
  CURB-65 score, 345-346, 346t
  definition of, 345
  diagnostic tests for, 346
  immunizations for, 202
  management of, 345-347
  mortality rate for, 345
  prevention of, 345
  Staphylococcus aureus as cause of, 403
  vaccinations for, 345
Compensatory emphysema, 180
Compensatory hyperinflation, 180
Complete blood count, 23
Complex sleep apnea syndrome, 237-238
Compression atelectasis, 245, 246f
Computed tomography
  bronchogenic cysts, 369, 369f
  chest, 133, 139
  description of, 133
  high-resolution. *See* High-resolution
    computed tomography
  parapneumonic pleural effusion, 279, 279f
  virtual bronchoscopy uses of, 166
Computed tomography angiography, 139
Conchae, 10
Conducting zone
  branching airways of, 31
  description of, 9, 31

Conduction, 114
Congenital anomalies
  larynx, 365-366, 366f
  trachea, 366-369, 367f-369f
Congenital bullous emphysema, 146
Congenital central alveolar hypoventilation
    syndrome, 238-239
Congenital cystic adenomatoid malformation,
    370f, 370-371
Congenital emphysematous bulla, 83
Congenital lobar emphysema, 180, 371
Congestive heart failure
  cardiac asthma manifestation of, 192
  chest x-rays of, 268f
  Cheyne-Stokes respiration caused by, 236
  left ventricular preload in, 56
  pulmonary edema caused by, 245
  transudative pleural effusion caused by,
    172, 277-278
Conjugated hyperbilirubinemia, 380
Connective tissue disorders, 215, 223-224, 226
Conscious sedation, 161
Consolidated lung tissue, 135
Constrictive pericarditis, 172
Continuous positive airway pressure
  central sleep apnea treated with, 236
  neonatal respiratory distress syndrome
    treated with, 389-390
  obstructive sleep apnea syndromes treated
    with, 233, 234f, 235t
  scuba diving and, 119
Contraction atelectasis, 245
Convection, 114
COPD. *See* Chronic obstructive pulmonary
    disease
Cor pulmonale, 202
Core temperature, 26
Corniculate cartilages, 13
Coronavirus, 341
Corticosteroids
  asthma treated with, 193-194
  excess, 155
  inhaled, 193-194
  interstitial lung diseases managed with, 228
  prenatal administration of, for neonatal
    respiratory distress syndrome, 390
Coryza, 338
Costophrenic angle, 134f, 135
Costophrenic sulcus, 276
Cough-variant asthma, 191
CPAP. *See* Continuous positive airway pressure
Crackles, 129, 221, 226
Crepitus, 207
"Crescendo-decrescendo" oscillations, 94, 94f
Cricoid cartilage, 13
Critical opening pressure, 39, 386
Cromolyn sodium, 194
Cromones, 194
Croup, 323, 400
Cryptococcus neoformans, 341, 342f
Cryptogenic fibrosing alveolitis. *See* Idiopathic
    pulmonary fibrosis
Cryptogenic organizing pneumonia, 213,
    215f, 221

CSA. *See* Central sleep apnea
C-shaped tracheal rings, 14
Cuffing, 59
Cuirass shell ventilator, 283, 284f
Cuneiform cartilages, 13
CURB-65 score, 345-346, 346t
Curschmann spirals, 184
Cushing syndrome, 314
Cyanomethemoglobin, 23
Cyanosis, 65
Cyclic AMP, 193
Cyclic AMP-dependent protein kinase, 375
Cyclical shear stress, 269
Cyclopropane, 65t
CYP4B1, 84
Cyst(s)
    bronchogenic, 369, 369f
    chest x-ray of, 138, 138f
Cysteinyl-leukotriene, 194
Cystic fibrosis
    antimicrobial agents in, 381
    azithromycin in, 382
    azoospermia associated with, 380
    clinical manifestations of, 376-377
    definition of, 359
    description of, 84
    distal intestinal obstruction syndrome in, 380
    endocrine features of, 380
    etiology of, 375-376
    exocrine pancreatic insufficiency in, 379
    gastrointestinal disease features of, 379-380
    hepatic dysfunction risks, 380
    high salt hypothesis of, 376
    historical descriptions of, 375
    infertility associated with, 380
    lung diseases associated with
        airway clearance methods, 381, 381f
        anti-inflammatory therapies for, 382
        description of, 379
        monitoring of, 382-383
        mucus removal techniques, 381, 381f
        pathogenesis of, 381f
        postural drainage techniques for, 381
        treatment of, 380-382
    lung transplantation for, 382-383
    newborn screening for, 377-378
    nonmycobacterial lung diseases in, 359-360
    organ system manifestations of, 379
    Pseudomonas aeruginosa infection in, 379, 381
    reproductive system defects in, 380
    screening for, 377-378
    signs and symptoms of, 376, 377t, 378f
    survival in, 383, 383f
    sweat chloride test for, 376
    sweat electrolyte abnormalities in, 375
Cystic Fibrosis Foundation, 381
Cystic fibrosis transmembrane conductance
        regulator, 359, 375-377, 376f
Cystic fibrosis-related diabetes mellitus, 380
Cytocentrifuge, 172
Cytokines, 84, 271
Cytologic atypia, 251
Cytomegalovirus, 338f

D

DAD. *See* Diffuse alveolar damage
DAH. *See* Diffuse alveolar hemorrhage
Dalton's law, 4, 24
D-dimer assay, 260
Dead space ventilation, 64t, 65
Dead space volume, 3
Decompression sickness, 119-120
Deep venous thrombosis
    description of, 255
    duplex ultrasonographic studies for, 261-262
Defense mechanisms
    mucociliary clearance, 83-84
    nasal cavity, 81
    oropharynx, 81-83
    respiratory parenchyma, 84-85
    sinuses, 81
Deoxygenated, 25
Dependent lung zones, 52, 52f
Descending aorta, 134, 134f
Detraining, 108
Diabetic ketoacidosis, 154
Diapedesis, 87
Diaphragm
    anatomy of, 48f, 94
    chest x-ray of, 134f, 135
Diaphragmatic hernia, 372
Diastolic pressure, 55
Diethyl ether, 65t
Diffuse alveolar damage
    crepitus associated with, 207
    definition of, 207
    description of, 222
    hyaline membranes associated with, 207
    lung findings, 207, 208f
    microscopic findings, 207, 209f, 389f
    pathogenesis of, 207
Diffuse alveolar hemorrhage
    bronchoalveolar lavage fluid
        findings in, 163
    chest x-ray findings, 225, 225f
    description of, 225
Diffuse interstitial lung diseases
    description of, 208
    flexible bronchoscopy indications for, 161
Diffuse interstitial pneumonitis, 213, 214f
Diffuse parenchymal lung disease, 140
Diffuse pulmonary hemorrhage syndromes, 249-251, 250f
Diffusion block, 387
Diffusion limited, 72, 73f, 115
Dipalmitoyl phosphatidylcholine, 41, 42t
2,3-Diphosphoglycerate
    hemoglobin-oxygen affinity affected by, 26, 26f
    hypoxia effects on, 115
Direct method, of percussion, 127
Directly observed therapy, 353, 357
Dissociation constant, 75
Distal acinar emphysema, 179, 181f
Distal intestinal obstruction syndrome, 380

Diving
    breath-hold, 118
    decompression sickness caused by, 119-120
    scuba, 118-119
Diving reflex, 81, 118
Diving response, 392
DL_{CO}. *See* Lung diffusing capacity for carbon
        monoxide
DM_{CO}, 148
Dorsal respiratory group, 95
Down syndrome, 231, 372
Dressler syndrome, 280
Drug-induced asthma, 184
Drug-induced pulmonary disease, 225
Ductus arteriosus
    description of, 57, 388
    patent, 58, 63, 74
DVT. *See* Deep venous thrombosis
Dynamic airway compliance, 48
Dynamic airway resistance
    description of, 35, 48
    work of breathing affected by, 35
Dynamic compliance maneuver, 49
Dynamic lung resistance, 50
Dyspnea, 35, 65, 93, 99-100

E

Early inspiratory crackles, 129
Eccrine glands, 11f
Eczema, 400
Effort-independent, 50
Egophony, 130
Electromagnetic navigational bronchoscopy, 166
Embolectomy, 264
Embryonic stage, 18, 18f
Emphysema
    bullous, 179, 181f
    centriacinar, 179, 180f
    compensatory, 180
    congenital lobar, 180, 371
    definition of, 179, 199
    description of, 40, 65, 86
    distal acinar, 179, 181f
    irregular, 179
    panacinar, 179, 181f, 199
    pathogenesis of, 179-180, 182f
    pathology of, 179-180, 180f-182f
    type A, 65
    type B, 65
Emphysema Severity Scores, 72f
Emphysematous blebs, 311f
Empyema, 173, 252, 279, 319, 347
Empyemic, 171
End-expiratory hold maneuver, 288
Endobronchial obstructing lesions, 162, 162f
Endobronchial tumors, 165
Endodermal, 18
Enflurane, 65t
Enoxaparin, 263
Environmental pollutants, 115
Environmental Protection Agency, 115

Environmental tobacco smoke
  chronic obstructive pulmonary disease risks, 200
  fetal lung function affected by, 189-190
  lung cancer risks, 307
Eosinophilic lung disorders
  acute eosinophilic pneumonia, 213
  characteristics of, 224, 224f
  pulmonary eosinophilia, 213, 213f
Eosinophilic pneumonia, 163
EPAP. *See* Expiratory positive airway pressure
Epiglottis
  bifid, 365
  description of, 12
  in laryngomalacia, 366, 366f
Epinephrine injection kit, 195
Epithelial type II cells, 41, 42t
Epithelioid histiocytes, 210, 211f, 339
Epstein-Barr virus, 322
Erythrocytes
  capillary transit times of, 71
  carbon dioxide transport role of, 27-28
  function of, 23
  indices of, 23-24
  life span of, 23
  oxygen transport role of, 24-25
Erythropoiesis, 117
Erythropoietin, 117
Esophageal atresia, 367
Esophageal manometry, 232
Esthesioneuroblastomas, 321, 322f
Ethambutol, 357
Ethane, 65t
ETS. *See* Environmental tobacco smoke
Eupnea, 93
Exacerbations
  asthma, 196
  chronic obstructive pulmonary disease, 203, 290
Exercise
  aerobic capacity improvements through, 109-110
  American College of Sports Medicine recommendations, 110, 110t
  Centers for Disease Control and Prevention recommendations, 110t
  in hot environment, 114
Exercise-induced arterial hypoxemia, 108
Exocrine pancreatic insufficiency, 379
Expiratory flow rate, 50
Expiratory flow-volume loop, 143, 144f
Expiratory positive airway pressure, 289
Expiratory reserve volume, 32, 33t
Extended spectrum beta-lactamase, 348
Extracellular fluid, 96
Extracorporeal membrane oxygenation, 366
Extrapulmonary shunts, 389, 389f
Extrinsic allergic alveolitis. *See* Hypersensitivity pneumonitis
Extrinsic asthma, 183-184
Exudative pleural effusions
  benign asbestos pleural effusion, 279
  causes of, 171, 278t
  characteristics of, 277t

Exudative pleural effusions (*Cont.*):
  description of, 171
  laboratory examination of, 172
  microscopic appearance of, 172, 173f
  transudative pleural effusions versus, 172, 277t

F

f. See Respiratory frequency
Facial muscles, 95
Factor V Leiden mutation, 256
False vocal chords, 13, 13f
Fat-soluble vitamins, 380
F$_e$NO. *See* Fractional excretion of nitric oxide
Ferruginous bodies, 217
Fetal reflexes, 392
Fetus
  environmental tobacco smoke exposure, 189-190
  lung maturity in, 385
FEV. *See* Forced expiratory volume
FEV$_1$. *See* Forced expiratory volume in 1 second
Fibrin, 271
Fibroma, 295
Fibrosarcoma, 302
Fick, Adolf Eugen, 104
Fick equation
  expression of, 103
  hot environment effects on, 114
  training effects on, 106t
Fine crackles, 129
F$_1$O$_2$. *See* Fractional concentration of oxygen in the inspired gas mixture
Fistula
  bronchopleural, 280
  tracheoesophageal, 368f, 368-369
Flail chest, 283
Flatness, 128
Flexible bronchoscopy, diagnostic
  alveolar macrophage studies with, 85
  biopsy forceps introduced through, 164, 164f
  bronchoalveolar lavage, 163-164
  bronchoscope used in
    description of, 159, 160f
    ultrasound-tipped, 165, 165f
  brushes used with, 164, 164f
  carina inspection using, 162f
  clinical uses of, 159
  computed tomography applications, 166
  conscious sedation for, 161
  contraindications, 161, 161t
  development of, 159
  electromagnetic navigation for, 166
  endobronchial tumor evaluations, 165
  equipment, 159, 160f
  fluoroscopy, 159, 164
  future of, 165-166
  indications for, 159-161, 160t
  interstitial lung disease evaluations, 227
  portable fluoroscopy "C-arm" unit, 159
  procedure, 161-163
  restrictive lung disease evaluations, 227

Flexible bronchoscopy, diagnostic (*Cont.*):
  suite for, 159, 160f
  topical anesthesia, 161
  tracheobronchial tree inspection using, 162, 162f
  transbronchial lung biopsy use of, 164, 164f, 227
  transbronchial needle aspiration use of, 164, 165f
  ultrasound-tipped bronchoscope, 165, 165f
  working channel of, 164, 164f-165f
Flow-volume loops
  expiratory, 143, 144f
  inspiratory, 143, 144f
  in obstructive airway diseases, 51, 52f
  shape of, during expiration, 143, 144f
Fluorescence polarization, 43
Fluoroquinolones, 347
Fluoroscopy, 159, 164
Flux equation, 48
Foam stability index, 43
Follicular tonsillitis, 321
Foramen ovale, 57, 388
Forced expiratory volume
  definition of, 32
  measurement of, 50
Forced expiratory volume in 1 second
  in obstructive airway diseases, 50
  spirometry measurement of, 143
Forced expiratory volume in 1 second/forced vital capacity ratio
  in asthma, 191, 192t
  calculation of, 191
  description of, 144
Forced vital capacity
  definition of, 32
  measurement of, 50
  spirometry measurement of, 143
Formoterol, 193
Four-ion anion gap, 153
Fractional concentration of oxygen in the inspired gas mixture, 4
Fractional excretion of nitric oxide, 192
FRC. *See* Functional residual capacity
Fremitus, 126-127
Functional residual capacity
  acute lung injury-related declines in, 269
  acute respiratory distress syndrome-related declines in, 269
  definition of, 32, 33t, 39
  measurement of, 33f
  physiology of, 35
  whole-body plethysmography measurement of, 146
Fungi, 338, 338f
FVC. *See* Forced vital capacity

G

Galen, Claudius, 283
Gas exchange, 71-73
Gas laws
  Boyle's law, 4, 118, 146
  Charles's law, 4-5

Gas laws (*Cont.*):
  Dalton's law, 4, 24
  general, 5
  Henry's law, 5, 64
Gas shadowing, subdiaphragmatic, 136, 137f
G551D, 380
General gas law, 5
Genioglossus muscle, 95
Genomovars, 379
Ghon complex, 339
Ghon focus, 339, 340f, 354
Giant cell carcinoma, 298
Global Initiative for Obstructive Lung Disease
      Guidelines, 199, 202t
Glucocorticoids, 202
Goblet cells
  description of, 9-10, 83f
  metaplasia of, 181, 183f
Goodpasture syndrome, 148, 227,
      249, 250f
Gram staining of sputum specimen, 169, 170f
Gram-negative pathogens, 397
Granulocyte-monocyte colony-stimulating
      factor, 214, 226
Granulomas
  necrotizing, 339f, 341f
  pulmonary necrotizing, 341f
  sarcoidosis, 210-211, 211f
Granulomatous infectious pneumonitis,
      339f-341f, 339-341
Ground-glass opacities, 140, 140f, 388
Group A *Streptococcus*, 403
Grunting, 387

H

Haemophilus influenzae
  antibiotic therapy for, 403t
  bacterial pneumonia caused by, 334
  description of, 169
  type B, 402-403
Hairy cell leukemia, 358
Haldane effect, 26, 28, 74
Hamman-Rich syndrome, 221
Hampton hump, 261
HAP. *See* Hospital-acquired pneumonia
Hard metal diseases, 218, 225
Harmonic mean, 71
Hay fever, 319
H_2CO_3. *See* Carbonic acid
Heart transplantation, 236
Heath and Edwards grading system,
      249, 249t
Helical computed tomographic angiography,
      261, 261f
Heliox mixtures, 34, 120, 196
Helium dilution technique, 33
Helminthic infections, 224
Hemacytometer, 23
Hemangioma, 295
Hemangiopericytoma, 302
Hematocrit
  description of, 23, 24f
  high altitude exposure effects on, 117

Hemidiaphragm
  percussion used to assess position of, 128
  phrenic nerve disruption as cause of, 313, 313f
  respiratory excursion of, 128
Hemoconcentration, 117
Hemoglobin
  description of, 5, 23
  molecular model of, 24f
  oxygen carrying capacity of, 24
  variants of, 26
Hemoglobin Capetown, 26
Hemoglobin concentration, 23
Hemoglobin Kansas, 26
Hemoglobin Rainier, 26
Hemoglobin-carbon monoxide accumulation, 148
Hemoglobin-oxygen affinity
  alkalosis effects on, 115
  color associated with, 27
  confounding variables of, 27
  core temperature effects on, 26
  2,3-diphosphoglycerate effects on, 26, 26f
  endogenous modulators of, 25-26
  features of, 25f
  genetic effects on, 26-27
  hypothermia effects on, 114
Hemoglobin-oxygen dissociation curve, 114
Hemoptysis, 250, 257, 360f
Hemorrhagic edema, 59, 60f
Hemothorax, 252, 280
Henderson-Hasselbalch equation
  derivation of, 151-153
  description of, 75-76
Henry's law, 5, 64
Heparin
  low-molecular-weight, 257, 263
  unfractionated, 263
Heparin-induced thrombocytopenia, 263
Hepatic hydrothorax, 278
Hering-Breuer reflex, 97, 238
High altitude
  acclimatization features, 117
  acute exposure to, 115
  arterial blood gases at, 116t
  interstitial edema caused by, 117
  lung function at, 115-118
  polycythemia and, 117
High altitude pulmonary edema, 60, 117
High-affinity IgE receptors, 194
High power field, 169
High-resolution computed tomography
  description of, 139
  diffuse parenchymal lung disease on, 140
  hypersensitivity pneumonia, 139f
  idiopathic pulmonary fibrosis findings,
      221, 222f
Hirschsprung disease, 238
Histoplasma capsulatum, 339
Histoplasmosis, 339-340, 341f
Hodgkin disease, 302
Hoover's sign, 200
Horner syndrome, 312, 312f
Hospital-acquired pneumonia
  antibiotics for, 348, 349t
  definition of, 345, 347

Hospital-acquired pneumonia (*Cont.*):
  management of, 347-349
  multidrug-resistant organisms that cause,
      348, 348t
  prevention of, 348
  ventilator-associated pneumonia, 347
Hot environments
  cardiopulmonary function in, 114-115
  cardiovascular shift in, 114
HRCT. *See* High-resolution computed
      tomography
HR_{max}. *See* Maximal heart rate
Human immunodeficiency virus, 353
Human papilloma virus, 307, 321
Humanized monoclonal antibody, 400
Hyaline membranes, 207, 338, 388
Hydrops fetalis, 370
Hydrostatic pressure, 58, 171
Hydrothorax, 252
Hydroxyl radical, 88
5-Hydroxytryptamine, 259
Hygiene Hypothesis, 190, 191f
Hyperbaric oxygen therapy, for decompression
      sickness, 120
Hypercarbia, 71
Hypercoagulable states, 247t
Hyperkeratosis, 324
Hyperoxia, 100
Hyperpnea, 93
Hyperresonance, 128
Hypersensitivity pneumonia
  high-resolution computed tomography of,
      139f
  sarcoidosis versus, 163
Hypersensitivity pneumonitis, 211-212, 212t,
      224, 359
Hypertonic saline, 380
Hyperventilation
  definition of, 93
  as metabolic acidosis response, 154
  respiratory alkalosis caused by, 155
Hypobaric hypoxia, 115
Hypocapnia, 100, 259
Hypochloridemia, 155
Hypochlorite ion, 88
Hypocrepitant, 338
Hypokalemia, 155
Hypopnea, 231, 234t
Hypothermia, 114
Hypothyroidism, 172, 231
Hypotonia, 99
Hypoventilation, 155
Hypoxemia
  description of, 71
  in neonatal respiratory distress syndrome,
      385, 388t
  pulmonary thromboembolism as cause of,
      247
  respiratory alkalosis caused by, 155
Hypoxemic hypoxia, 7
Hypoxia
  blunted ventilatory response to, 117
  hypobaric, 115
  hypoxemic, 7

Hypoxia (*Cont.*):
  hypoxic, 6
  pulmonary embolism, 259
  serum lactate increases during, 154
Hypoxic hypoxia, 6
Hysteresis, 39

I

Iatrogenic lung diseases, 251, 251t
Ibuprofen, 382
Idiopathic acute lung injury-diffuse alveolar
    damage. *See* Acute interstitial
    pneumonia
Idiopathic chronic eosinophilic pneumonia,
    213
Idiopathic interstitial pneumonias, 221-222,
    222t. *See also specific pneumonia*
Idiopathic pulmonary fibrosis, 208-209, 209f,
    221-222, 222f
Idiopathic pulmonary hemosiderosis, 250-251
IgE-blocking antibodies, 194
Immotile cilia syndrome, 83, 331
Immune reconstitution syndrome, 357
Immunizations
    in asthma patients, 196
    in chronic obstructive pulmonary disease
        patients, 202
Immunoglobulin G autoantibodies, 249
Immunoreactive trypsinogen, 377-378
Immunotherapy, for asthma, 194-195
Impaction, 82
Indirect method, of percussion, 127
Inducible nitric oxide synthase, 88
Inert gas narcosis. *See* Nitrogen narcosis
Infants
    bronchial development defects in, 369, 369f
    cystic fibrosis screening in, 377-378
    laryngeal anomalies in, 365-366, 366f
    respiratory parenchyma defects in, 369-372,
        370f-372f
    tracheal anomalies in, 366-369, 367f-369f
Infectious Disease Society of America, 346-
    347
Infectious interstitial pneumonitis, 338, 338f
Inferior vena cava, 134f, 135
Inferior vena cava filters, 264
Inflammatory pseudotumor, 295
Influenza virus
    epidemic outbreaks of, 401
    lower respiratory tract infections caused by,
        400-401
    vaccinations against
        in asthmatics, 196
        community-acquired pneumonia
            prevention use of, 345
Infraglottic, 13
Infrahilar window, 134f, 135
Inhalational injuries, 161
Inhaled corticosteroids
    asthma treated with, 193-194
    side effects of, 193-194
Injection allergen immunotherapy, 194-195
Innate immunity, 82

Inspection
    accessory muscles, 125
    chest expansion, 126, 126f
    tracheal position, 126
Inspiratory capacity, 33t
Inspiratory flow-volume loop, 143, 144f
Inspiratory positive airway pressure, 289
Inspiratory reserve volume, 32, 33t
Inspiratory time/expiratory time ratio, 285
Intercostal muscles, 94
Interferon-γ, 354
Interlobular septum, 16, 17f, 139
Intermittent asthma, 194
International Association of Lung Cancer, 315
Interstitial edema, 58, 117
Interstitial emphysema, 180
Interstitial fibrosis, 208
Interstitial lung diseases. *See also* Chronic
    restrictive lung diseases
    bibasilar inspiratory crackles associated
        with, 226
    chest x-rays, 227
    clinical features of, 221, 226
    connective tissue disorders and, 215,
        223-224, 226
    corticosteroids for, 228
    definition of, 221
    diagnostic approach, 226-228
    eosinophilic lung disorders, 224, 224f
    high-resolution computed tomography of,
        139, 139f
    laboratory tests for, 226-227
    lung biopsy for, 227-228, 228t
    lung transplantation for, 228-229
    lymphangioleiomyomatosis, 226-227, 227f
    pneumoconioses manifesting as. *See*
        Pneumoconioses
    pulmonary alveolar proteinosis, 226, 226f
    pulmonary function testing for, 227
    pulmonary Langerhans cell histiocytosis,
        226, 228f
    pulmonary rehabilitation for, 228
    pulmonary vasculitides and, 224-225
    radiological studies, 227
    respiratory bronchiolitis-associated, 213
    surgical lung biopsy for, 227-228, 228t
    treatment of, 228-229
Interstitial opacities
    chest x-ray of, 137, 137f
    linear, 137, 137f
Interstitial pneumonia
    lymphocytic, 302
    nonspecific, 209, 211f, 221, 224
    usual, 209, 210f, 221
Interstitial pneumonitis
    diffuse, 213, 214f
    infectious, 338, 338f
Interval training, 110
Intrapleural pressure, 34, 36, 145f
Intrapulmonary hemorrhage, 148
Intrapulmonary shunts, 389, 389f
Intrathecal pressure, 34
Intratracheal pressure, 367
Intravascular thromboembolism, 258

Intrinsic asthma, 184
Intrinsic positive end-expiratory pressure, 288
Invasive carcinoma, 324
Inverse-ratio pressure control ventilation, 285
Ionizing radiation, 251, 252f
IPAP. *See* Inspiratory positive airway pressure
Ipratropium, 193
Iron lung, 283, 284f
Irregular emphysema, 179
Irritant receptors, 81, 97
Irritant-induced occupational asthma, 190
Isoniazid, 357

J

Juvenile laryngeal papillomatosis, 324, 325f

K

Kaposi sarcoma, 161f
Kartagener syndrome, 320, 331
Keratin pearl, 296f
Keratinizing squamous cell carcinoma, 322,
    323f
Klebsiella pneumoniae, 334
Kölliker-Fuse area, 95, 96f
Kwashiorkor, 58

L

Ladder pattern, for percussion, 127, 128f
Lady Windermere syndrome, 359, 359f
Lambert-Eaton myasthenic syndrome, 314
Lamellar bodies, 43
Lamellar body count, 43
Laminar flow, 50f
Large cell carcinoma, 298, 298f
Laryngeal atresia, 365
Laryngeal chemoreceptor reflex, 392
Laryngeal dysplasia, 324
Laryngeal keratosis, 324
Laryngeal muscles, 95
Laryngeal ventricles, 13
Laryngeal webs, 365, 366f
Laryngitis, 323
Laryngomalacia, 366, 366f
Laryngoscopy, 192
Laryngotracheitis, 400
Laryngotracheobronchitis, 323
Laryngotracheoesophageal clefts, 365-366
Larynx
    anatomy of, 10t, 12-13, 13f
    congenital defects of, 365-366, 366f
    infections of, 323-324
    nodules of, 323-324, 324f
    papillomas of, 324
    papillomatosis of, 324, 325f
    precancerous lesions of, 324-326
    respiratory epithelium of, 13
    sensory innervation of, 98
    squamous cell carcinoma of, 325f, 325-326,
        326f
    tumors of, 324-326
Late inspiratory crackles, 129

Neonatal respiratory distress syndrome (*Cont.*):
prematurity as risk factor for, 385
prenatal corticosteroid administration for, 390
presentation of, 386
preterm delivery prevention, 390
prognosis for, 390-391
radiographic findings in, 388, 388f
right-to-left shunting correction in, 389, 389f
risk factors for, 387, 387t
surfactant in
production deficiency of, 386
replacement of, 390
treatment of, 389-390
ventilation/perfusion mismatch in, 388
Nephrotic syndrome, 172, 278, 278f
Neuroendocrine cells, 10
Neurofilaments, 322
Neuron-specific enolase, 321-322
Neutrophil elastase, 199
Neutrophils
bronchoalveolar lavage fluid level of, 163, 271
respiratory parenchyma recruitment of, 88, 88f
Nicotine replacement therapies, 201
Nitric oxide, 88, 390
Nitrogen narcosis, 120
Nitrogen washout, 34, 34f
Nocardia asteroides, 334f, 334-335
Nodules
chest x-ray of, 137, 138f
description of, 140
Nomogram, 130f
Nonanion gap metabolic acidosis, 154
Non-atopic asthma, 184
Noncardiogenic pulmonary edema, 59, 268-269
Noncaseating granulomas, 210, 211f
Nondegradable materials, 89
Non-Hodgkin lymphoma, 174f, 302
Non-invasive positive pressure ventilation, 289-290, 290t
Nonkeratinizing squamous cell carcinoma, 323, 323f
Nonshivering thermogenesis, 114
Nonspecific interstitial pneumonia, 209, 211f, 221, 224
Nontuberculous mycobacterial infection, 357-360, 358t
Nonvolatile acids, 151
Normal saline, 39
Nortriptyline, 202
Nose
infections of, 319-321
tumors of, 321-323
Nucleotide binding domains, 375
Nucleus accumbens, 201
Nucleus ambiguus, 95
Nucleus tractus solitarii, 96f

O

O_2. *See* Oxygen
Obesity-hypoventilation syndrome, 239
Obstruction atelectasis, 245

Obstructive airway diseases. *See also* Obstructive lung diseases
characteristics of, 50
description of, 3
flow-volume loops in, 51, 52f
forced expiratory volume in 1 second in, 50
forced vital capacity in, 50
types of, 50
Obstructive chronic bronchitis, 181
Obstructive expiratory apnea, 99
Obstructive hypoventilation, 99
Obstructive lung diseases. *See also* Obstructive airway diseases
asthma. *See* Asthma
bronchiectasis. *See* Bronchiectasis
bronchiolar edema as, 59
characteristics of, 179
chronic bronchitis. *See* Chronic bronchitis
emphysema. *See* Emphysema
pulmonary diffusing capacity for carbon monoxide reductions in, 148
Obstructive overinflation, 180
Obstructive sleep apnea syndromes
adenoidectomy for, 234
adverse health effects caused by, 231-232, 232t
atonia as cause of, 99
body mass index and, 231
in children, 233-234
continuous positive airway pressure for, 233, 234f, 235t
description of, 231
diagnosis of, 232, 233f, 234t
epidemiology of, 231
flexible bronchoscopy contraindications in, 161
neurocognitive dysfunction in, 232
oral appliances for, 233-234
pathophysiology of, 231
polysomnogram evaluation, 232, 233f
positional, 233
respiratory effort-related arousals associated with, 232, 233f, 234t
risk factors for, 231, 232t
surgical techniques for, 234, 235t
tonsillectomy for, 234
treatment of, 233-234
uvulopalatopharyngoplasty for, 234, 235t
Occupational asthma, 183, 190
Ohm's law, 4, 48, 57, 72f
Olfactory cells, 10
Olfactory epithelium, 11, 12f
Olfactory neuroblastomas, 321
Oligohydramnios, 372
Omalizumab, 194
Oncogenes, 295
Ondine's curse, 99, 238
$1/DM_{CO}$. *See* Membrane diffusive resistance
Opitz G/BBB syndrome, 366
Oropharynx
anatomy of, 11
defense mechanisms of, 81-83
OSAS. *See* Obstructive sleep apnea syndromes
Oxidants, 271

Oxygen carrying capacity, 24
Oxygen consumption
description of, 28
Fick equation used to estimate, 104-108
Oxygen delivery
cold environment effects on, 114
estimating of, 73-74
measurement of, 104
Oxygen dissociation curve, 25
Oxygen extraction, 104
Oxygen hood, 385, 386f
Oxygen therapy
chronic obstructive pulmonary disease managed with, 202
neonatal respiratory distress syndrome treated with, 385-386, 386f, 389
Oxygen transport
cascade of, 3, 4f
erythrocytes' role in, 24-25
Oxyradicals, 271
Ozone, 115

P

P_{50}, 25-26
P_A. *See* Alveolar pressure
$P_A{CO_2}$. *See* Carbon dioxide partial pressure of alveolar gas
Palivizumab, 400
Palpation, 126-127, 127f
Panacinar emphysema, 179, 181f, 199
Pancoast tumor, 140, 312, 313f
Panting, 93
$P_A{O_2}$. *See* Alveolar partial pressure of oxygen
Papillomas
laryngeal, 324
sinonasal, 321, 321f
tracheal, 324
Parabrachial nucleus, 95
Paradoxic embolism, 247
Parainfluenza viruses, 400
Paranasal sinuses, 11
Paraneoplastic syndromes, 312, 314, 314t
Parapneumonic pleural effusions, 278-280, 279f, 347, 402
Parietal pleura
description of, 9, 170
hydrostatic pressure of capillaries in, 171
lymphatic stroma, 275, 276f
pleural fluid reabsorption, 275, 276f
Partial pressure of carbon dioxide, 25
Passive atelectasis, 245
Patent ductus arteriosus, 58, 63, 74
Patent foramen ovale
description of, 58, 63, 74
paradoxic embolism secondary to, 247
P_B. *See* Barometric pressure
$P{CO_2}$. *See* Partial pressure of carbon dioxide
P_{CO}. *See* Critical opening pressure
Peak airway pressure, 287, 288f
Peak expiratory flow rate
in asthma, 191
description of, 118
Pectoriloquy, 130

PEEP. *See* Positive end-expiratory pressure
Percussion, 127-128, 128f
Perforated viscus, 136, 137f
Perfusion limited, 72, 73f
Peribronchial thickening, 399
Periciliary layer, 376
Periodic acid-Schiff reagent, 226
Periodic breathing, 99-100
Peripheral blood neutrophilia, 226
Peripheral chemoreceptors, 96
Peripheral gas trapping, 36
Peripheral sensory receptors, 98
Permissive hypercapnia, 155, 196, 272, 287
Peroxynitrite anion, 88
Persistent asthma, 194
Pharyngitis, 321
Pharynx
    anatomy of, 10t, 11
    muscles of, 95
Phosphatidylglycerol, 43
Phospholipids, 41
PHOX2B gene, 239
Physiological dead space
    description of, 63, 64f
    equation for, 66-67
Physiological shunts
    cyanosis caused by, 65
    description of, 5, 17, 63, 64f
    measurement of, 74f
    in pulmonary circulation, 74
    reporting methods for, 74
    venous admixture, 73
Pickwickian syndrome, 239
PiMM phenotype, 199
Pink puffer, 65, 66f
P_{IP}. *See* Intrapleural pressure
PiZZ phenotype, 199
Plasmacytomas, 323
Plasmapheresis, 250
Plateau airway pressure, 287, 288f
Platelet activating factor, 207
Platelet-derived growth factor, 207
Pleura
    calcifications of, 139
    diseases of, 138-139, 139f. *See also specific disease*
    parietal. *See* Parietal pleura
    thickening of, 138-139
    tumors of, 302, 302f-303f
    visceral. *See* Visceral pleura
Pleural effusions
    breast carcinoma cells in, 174f
    causes of, 171
    chest examination findings, 131
    chest x-rays of, 138, 139f, 276-277, 277f
    clinical manifestations of, 275-277
    diagnostic algorithm for, 173f, 277
    empyemic, 171
    exudative
        benign asbestos pleural effusion, 279
        causes of, 171, 278t
        characteristics of, 277t
        description of, 171
        laboratory examination of, 172

Pleural effusions (*Cont.*):
        microscopic appearance of, 172, 173f
        transudative pleural effusions versus, 172, 277t
    fremitus decreases associated with, 127
    macroscopic and microscopic evaluation of, 173-174, 174f-175f
    malignant causes of, 279t
    in non-Hodgkin lymphoma, 174f
    parapneumonic, 278-280, 279f, 347, 402
    pathophysiology of, 275, 276t
    sample collection, 171-172
    symptoms of, 275-276
    thoracentesis for, 171, 171f, 402
    transudative
        causes of, 278t
        congestive heart failure as cause of, 277-278
        description of, 171-172, 277-278
        exudative pleural effusions versus, 172, 277t
        microscopic appearance of, 172, 173f
        nephrotic syndrome and, 278, 278f
        pathophysiology of, 277
    treatment of, 280
Pleural fibroma, 302
Pleural fluid
    characteristics of, 170-171
    colloid osmotic pressure elevation effects on, 171
    flow rate for, 275
    formation of, 171
    laboratory analysis of, 170-172
    leukocyte count in, 173
    macrophages in, 174f
    metastatic adenocarcinoma cells in, 175f
    reabsorption of, 275, 276f
Pleural friction rub, 258
Pleural plaques, 217, 218f
Pleural rub, 129
Pleural space
    air detection in, 135-136
    anatomy of, 171f
    definition of, 275
    physiology of, 171, 275
    as potential space, 170
Pleural space diseases
    description of, 275
    effusions. *See* Pleural effusions
    hemothorax, 280
    pneumothorax. *See* Pneumothorax
Pleuritic chest pain, 36, 258
Pleximeter, 127
PMN. *See* Polymorphonuclear neutrophils
P_{MV}. *See* Hydrostatic pressure
Pneumatic caisson, 119, 119f
Pneumatocele, 399, 403
Pneumococcal conjugate vaccine, 397, 401
Pneumococcal pneumonia, 399
Pneumococcal polysaccharide vaccine, 202
Pneumoconioses
    asbestosis, 217, 217f, 225, 225t, 304
    berylliosis, 218, 223, 225t
    coal worker's, 215, 216f, 225t
    definition of, 215
    silicosis, 216f, 216-217

Pneumoconioses (*Cont.*):
    talcosis, 217-218
    welder's, 218
Pneumocystis jiroveci pneumonia, 227, 343, 343f
Pneumonectomy, 316
Pneumonia
    acute, 333f
    aspiration, 335, 335f
    atypical, 338
    bacterial. *See* Bacterial pneumonia
    bronchopneumonia, 332, 334f
    classification of, 332t
    community-acquired. *See* Community-acquired pneumonia
    fremitus increases associated with, 127
    hospital-acquired. *See* Hospital-acquired pneumonia
    phases of, 333f
    pneumococcal, 399
    Pneumocystis jiroveci, 227, 343, 343f
    primary atypical, 401
    tachypnea in, 399
Pneumonitis
    definition of, 331
    diffuse interstitial, 213, 214f
    hypersensitivity, 211-212, 212t
    infectious interstitial, 338, 338f
Pneumotachometer, 146
Pneumothorax
    in acute lung injury/acute respiratory distress syndrome patients, 272
    bilateral, 47
    chest x-ray findings, 135-136
    definition of, 39, 252, 280
    flexible bronchoscopy contraindications, 161
    fremitus decreases associated with, 127
    primary spontaneous, 280, 280f
    resolution rate for, 280-281
    spontaneous, 136, 136f, 280, 280f
    sterile wound created by, 83
    tension, 136, 252, 281
Poiseuille equation, 48
Polycythemia, 117
Polymorphonuclear neutrophils
    bronchoalveolar lavage fluid level of, 163, 271
    respiratory parenchyma recruitment of, 88, 88f
Polyps, nasal, 319, 320f
Polysomnogram
    obstructive sleep apnea syndrome evaluations, 232, 233f
    sleep-related hypoventilation/hypoxemic syndrome criteria, 239t
Pons, 95, 96f
Pontine pneumotaxic center, 95
Pores of Kohn, 15
Portable fluoroscopy "C-arm" unit, 159
Positional obstructive sleep apnea, 233
Positive end-expiratory pressure
    acute lung injury treated with, 267
    acute respiratory distress syndrome treated with, 267
    auto-PEEP, 288, 289f
    description of, 52, 74, 119

Positive end-expiratory pressure (*Cont.*):
extrinsic, 288
intrinsic, 288
Positive likelihood ratio, 130
Positive pressure ventilation
invasive, 284-287, 285f
non-invasive, 289-290, 290t
Posterior chest wall
hemidiaphragm position, 128
inspection of, 125
percussion of, 127
Posterior costophrenic angles, 134f, 135
Postpericardial injury syndrome, 280
Posttest probability, 130
Potential space, 170
P_{PEAK}, 287
P_{PLAT}, 287
PPV. *See* Positive pressure ventilation
P_{PV}. *See* Pulmonary venous pressure
P_{PW}. *See* Pulmonary wedge pressure
Pre-Bötzinger complex, 93, 95
Predicted body weight, 272
Prednisone, 228
Premature infants
neonatal respiratory distress syndrome
risks. *See* Neonatal respiratory distress
syndrome
periodic breathing in, 100
Pressure support ventilation, 285, 287f
Pressure-controlled ventilation, 285, 286f
Pretest probability, 130
Primary atypical pneumonia, 401
Primary bronchi, 14
Primary ciliary dyskinesia, 83
Primary spontaneous pneumothorax, 280, 280f
Primary tuberculosis, 339, 340f, 354
Progressive massive fibrosis, 215
Progressive primary tuberculosis, 354
Progressive pulmonary tuberculosis, 339
Progressive systemic sclerosis, 215
Proliferative glomerulonephritis, 249
Prospective Investigation of Pulmonary
Embolism Diagnosis, 257
Proteases, 271
Protein C, 264
Protein kinase A, 193
Protein S, 264
Proton acceptor, 28
Proximal left pulmonary artery, 134, 134f
Pseudoglandular stage, of lung development,
18, 19f
Pseudohyphae, 335, 336f
Pseudolymphoma, 302
Pseudomonas aeruginosa, 334, 376, 379, 381
Pseudo-stratified epithelium, 11, 11f
PSG. *See* Polysomnogram
Psychogenic stress, 190
Pulmonary abscess, 335, 336f, 402, 402f
Pulmonary agenesis, 369-370, 370f
Pulmonary alveolar proteinosis, 214, 215f,
226, 226f
Pulmonary amyloidosis, 213, 214f
Pulmonary angiography, 262, 262f
Pulmonary aplasia, 369

Pulmonary arterial blood pressure, 55
Pulmonary arteries
chest x-ray of, 134f, 134-135
description of, 9, 17
functions of, 17
Pulmonary artery catheters, 55, 56f, 272
Pulmonary capillary fluid balance, 58-60
Pulmonary circulation
description of, 55
features of, 56f
perfusion pressures in, 56f
Pulmonary diffusing capacity for carbon
monoxide
American Thoracic Society/European
Respiratory Society severity criteria, 149t
definition of, 147
description of, 73
equation for calculating, 148
high altitude effects, 117
measurement of, 147-148, 149t
single-breath method, 147, 147f
Pulmonary disease. *See also specific disease*
chest x-ray localization of, 135-139
Mycobacterium avium complex-related, 358
Pulmonary edema
categories of, 59t
causes of, 60, 60t
clinical manifestations of, 245-246
congestive heart failure as cause of, 245
high altitude, 60, 117
microscopic findings, 245-246, 246f
noncardiogenic, 268-269
reexpansion, 281
Pulmonary embolism
acute, 257, 262f
anticoagulation therapies for, 263-264
brain natriuretic peptide levels, 260
cardiovascular manifestations of, 257-258
chest examination findings, 131
chest x-ray findings, 261
clinical presentation of, 257-258
clinical probability model of, 259, 260t
computed tomography angiography of, 139,
139f, 257, 257f, 261f
D-dimer assay for, 260
differential diagnosis of, 258, 258t
electrocardiogram evaluations, 260, 260f
embolectomy for, 264
epidemiology of, 255
etiology of, 255
helical computed tomographic angiography
of, 261, 261f
hypercapnia in, 259
hypocapnia in, 259
hypoxia in, 259
imaging of, 261f, 261-262
inferior vena cava filters for, 264
laboratory evaluation of, 259-261
low-molecular-weight heparin for, 257, 263
lung infarction secondary to, 258
mortality rates, 255, 256f
pathophysiology of, 258-259, 259f
prognosis for, 264
pulmonary angiography evaluations, 262, 262f

Pulmonary embolism (*Cont.*):
risk factors for, 246, 255-257, 257t
risk stratification, 262, 263f
thromboembolism caused by, 246
thrombolytic therapy for, 264
treatment of, 262-264
unfractionated heparin for, 263
ventilation/perfusion matching inequalities
caused by, 65, 66f
ventilation/perfusion scan of, 261, 262f
warfarin for, 264
Pulmonary eosinophilia, 213, 213f
Pulmonary fibrosis, idiopathic, 208-209, 209f,
221-222, 222f
Pulmonary function testing
advanced, 145-146
chronic obstructive pulmonary disease
diagnosis using, 201
description of, 4, 34, 143
interstitial lung diseases, 221-222, 227
reasons for, 144t
restrictive lung diseases, 221-222, 227
spirometry, 143-145
Pulmonary hamartoma, 295, 296f
Pulmonary hypertension
bone morphogenetic protein receptor type
2, 248
definition of, 248
description of, 57, 135
Heath and Edwards grading system for,
249, 249t
high altitude and, 117
magnetic resonance imaging of, 140, 140f
morphologic findings in, 249, 249f
pathogenesis of, 248
Rabinovitch-Reid grading of, 249, 249t
secondary, 248t, 248-249
Pulmonary hypoplasia, 371-372, 372f
Pulmonary infarction, 247, 248f, 258
Pulmonary Langerhans cell histiocytosis,
226, 228f
Pulmonary lymphoma, 163
Pulmonary rehabilitation
chronic obstructive pulmonary disease
managed with, 203
interstitial lung diseases managed with, 228
Pulmonary sequestrations, 371
Pulmonary thromboembolism, 246-248, 247f,
278. *See also* Pulmonary embolism;
Venous thromboembolism
Pulmonary vascular resistance, 4, 55, 390
Pulmonary vasculitides, 224-225
Pulmonary veins
chest x-ray of, 134f, 135
description of, 9
Pulmonary venous blood oxygen content, 63
Pulmonary venous pressure, 55
Pulmonary wedge pressure, 55
Pulse oximetry, 348
Purified protein derivative, 356
Purulent specimen, 169
PVT. *See* Pulmonary vascular resistance
Pyrazinamide, 357
Pyruvate, 154

Q

Q_{max}
aerobic training effects on, 105f
in elite athletes, 108
stroke volume effects on, 106f
Qs. *See* Physiological shunts
Quintile, 104

R

Rabinovitch-Reid grading, of pulmonary
hypertension, 249, 249t
Radiation pneumonitis, 251, 252f
Radiographic densities, 133, 134f
Radiosurgery, 316
Radon exposure, 307
Rales, 129
Rapid shallow breathing index, 289
Rapidly adapting pulmonary stretch receptors,
97-98, 98t
Raptures of the deep. *See* Nitrogen narcosis
Reactivation tuberculosis, 355, 355f
Reactive amyloidosis, 335
Reactive nitrogen species, 88
Reactive oxygen species, 88
Recombinant tissue plasminogen activator, 264
Red blood cell count, 23
Red blood cells. *See* Erythrocytes
Reed-Sternberg cells, 302
Reexpansion pulmonary edema, 281
Reid Index, 181, 183f
Relative humidity, 5
Relaxation atelectasis, 245
Relaxation pressure-volume maneuver, 47, 49f
Rescue bronchodilator, 193
Residual volume, 32, 33t
Resonance, 128
Resorption atelectasis, 245
Respiration
brainstem integration of, 96
central control mechanisms of, 99f
control of. *See* Respiratory control
cranial striated muscles involved in, 95
patterns of, 93-94
peripheral control mechanisms of, 99f
physiology of, 283
rhythm of, 93
sensory modulation of, 96, 97f
Respiratory acidosis
acute, 76
causes of, 151, 152f
compensatory responses for, 152t
criteria for, 154
description of, 76
pathophysiology of, 155
Respiratory alkalosis
acute hypoxic pressor response as cause of,
115
causes, 115, 151, 152f, 155
causes of, 76
compensatory responses for, 152t
criteria for, 154
hemoglobin-oxygen affinity affected by, 115

Respiratory alkalosis (*Cont.*):
in interstitial lung diseases, 227
pathophysiology of, 155
Respiratory arrest, 94
Respiratory bronchiole, 15, 16f
Respiratory bronchiolitis-associated interstitial
lung disease, 213
Respiratory compliance, 51-52
Respiratory control
central pattern generator, 93
central rhythm generator, 93
description of, 93
during sleep, 99
Respiratory distress syndrome. *See* Acute
respiratory distress syndrome; Neonatal
respiratory distress syndrome
Respiratory disturbance index, 232, 234t
Respiratory effort-related arousals, 232, 233f,
234t
Respiratory epithelium, 9
Respiratory excursion of hemidiaphragm, 128
Respiratory frequency, 3, 31
Respiratory function, 99
Respiratory motor neurons, 94-95
Respiratory mucosa
airway diameter and, correlation between,
84, 84f
description of, 9
Respiratory muscles
accessory, 95, 125
anatomy of, 48f
description of, 94
fatigue of, 35
Respiratory parenchyma
alveolar macrophages in, 180
anatomy of, 9, 16f, 31
in cigarette smokers, 180
circulating leukocyte recruitment into, 86-89
congenital defects of, 369-372, 370f-372f
defense mechanisms of, 84-85
injury of, 402
surfactant-associated proteins in, 86
Respiratory quotient, 28
Respiratory syncytial virus, 321, 400
Respiratory system. *See also specific anatomy*
conducting zone of, 9
congenital anomalies of. *See* Congenital
anomalies
connective tissue of, 9
development of, 18, 18f-19f
nomenclature of, 3-4
radiographic densities of, 133, 134f
Respiratory tract
congenital anomalies of, 365-372
lower. *See* Lower respiratory tract infections
nasal cavities, 9-11
paranasal sinuses, 11
sections of, 9-15, 10f
structural changes in, 10t
Respiratory-related neurons, 95
Restrictive lung diseases
acute, 207-208, 208f-209f, 208t
bibasilar inspiratory crackles associated
with, 226

Restrictive lung diseases (*Cont.*):
causes of, 207
characteristics of, 50, 207
chronic. *See* Chronic restrictive lung
diseases
cigarette smoking-related, 213, 214f
clinical features of, 221, 226
definition of, 221
description of, 3
diagnostic approach, 226-228
fiberoptic bronchoscopy for, 227
laboratory tests for, 226-227
management of, 221-229
pulmonary edema as, 59
pulmonary function testing findings,
221-222
residual volume in, 51
treatment of, 228-229
Retrosternal space, 134f, 135
Rheumatoid arthritis, 215
Rheumatoid nodules, 324
Rhinitis, 319
Rhinorrhea, 319
Rhonchus, 129
Ribavirin, 400
Rifampin, 357
Right atrium, 134f, 135
Right diaphragm, 134f, 135
Right interlobar pulmonary artery, 134, 134f
Right paratracheal stripe, 134, 134f
Right pulmonary artery, 134f, 135
Right upper lobe, 134f, 135
Right ventricle, 134f, 135
Right ventricular dysfunction, 262
Right-to-left shunting, 389, 389f
Rigid bronchoscope, 159
Rostral ventral respiratory group, 95
RSBI. *See* Rapid shallow breathing index

S

Saccular stage, of lung development, 18, 19f
"Saddle embolus," 247, 258
Salmeterol, 193
Samter triad, 190
Sarcoidosis
bronchoalveolar lavage fluid analysis in, 163
characteristics of, 209-210
chest x-ray findings, 222, 223f-224f, 223t
definition of, 222
granulomata associated with, 210-211, 211f
high-resolution computed tomography of,
140f
hypersensitivity pneumonia versus, 163
pathogenesis of, 210, 222
prednisone for, 228
presentation of, 211
T-helper cell lymphocyte-mediated
inflammation associated with, 222
treatment of, 228
SARs. *See* Slowly adapting pulmonary stretch
receptors
Schaumann bodies, 211, 211f
Scleroderma, 215

Scuba diving, 118-119
Secondary chronic pulmonary eosinophilia, 213
Secondary tuberculosis, 339, 340f
Sedimentation, 82
Sensitizer-induced occupational asthma, 190
Sensory receptors
  of lower airways, 97-98, 98t
  peripheral, 98
  of upper airways, 98
Septic embolism, 335
Severe acute respiratory syndrome, 341-342
Shivering thermogenesis, 114
Short-acting β_2-agonists, 193, 196
Shunt equation, 74
Sickle cell hemoglobin, 26
Siderophages, 246
Silhouette sign, 135, 136f
Silicosis, 216f, 216-217
Simple chronic bronchitis, 181
Simple ciliated columnar epithelium, 15
Simple ciliated cuboidal epithelium, 15
Simple pulmonary eosinophilia, 213, 224
Singer's nodules/polyps, 323-324
Single-breath method, for pulmonary diffusing
    capacity for carbon monoxide, 147,
    147f
Sinonasal papillomas, 321, 321f
Sinus bradycardia, 237
Sinuses
  defense mechanisms of, 81
  description of, 11
  tumors of, 321-323
Sinusitis, 319-320, 320f
Situs inversus, 136, 320
Six-minute walk test, 222
Sleep, 99
Sleep apnea
  central. See Central sleep apnea
  complex sleep apnea syndrome, 237-238
  obstructive. See Obstructive sleep apnea
    syndromes
  prevalence of, 100
Sleep Heart Health Study, 232
Sleep-related breathing disorders
  central sleep apnea. See Central sleep apnea
  complex sleep apnea syndrome, 237-238
  obstructive sleep apnea syndromes, Se
    Obstructive sleep apnea syndromes
  types of, 231
Sleep-related hypoventilation/hypoxemic
    syndrome
  bilevel positive airway pressure for, 203
  classification of, 238t
  definition of, 238
  polysomnogram criteria for, 239t
Slowly adapting pulmonary stretch receptors,
    97, 98t
Small cell carcinoma, 298, 299f, 311-312,
    312f, 316
Smoking. See Cigarette smoking; Tobacco
    smoking
Snorkeling, 118
Solitary fibrous tumor, 302, 302f

Solution, 24
Sphingomyelin, 43
Spinal cord respiratory motor neurons, 94-95
Spindle cell carcinoma, 298
Spirometry
  American Thoracic Society/European
    Respiratory Society, 144t-145t
  asthma diagnosis using, 191
  description of, 143-145
  elements of, 34
  false positives, 145
  lung volume measurements using, 32,
    143-147
  variation in results of, 145
Splanchnic mesoderm, 18
Splinting, 399
Spontaneous breathing trial, 289
Spontaneous patient-initiated breath, 286
Spontaneous pneumothorax, 136, 136f, 280,
    280f
Sputum induction, 169
Sputum sample
  bronchogenic carcinoma diagnosis, 298
  collection of, 169
  culturing of, 169-170, 170f
  cytological examination, 170, 170f
  Gram staining of, 169, 170f
  spontaneous expectoration of, 169
Squamous cell carcinoma
  bronchiogenic, 295, 296f
  keratinizing, 322, 323f
  laryngeal, 325f, 325-326, 326f
  lung cancer, 310, 312f
  nonkeratinizing, 323, 323f
  tracheal, 326
Squamous metaplasia, 181
Staphylococcus aureus
  bacterial pneumonia caused by, 334, 334f
  community-acquired pneumonia caused by,
    403
  methicillin-resistant, 348-349, 379, 403t
Starling's equation
  description of, 59, 268, 275
  pulmonary edema causes based on, 60t
Starling's law, 58
Static compliance, 39
Static elements of lung resistance and
    compliance, 35
Static lung recoil, 39
Static lung resistance, 50
Status asthmaticus, 184, 194, 196
Stenotrophomonas maltophilia, 379
Stepwise exercise stress test, 106
STPD, 5
Stratified squamous epithelium, 11f, 12, 321f
Streptococcus pneumoniae, 333-334, 346, 348,
    399, 401-402, 403t
Streptokinase, 264
Stridor, 129
Stroke volume
  Q_{max} declines affected by, 106f
  thermal stress effects on, 114
Subcutaneous emphysema, 180
Subdiaphragmatic gas shadows, 136, 137f

Sublingual allergen immunotherapy, 195
Sudden infant death syndrome, 391t, 391-392,
    393f-394f
Sulfur granules, 335
Sulfur hexafluoride, 65t
Superior sulcus tumors, 312-313
Superior vena cava, 134, 134f
Superior vena cava syndrome, 140, 313
Superoxide anion, 88
Suppurative bacterial pneumonia, 331-338,
    333f
Suppurative granulomatous inflammation, 340,
    341f
Supraglottic, 13
Surface tension recoil, 34, 39, 41
Surfactant
  deficiency of, 42, 386
  description of, 15
  developmental biology of, 42-43
  laboratory evaluation of, 43
  primary deficiency of, 42
  role of, 41
  secondary deficiency of, 42
Surfactant proteins, 42, 86
$S_{\bar{v}}O_2$. *See* Mixed venous % oxygenation or
    saturation
Swallowing, 12
Sweat chloride test, 376
Synchronized intermittent mandatory
    ventilation, 286-287, 288f
Syndrome of inappropriate antidiuretic
    hormone hypersecretion, 314
Systemic lupus erythematosus, 215
Systemic vascular resistance, 55
Systolic pressure, 55

T

T_A. *See* Ambient temperature
Tachypnea, 65, 93, 257, 387, 399
Tactile fremitus, 126
Talcosis, 217-218
T_B. *See* Body temperature
T-bet, 183
Temazepam, 237
Tension pneumothorax, 136, 252, 281
Tension recoil, 34, 39
Terminal bronchiole, 15, 16f
T_H1 cells, 183, 190
T_H2 cells, 183-184, 190
Theophylline, 194, 236
Thermal dilution, 55
Thermogenesis, 114
Thin layer chromatography, 43
Thoracentesis
  definition of, 171
  pleural effusion treated with, 171, 171f, 402
  spontaneous pneumothorax after, 136
Thoracic empyema, 279
Thorax
  elastic properties of, 47-48
  trauma of, flexible bronchoscopy indications
    for, 161
Thrombocytopenia, 380

Thrombolytic therapy, 264
Thrombophilias, 256
Thromboxane A$_2$, 259
Thyroid cartilage, 13
Tidal ventilation, 9
Tidal volume, 3, 31, 33t
Tissue elastic recoil, 34, 41
Tissue plasminogen activator, 402
Tissue viscous drag, 50
TLC. *See* Total lung capacity
TNM staging system
  laryngeal carcinoma staging using, 326
  lung cancer staging using, 315t, 315-316,
    316f
  tracheal carcinoma staging using, 326
Tobacco smoking
  asthma and, 190
  bupropion for cessation of, 201-202
  cessation of, 201-202
  chronic obstructive pulmonary disease risks,
    200
  lung cancer risks associated with, 307, 310f
  nicotine replacement therapies for, 201
  respiratory parenchyma effects, 180
  restrictive lung diseases caused by, 213, 214f
  varenicline for cessation of, 202
Tobramycin, 381
Tocolytic agents, 390
Tongue muscles, 95
Tonsillectomy, 234
Tonsillitis, 321
Tonsils, 81-82
Total lung capacity
  definition of, 32, 33t
  measurement of, 33f, 146
Total ventilation, 31
Total work of breathing, 50
Trachea
  agenesis of, 366
  anatomy of, 10t, 13-14
  chest x-ray of, 134f, 135
  congenital anomalies of, 366-369,
    367f-369f
  flexible bronchoscopy inspection of, 161f,
    161-162
  infections of, 323-324
  inspection of, 126
  obstruction of, 161
  papilloma of, 324
  position of, 126
  precancerous lesions of, 324-326
  squamous cell carcinoma of, 326
  stenosis of, 160, 367, 367f
  tumors of, 324-326
Tracheal bronchus, 367, 367f
Tracheal papillomatosis, 324
Tracheobronchial C-fibers, 98
Tracheobronchial tree, 162, 162f
Tracheoesophageal fistulae, 368f, 368-369
Tracheomalacia, 160-161, 367f, 367-368
Tracheopathia osteoplastica, 324
Transbronchial lung biopsy
  flexible bronchoscopy for, 164, 164f, 227
  respiratory conditions diagnosed with, 165t

Transbronchial needle aspiration
  description of, 163
  flexible bronchoscopy for, 164, 164f, 227
Transforming growth factor-beta, 207
Transfusion-related acute lung injury, 271
Transitional flow, 50f
Transjugular intrahepatic portosystemic shunt,
    278
Transudative pleural effusion
  causes of, 278t
  congestive heart failure as cause of,
    277-278
  description of, 171-172, 277-278
  exudative pleural effusions versus, 172, 277t
  microscopic appearance of, 172, 173f
  nephrotic syndrome and, 278, 278f
  pathophysiology of, 277
Trapped lung, 279
Tropical eosinophilia, 213
Troponins, 260
True vocal chords, 13, 13f
Tuberculin skin testing, 356, 356t
Tuberculosis
  acid-fast bacilli smear, 353, 354f
  chest x-rays of, 355, 355f
  clinical manifestations of, 353-355
  course of, 354f
  description of, 339, 340f
  diagnostic tests for, 356
  directly observed therapy for, 353, 357
  ethambutol for, 357
  extrapulmonary, 355
  in HIV-infected patients, 356
  incidence of, 353
  isoniazid for, 357
  latent, 354, 357
  miliary, 339
  multidrug-resistant, 357
  pathogenesis of, 353-355
  primary, 339, 340f, 354
  progression of, 355t
  progressive primary, 354
  progressive pulmonary, 339
  pyrazinamide for, 357
  reactivation, 355, 355f
  rifampin for, 357
  secondary, 339, 340f
  transmission of, 353
  treatment of, 356-357
  tuberculin skin test reactivity, 356, 356t
Tumors
  laryngeal, 324-326
  lung. *See* Lung tumors
  nasal, 321-323
  sinus, 321-323
  tracheal, 324-326
Turbulent flow, 50f
23-valent pneumococcal vaccine, 196
Tympany, 127
Type 1 pneumocytes, 15
Type 2 pneumocytes, 15
Type I hypersensitivity reaction, 183
Type III hypersensitivity reaction, 211-212
Type IV hypersensitivity reaction, 210, 212

U

Ultrafiltration, 58
Ultrasound-tipped bronchoscope, 165, 165f
Undifferentiated carcinomas, 323, 323f
Unfractionated heparin, 263
Upper airways
  defense mechanisms of, 81-83
  sensory receptors of, 98
Urokinase, 264
Usual interstitial pneumonia, 209, 210f, 221
Uvulopalatopharyngoplasty, 234, 235t

V

V$_A$. *See* Alveolar volume
Valsalva maneuver, 93, 147
VAP. *See* Ventilator-associated pneumonia
V̇$_A$/Q̇. *See* Alveolar ventilation/perfusion ratio
Varenicline, 202
"Vascular waterfall" model, 57, 57f
VATS. *See* Video-assisted thoracoscopic
    surgery
VC. *See* Vital capacity
V$_D$. *See* Anatomical dead space; Dead space
    volume
V$_E$. *See* Total ventilation
Venous admixture, 73
Venous blood
  carbon dioxide content of, 28t
  oxygen content for, 28t
Venous thromboembolism. *See also* Pulmonary
    embolism
  definition of, 255
  inferior vena cava filters for, 264
  intravascular, 258
  lower extremity orthopedic surgery and, 255
  natural history of, 258
  prognosis for, 264
  risk factors for, 255-256, 257t
  sudden cardiac death from, 258
  thrombophilias as risk factor for, 256
Ventilation
  cardiovascular effects of, 36
  definition of, 31
  mechanical. *See* Mechanical ventilation
  regional lung differences in, 51-52
Ventilation-associated lung injury, 269
Ventilation/perfusion matching
  abnormalities in, 64-66
  inequalities in, 63
  multiple inert gas technique, 64, 65t
  overview of, 63-64
  pulmonary embolism effects on, 65, 66f
  working definitions of, 64
Ventilation/perfusion mismatch, 388
Ventilation/perfusion scan, 261, 262f
Ventilator-associated pneumonia
  description of, 271-272, 347
  pressure-controlled ventilation for, 285
Ventral horn, 94
Ventral respiratory column, 95
Verrucous carcinoma, 326
Vesicular breath sounds, 129

Vestibule, 9, 11f
Vibrissae, 9, 81
Video-assisted thoracoscopic surgery
  biopsy uses of, 228
    intrapleural adhesions removed
      with, 280
    pleural fluid evacuation using, 402
Virchow's triad, 255
Virtual bronchoscopy, 166
Visceral pleura, 9, 170
Viscous tissue drag, 36
Viscus perforation, 136, 137f
Vital capacity
  definition of, 32, 33t
  measurement of, 33f
VO$_2$. *See* Oxygen consumption
Vocal chord dysfunction syndrome, 192
Vocal chords, 13, 13f
Vocal fremitus, 126
Vocalis muscle, 13
Voice sound transmission, 129-130
Volume-controlled ventilation, 285, 286f
Volume-dependent airway compression, 50
Volutrauma, 269
VO$_{2max}$. *See* Maximal oxygen consumption

V$_T$. *See* Tidal volume
VTE. *See* Venous thromboembolism
VX770, 380
VX889, 380

W

Wakefulness stimulus, 99
Warfarin, 264
Wegener granulomatosis, 224, 226, 250,
      250f, 320
Weight-adjusted aerobic capacity, 103
Welder's pneumoconiosis, 218
Westermark sign, 261
Wheeze/wheezing
  airway obstruction, 192
  description of, 129
  in respiratory syncytial virus bronchiolitis,
      400
Whispered pectoriloquy, 130
Whole-body plethysmograph,
      146, 146f
Whole-body plethysmography
  Boyle's law and, 146
  Charles's law and, 4

Whole-body plethysmography (*Cont.*):
  description of, 47
  functional residual capacity measurements
      using, 146
  intra-thoracic air volume estimates using, 146
  procedure for, 146-147
  relaxation pressure-volume curves and, 49f
Work of breathing
  description of, 3, 35
  dynamic airway resistance effects on, 35
  total, 50
Wuchereria bancrofti, 173f

X

^{133}Xenon, 51-52, 57, 261
X-rays. *See* Chest x-rays

Z

Zafirlukast, 194
Ziehl-Neelsen stain, 170f
Zileuton, 194
Zolpidem, 237
Zygomycetes, 337, 338f